Natural Medicine in Therapy

Natural Medicine in Therapy

Editor

Raffaele Capasso

MDPI • Basel • Beijing • Wuhan • Barcelona • Belgrade • Manchester • Tokyo • Cluj • Tianjin

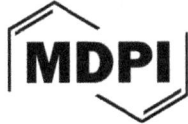

Editor
Raffaele Capasso
University of Naples Federico II
Italy

Editorial Office
MDPI
St. Alban-Anlage 66
4052 Basel, Switzerland

This is a reprint of articles from the Special Issue published online in the open access journal *Biomedicines* (ISSN 2227-9059) (available at: https://www.mdpi.com/journal/biomedicines/special_issues/natural_medicine).

For citation purposes, cite each article independently as indicated on the article page online and as indicated below:

LastName, A.A.; LastName, B.B.; LastName, C.C. Article Title. *Journal Name* **Year**, *Volume Number*, Page Range.

ISBN 978-3-0365-2914-1 (Hbk)
ISBN 978-3-0365-2915-8 (PDF)

© 2022 by the authors. Articles in this book are Open Access and distributed under the Creative Commons Attribution (CC BY) license, which allows users to download, copy and build upon published articles, as long as the author and publisher are properly credited, which ensures maximum dissemination and a wider impact of our publications.

The book as a whole is distributed by MDPI under the terms and conditions of the Creative Commons license CC BY-NC-ND.

Contents

Giuseppe Lucariello, Donatella Cicia and Raffaele Capasso
Pharmacological Studies on Traditional Plant-Based Remedies
Reprinted from: *Biomedicines* 2021, 9, 315, doi:10.3390/biomedicines9030315 1

Millena S. Cordeiro, Daniel L. R. Simas, Juan F. Pérez-Sabino, Max S. Mérida-Reyes,
Manuel A. Muñoz-Wug, Bessie E. Oliva-Hernández, Antônio J. R. da Silva,
Patricia D. Fernandes and Thais B. S. Giorno
Characterization of the Antinociceptive Activity from *Stevia serrata* Cav
Reprinted from: *Biomedicines* 2020, 8, 79, doi:10.3390/biomedicines8040079 5

Md. Adnan, Md. Nazim Uddin Chy, A.T.M. Mostafa Kamal, Md. Obyedul Kalam Azad,
Kazi Asfak Ahmed Chowdhury, Mohammad Shah Hafez Kabir, Shaibal Das Gupta,
Md. Ashiqur Rahman Chowdhury, Young Seok Lim and Dong Ha Cho
Comparative Study of *Piper sylvaticum* Roxb. Leaves and Stems for Anxiolytic and Antioxidant
Properties Through In Vivo, In Vitro, and In Silico Approaches
Reprinted from: *Biomedicines* 2020, 8, 68, doi:10.3390/biomedicines8040068 15

Thaarvena Retinasamy, Mohd. Farooq Shaikh, Yatinesh Kumari,
Syafiq Asnawi Zainal Abidin and Iekhsan Othman
Orthosiphon stamineus Standardized Extract Reverses Streptozotocin-Induced Alzheimer's
Disease-Like Condition in a Rat Model
Reprinted from: *Biomedicines* 2020, 8, 104, doi:10.3390/biomedicines8050104 31

Bernhard P. Kaltschmidt, Inga Ennen, Johannes F. W. Greiner, Robin Dietsch, Anant Patel,
Barbara Kaltschmidt, Christian Kaltschmidt and Andreas Hütten
Preparation of Terpenoid-Invasomes with Selective Activity against *S. aureus* and
Characterization by Cryo Transmission Electron Microscopy
Reprinted from: *Biomedicines* 2020, 8, 105, doi:10.3390/biomedicines8050105 47

Dayana da Costa Salomé, Natália de Moraes Cordeiro, Tayná Sequeira Valério,
Darlisson de Alexandria Santos, Péricles Barreto Alves, Celuta Sales Alviano,
Daniela Sales Alviano Moreno and Patricia Dias Fernandes
Aristolochia trilobata: Identification of the Anti-Inflammatory and Antinociceptive Effects
Reprinted from: *Biomedicines* 2020, 8, 111, doi:10.3390/biomedicines8050111 65

Javed Iqbal, Banzeer Ahsan Abbasi, Riaz Ahmad, Mahboobeh Mahmoodi, Akhtar Munir,
Syeda Anber Zahra, Amir Shahbaz, Muzzafar Shaukat, Sobia Kanwal, Siraj Uddin,
Tariq Mahmood and Raffaele Capasso
Phytogenic Synthesis of Nickel Oxide Nanoparticles (NiO) Using Fresh Leaves Extract of
Rhamnus triquetra (Wall.) and Investigation of Its Multiple In Vitro Biological Potentials
Reprinted from: *Biomedicines* 2020, 8, 117, doi:10.3390/biomedicines8050117 83

Solomon Habtemariam
Trametes versicolor (Synn. *Coriolus versicolor*) Polysaccharides in Cancer Therapy: Targets
and Efficacy
Reprinted from: *Biomedicines* 2020, 8, 135, doi:10.3390/biomedicines8050135 99

Jinbong Park
Anti-Anaphylactic Activity of Isoquercitrin (Quercetin-3-O-β-D-Glucose) in the Cardiovascular
System of Animals
Reprinted from: *Biomedicines* 2020, 8, 139, doi:10.3390/biomedicines8050135 125

Giacomo Picciolo, Giovanni Pallio, Domenica Altavilla, Mario Vaccaro, Giacomo Oteri, Natasha Irrera and Francesco Squadrito
β-Caryophyllene Reduces the Inflammatory Phenotype of Periodontal Cells by Targeting CB2 Receptors
Reprinted from: Biomedicines 2020, 8, 164, doi:10.3390/biomedicines8060164 137

Nobutomo Ikarashi, Motohiro Hoshino, Tetsuya Ono, Takahiro Toda, Yasuharu Yazawa and Kiyoshi Sugiyama
A Mechanism by which Ergosterol Inhibits the Promotion of Bladder Carcinogenesis in Rats
Reprinted from: Biomedicines 2020, 8, 180, doi:10.3390/biomedicines8070180 149

Ani Georgieva, Katerina Todorova, Ivan Iliev, Valeriya Dilcheva, Ivelin Vladov, Svetlozara Petkova, Reneta Toshkova, Lyudmila Velkova, Aleksandar Dolashki and Pavlina Dolashka
Hemocyanins from *Helix* and *Rapana* Snails Exhibit in Vitro Antitumor Effects in Human Colorectal Adenocarcinoma
Reprinted from: Biomedicines 2020, 8, 194, doi:10.3390/biomedicines8070194 161

Milad Ashrafizadeh, Masoud Najafi, Sima Orouei, Amirhossein Zabolian, Hossein Saleki, Negar Azami, Negin Sharifi, Kiavash Hushmandi, Ali Zarrabi and Kwang Seok Ahn
Resveratrol Modulates Transforming Growth Factor-Beta (TGF-β) Signaling Pathway for Disease Therapy: A New Insight into Its Pharmacological Activities
Reprinted from: Biomedicines 2020, 8, 261, doi:10.3390/biomedicines8080261 175

Francisco Javier Álvarez-Martínez, Enrique Barrajón-Catalán and Vicente Micol
Tackling Antibiotic Resistance with Compounds of Natural Origin: A Comprehensive Review
Reprinted from: Biomedicines 2020, 8, 405, doi:10.3390/biomedicines8100405 201

Giovanna Casili, Alessio Ardizzone, Marika Lanza, Enrico Gugliandolo, Marco Portelli, Angela Militi, Salvatore Cuzzocrea, Emanuela Esposito and Irene Paterniti
Treatment with Luteolin Improves Lipopolysaccharide- Induced Periodontal Diseases in Rats
Reprinted from: Biomedicines 2020, 8, 442, doi:10.3390/biomedicines8100442 231

Md. Ataur Rahman, MD. Hasanur Rahman, Md. Shahadat Hossain, Partha Biswas, Rokibul Islam, Md Jamal Uddin, Md. Habibur Rahman and Hyewhon Rhim
Molecular Insights into the Multifunctional Role of Natural Compounds: Autophagy Modulation and Cancer Prevention
Reprinted from: Biomedicines 2020, 8, 517, doi:10.3390/biomedicines8110517 245

Giulia Sbrini, Paola Brivio, Enrico Sangiovanni, Marco Fumagalli, Giorgio Racagni, Mario Dell'Agli and Francesca Calabrese
Chronic Treatment with a Phytosomal Preparation Containing *Centella asiatica* L. and *Curcuma longa* L. Affects Local Protein Synthesis by Modulating the BDNF-mTOR-S6 Pathway
Reprinted from: Biomedicines 2020, 8, 544, doi:10.3390/biomedicines8120544 273

Tapan Behl, Aditi Sharma, Lalit Sharma, Aayush Sehgal, Gokhan Zengin, Roxana Brata, Ovidiu Fratila and Simona Bungau
Exploring the Multifaceted Therapeutic Potential of Withaferin A and Its Derivatives
Reprinted from: Biomedicines 2020, 8, 571, doi:10.3390/biomedicines8120571 287

Jung-Yeon Kim, Jungmin Jo, Jaechan Leem and Kwan-Kyu Park
Kahweol Ameliorates Cisplatin-Induced Acute Kidney Injury through Pleiotropic Effects in Mice
Reprinted from: Biomedicines 2020, 8, 572, doi:10.3390/biomedicines8120572 311

Shara Francesca Rapa, Rosanna Di Paola, Marika Cordaro, Rosalba Siracusa, Ramona D'Amico, Roberta Fusco, Giuseppina Autore, Salvatore Cuzzocrea, Hermann Stuppner and Stefania Marzocco
Plumericin Protects against Experimental Inflammatory Bowel Disease by Restoring Intestinal Barrier Function and Reducing Apoptosis
Reprinted from: *Biomedicines* **2021**, *9*, 67, doi:10.3390/biomedicines9010067 . . . . **325**

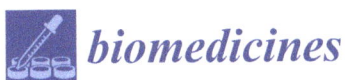

Editorial

Pharmacological Studies on Traditional Plant-Based Remedies

Giuseppe Lucariello [1], Donatella Cicia [1] and Raffaele Capasso [2,*]

1. Department of Pharmacy, School of Medicine and Surgery, University of Naples Federico II, 80131 Naples, Italy; giuseppe.lucariello@unina.it (G.L.); donatella.cicia@unina.it (D.C.)
2. Department of Agricultural Sciences, University of Naples Federico II, 80055 Portici, Italy
* Correspondence: rafcapas@unina.it

Citation: Lucariello, G.; Cicia, D.; Capasso, R. Pharmacological Studies on Traditional Plant-Based Remedies. *Biomedicines* 2021, *9*, 315. https://doi.org/10.3390/biomedicines9030315

Received: 15 March 2021
Accepted: 17 March 2021
Published: 19 March 2021

Publisher's Note: MDPI stays neutral with regard to jurisdictional claims in published maps and institutional affiliations.

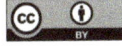

Copyright: © 2021 by the authors. Licensee MDPI, Basel, Switzerland. This article is an open access article distributed under the terms and conditions of the Creative Commons Attribution (CC BY) license (https://creativecommons.org/licenses/by/4.0/).

For years, plant-based remedies have been used as a traditional practice to treat and prevent a broad range of diseases. During the past decade, natural therapies have regained public attention, and, to date, great interest has caught on, as demonstrated by the elevated number of new studies concerning this topic, and by the high funds earmarked every year on medicinal plants. Several reasons contribute to this renovated attention on herbal remedies, among which we can include: the prospect to study a high quantity of unexplored botanicals species; an eco-friendly and cost-efficient approach in terms of research, isolation, and production; the possibility to discover new antimicrobial natural products, that can face the current spreading of antibiotic resistance; the demanding need to reveal potential side effects and interactions of the most widely used natural products with concomitant drug therapies.

In this editorial, we have compiled 20 articles about this study area, summarized as below.

Cordeiro et al. studied the antinociceptive and anti-inflammatory effects of *Stevia serrata* Cav. (Asteraceae) essential oil (EO) and the mechanism of action using opioid and cholinergic antagonists (naloxone and atropine, respectively) and the nitric oxide synthase inhibitor (N-omega-nitro-L-arginine methyl ester, L-NAME).Their work suggests that essential oil of *S. serrata* presents an antinociceptive effect mediated, at least in part, through activation of opioid, cholinergic and nitrergic pathways [1]. *Piper sylvaticum* Roxb, is traditionally used by the indigenous people of tropical and subtropical countries like Bangladesh, India, and China for a variety of chronic diseases. Adnan et al. in their study tested the metabolites extracted (methanol) from the leaves and stems of *P. sylvaticum*, showing a reduction of anxiety-like behavior in vivo and a moderate antioxidant activity in vitro [2]. The Malaysian herb *Orthosiphon stamineus* is a traditional remedy that possesses anti-inflammatory, anti-oxidant, and free-radical scavenging abilities, all of which are known to protect against Alzheimer's disease (AD). With their research, Retinasamy et al. demonstrated an improved effect of *O. stamineus* ethanolic extract on memory in rat, and hence, could serve as a potential therapeutic target for the treatment of neurodegenerative diseases such as AD [3]. Terpenoids are natural plant-derived products that are used to treat a broad range of human diseases, including airway infections and inflammation. However, pharmaceutical applications of terpenoids against bacterial infection remain challenging due to their poor water solubility. Kaltschmidt et al. perfectioned the preparation of terpenoid-invasomes with selective activity against *S. Aureus*. They also performed characterization by cryo-transmission electron microscopyand demonstrated that, particularly thymol-invasomes, show a strong selective activity against Gram-positive bacteria [4]. Salomè et al. evaluated the antinociceptive and anti-inflammatory activities of the essential oil (EO) of *Aristolochia trilobata* and its main ingredient the sulcatyl acetate (SA), they studied the mechanism of antinociceptive activity being evaluated in presence of opioid, cholinergic receptor antagonists (naloxone and atropine), or nitric oxide synthase inhibitor (L-NAME). EO and SA present peripheral and central antinociceptive and anti-inflammatory effects, mediated by inhibition of inducible nitric oxide synthase (iNOS) and spleen tyrosine kinases (Syk) expression [5]. Chemically nickel oxide nanoparticles (NiONP) involve the synthesis of some toxic products for different microbial agents and microalgae by producing reactive oxygen species (ROS), inducing oxidative stress and releasing (Ni^{2+}) inside the cell, which restrict their biological applications. Iqbal et al. developed a chemistry method for the fabrication of NiONPs using fresh leaf broth of *Rhamnus triquetra* (RT), making them an attractive and eco-friendly alternative, that also showed potential in vitro biological activities [6].In his review, Habtemariam scrutinizedin vitro, in vivo, and clinical outcomes of *Trametes versicolor (L.)* polysaccharides which are thought to being useful as adjuvant therapy for cancer [7].Park study related about anti-anaphylactic activity of isoquercitin (Quercetin-3-O-β-d-Glucose) (IQ) in cardiovascular systems of experimental animals, like rats and pigs. Overall, this study provided evidence for the beneficial effect of IQ on cardiac anaphylaxis, thus suggesting its potential applications in the treatment and prevention of related diseases [8]. Picciolo et al. evaluated the therapeutic potential of β-Caryophyllene (BCP), a cannabinoid receptor 2 (CB2) agonist, in an in vitro model of oral mucositis, exploring the human gingival fibroblasts (GF), and human oral mucosa epithelial cells (EC) with an inflammatory phenotype representing a valuable experimental paradigm. BCP blunted the lipopolysaccharides (LPS)-induced inflammatory phenotype and this effect was reverted by the CB2 antagonist AM630. These results suggest that CB2 receptors are an interesting target to develop innovative strategies for oral mucositis [9]. Ikarashi et al., starting from previously data that suggest an inhibitory effect byergosterol on bladder carcinogenesis, elucidated its molecular mechanism using a rat model of N-butyl-N-(4-hydroxybutyl)-nitrosamine-induced bladder cancer. They also analyzed various aspects of the cell cycle, inflammation-related signaling, and androgen signaling, suggesting that ergosterol inhibits bladder carcinogenesis [10]. Georgieva et al. demonstrated that hemocyanins isolated from *H. aspersa*, *H. lucorum*, and *R. venosa*, as well as the mucus from *H. aspersa* exert an antitumor activity in vitro against colorectal carcinoma cell line HT-29, reducing cell viability with a mechanism that includes the induction of apoptosis [11]. Ashrafizadeh et al. reviewed the therapeutic effects of resveratrol, shading light on its possible impact on the tumor growth factor beta (TGF-beta) signaling pathway. Interestingly, resveratrol inhibits both upstream (such as microRNAs (miR)) and downstream mediators of TGF-beta signaling (small mother against decapentaplegic (SMAD), programmed cell death protein 1 (known asPD-1) andepithelial mesenchymal transition (EMT)). Via the down regulation of this pathway, resveratrol exerts its anti-fibrotic, anti-tumor, neuroprotective, lung protective, and anti-diabetics effects [12]. Álvarez-Martínez et al. reviewed the activity of the most representative antimicrobial products of natural origin. Mostnatural products (NP), do not have sufficient therapeutic power to be used in monotherapy against antibiotic resistant bacteria, but some of them have shown synergistic capacity with traditional antibiotics [13]. Casili et al. demonstrated anti-inflammatory properties of luteolin in a model of periodontitis induced by LPS in rats. Based on these results, luteolin implementation could represent a support to the traditional pharmacological approach for periodontitis [14]. Rahman et al. analyzed the role of natural compounds in the modulation of autophagy pathway in cancer prevention and treatment, neurodegenerative and cardiovascular diseases. Mammalian target of rapamycin (mTOR) and adenosine monophosphate-activated protein kinase (AMPK) are the leading regulatory path way of autophagy and they are known targets for natural compounds such as resveratrol, curcumin, antroquinonol and many others [15]. Sbrini et al. investigated the effect of the chronic oral treatment for 10 days with a phytosomal preparation containing *Centellaasiatica* and *Curcumalonga* on brain-derived neurotrophic factor (BDNF) levels in prefrontal cortex of adult rats. The phytosome ameliorates brain plasticity, enhancing mTOR-S6 regulated transcription of proteins involved in memory processes, suggesting that this preparation can be used as a supporting therapy in subjects with memory and cognitive disfunction [16]. Behl et al. discussed withaferin A (WA) pharmacokinetics, synergistic combination, and biological activities. This review highlighted that WA is a promising anticancer compound, but its benefits include also AD, cardioprotective, neuroprotective, osteoporotic, and antiviral effects. Moreover, according to pharmacokinetics studies, it can be used to design drug delivery systems [17]. Kim et al. investigated whether kahweol exerts a protective effect against cisplatin-induced renal injury. The results show that kahweol inhibits immune cell accumulation presumably through down regulation of vascular adhesion molecules, suggesting that it can be a potential preventive agent against cisplatin-induced acute kidney injury, enabling the use of a high dose of cisplatin [18]. Rapa et al. evaluated the effect of plumericin to improve intestinal epithelial barrier function both in intestinal epithelial cells in vitro, and in vivo in a model of dinitrobenzene sulfonic acid (DNBS) induced colitis. This study provided evidence that plumericin improves the expression of junctions' proteins in the epithelial cells, reducing also apoptotic parameters, and enhancing actin cytoskeleton rearrangement. In vivo experiments sustain this evidence, thus supporting the pharmacological potential of plumericin as an adjuvant in inflammatory bowel diseases (IBD) [19].In their review, Devi et al. provided an insight into the potential role of flavonoids against cellular stress response in neurodegenerative disorders. Flavonoids have the potential to reduce these exaggerated cellular stress responses in-turn preventing cell death. Further studies are needed to determine their clinical acceptance [20].

Institutional Review Board Statement: Not applicable.

Informed Consent Statement: Not applicable.

Data Availability Statement: Not applicable.

Conflicts of Interest: The authors declare no conflict of interest.

References

1. Cordeiro, M.S.; Simas, D.L.R.; Pérez-Sabino, J.F.; Mérida-Reyes, M.S.; Muñoz-Wug, M.A.; Oliva-Hernández, B.E.; Da Silva, A.J.R.; Fernandes, P.D.; Giorno, T.B.S. Characterization of the Antinociceptive Activity from Stevia serrata Cav. *Biomedicines* **2020**, *8*, 79. [CrossRef]
2. Adnan, M.; Kamal, A.M.; Azad, O.K.; Chowdhury, K.A.A.; Kabir, M.S.H.; Das Gupta, S.; Chowdhury, A.R.; Lim, Y.S.; Cho, D.H. Comparative Study of Piper sylvaticum Roxb. Leaves and Stems for Anxiolytic and Antioxidant Properties Through in vivo, in vitro, and in silico Approaches. *Biomedicines* **2020**, *8*, 68. [CrossRef] [PubMed]
3. Retinasamy, T.; Shaikh, M.F.; Kumari, Y.; Abidin, S.A.Z.; Othman, I. Orthosiphon stamineus Standardized Extract Reverses Streptozotocin-induced Alzheimer's Disease-Like Condition in a Rat Model. *Biomedicines* **2020**, *8*, 104. [CrossRef] [PubMed]
4. Kaltschmidt, B.P.; Ennen, I.; Greiner, J.F.; Dietsch, R.; Patel, A.; Kaltschmidt, B.; Kaltschmidt, C.; Hütten, A. Preparation of Terpenoid-Invasomes with Selective Activity against S. aureus and Characterization by Cryo Transmission Electron Microscopy. *Biomedicines* **2020**, *8*, 105. [CrossRef] [PubMed]
5. Salome, D.D.C.; Cordeiro, N.D.M.; Valério, T.S.; Santos, D.D.A.; Alves, P.B.; Alviano, C.S.; Moreno, D.S.A.; Fernandes, P.D. Aristolochia trilobata: Identification of the Anti-Inflammatory and Antinociceptive Effects. *Biomedicines* **2020**, *8*, 111. [CrossRef] [PubMed]
6. Iqbal, J.; Abbasi, B.A.; Ahmad, R.; Mahmoodi, M.; Munir, A.; Zahra, S.A.; Shahbaz, A.; Shaukat, M.; Kanwal, S.; Uddin, S.; et al. Phytogenic Synthesis of Nickel Oxide Nanoparticles (NiO) Using Fresh Leaves Extract of Rhamnus triquetra (Wall.) and Investigation of Its Multiple In Vitro Biological Potentials. *Biomedicines* **2020**, *8*, 117. [CrossRef] [PubMed]
7. Habtemariam, S. Trametes versicolor (Synn. Coriolus versicolor) Polysaccharides in Cancer Therapy: Targets and Efficacy. *Biomedicines* **2020**, *8*, 135. [CrossRef] [PubMed]
8. Park, J. Anti-Anaphylactic Activity of Isoquercitrin (Quercetin-3-O-beta-d-Glucose) in the Cardiovascular System of Animals. *Biomedicines* **2020**, *8*, 139. [CrossRef] [PubMed]
9. Picciolo, G.; Pallio, G.; Altavilla, D.; Vaccaro, M.; Oteri, G.; Irrera, N.; Squadrito, F. beta-Caryophyllene Reduces the Inflammatory Phenotype of Periodontal Cells by Targeting CB2 Receptors. *Biomedicines* **2020**, *8*, 164. [CrossRef] [PubMed]
10. Ikarashi, N.; Hoshino, M.; Ono, T.; Toda, T.; Yazawa, Y.; Sugiyama, K. A Mechanism by which Ergosterol Inhibits the Promotion of Bladder Carcinogenesis in Rats. *Biomedicines* **2020**, *8*, 180. [CrossRef] [PubMed]
11. Georgieva, A.; Todorova, K.; Iliev, I.; Dilcheva, V.; Vladov, I.; Petkova, S.; Toshkova, R.; Velkova, L.; Dolashki, A.; Dolashka, P. Hemocyanins from Helix and Rapana Snails Exhibit in Vitro Antitumor Effects in Human Colorectal Adenocarcinoma. *Biomedicines* **2020**, *8*, 194. [CrossRef] [PubMed]
12. Ashrafizadeh, M.; Najafi, M.; Orouei, S.; Zabolian, A.; Saleki, H.; Azami, N.; Sharifi, N.; Hushmandi, K.; Zarrabi, A.; Ahn, K.S. Resveratrol Modulates Transforming Growth Factor-Beta (TGF-beta) Signaling Pathway for Disease Therapy: A New Insight into Its Pharmacological Activities. *Biomedicines* **2020**, *8*, 261. [CrossRef]

13. Alvarez-Martinez, F.J.; Barrajon-Catalan, E.; Micol, V. Tackling Antibiotic Resistance with Compounds of Natural Origin: A Comprehensive Review. *Biomedicines* **2020**, *8*, 405. [CrossRef]
14. Casili, G.; Ardizzone, A.; Lanza, M.; Gugliandolo, E.; Portelli, M.; Militi, A.; Cuzzocrea, S.; Esposito, E.; Paterniti, I. Treatment with Luteolin Improves Lipopolysaccharide-Induced Periodontal Diseases in Rats. *Biomedicines* **2020**, *8*, 442. [CrossRef]
15. Rahman, M.A.; Rahman, M.D.; Hossain, M.; Biswas, P.; Islam, R.; Uddin, M.J.; Rhim, H. Molecular Insights into the Multifunctional Role of Natural Compounds: Autophagy Modulation and Cancer Prevention. *Biomedicines* **2020**, *8*, 517. [CrossRef] [PubMed]
16. Sbrini, G.; Brivio, P.; Sangiovanni, E.; Fumagalli, M.; Racagni, G.; Dell'Agli, M.; Calabrese, F. Chronic Treatment with a Phytosomal Preparation Containing Centella asiatica L. and Curcuma longa L. Affects Local Protein Synthesis by Modulating the BDNF-mTOR-S6 Pathway. *Biomedicines* **2020**, *8*, 544. [CrossRef]
17. Behl, T.; Sharma, A.; Sharma, L.; Sehgal, A.; Zengin, G.; Brata, R.; Fratila, O.; Bungau, S. Exploring the Multifaceted Therapeutic Potential of Withaferin A and Its Derivatives. *Biomedicines* **2020**, *8*, 571. [CrossRef]
18. Kim, J.Y.; Jo, J.; Leem, J.; Park, K.-K. Kahweol Ameliorates Cisplatin-Induced Acute Kidney Injury through Pleiotropic Effects in Mice. *Biomedicines* **2020**, *8*, 572. [CrossRef]
19. Rapa, S.F.; Di Paola, R.; Cordaro, M.; Siracusa, R.; D'Amico, R.; Fusco, R.; Autore, G.; Cuzzocrea, S.; Stuppner, H.; Marzocco, S. Plumericin Protects against Experimental Inflammatory Bowel Disease by Restoring Intestinal Barrier Function and Reducing Apoptosis. *Biomedicines* **2021**, *9*, 67. [CrossRef] [PubMed]
20. Devi, S.; Kumar, V.; Singh, S.; Dubey, A.; Kim, J.-J. Flavonoids: Potential Candidates for the Treatment of Neurodegenerative Disorders. *Biomedicines* **2021**, *9*, 99. [CrossRef] [PubMed]

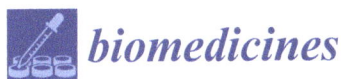

Article

Characterization of the Antinociceptive Activity from *Stevia serrata* Cav

Millena S. Cordeiro [1], Daniel L. R. Simas [2], Juan F. Pérez-Sabino [3], Max S. Mérida-Reyes [3], Manuel A. Muñoz-Wug [3], Bessie E. Oliva-Hernández [3], Antônio J. R. da Silva [2], Patricia D. Fernandes [1] and Thais B. S. Giorno [1,*]

[1] Institute of Biomedical Sciences, Federal University of Rio de Janeiro, Rio de Janeiro 21941-902, Brazil
[2] Institute of Natural Products Research, Federal University of Rio de Janeiro, Rio de Janeiro 21941-902, Brazil
[3] School of Chemistry, Faculty of Chemical Sciences and Pharmacy, University of San Carlos of Guatemala, Guatemala 01012, Guatemala
* Correspondence: thais.sardella.farma@hotmail.com; Tel.: +55-21-3938-6442

Received: 3 March 2020; Accepted: 31 March 2020; Published: 7 April 2020

Abstract: Background: *Stevia serrata* Cav. (Asteraceae), widely found in Guatemala, is used to treat gastrointestinal problems. The aim of this study was to demonstrate the antinociceptive and anti-inflammatory effects of the essential oil (EO) and the mechanism of action. Methods: EO was tested in chemical (capsaicin- and glutamate-induced licking response) or thermal (hot plate) models of nociception at 10, 30 or 100 mg/kg doses. The mechanism of action was evaluated using two receptor antagonists (naloxone, atropine) and an enzyme inhibitor (L-NAME). The anti-hyperalgesic effect was evaluated using carrageenan-induced nociception and evaluated in the hot plate. Results: All three doses of EO reduced licking response induced by glutamate, and higher doses reduced capsaicin-induced licking. EO also increased area under the curve, similar to the morphine-treated group. The antinociceptive effect induced by EO was reversed by pretreatment of mice with naloxone (1 mg/kg, ip), atropine (1 mg/kg, ip) or L-NAME (3 mg/kg, ip). EO also demonstrated an anti-hyperalgesic effect. The 100 mg/kg dose increased the latency time, even at 1 h after oral administration and this effect has been maintained until the 96th hour, post-administration. Conclusions: Our data suggest that essential oil of *S. serrata* presents an antinociceptive effect mediated, at least in part, through activation of opioid, cholinergic and nitrergic pathways.

Keywords: *Stevia serrata*; essential oil; inflammation; antinociception; pain

1. Introduction

Stevia serrata Cav. is a plant of the Asteraceae family (Asteroideae) that grows in Central America and Mexico, usually over 1500 m, and in northern South America at higher altitudes. In Guatemala it is found in the regions of Chimaltenango, Huehuetenango, El Quiche, Sacatepéquez and Sololá, near pine and oak forests in sunny sites [1]. This plant grows as a perennial herb, from 0.6–1 m tall, with stems puberulent to densely pilose, linear-spatulate to oblanceolate leaves, an apex rounded to acute, 2–6 cm long and 0.2–1.5 cm wide blades [2]. This plant has the following synonymia: *Ageratum punctatum* Ortega, *Stevia ivifolia* Willd., *Stevia pubescens* Kunth, *Stevia punctata* (Ortega) Pers., *Stevia serrata* var. *ivifolia* (Willd.) B.L. Rob., *Stevia virgata* Kunth [2].

Recently, it has been demonstrated that chamazulene, a sesquiterpene, is the major component of the essential oil (60.1%) and suggested that essencial oil (EO) reduced the time that mice spent licking the formalin-injected paw [3]. However, in the paper, neither the possible effects of the EO in other models of nociception, nor the mechanism of action was studied. In this regard, the aim of the present paper was to evaluate the antinociceptive effect of EO in other models of nociception, i.e., capsaicin-

and glutamate-induced licking, hot plate and carrageenan-induced hyperalgesia, and to identify the mechanism by which *S. serrata* exerts its effect.

2. Materials and Methods

2.1. Plant Material and Extraction

Aerial parts of *S. serrata* were collected in September 2014, from a population found in San José Chacayá, province of Sololá, west from Guatemala City. A voucher specimen was kept at the Herbarium of the Faculty of Chemistry and Pharmacy of the University of San Carlos, Guatemala (BIGU 72832). The oil from 40 g of aerial parts of *S. serrata* was extracted by hydro distillation using a clevenger-type apparatus for 2 h. A yield of 0.2% (w/w) was obtained. Essential oil (EO) was maintained at $-20\ °C$ until use.

2.2. Essential Oil Chemical Composition

The essential oil was analyzed by gas chromatography/-mass spectrometry (GC-MS) according to Simas et al. (2017). The identification of the EO components was made by comparison of their mass spectra and retention indexes with data from the literature [4]. The compounds found in higher concentrations were the sesquiterpenes chamazulene (60.1%), (E)-nerolidol (7.3%), caryophyllene oxide (6.3%) and germacrene D (5.4%).

2.3. Animals

Swiss *Webster* mice (20–25 g, 8–10 weeks, 200 animals) of both sexes were donated by the Institute Vital Brazil (Niteroi, RJ, Brazil). Animals have been housed in a temperature-controlled room at $22 \pm 2\ °C$ with a 12 h light/dark cycle and free access to pelleted food (Nutrilab, Belo Horizonte, MG, Brazil) and water. Twelve hours before each experiment, the animals received only water in order to avoid food interference with substance absorption. The experimental protocols used in this work followed the rules advocated by Law 11,794, from October 8th 2008 by the National Council of Animal Experimentation Control (CONCEA) and were approved by the Ethics Committee of Animal Use (CEUA), Science Centre Health/UFRJ (DFBCICB015-04/16).

2.4. Drugs, Reagents and Treatments

All solvents were chromatographic grade (Tedia, Rio de Janeiro, RJ, Brazil). Carrageenan, glutamic acid, atropine, Nω-nitro-L-arginine methyl ester (L-NAME) were purchased from Sigma-Aldrich (St. Louis, MO, USA). Formalin was purchased from Merck (Darmstadt, Germany). Cristália (São Paulo, Brazil) kindly provided morphine sulphate and naloxone hydrochloride. Capsaicin was purchased from Galena (Campinas, SP, Brazil). A stock solution at 100 mg/mL in extrapure oil was prepared with the essential oil (EO). This EO was administered to mice by oral gavage, at doses of 10 to 100 mg/kg, in a final volume of 0.1 mL, 60 min prior to experiments. Morphine (5 mg/kg, p.o.) was diluted in extrapure oil just before use and was used as a reference drug. The control group received vehicle (extrapure oil) by oral gavage.

2.5. Capsaicin- and Glutamate-Induced Nociception

Animals received oral administration of EO (10, 30 or 100 mg/kg) one hour before intraplantar injection of capsaicin (20 μL, 1.6 μg/paw). Mice were individually placed in a transparent glass observation chamber. Based on Giorno et al. [5], nociception was assessed immediately after injection and quantified by paw licking time during a period of 5 min.

In the glutamate-induced licking test, the mice were orally treated with the EO (10, 30 and 100 mg/kg), 60 min before intraplantar injection of glutamate (20 μL, 3.7 ng/paw). Immediately after the injection, the animals were individually placed in a transparent glass observation chamber.

The nociception was considered as the total time (recorded with a chronometer) the animals remained licking the injected paw [5].

2.6. Formalin-Induced Nociception

This assay was performed as described by Sakurada et al. [6] and adapted by Giorno et al. [5]. After an intraplantar injection of formalin (20 µL, 2.5% v/v), the period during which mice remained licking the injected paw was immediately recorded. This response has been divided in two phases: The first one, between the injection and 5 min (neurogenic phase) and the second one, between 15–30 min post-formalin injection (inflammatory phase). EO or vehicle was administered 60 min before the injection of formalin.

2.7. Hot Plate Test

According to the method described previously [7] and adapted by Matheus et al. [8], the animals were placed in a glass cylinder on a heated metal plate maintained at 55 ± 1 °C every 30 min after administration of EO (10, 30 and 100 mg/kg) until 180 min. The latency of nociceptive responses, such as jumping or licking of the hind paws, was recorded with a stopwatch. Two measurements were taken 30 and 60 min before the treatment of animals and the average of these measurements was referred to as "baseline".

2.8. Thermal Hyperalgesia

The methodology described by Sammons et al. [9], with some modifications, was used. Briefly, the hyperalgesia was induced by carrageenan (2%, 25 µL) injection in the right hind paw, 30 min after oral treatment with EO (10, 30 and 100 mg/kg) or vehicle. The animals were individually placed in a hot plate apparatus (55 ± 1 °C). At intervals of 1, 2, 4, 6, 24, 48, 72 and 96 h after the treatment, the time period (in seconds) necessary for animals to jump or lick the carrageenan-injected paw was recorded.

2.9. Mechanism of Action

For the study of the possible mechanism of action of *S. serrata*, mice received intraperitoneal injection of naloxone (a non-selective opioid receptor antagonist, 1 mg/kg), atropine (non-selective muscarinic receptor antagonist, 1 mg/kg) or L-NAME (inhibitor of nitric oxide synthase enzyme, 3 mg/kg) 15 min prior to oral administration of *S. serrata* EO (100 mg/kg). Antinociception was evaluated in the hot plate test, as previously described (Section 2.7.). The doses of antagonists and inhibitor were chosen based on previous data described in the literature [10,11]. The experiments conducted in our laboratory and dose response curves for each antagonist were previously constructed, and the dose that reduced 50% of the responses of the agonist was chosen for these assays [12,13].

2.10. Locomotor Performance and Spontaneous Activity Evaluation

To exclude a possible central effect, both the spontaneous activity and the locomotor performance have been evaluated as adapted by Barros et al. [14]. Each animal received oral administration of *S. serrata* EO (100 mg/kg). They have been immediately placed in a chamber with the floor divided into 50 squares (5 cm × 5 cm). The total number of squares in which mice walked has been counted. For locomotor evaluation, mice were trained in apparatus (rotarod; 3.7 cm in diameter, 8 r.p.m) until they remained in for 60 s without falling. On the day of the experiment, mice were treated with EO (100 mg/kg) and the total number of falls was recorded. In both protocols, mice were evaluated at 30, 60, 150 and 240 min after administration.

2.11. Statistical Analysis

Each group was composed by 6 animals, randomly divided. The results are presented as the average ± standard deviation (S.D.). Statistical analyses were performed using analysis of variance (ANOVA) followed by Bonferroni test using Prism Software 5.0 (Graph-Pad Software, La Jolla, CA, USA). The p values of 0.05 have been considered as indicative of significance.

3. Results

3.1. Effect of Essential Oil of Stevia Serrata on Capsaisin and Glutamate Induced-Licking

Previous results from our group indicated that EO from *S. serrata* reduced formalin-induced licking response in a dose response manner, to doses of 10, 30 and 100 mg/kg [3]. In view of these previous results, we decided to further investigate whether EO from *S. serrata* could present a central antinociceptive effect, and the possible mechanism of action.

Figure 1 shows the nociception after capsaicin or glutamate intraplantar injection and the effects observed after pretreatment of mice with increasing doses of EO. It could be noted that 30 and 100 mg/kg doses of EO significantly reduced licking induced by capsaicin (56.8% and 68.7% of inhibition, respectively) while all three doses (10, 30 and 100 mg/kg) reduced the response induced by glutamate (75.4%, 41.3% and 58.7% inhibition, to 10, 30 and 100 mg/kg, respectively).

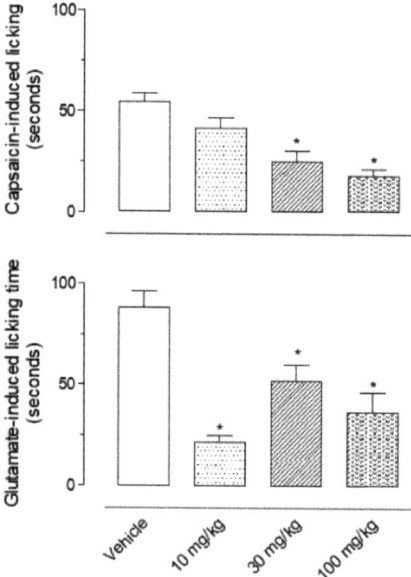

Figure 1. Effect of essential oil of *Stevia serrata* in the capsaicin- and glutamate-induced licking response. The animals have been orally pretreated with the vehicle or essential oil (10, 30, 100 mg/kg) 1 h before the injection of capsaicin (1.6 µg/paw) or glutamate (3.7 ng/paw). Results are expressed as mean ± S.D. (n = 6). Data have been analyzed by ANOVA, followed by Bonferroni post-test, * $p < 0.05$ has been considered as significant when compared to the vehicle-treated groups.

3.2. Effect of Essential Oil of Stevia Serrata on the Hot Plate Test

We also evaluated if EO could present central antinociceptive activity using the hot plate test. Increasing doses of orally administered EO presented antinociceptive activity, similar to data obtained after pretreatment of mice with morphine (an opioid agonist), the positive control drug. Values of area under the curve obtained with all doses of EO varied between 1500 and 2000 arbitrary units, and after morphine, pretreatment values were almost 2000 (Figure 2A). To investigate the possible mechanism of antinociception induced by *S. serrata* essential oil, mice have been pretreated with naloxone (an opioid receptor antagonist, 1 mg/kg, i.p.), atropine (a cholinergic receptor antagonist, 1 mg/kg, i.p) or L-NAME (inhibitor of nitric oxide synthase enzyme, 3 mg/kg, i.p.) 15 min before oral administration of EO (100 mg/kg). Data in Figure 2B shows that both the antagonists, naloxone and atropine, as well the enzyme inhibitor partially reversed the effect caused by EO and reduced its antinociceptive activity in almost 50% of cases.

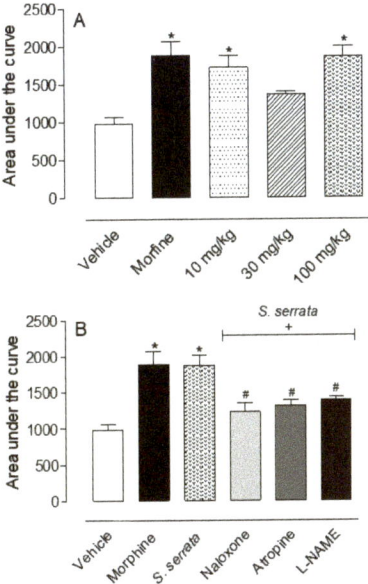

Figure 2. Effects of essential oil of *Stevia serrata* and different antagonists in the thermal nociception model (hot plate). The mice were pretreated orally with the vehicle, essential oil (10, 30, 100 mg/kg) or morphine (2.5 mg/kg) and nociceptive effect was evaluated in the hot plate model (**A**). The animals have been pretreated with naloxone (1 mg/kg, i.p.), atropine (1 mg/kg, i.p.) or L-NAME (3 mg/kg, i.p.) 15 min before oral administration of EO (100 mg/kg) or vehicle (**B**). Results are expressed as mean ± S.D. ($n = 6$) of area under the curve calculated by GraphPad Prism Software 5.0. Data have been analyzed by ANOVA, followed by Bonferroni post-test. * $p < 0.05$ has been considered as significant when compared to the vehicle-treated group and # $p < 0.05$ when comparing with *S. serrata*-treated group.

3.3. Effect of Essential Oil of Stevia Serrata on Formalin Induced-Licking

Sequentially, whether the same antagonists would also have activity in the formalin-induced licking response was also evaluated. As can be observed in Figure 3, none of the antagonists and enzyme inhibitors demonstrated an effect in the first phase of the licking response. However, all three drugs almost completely reversed the antinociceptive effect of EO in the second phase of the model.

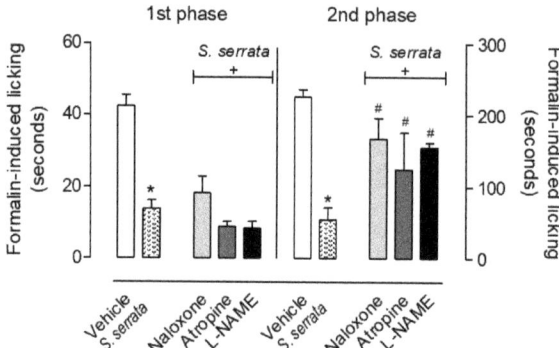

Figure 3. Effects of different antagonists on the antinociceptive activity of the essential oil of *Stevia serrata* in the formalin-induced licking response. Mice received intraperitoneal injection of naloxone (1 mg/kg), atropine (1 mg/kg) or L-NAME (3 mg/kg) 15 min prior to oral administration with the vehicle or essential oil (100 mg/kg). After 60 min, mice received an intraplantar injection of formalin (20 µL, 2.5%). Results are expressed as mean ± S.D. ($n = 6$). Data have been analyzed by ANOVA, followed by Bonferroni post-test. * $p < 0.05$ has been considered as significant when compared to the vehicle-treated groups and # $p < 0.05$ when comparing with *S. serrata*-treated group.

3.4. Effect of Essential Oil of Stevia Serrata in the Thermal Hyperalgesia Model

As the essential oil of *Stevia serrata* presented a significant antinociceptive effect in the inflammatory (formalin-induced licking) and thermal models (hot plate) of nociception, we further decided to analyze if it could present activity in a model of hyperalgesia. In this regard, carrageenan was injected in the paws of mice previously treated with increasing doses (10, 30 or 100 mg/kg) of the essential oil. As the time passes after intraplantar injection of carrageenan, a reduction of latency time could be observed. Even at 96 h post-carrageenan injection, a reduction in latency time could be observed. At the 4th hour after oral treatment, higher doses (30 and 100 mg/kg) of EO significantly increased the latency time. And at the 6th hour, all three doses presented capacity in increasing the period necessary for animals to respond to the hyperalgesic stimulus. It is important to report that the dose of 100 mg/kg presented a significant anti-hyperalgesic effect during the entire assay. Increased latency time was observed from 1 to 96 h post-oral administration of EO (at 100 mg/kg) (Figure 4).

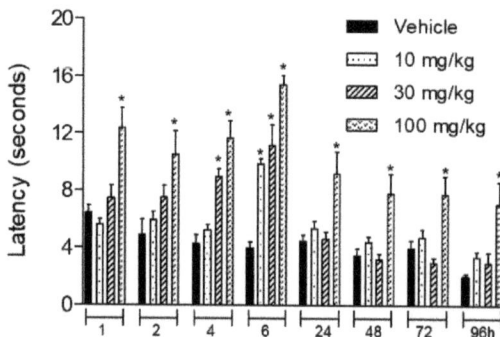

Figure 4. Effect of essential oil of *Stevia serrata* in the hyperalgesic effect induced by carrageenan. The animals have been pretreated orally with the vehicle or essential oil (10, 30, 100 mg/kg) 1 h before intraplantar injection of carrageenan (1%/paw). Hyperalgesia has been evaluated in the hot plate model. Results are expressed as mean ± S.D. ($n = 6$). Data have been analyzed by ANOVA, followed by Bonferroni post-test, * $p < 0.05$ has been considered as significant when compared to the vehicle-treated groups.

4. Discussion

In the present work, it has been demonstrated that the essential oil obtained from aerial parts of *Stevia serrata* presents significant antinociceptive activity in thermal (hot plate) and capsaicin and glutamate-induced licking. It has also been demonstrated that these effects are partially mediated through opioid, muscarinic and nitrergic pathways.

The effect of *S. serrata* against glutamate and capsaicin-induced algesia is of great interest because both agonists play an important participation in central and peripheral nociceptive processes [15–18]. Glutamate is the main mediator of excitatory synaptic transmission in the central nervous system and activates several intracellular events, such as alteration in intracellular calcium levels, activation of cellular mediators and opening of ion channels [18,19]. It also induces the release of excitatory amino acids, PGE2, NO and kinins [6,20] and promotes the activation of sensitive fibers that induce the release of several substances in the dorsal horn, which can also activate the TRPV1 receptor in the spinal cord [19,21]. Capsaicin is an agonist of vanilloid receptor type-1 (TRPV1) receptors and can activate nociceptive fibers [22]. The activation of TRPV1 receptors is also mediated by the release of neurotransmitters (i.e., glutamate and substance P), an effect that can participate in nociceptive processing [23,24]. *S. serrata* EO significantly reduced the licking time induced by glutamate and capsaicin. Results with EO against capsaicin- and glutamate-induced nociception corroborate each other. These findings suggest that, at least part of the antinociceptive effect of EO is mediated by the glutamatergic pathway. We can also infer that TRPV1 receptors could be involved, thus contributing to the modulation of the antinociceptive effect of EO.

Our data of capsaicin and glutamate-induced licking can complete previous results from our group in formalin-induced-licking. This model is a biphasic model with involvement of a neurogenic pain (first phase) and inflammatory pain (second phase) [25]. EO from *S. serrata* reduced both phases of this model suggesting the involvement of inflammatory mediators as well as algesic pathways. Therefore, reduction previously observed in formalin-induced licking could be due, at least in part, to a blockage in TRPV1 and/or glutamate receptors.

It has also been demonstrated that naloxone partially reverted the antinociceptive effect of *S. serrata*. Naloxone is an antagonist of opioid receptors, widely distributed in the body. Activation of these receptors by its agonist, morphine, induces several effects, analgesia being one of the most prominent [26,27]. It is possible that different substances present in the EO can act in different pathways acting together amplifying the antinociceptive response.

EO also increased the time period of response in the carrageenan-induced hyperalgesia. It is well known that carrageenan is a phlogistic agent that induces mouse paw inflammation with a biphasic profile. Its response includes a first peak at the 4th hour and a second one at 72 h post-injection. Phase one and phase two were mediated by migration of neutrophils and lymphocytes, respectively, and with liberation of several mediators [28]. It can explain the fact that all three doses of EO increased the time period of response at the 6th hour after treatment. During this period there is an increase in inflammatory mediators (i.e., histamine, prostaglandins) induced by carrageenan in mouse paws. The diversity of substances that can be found in the essential oil may be acting by inhibiting different mediators that are liberated in the paw. The sum of the effects produces an increase in the antinociceptive response.

In this study the oral administration of EO did not affect motor performance evaluated by either forced locomotion in the rotarod or spontaneous locomotion in the open-field test. Thus, the possibility that the antinociceptive effect of the compounds tested is due to any degree of motor impairment or sedation is very low.

It has been previously reported that the compounds found in higher concentration of EO were the sesquiterpenes chamazulene (60.1%), (*E*)-nerolidol (7.3%), caryophyllene oxide (6.3%) and germacrene D (5.4%) [3]. The concentration of chamazulene found in this EO was almost 10 times higher than in oil of chamomile flowers [29,30]. As observed in chamomile, chamazulene is formed during the steps of the essential oil production, being an artifact. The precursor of chamazulene in chamomile is matricin, a sesquiterpene, which suffers a fast degradation to chamazulene via the intermediate chamazulene carboxylic acid [31]. Calderon et al. [32] reported the formation of chamazulene in the course of the column chromatographic separation of the pro-chamazulene components from *Stevia serrata* Cav. of silica gel column. Safayhi et al. [33] studied the effect of chamazulene on the leukotriene production in neutrophilic granulocytes and demonstrated that chamazulene inhibited the formation of leukotriene B4 in intact cells and in the supernatant fraction in a concentration-dependent manner. The second most abundant component in the OE is nerolidol that exhibits antinociceptive and anti-inflammatory activity, involving the GABAergic system and proinflammatory cytokines [34]. On the other hand, it is well known that caryophyllene oxide presents anti-inflammatory and antinociceptive effects [35–37]. Thus, the anti-inflammatory effect observed in the present work can be explained, at least in part, by the presence of cariophyllene oxide, chamazulene and nerolidol. It is well known that this sesquiterpene presents anti-inflammatory and antinociceptive effects [35–38], thus suggesting the effect of the EO tested.

5. Conclusions

To the best of our knowledge, this paper is the first to suggest the possible mechanism of action of the essential oil of *Stevia serrata* Cav. and demonstrate its antinociceptive activity.

Author Contributions: Conceptualization, P.D.F. and T.B.S.G.; Methodology, M.S.C., T.B.S.G., D.L.R.S., J.F.P.-S., M.S.M.-R., M.A.M.-W., B.E.O.-H. and A.J.R.d.S.; Formal analysis, M.S.C. and T.B.S.G.; Investigation, M.S.C. and T.B.S.G.; Resources, P.D.F.; Data curation, M.S.C. and T.B.S.G.; Writing—original draft preparation, T.B.S.G.; Writing—review and editing, T.B.S.G.; Supervision, P.D.F. and T.B.S.G.; Project administration, P.D.F.; Funding acquisition, P.D.F. All authors have read and agreed to the published version of the manuscript.

Funding: This research was funded by Coordenação de Aperfeiçoamento de Pessoal de Nível Superior (CAPES), Conselho Nacional de Desenvolvimento Científico e Tecnológico (CNPq), Fundação de Amparo à Pesquisa do Estado do Rio de Janeiro (FAPERJ, fellowship to T.B.S.G.) and CONCYT (FINDECYT/FODECYT 17-2017, Guatemala).

Acknowledgments: We would like to thank the Vital Brazil Institute for animal donation and Alan Minho for technical assistance.

Conflicts of Interest: The authors declare no conflict of interest.

References

1. Nash, D.L.; Williams, L.O. *Flora of Guatemala*. Fieldiana: Botany, Field Mus. *Nat. Hist.* **1976**, *24*, 125–126.
2. Pruski, J.F.; Robinson, H. Asteraceae Bercht. & J. Presl, nom. cons. (Compositae Giseke, nom. alt.). *Flora Mesoam.* **2015**, *5*, 554–571.
3. Simas, D.L.R.; Mérida-Reyes, M.S.; Muñoz-Wug, M.A.; Cordeiro, M.S.; Giorno, T.B.S.; Taracena, E.A.; Oliva-Hernández, B.E.; Martínez-Arévalo, J.V.; Fernandes, P.D.; Pérez-Sabino, J.F.; et al. Chemical composition and evaluation of antinociceptive activity of the essential oil of Stevia serrata Cav. from Guatemala. *Nat. Prod. Res.* **2017**, *13*, 1–3. [CrossRef]
4. Adams, R.P. *Identification of Essential Oil Components by Gas Chromatography/Quadrupole Mass Spectroscopy*; Allured Publ. Corp.: Carol Stream, IL, USA, 2001.
5. Giorno, T.B.S.; Ballard, Y.L.L.; Cordeiro, M.S.; Silva, B.V.; Pinto, A.C.; Fernandes, P.D. Central and peripheral antinociceptive activity of 3-(2-oxopropyl)-3-hydroxy-2-oxindoles. *Pharmacol. Biochem. Behav.* **2015**, *135*, 13–19. [CrossRef]
6. Sakurada, T.; Sugiyama, A.; Sakurada, C.; Tanno, K.; Sakurada, S.; Kisara, K.; Hara, A.; Abiko, Y. Involvement of nitric oxide in spinally mediated capsaicin- and glutamate-induced behavioural responses in the mouse. *Neurochem. Int.* **1996**, *29*, 271–278. [CrossRef]
7. Sahley, T.L.; Berntson, G.G. Antinociceptive effects of central and systemic administration of nicotine in the rat. *Psychopharmacology* **1979**, *65*, 279–283. [CrossRef]
8. Matheus, M.E.; Berrondo, L.F.; Vieitas, E.C.; Menezes, F.S.; Fernandes, P.D. Evaluation of the antinociceptive properties from Brillantaisia palisotii Lindau stems extracts. *J. Ethnopharmacol.* **2005**, *102*, 377–381. [CrossRef]

9. Sammons, M.J.; Raval, P.; Davey, P.T.; Rogers, D.; Parson, A.A.; Bingham, S. Carrageenan-induced thermal hyperalgesia in the mouse: Role of nervegrowth factor and the mitogen-activated protein kinase pathway. *Brain Res.* **2000**, *876*, 48–54. [CrossRef]
10. Otuki, M.F.; Ferreira, J.; Lima, F.V.; Meyre-Silva, C.; Malheiros, A.; Muller, L.A.; Cani, G.S.; Santos, A.R.; Yunes, R.A.; Calixto, J.B. Antinociceptive properties of mixture of alphaamyrin and beta-amyrin triterpenes: Evidence for participation of protein kinase C and protein kinase A pathways. *J. Pharmacol. Exp. Ther.* **2005**, *313*, 310–318. [CrossRef]
11. Tabarelli, Z.; Berlese, D.B.; Sauzem, P.D.; Rubin, M.A.; Missio, T.P.; Teixeira, M.V.; Sinhorin, A.P.; Martins, M.A.P.; Zanatta, N.; Bonacorso, H.G.; et al. Antinociceptive effect of novel pyrazolines in mice. *Braz. J. Med. Biol. Res.* **2004**, *37*, 1531–1540. [CrossRef]
12. Pinheiro, M.M.G.; Bessa, S.O.; Fingolo, C.E.; Kuster, R.M.; Matheus, M.E.; Menezes, F.S.; Fernandes, P.D. Antinociceptive activity of fractions from Couroupita guianensis Aubl. leaves. *J. Ethnopharmacol.* **2010**, *127*, 407–413. [CrossRef]
13. Pinheiro, M.M.G.; Radulović, N.S.; Miltojević, A.B.; Boylan, F.; Fernandes, P.D. Antinociceptive esters of N-methylanthranilic acid: Mechanism of action in heat-mediated pain. *Eur. J. Pharmacol.* **2014**, *727*, 106–114. [CrossRef]
14. Barros, H.M.T.; Tannhauser, M.A.L.; Tannhauser, S.L.; Tannhauser, M. Enhanced detection of hyperactivity after drug withdrawal with a simple modification of the open-field apparatus. *J. Pharmacol. Methods* **1991**, *26*, 269–275. [CrossRef]
15. Carsten, E. Responses of rat spinal dorsal horn neurons to intracutaneous microinjection of histamine, capsaicin, and other irritants. *J. Neurophysiol.* **1997**, *77*, 2499–2514. [CrossRef]
16. Carnevale, V.; Rohacs, T. TRPV1: A Target for Rational Drug Design. *Pharmaceuticals* **2016**, *9*, 52. [CrossRef]
17. Hong, Y.; Abbott, F.V. Behavioural effects of intraplantar injection of inflammatory mediators in the rat. *Neuroscience* **1994**, *63*, 827–836. [CrossRef]
18. Zhuo, M. Ionotropic glutamate e receptors contribute to pain transmission and chronic pain. *Neuropharmacology* **2017**, *112*, 228–234. [CrossRef]
19. Millan, M.J. The induction of pain: An integrative review. *Prog. Neurobiol.* **1999**, *57*, 1–164. [CrossRef]
20. Beirith, A.; Santos, A.R.S.; Calixto, J.B. Mechanisms underlying the nociception and paw oedema caused by injection of glutamate into the mouse paw. *Brain Res.* **2002**, *924*, 219–228. [CrossRef]
21. Julius, D.; Basbaum, A. Molecular mechanisms of nociception. *Nature* **2001**, *413*, 203–210. [CrossRef]
22. Szallasi, A.; Blumberg, P.M. Vanilloid (capsaicin) receptors and mechanisms. *Pharmacol. Rev.* **1999**, *51*, 159–212.
23. Afrah, A.W.; Stiller, C.O.; Olgart, L.; Brodin, E.; Gustafsson, H. Involvement of spinal Nmethyl- D-aspartate receptors in capsaicin-induced in vivo release of substance P in the rat dorsal horn. *Neurosci. Lett.* **2001**, *316*, 83–86. [CrossRef]
24. Medvedeva, Y.V.; Kim, M.S.; Usachev, Y.M. Mechanisms of prolonged presynaptic Ca^{2+} signaling and glutamate release induced by TRPV1 activation in rat sensory neurons. *J. Neurosci.* **2008**, *28*, 5295–5311. [CrossRef]
25. Rosland, J.H.; Tjolsen, A.; Maehle, B.; Hole, D.K. The formalin test in mice. Effect of the formalin concentration. *Pain* **1990**, *42*, 235–242. [CrossRef]
26. Matthes, H.W.; Maldonado, R.; Simonin, F.; Valverde, O.; Slowe, S.; Kitchen, I.; Befort, K.; Dierich, A.; Le Meur, M.; Dollé, P.; et al. Loss of morphine-induced analgesia, reward effect and withdrawal symptoms in mice lacking the m-opioid-receptor gene. *Nature* **1996**, *383*, 819–823. [CrossRef]
27. Romberg, R.; Sarton, E.; Teppema, L.; Matthes, H.W.; Kieffer, B.L.; Dahan, A. Comparison of morphine-6-glucuronide and morphine on respiratory depressant and antinociceptive responses in wild type and m-opioid receptor deficient mice. *Br. J. Anaesth.* **2003**, *91*, 862–870. [CrossRef]
28. Henriques, M.G.M.O.; Silva, P.M.R.; Martins, M.A.; Flores, C.A.; Cunha, F.Q.; Assreuy-Filho, J.; Cordeiro, R.S.B. Mouse paw edema. A new model for inflammation. *Bras. J. Med. Biol. Res.* **1987**, *20*, 243–249.
29. Orav, A.; Raal, A.; Arak, E. Content and composition of the essential oil of *Chamomilla recutita* (L.) Rauschert from some European countries. *Nat. Prod. Res.* **2010**, *24*, 48–55. [CrossRef]
30. Raal, A.; Orav, A.; Püssa, T.; Valner, C.; Malmiste, B.; Arak, E. Content of essential oil, terpenoids and polyphenols in commercial chamomile (*Chamomilla recutita* L. Rauschert) teas from different countries. *Food Chem.* **2012**, *131*, 632–638. [CrossRef]

31. Flemming, M.; Kraus, B.; Rascle, A.; Jürgenliemk, G.; Fuchs, S.; Fürst, R.; Heilmann, J. Revisited anti-inflammatory activity of matricine in vitro: Comparison with chamazulene. *Fitoterapia* **2015**, *106*, 122–128. [CrossRef]
32. Calderón, J.S.; Quijano, L.; Gómez, F.; Ríos, T. Prochamazulene sesquiterpene lactones from *Stevia serrata*. *Phytochemistry* **1989**, *28*, 3526–3527. [CrossRef]
33. Safayhi, H.; Sabieraj, J.; Sailer, E.R.; Ammon, H.P. Chamazulene: An antioxidant-type inhibitor of leukotriene B4 formation. *Planta Med.* **1994**, *60*, 410–413. [CrossRef] [PubMed]
34. Fonsêca, D.V.; Salgado, P.R.R.; Carvalho, F.L.; Salvadori, M.G.S.S.; Antonia Penha, A.R.S.; Leite, F.C.; Borges, C.J.S.; Piuvezam, M.R.; Pordeus, L.C.M.; Damiao, P.; et al. Nerolidol exhibits antinociceptive and anti-inflammatory activity: Involvement of the GABAergic system and proinflammatory cytokines. *Fund Clin. Pharmacol.* **2016**, *30*, 14–22. [CrossRef] [PubMed]
35. Basile, A.C.; Sertie, J.A.; Freitas, P.C.D.; Zanini, A.C. Anti-inflammatory activity of oleoresin from Brazilian Copaiba. *J. Ethnopharmacol.* **1988**, *22*, 101–109. [CrossRef]
36. Gomes, N.M.; Rezende, C.M.; Fontes, S.P.; Matheus, M.E.; Fernandes, P.D. Antinociceptive activity of Amazonian Copaiba oils. *J. Ethnopharmacol.* **2007**, *109*, 486–492. [CrossRef]
37. Paiva, L.A.F.; Gurgel, L.A.; Silva, R.M.; Tome, A.R.; Gramosa, N.V.; Silveira, E.R.; Santos, F.A.; Rao, V.S.N. Anti-inflammatory effect of kaurenoic acid, a diterpene from *Copaifera langsdorfii* on acetic acid-induced colitis in rats. *Vasc. Pharmacol.* **2004**, *39*, 303–307. [CrossRef]
38. Gomes, N.M.; Rezende, C.R.; Fontes, S.P.; Matheus, M.E.; Pinto, A.C.; Fernandes, P.D. Characterization of the antinociceptive and anti-inflammatory activities of fractions obtained from Copaifera multijuga Hayne. *J. Ethnopharmacol.* **2010**, *128*, 177–183. [CrossRef]

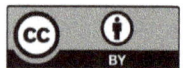

© 2020 by the authors. Licensee MDPI, Basel, Switzerland. This article is an open access article distributed under the terms and conditions of the Creative Commons Attribution (CC BY) license (http://creativecommons.org/licenses/by/4.0/).

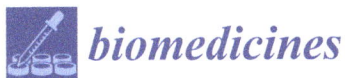

Article

Comparative Study of *Piper sylvaticum* Roxb. Leaves and Stems for Anxiolytic and Antioxidant Properties Through In Vivo, In Vitro, and In Silico Approaches

Md. Adnan [1,†], Md. Nazim Uddin Chy [2,3,†], A.T.M. Mostafa Kamal [2,*], Md Obyedul Kalam Azad [1], Kazi Asfak Ahmed Chowdhury [2], Mohammad Shah Hafez Kabir [2,3,4], Shaibal Das Gupta [3,5], Md. Ashiqur Rahman Chowdhury [3,6], Young Seok Lim [1,*] and Dong Ha Cho [1,*]

1. Department of Bio-Health Technology, Kangwon National University, Chuncheon 24341, Korea; mdadnan1991.pharma@gmail.com (M.A.); azadokalam@gmail.com (M.O.K.A.)
2. Department of Pharmacy, International Islamic University Chittagong, Chittagong 4318, Bangladesh; nazim107282@gmail.com (M.N.U.C.); ashfak4u_ctg@yahoo.com (K.A.A.C.); mohammadshahhafezkabir@yahoo.com (M.S.H.K.)
3. Drug Discovery, GUSTO A Research Group, Chittagong 4000, Bangladesh; shaibaldasgupta88@gmail.com (S.D.G.); ashiq.ctgcu@gmail.com (M.A.R.C.)
4. Department of Chemistry, Wayne State University, Detroit, MI 48202, USA
5. Department of Pharmacy, University of Science and Technology Chittagong, Chittagong 4202, Bangladesh
6. Department of Chemistry, University of Chittagong, Chittagong 4331, Bangladesh
* Correspondence: mostafa@pharm.iiuc.ac.bd (A.T.M.M.K.); potatoschool@kangwon.ac.kr (Y.S.L.); chodh@kangwon.ac.kr (D.H.C.)
† These authors contributed equally to this work.

Received: 2 March 2020; Accepted: 21 March 2020; Published: 25 March 2020

Abstract: *Piper sylvaticum* Roxb. is traditionally used by the indigenous people of tropical and subtropical countries like Bangladesh, India, and China for relieving the common cold or a variety of chronic diseases, such as asthma, chronic coughing, piles, rheumatic pain, headaches, wounds, tuberculosis, indigestion, and dyspepsia. This study tested anxiolytic and antioxidant activities by *in vivo*, *in vitro*, and *in silico* experiments for the metabolites extracted (methanol) from the leaves and stems of *P. sylvaticum* (MEPSL and MEPSS). During the anxiolytic evaluation analyzed by elevated plus maze and hole board tests, MEPSL and MEPSS (200 and 400 mg/kg, body weight) exhibited a significant and dose-dependent reduction of anxiety-like behavior in mice. Similarly, mice treated with MEPSL and MEPSS demonstrated dose-dependent increases in locomotion and CNS simulative effects in open field test. In addition, both extracts (MEPSL and MEPSS) also showed moderate antioxidant activities in DPPH scavenging and ferric reducing power assays compared to the standard, ascorbic acid. In parallel, previously isolated bioactive compounds from this plant were documented and subjected to a molecular docking study to correlate them with the pharmacological outcomes. The selected four major phytocompounds displayed favorable binding affinities to potassium channel and xanthine oxidoreductase enzyme targets in molecular docking experiments. Overall, *P. sylvaticum* is bioactive, as is evident through experimental and computational analysis. Further experiments are necessary to evaluate purified novel compounds for the clinical evaluation.

Keywords: *Piper sylvaticum*; anxiolytic; antioxidant; molecular docking; phytochemistry

1. Introduction

Human neurological disarrays have instigated as ever-growing intimidation in the public health sector and significantly affected the function and quality of life [1]. Anxiety is a regular emotion but becomes appalling when it transpires too often and turns to a terrible psychiatric disorder [2]. Perhaps stress plays a vital part in the pathogenesis of anxiety. Moreover, the stressful state leads to oxidative stress, which has been described as a potential contributor to the pathogenesis of several chronic diseases, such as diabetes, liver damage, inflammation, aging, neurological disorders, and cancer [3,4]. To treat such chronic diseases, medicinal plants derived natural products have been used around the globe clinically, even for the management of normal fever to life-threatening conditions [5]. The rural people of Bangladesh consume medicinal plants as a primary source of health-care, so they play a pivotal role in treating a large number of diseases [6]. However, the folkloric practice of medicinal plants is mainly based on empirical shreds of evidence which need proper rationalization on scientific grounds.

Piper sylvaticum (Roxb.) belongs to the Piperaceae family; is a climbing herb, commonly known as pahari pipul (Hindi), pahaari peepal (Folk medicine), vana-pippali (Ayurveda), chang bing hu jiao (China), or the mountain long pepper (English). It is widely distributed in the tropical and subtropical countries such as India, Bangladesh, China, and Myanmar. The plant has several parts, such as leaves, the stem, roots, fruits, and seeds, and most of them have wide traditional uses for the treatment of various diseases such as rheumatic pain, headaches, chronic cough, cold, asthma, piles, diarrhea, wounds in lungs, tuberculosis, indigestion, dyspepsia, hepatomegaly, and pleenomegaly [7–9]. Besides, the root of this plant is used as carminative, and the aerial parts have diuretic actions [10]. The preliminary qualitative phytochemical analysis of this plant (leaves and stem) revealed the presence of several phytochemicals, including alkaloids, flavonoids, carbohydrates, tannins, and saponins. Additionally, an earlier quantitative phytochemical study of this plant reported that the plant contains substantial amounts of phenols (65.83 and 93.39 mg GAE/g dried extract), flavonoids (102.56 and 53.74 mg QE/g dried extract), and condensed tannins (89.32 and 55.82 mg CE/g dried extract) in the leaves and stem [9,11]. Besides, several phytoconstituents have been isolated from this plant, such as piperine, piperlonguminine, sylvamide, sylvatesmin, sylvatine, sylvone, piperic acid, sesamin, and beta-sitosterol; most of them are fall into the categories of alkaloids, alkamides, flavone, and lignins [9,12]. In addition, several pharmacological activities of this plant (leaf, stem, and root) have been reported previously. Kumar et al. reported antioxidant activity of the roots and fruits [13]. Paul et al. reported the anthelmintic activity of stem [14] and Haque et al. described the antidiarrheal activity of the stem [15]. Chy et al. stated that the plant (stem) has anti-nociceptive and anti-inflammatory properties [11]. Chy et al. also reported antibacterial, anthelmintic, and analgesic activities of the leaf part [9].

Even though the plant (*P. sylvaticum*) has numerous significant medicinal properties, hitherto, no studies have been performed to determine the anxiolytic and antioxidant activities of the leaf and stem parts. Therefore, this study aimed to investigate the anxiolytic and antioxidant activities of the methanol extracts of *P. sylvaticum* leaves and stems (MEPSL and MEPSS) in several experimental models, and an *in silico* molecular docking study was performed to identify the potential lead compounds of this plant for the aforementioned activity.

2. Materials and Methods

2.1. Drugs and Chemicals

Methanol, potassium ferricyanide, phosphate buffer, and ferric chloride ($FeCl_3$), were obtained from Merck (Darmstadt, Germany). 1,1-diphenyl-2-picrylhydrazyl radical (DPPH) and trichloroacetic acid (TCA) were obtained from Sigma Chemicals Co. (St. Louis, MO, USA), and ascorbic acid from BDH Chemicals Ltd. (Poole, UK). Diazepam was obtained from Square Pharmaceuticals Ltd (Dhaka, Bangladesh). All other chemicals used in this study were of analytical reagent grade unless unless specified with an additional reference.

2.2. Plant Material Collection and Identification

The leaves and stems of *Piper sylvaticum* (Roxb.) were collected from Sita Pahar area of Kaptai, Rangamati district, Chittagong division (22°28′45″N 92°13′22″E and altitude: 14 m (49 feet), Bangladesh in October 2014, and the plant was identified by Dr. Shaikh Bokhtear Uddin, Taxonomist and Professor,

Department of Botany, University of Chittagong. A voucher specimen number (SUB 3217) has been deposited at the Department of Pharmacy, International Islamic University, Chittagong, Bangladesh, and also in the Herbarium of the University of Chittagong for future reference.

2.3. Preparation of Extract

Approximately 400 g (leaves) and 220 g (stem) of the powdered materials were soaked in 700 and 900 mL of methanol, respectively at room temperature for 14 days with occasional stirring and shaking. Finally, the resultant mixture was filtered through a cotton plug, followed by Whatman No.1 filter paper (Sigma-Aldrich, St. Louis, MO, USA), and the filtrate solution evaporated to yield the methanol extract of *P. sylvaticum* leaves and stems (MEPSL and MEPSS). The detailed procedure was described in our previous articles—see materials and methods sections [9,11].

2.4. Experimental Animals and Ethical Statements

Swiss albino mice of both sexes (weighing about, 20–25 g) were collected from Jahangir Nagar University, Savar, Dhaka, Bangladesh. The animals were sheltered in polypropylene cages by maintaining suitable laboratory conditions (room temperature 25 ± 2 °C; relative humidity 55–60%; 12 h light/dark cycle) along with standard laboratory food and distilled water ad libitum. All the experimental works were conducted in noiseless conditions and the animals were acclimatized to laboratory conditions for 10 days before experimentation. This study was carried out in accordance with the internationally accepted principles for proper use of laboratory animal's; namely, those of the National Institutes of Health (NIH) and the International Council for Laboratory Animal Science (ICLAS). The present study protocol was reviewed and approved by the "P&D committee" of the Department of Pharmacy, International Islamic University Chittagong, Bangladesh with a reference number: Pharm-P&D-61/08'16-125 (25/08/2016).

2.5. In vivo Study: Anxiolytic Activity

2.5.1. Dosing Groups

In the present study, mice were randomly divided into six groups, and each group consisted of six mice ($n = 6$). Here, the control group received 1% Tween-80 in distilled water (Sigma-Aldrich, St. Louis, MO, USA); the positive control group received reference drug diazepam (1 mg/kg, body weight), whereas the remaining groups were given 200 and 400 mg/kg body weight of the MEPSL and MEPSS, individually.

2.5.2. Elevated Plus Maze Test (EPM) in Mice

To prove the presence of anxiolytic compounds, a commonly known methodological tool is elevated plus maze (EPM), a rodent/experimental animal model which is used for the test [16]. With a height of 40 cm above from the ground, the design of the instrument is plus-shaped (+) with two opens arms (5 × 10 cm) and two closed arms (5 × 10 × 15 cm) diverging from a common point (5 × 5 cm). To avoid the occurrence of dropping down of the mice from the instrument, the open and the closed arms edges were kept 0.5 cm and 15 cm in height, respectively. After counting 30 min from the administration period of the test drug, each animal facing any of the enclosed arms was plotted in the middle of this instrument. Then total counting was noted in the open and closed entries for 5 min. When there was a sign of four paws in a single arm then that particular entry was recorded. The whole operation was conducted in a sound-proof room or equivalent by keeping eye on it from the nearby corner.

2.5.3. Hole-Board Test in Mice

The hole board test is the widely used valid pharmacological method for assessing anxiolytic and/or anxiogenic activity [17]. The hole board apparatus consists of a wooden box (40 cm × 40 cm × 25 cm) with sixteen equidistant holes (diameter 3 cm) evenly distributed on the base of the box.

The apparatus was elevated 25 cm above the floor. After 30 min of oral administration of treatments, each mouse was placed individually on the center of the board (facing away from the observer). Finally, the numbers of heads dipping in a period of 5 min were counted.

2.5.4. Open Field Test in Mice

The spontaneous locomotor activities were assessed using the open field test [18]. Test animals were kept in the test room at least 1 h before each open field test for habituation. The apparatus comprised of a wood square box (50 cm × 50 cm × 40 cm) with the floor divided into twenty-five small squares of equal dimensions (10 cm × 10 cm) marked by black and white color. In this study, each test animal was placed individually at the center of the apparatus and observed for 5 min to record the number of squares crossed by the animal with its four paws. The open field arena was thoroughly cleaned by using isopropyl alcohol (70%) between each test to prevent each mouse from being influenced by the odors of urine and feces from the previous mouse.

2.6. In vitro Study: Antioxidant Activity

DPPH Free Radical Scavenging and Ferric Reducing Power Assays

The DPPH (1,1-diphenyl-1-picrylhydrazyl) free radical scavenging activities of the MEPSL and MEPSS were determined as described previously [19], and results were expressed as μg/mL in compared to reference standard ascorbic acid. Then, the reducing power assay of the both extract was determined based on the previously reported method [20,21], using ferric ion reducing antioxidant power, and the results were expressed as mean ± standard error mean (SEM). In both assays, change in absorbance was taken using UV–VIS Spectrophotometer (UVmini-1240, Shimadzu, Shimadzu Corporation, Kyoto, Japan).

2.7. Chemical Compounds Studied in this Article

Piperine ($C_{17}H_{19}NO_3$), piperlonguminine ($C_{16}H_{19}NO_3$), sylvamide ($C_{14}H_{27}NO_3$), sylvatine ($C_{24}H_{33}NO_3$), sylvatesmin ($C_{21}H_{24}O_6$), and sylvone ($C_{23}H_{28}O_8$) were selected through literature study, and the chemical structures of the compounds were downloaded from the PubChem compound repository: piperine (PubChem CID: 638024); piperlonguminine (PubChem CID: 5320621); sylvamide (PubChem CID: 21580215); sylvatine (PubChem CID: 90472536); sylvatesmin (PubChem CID: 3083590); and sylvone (PubChem CID: 15043005).

2.8. In silico Study: Molecular Docking Study

2.8.1. Ligand and Protein Preparation

The chemical structures of six major compounds of *P. sylvaticum* were obtained from PubChem database (https://pubchem.ncbi.nlm.nih.gov/); then to prepare the ligand it was neutralized at pH 7.0 ± 2.0 and minimized by LigPrep tool (force field OPLS_2005) embedded in Schrödinger suite-Maestro version 10.1. Alternatively, three-dimensional crystallographic structures were retrieved from the Protein Data Bank RCSB PDB [22]: potassium channel (PDB: 4UUJ) [23] and xanthine oxidoreductase (PDB: 1R4U) [24]. These proteins were prepared for the docking experiment by Protein Preparation Wizard embedded in Schrödinger suite-Maestro version 10.1 (Schrödinger, LLC New York, NY, USA) as in the previously described method [5].

2.8.2. Glide Standard Precision Docking Procedure

Molecular docking studies were performed to elucidate the possible mechanisms of the selected compounds against potassium channel and xanthine oxidoreductase receptors for anxiolytic and antioxidant activities. In this study, molecular docking experiments were carried out using Glide embedded in Maestro by standard precision scoring function, as in the previously described method [5].

2.9. Statistical Analysis

SPSS version 20 (Statistical package for the social sciences) software (Schrödinger, LLC New York, NY, USA) was used for data analysis and all comparisons were made by using one-way ANOVA followed by Dunnett's test. Values were expressed as means ± SEM (standard errors of means) and standard deviations (SD), for which the *P*-values less than 0.05, 0.01, and 0.001 were considered statistically significant.

3. Results and Discussion

The present study was carried out to investigate the anxiolytic and antioxidant activities of the methanol extract of *P. sylvaticum* leaves and stem (MEPSL and MEPSS) through *in vivo*, *in vitro*, and *in silico* approaches. An earlier preliminary qualitative phytochemical study of this plant (both leaves and stem) reported that the plant contains numerous phytochemicals, such as alkaloids, flavonoids, carbohydrates, tannins, and saponins. Additionally, a quantitative phytochemical analysis of MEPSL also reported that it contains substantial amounts of phenol (65.83 mg gallic acid equivalent/g dried extract), flavonoids (102.56 mg quercetin equivalent/g dried extract), and condensed tannins (89.32 mg catechin equivalent/g dried extract). Furthermore, MEPSS contains significant amounts of phenol (93.39 mg), flavonoids (53.74 mg), and condensed tannins (55.82 mg) [9,11,14]. On the other hand, a previous acute toxicity study described that the plant had no mortality, abnormal behavior, and neurological changes up to 2000 mg/kg dose, which is a clear indication that the plant extract has low toxicity profile and is safe for a therapeutic dose [11].

Medicinal plants are the innumerable resources of pharmacologically active components. Plant-derived drugs have been demanding a very potential position due to their role as safer, cheaper, and effective drugs in the present world [25]. However, to develop a potential lead compound from a medicinal plant having multifarious pharmacological activities, various animal models and well-validated tests are inevitable in order to get a consistent preclinical and clinical decision [26]. In this study, we have presented a comparative pharmacological evaluation of *Piper sylvaticum*, to find whether leaves and stems of *P. sylvaticum* (MEPSL and MEPSS) have manifold pharmacological effects toward mitigating the anxiety disorder—the ultimate aim of our research. Then, we also explored the potentials of MEPSL and MEPSS for antioxidant activity, and finally a molecular docking study was performed to identify the possible lead compounds for the anxiolytic and antioxidant activity.

Both extracts of *P. sylvaticum* were evaluated for anxiolytic activity by employing the elevated plus maze (EPM) animal model, which is very popular due to the rapid assessment of the anxiety modifying reactions in mice [27]. The typical EPM tool has two opposite open and two bounded arms, whereas the open arena is thought to be more abysmal for the animals, and an anxiolytic agent can motivate the mice toward open arm exploration [28]. Table 1 demonstrated the anxiolytic activity of MEPSL and MEPSS in the EPM test. Administration of MEPSL and MEPSS (400 and 200 mg/kg, body weight) revealed a dose dependent increase in locomotion. Particularly, 400 mg/kg significantly ($P < 0.01$) elevated the amount of time spent in the open arms. Among both extracts, MEPSL was very effective, and 400 mg/kg remarkably enhanced spending time (109.65 ± 4.88) ($P < 0.01$) and the number of entries (11.33 ± 1.33) ($P < 0.001$) in the open arms. Similarly, 200 mg/kg showed a moderate (82.73 ± 3.03) but significant ($P < 0.01$) anxiolytic effect compared to the control group (78.50 ± 4.75). In addition, reference drug (diazepam at 1 mg/kg, i.p.) treated mice exposed an obvious provocation in the time spent and number of entries in the open arms.

Table 1. Anxiolytic effects of MEPSL, MEPSS, and diazepam on behavior of mice in elevated plus-maze model test in mice.

Treatment (mg/kg)	Time Spent in Open Arm (sec)	No. of Entry in Open Arm
Control	78.50 ± 4.75	9.50 ± 1.96
RSD 1	119.16 ± 5.45	13.83 ± 1.25 *
MEPSL 200	82.73 ± 3.03 **	9.66 ± 1.42 *
MEPSS 200	69.93 ± 3.65	6.83 ± 1.60 *
MEPSL 400	109.65 ± 4.88 **	11.33 ± 1.33 ***
MEPSS 400	93.89 ± 3.66 **	7.33 ± 1.49

Each value is expressed as mean ± SEM ($n = 6$). * $P < 0.05$, ** $P < 0.01$, and *** $P < 0.001$ compared with the control group (Dunnett's test). MEPSL, methanol extract of *Piper sylvaticum* leaves; MEPSS, methanol extract of *Piper sylvaticum* stem; RSD: reference standard drug (Diazepam, 1 mg/kg).

In the same way, with the hole board test (HBT) we intended to determine the exploratory responses as well as numerous extents of the undefined behavior of a mouse to an unacquainted atmosphere [29]. The demonstration of hole poking (head dipping) inclination specifies a high level of anxiolytic activity, while reluctance of the hole visiting indicates high level of anxiety [30]. In this test, mice treated with MEPSL and MEPSS (200 and 400 mg/kg, body weight) displayed noteworthy exploratory behavior in a dose dependent way (Table 2). The treatment of 400 mg/kg exposed significant hole poking tendencies for both extracts; a higher number of head dips resulted with 200 mg/kg. In addition, the positive control diazepam (1 mg/kg, i.p.) also manifested more head dipping compared to the control group.

Table 2. Anxiolytic effects of MEPSL, MEPSS, and diazepam in hole board test in mice.

Treatment (mg/kg)	No. of Head Dipping	Latency to the First Head Dipping (sec)
Control	31.16 ± 3.12	20.83 ± 1.52
RSD 1	67.66 ± 1.90	2.46 ± 0.42 **
MEPSL 200	41.16 ± 2.53 ***	8.91 ± 0.16 **
MEPSS 200	37.33 ± 2.10 *	6.95 ± 1.07
MEPSL 400	56.16 ± 4.70 *	5.28 ± 0.27 ***
MEPSS 400	49.83 ± 3.98 **	3.35 ± 1.02 **

Each value is expressed as mean ± SEM ($n = 6$). *$P < 0.05$, ** $P < 0.01$, and *** $P < 0.001$ compared with the control group (Dunnett's test). MEPSL, methanol extract of *Piper sylvaticum* leaves; MEPSS, methanol extract of *Piper sylvaticum* stem; RSD: reference standard drug (Diazepam, 1 mg/kg).

Further we confirmed the possibility of locomotor and exploratory activity of MEPSL and MEPSS through open field assay. The conditions of this test were highly anxiogenic, for which most standard anxiolytic agents are identified from this assessment [31]. In our study, dose (MEPSL and MEPSS at 200 and 400 mg/kg, body weight) administration significantly stimulated locomotion and exploration tendency in mice (Table 3). In this test, the lower dose (200 mg/kg) exhibited maximum agility and CNS (central nervous system) exciting effects, while exploration and locomotion of MEPSL at both doses were almost identical at all intervals over 120 min. It was reported that anxiolytics with low doses improved the anxiety state by altering motor activity followed by suppressing the muscle relaxation [31]. In contrast, the reference drug (diazepam, 1 mg/kg) produced quietness or CNS depressant-like activity. Importantly, CNS depressant-drug-like benzodiazepines inhibit excitation and curiosity in mice against the new ambient which decreases their locomotion tendency in consequence [32]. The neurobiological mechanism of anxiety is the result of either an imbalance of neurotransmitter (dopamine, GABA, and serotonin) function or dysregulation of glutamatergic, serotonergic, GABA-ergic, and noradrenergic transmission [33]. In our experiment, extracts of *P. sylvaticum* may exert anxiolytic actions by modifying neurotransmitter synthesis and functions. It is supposed that active components of *P. sylvaticum* interact with the neurotransmitter or neuromodulator receptors, which regulate the neuronal communication, stimulate the CNS activity, and improve the function of endocrine systems [34]. Additionally, it has been previously reported that the plant contains flavonoids, saponins, and tannins that are responsible for the anxiolytic activity [35], and our earlier qualitative and quantitative phytochemical studies revealed that the plant contains alkaloids, flavonoids, phenol, tannins, and saponins [9,11]. Thus, the anxiolytic activities of the MEPSL and MEPSS might be due to the binding of any of these phytochemicals to the GABAA-BZDs complex.

Table 3. Anxiolytic effects of MEPSL, MEPSS, and diazepam on a number of movements in open field test in mice.

Treatment (mg/kg)	No. of movements				
	0 min	30 min	60 min	90 min	120 min
Control	86.16 ± 4.59	71.83 ± 3.82	67.66 ± 4.25	60.50 ± 3.58	54.83 ± 5.23
RSD 1	79.16 ± 5.32	46.83 ± 4.26 **	35.66 ± 4.21	17.50 ± 3.25*	11.33 ± 2.36 ***
MEPSL 200	76.50 ± 2.48	58.83 ±6.56*	43.83 ±7.40	37.66 ±7.05*	28.83 ± 2.32 *
MEPSS 200	85.50 ± 6.69	51.16 ± 5.52	34.83 ± 5.90 **	22.33 ± 5.01	18.33 ± 1.45 **
MEPSL 400	91.50 ± 2.01	63.83 ± 2.93 ***	48.83 ± 2.49	36.33 ± 1.72 *	32.16 ± 1.47 **
MEPSS 400	79.33 ± 6.57	56.83 ± 3.44*	38.83 ± 3.74 **	31.66 ±2.23 **	20.16 ± 5.61

Each value is expressed as mean ± SEM ($n = 6$). * $P < 0.05$, ** $P < 0.01$, and *** $P < 0.001$ compared with the control group (Dunnett's test). MEPSL, methanol extract of *Piper sylvaticum* leaves; MEPSS, methanol extract of *Piper sylvaticum* stem; RSD: reference standard drug (Diazepam, 1 mg/kg).

Stressful conditions, such as EPM, HC, and OP tests, can boost up the production of reactive oxygen species (ROS) in mice and prevails over their brain defenses. However, the interplay relationship between oxidative stress (OS) and neurological disorders is not surprising [36]. *Rammal H* et al. 2008 revealed a clear interlink between anxiety and OS wherein such an imbalance of the redox system in mice led to the development of neuro-degeneration and chronic inflammation [37]. In this regard, antioxidant therapy may improve the neuronal functions and OS by inhibiting ROS formation. As shown in Figure 1, free radical scavenging capacity of MEPSL and MEPSS were concentration dependent, wherein the highest DPPH scavenging capacity was observed for MEPSL at highest concentration (100 μg/mL). In addition, 50% inhibitory concentration (IC$_{50}$) values were found 288.39 μg/mL for MEPSL and 476.97 μg/mL for MEPSS, respectively, while ascorbic acid showed 6.87 μg/mL.

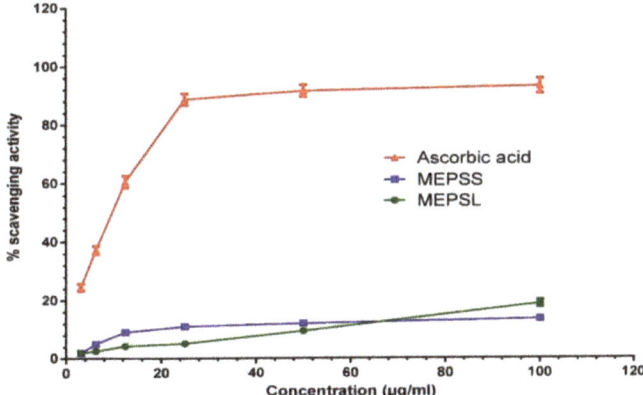

Figure 1. DPPH free radical scavenging activities of MEPSL and MEPSS compared with the reference standard ascorbic acid. Percentage of DPPH free radical scavenging activity by different concentrations of the MEPSL, MEPSS, and reference standard ascorbic acid. Values are expressed as mean ± SD ($n = 3$). MEPSL, methanol extract of *Piper sylvaticum* leaves; MEPSS, methanol extract of *Piper sylvaticum* stem.

To reassess the antioxidant ability of MEPSL and MEPSS in reducing Fe^{3+} to Fe^{2+} ions, we conducted ferric reducing antioxidant power assay (FRAP). Both extracts were found as strong antioxidant, confirmed by color change from yellow (test solution) to green and prussian blue, indicating reduction of Fe^{3+} to Fe^{2+} ions. The reduction was also monitored by UV-vis analysis at 700 nm, as increased absorbance is proportional to higher reduction of Fe^{3+} ions [38]. Data for the reducing power of MEPSL and MEPSS was shown in Figure 2, and a dose-dependent reducing capability was observed compared to reference standard ascorbic acid. Scientific investigations have been reported previously that phenolic compounds are responsible for the free radical scavenging effect of the plant and also could play an essential role in the reducing power of the plant extract [39–41]. An earlier quantitative phytochemical study of this plant revealed that it contains a considerable amount of polyphenols such as flavonoids, phenols, and condensed tannins [9,11]. Thus, it might be possible that the presence of such phytochemicals could be responsible for the free radical scavenging activity and ferric reducing power capacity of both extract.

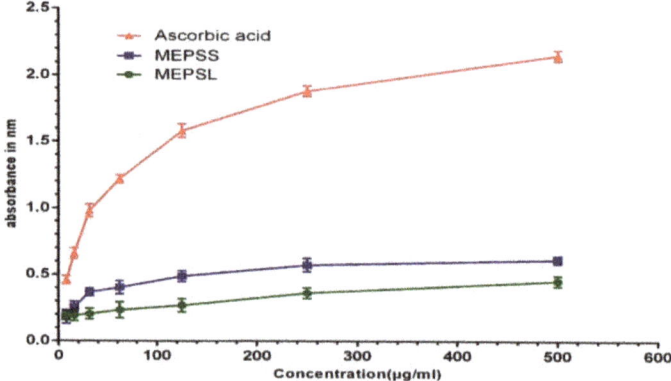

Figure 2. Reducing power capacity of MEPSL and MEPSS compared with the reference standard ascorbic acid. Values are expressed as mean ± SEM (n = 3). MEPSL, methanol extract of *Piper sylvaticum* leaves; MEPSS, methanol extract of *Piper sylvaticum* stem.

The previous phytochemical study revealed the presence of various phytochemicals in the MEPSL and MEPSS like alkaloids, flavonoids, carbohydrates, tannins, and saponins. In addition, an earlier quantitative phytochemical analysis of this plant indicated the highest amount of polyphenols contents in the both plant extract [9,11]. Furthermore, piperine, piperlonguminine, sylvamide, sylvatine, sylvatesmin, and sylvone were selected based on the availability as major compounds through literature review where most of them are fall in the categories of flavones, lignans, amide alkaloids, and alkaloids [9,12]. After the selection of compounds, an *in silico* molecular docking study was performed. Molecular docking is a key tool which has been widely used for the drug development process. It is a form of structure-based process that measures the binding affinities between small molecules and macromolecular targets like proteins. Moreover, it is also used to understand the possible molecular mechanism of action of various pharmacological responses [5,42]. From this understanding, this study was performed to comprehend the molecular mechanism of action better and to correlate their findings with the experimental results. In the present study, six major selected phytocompounds of *P. sylvaticum* were docked against two target enzyme or receptor, viz. the potassium channel receptor (PDB: 4UUJ), and xanthine oxidoreductase (PDB ID: 1R4U) enzyme, and the docking scores obtained for all compounds have been reported in Table 4.

Table 4. Docking scores and binding interactions of the selected compounds with xanthine oxidoreductase (PDB: 1R4U) and potassium channel (PDB: 4UUJ) for antioxidant and anxiolytic activity respectively.

Compounds	Docking score (kcal/mol)	Hydrogen bond interactions		Hydrophobic interactions	
		Amino acid residue	Distance (Å)	Amino acid residue (bond)	Distance (Å)
Antioxidant activity: Xanthine oxidoreductase (PDB: 1R4U)					
Piperine	−3.43	-	-	Ile288 (Alkyl)	5.09
				Phe159 (Pi-Alkyl)	4.95
				Arg176 (Pi-Alkyl)	5.46
Piperlonguminine	−2.65	Arg176	2.35	Phe162 (Pi-Pi Stacked)	5.83
				Ile288 (Alkyl)	4.48
				His256 (Pi-Alkyl)	4.93
Sylvamide	+1.33	Arg176	2.03	Val227 (Alkyl)	3.89
		Arg176	2.60	Ile288 (Alkyl)	4.43
		His256	2.86		
		His256	2.87	Phe159 (Pi-Alkyl)	5.22
		His256	2.75		
		Ile288	3.59		
Sylvatine	−1.15	Arg176	2.06	Leu163 (Alkyl)	4.88
		Asp165	2.20		
Sylvatesmin	-	-	-	-	-
Sylvone	-	-	-	-	-
Ascorbic acid (standard)	−5.13	Arg176	2.34	-	-
		Arg176	2.16		
		Val227	2.14		
		His256	2.07		
		His256	2.56		
		Asn254	1.99		
		Gln228	2.13		
Anxiolytic activity: Potassium channel (PDB: 4UUJ)					
Piperine	−4.12	Asp165	2.45	Lys142 (Pi-Alkyl)	4.11
		Asp143	2.82		
		Asn145	2.38		
		Asn145	2.75		
		Asp165	3.02		
Piperlonguminine	−4.03	Ile144	2.34	Trp163 (Pi-Pi Stacked)	4.41
		Asp143	2.57	Trp163 (Pi-Pi Stacked)	5.20
		Asp165	2.63		
		Ile144	2.48	Pro172 (Alkyl)	5.08
		Asn145	2.68		
Sylvamide	−0.59	Lys142	2.31	Lys142 (Alkyl)	3.88
		Glu105	1.91	Pro172 (Alkyl)	4.96
		Asp165	1.84	Pro172 (Alkyl)	4.27
		Asp165	2.54	Trp163 (Pi-Alkyl)	4.13
Sylvatine	−2.53	Lys199	2.88	-	-
Sylvatesmin	-	-	-	-	-
Sylvone	-	-	-	-	-
Diazepam (standard)	−3.81	Thr164	2.50	Lys103 (Pi-Cation)	4.86
				Asp165 (Pi-Anion)	4.50
				Trp163 (Pi-Sigma)	2.76
				Pro172 (Alkyl)	5.02
				Trp163 (Pi-Alkyl)	4.13

In the case of antioxidant docking study, the six selected phytocompounds of *P. sylvaticum* were docked against xanthine oxidoreductase (PDB ID: 1R4U) and showed docking scores ranging from +1.33 to −3.43 kcal/mol. The result of the docking study is shown in Table 4, and the docking figure is presented in Figures 3 and 4. From the results, it is clear that the phytocompounds piperine (−3.43 kcal/mol) displayed the highest scores against target enzyme, followed by piperlonguminine (−2.65 kcal/mol), sylvatine (−1.15 kcal/mol), and sylvamide (+1.33 kcal/mol). Here, piperine interacts with the target enzyme through two pi-alkyl interactions with Phe159 and Arg176, and one alkyl interaction with Ile288. Piperlonguminine interacted with the same enzyme by forming one hydrogen bond with Arg176, one alkyl bond with Ile288, one pi-alkyl bond with His256, and one pi-pi stacked with Phe162. Sylvatine showed the interactions forming two hydrogen bond with Arg176 and Asp165, and one alkyl interaction with Leu163 while sylvamide showed five hydrogen bond interactions with Arg176 (two interactions), His256 (two interactions), and Ile288, and three hydrophobic interactions with Val227, Ile288, and Phe159. The reference drug, ascorbic acid showed seven hydrogen bond interactions with Arg176 (two interactions), Val227, His256 (two interactions), Asn254, and Gln228. However, sylvatesmin and sylvone did not dock with the target receptor/enzyme at all.

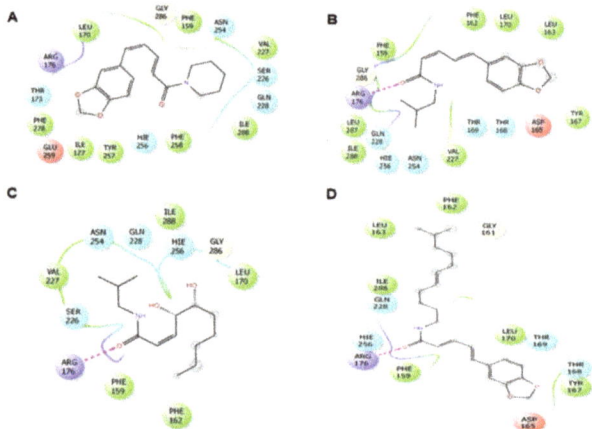

Figure 3. 2D interactions of the piperine (**A**), piperlonguminine (**B**), sylvamide (**C**), and sylvatine (**D**) with the active site of xanthine oxidoreductase (PDB: 1R4U). Colors indicate the residue (or species) type: Red—acidic (Asp, Glu), green—hydrophobic (Ala, Val, Ile, Leu, Tyr, Phe, Trp, Met, Cys, Pro), purple—basic (Hip, Lys, Arg), blue—polar (Ser, Thr, Gln, Asn, His, Hie, Hid), light gray—other (Gly, water), and darker gray—metal atoms. Interactions with the protein are marked with lines between ligand atoms and protein residues: Solid pink: H—bonds to the protein backbone, Dotted pink: H-bonds to protein side chains, Green: pi-pi stacking interactions, Orange: pi-cation interactions. Ligand atoms exposed to solvent are marked with gray spheres. The protein "pocket" is displayed with a line around the ligand, colored with the color of the nearest protein residue. The gap in the line shows the opening of the pocket.

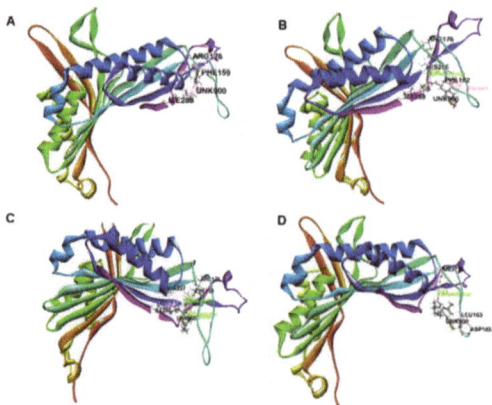

Figure 4. Best ranked pose of piperine (**A**), piperlonguminine (**B**), sylvamide (**C**), and sylvatine (**D**) in the binding pocket of xanthine oxidoreductase (PDB: 1R4U).

In the case of anxiolytic docking study, results are shown in Table 4, and the most representative interactions between ligands and receptors have been presented in Figures 5 and 6. Our study showed that piperine and sylvamide have shown the highest and lowest binding affinities against the potassium channel (PDB: 4UUJ) with docking scores of −4.12 kcal/mol and −0.59 kcal/mol respectively. The ranking order of docking score for anxiolytic effect is given below: piperine > piperlonguminine > sylvatine > sylvamide.

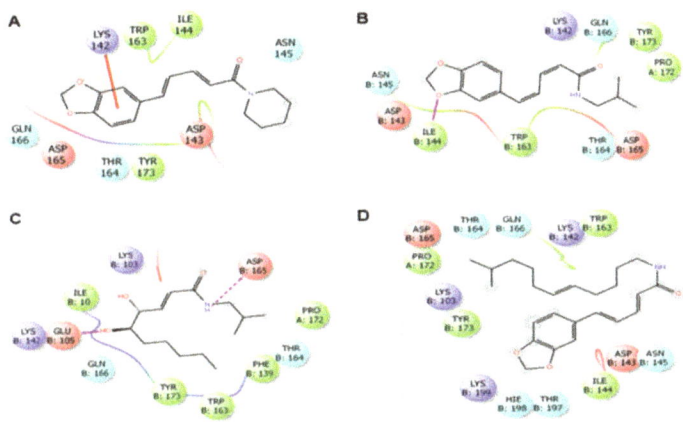

Figure 5. 2D interactions of the piperine (**A**), piperlonguminine (**B**), sylvamide (**C**), and sylvatine (**D**) with the active site of potassium channel (PDB: 4UUJ).

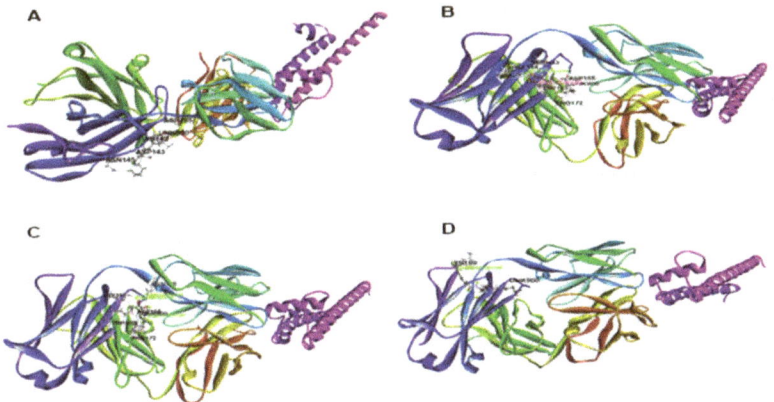

Figure 6. Best ranked pose of piperine (**A**), piperlonguminine (**B**), sylvamide (**C**), and sylvatine (**D**) in the binding pocket of potassium channel (PDB: 4UUJ).

The molecular docking study of each compound displayed several binding interactions between the ligands and the target receptor. Here, piperine interacts with the potassium channel (PDB: 4UUJ) receptor through five hydrogen bonds to Asp165 (two interactions), Asn145 (two interactions), Asp143, and one pi-alkyl interaction with Lys142. Piperlonguminine interacted with the same receptor by forming five hydrogen bonds to Ile144 (two interactions), Asp143, Asp165, and Asn145; two pi-pi stacked interactions with Trp163; and one alkyl interaction with Pro172, whereas sylvatine showed only one hydrogen bond interaction with Lys199. Besides, sylvamide interacted with the same receptor by forming four hydrogen bonds to Lys142, Glu105, and Asp165 (two interactions); three alkyl interactions with Pro172 (two interactions) and Lys142; and one pi-alkyl interaction with Trp163. The standard drug (Table 4 and Figure 7), diazepam showed one hydrogen bond interaction with Thr164 and five hydrophobic interactions with Lys103, Asp165, Trp163 (two interactions), and Pro172. However, sylvatesmin and sylvone did not dock with the target receptor/enzyme.

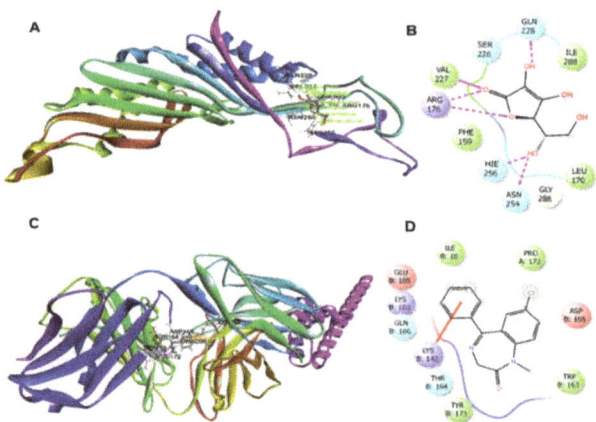

Figure 7. (**A**) Best ranked pose and (**B**) 2D interaction diagram of ascorbic acid docked at the binding pocket of xanthine oxidoreductase (PDB: 1R4U). (**C**) Best ranked pose and (**D**) 2D interaction diagram of diazepam docked at the binding pocket of potassium channel (PDB: 4UUJ).

From these results, we can conclude that the studied phytocompounds, particularly piperine, piperlonguminine, sylvamide, and sylvatine, may in part be responsible for the anxiolytic and antioxidant activities of the plant extract through interactions with these target enzyme or receptor. It has been previously reported that piperine has anxiolytic [43] and antioxidant [44] activities. Another phytoconstituent, piperlonguminine, has been reported to have multifarious pharmacological potentials, including anticancer, analgesic, cytotoxic, antioxidant, anxiolytic, and antidepressant ones [45,46]. In addition, sylvamide possesses a wide range of pharmacological effects, such as antimicrobial, neuropharmacological, antioxidant, anxiolytic, and hepatoprotective ones. This compound is also used to treat cognitive disorders [47].

4. Conclusions

In summary, results of the present study revealed that both extracts (MEPSL and MEPSS) possesses significant anxiolytic and antioxidant activities. These activities might be due to the presence of high polyphenol content in both extracts and could be due to the individual or synergistic effects of different phytochemicals, such as alkaloids, flavonoids, saponins, tannins, and phenols. Additionally, our molecular docking study unveiled that piperine, piperlonguminine, sylvamide, and sylvatine have higher binding affinities towards the target receptor/enzymes for anxiolytic and antioxidant activity, respectively. It might be possible that, for these four phytocompounds responsible for the observed pharmacological responses, further study is still necessary to elucidate their in-depth molecular mechanisms of action in animal models.

Author Contributions: M.A. and M.N.U.C. conceived and designed the experiments, prepared the plant extract, carried out all the experimental works, and collected and analyzed the data. M.A. drafted the final manuscript. M.N.U.C. and M.A. performed the in silico studies. K.A.A.C., M.O.K.A., M.S.H.K., S.D.G., and M.A.R.C. revised and improved the manuscript. A.T.M.M.K. and Y.S.L. validated all the protocols and co-supervised this study, and D.H.C. supervised the study. All authors read and approved the final manuscript.

Funding: This research did not receive any specific grant from funding agencies in the public, commercial, or not-for-profit sectors.

Acknowledgments: This research was supported by the Department of Pharmacy, International Islamic University Chittagong 4318, Bangladesh and Kangwon National University, Chuncheon, 24341, Republic of Korea.

Conflicts of Interest: The authors declare that they have no conflict of interest.

Abbreviations

MEPSL	Methanol extract of *Piper sylvaticum* leaves
MEPSS	Methanol extract of *Piper sylvaticum* stem
PDB	Protein data bank
OPLS	Optimized potentials for liquid simulations
RMSD	Root-mean-square deviation
SPSS	Statistical package for the social sciences
SEM	Standard error of the mean
BZDs	Benzodiazepines
GAE	Gallic acid equivalent
QE	Quercetin equivalent
CE	Catechin equivalent

References

1. Möller, H.-J.; Bandelow, B.; Volz, H.-P.; Barnikol, U.B.; Seifritz, E.; Kasper, S. The relevance of 'mixed anxiety and depression'as a diagnostic category in clinical practice. *Eur. Arch. Psychiatry Clin. Neurosci.* **2016**, *266*, 725–736. [CrossRef] [PubMed]
2. Kara, S.; Yazici, K.M.; Güleç, C.; Ünsal, I. Mixed anxiety–depressive disorder and major depressive disorder: comparison of the severity of illness and biological variables. *Psychiatry Res.* **2000**, *94*, 59–66. [CrossRef]
3. Hassan, W.; Eduardo Barroso Silva, C.; Mohammadzai, I.U.; Batista Teixeira da Rocha, J.; Landeira-Fernandez, J. Association of oxidative stress to the genesis of anxiety: implications for possible therapeutic interventions. *Curr. Neuropharmacol.* **2014**, *12*, 120–139. [CrossRef] [PubMed]
4. Salim, S. Oxidative stress and psychological disorders. *Curr. Neuropharmacol.* **2014**, *12*, 140–147. [CrossRef] [PubMed]
5. Adnan, M.; Nazim Uddin Chy, M.; Mostafa Kamal, A.T.M.; Azad, M.O.K.; Paul, A.; Uddin, S.B.; Barlow, J.W.; Faruque, M.O.; Park, C.H.; Cho, D.H. Investigation of the biological activities and characterization of bioactive constituents of ophiorrhiza rugosa var. prostrata (D.Don) & Mondal leaves through in vivo, in vitro, and in silico approaches. *Molecules* **2019**, *7*, 1367. [CrossRef]
6. Adnan, M.; Chy, M.N.U.; Kamal, A.T.M.M.; Barlow, J.W.; Faruque, M.O.; Yang, X.; Uddin, S.B. Evaluation of anti-nociceptive and anti-inflammatory activities of the methanol extract of Holigarna caustica (Dennst.) Oken leaves. *J. Ethnopharmacol.* **2019**, *26*, 401–411. [CrossRef]
7. Quattrocchi, U. *CRC World Dictionary of Medicinal and Poisonous Plants: Common Names, Scientific Names, Eponyms, Synonyms, and Etymology (5 Volume Set)*; CRC Press: Boca Raton, FL, USA, 2012; ISBN 142008044X.
8. *Knowledge of Herbs*, 1st ed.; Sai ePublications: Andhra Pradesh, India, 2013; ISBN 9781301080786.
9. Chy, M.N.U.; Chakrabarty, N.; Roy, A.; Paul, A.; Emu, K.A.; Dutta, T.; Dutta, E.; Ferdous, I.; Das, R.; Hasan, M.J. Antibacterial, anthelmintic, and analgesic activities of Piper sylvaticum (Roxb.) leaves and in silico molecular docking and PASS prediction studies of its isolated compounds. *J. Complement. Integr. Med.* **2019**, *16*. [CrossRef]
10. Khare, C.P. *Piper sylvaticum Roxb. BT—Indian Medicinal Plants: An Illustrated Dictionary*; Khare, C.P., Ed.; Springer: New York, NY, USA, 2007; pp. 61–91. ISBN 978-0-387-70638-2.
11. Chy, M.N.U.; Adnan, M.; Rauniyar, A.K.; Amin, M.M.; Majumder, M.; Islam, M.S.; Afrin, S.; Farhana, K.; Nesa, F.; Sany, M.A. Evaluation of anti-nociceptive and anti-inflammatory activities of Piper sylvaticum (Roxb.) stem by experimental and computational approaches. *Orient. Pharm. Exp. Med.* **2019**, 1–15. [CrossRef]
12. Parmar, V.S.; Jain, S.C.; Bisht, K.S.; Jain, R.; Taneja, P.; Jha, A.; Tyagi, O.D.; Prasad, A.K.; Wengel, J.; Olsen, C.E. Phytochemistry of the genus Piper. *Phytochemistry* **1997**, *46*, 597–673. [CrossRef]
13. Kumar, K.; Kumar, D.; Jindal, D.K.; Yadav, M.; Sharma, N.; Gupta, R. Comparative antioxidant activity of roots and fruits of Piper sylvaticum Roxb. *J. Compr. Pharm.* **2016**, *3*. [CrossRef]

14. Paul, A.; Adnan, M.; Majumder, M.; Kar, N.; Meem, M.; Rahman, M.S.; Rauniyar, A.K.; Rahman, N.; Chy, M.N.U.; Kabir, M.S.H. Anthelmintic activity of Piper sylvaticum Roxb.(family: Piperaceae): In vitro and in silico studies. *Clin. Phytoscience* **2018**, *4*, 17. [CrossRef]
15. Haque, M.T.; Ershad, M.; Kabir, M.A.; Shams, M.R.; Tahsin, F.; Milonuzzaman, M.; Al Haque, M.M.; Hasan, M.Z.; Al Mahabub, A.; Rahman, M.M. Antidiarrheal activity of methanol extract of Piper sylvaticum (roxb.) stem in mice and in silico molecular docking of its isolated compounds. *Discov. Phytomed.* **2019**, *6*, 92–98.
16. Pellow, S.; File, S.E. Anxiolytic and anxiogenic drug effects on exploratory activity in an elevated plus-maze: a novel test of anxiety in the rat. *Pharmacol. Biochem. Behav.* **1986**, *24*, 525–529. [CrossRef]
17. Takeda, H.; Tsuji, M.; Matsumiya, T. Changes in head-dipping behavior in the hole-board test reflect the anxiogenic and/or anxiolytic state in mice. *Eur. J. Pharmacol.* **1998**, *350*, 21–29. [CrossRef]
18. Gupta, B.D.; Dandiya, P.C.; Gupta, M.L. A psycho-pharmacological analysis of behaviour in rats. *Jpn. J. Pharmacol.* **1971**, *21*, 293–298. [CrossRef]
19. Adnan, M.; Azad, M.O.K.; Ju, H.S.; Son, J.M.; Park, C.H.; Shin, M.H.; Alle, M.; Cho, D.H. Development of biopolymer-mediated nanocomposites using hot-melt extrusion to enhance the bio-accessibility and antioxidant capacity of kenaf seed flour. *Appl. Nanosci.* **2020**, *10*, 1305–1317. [CrossRef]
20. Shoibe, M.; Chy, M.N.U.; Alam, M.; Adnan, M.; Islam, M.Z.; Nihar, S.W.; Rahman, N.; Suez, E. In Vitro and In Vivo Biological Activities of Cissus adnata (Roxb.). *Biomedicines* **2017**, *5*. [CrossRef]
21. Oyaizu, M. Studies on products of browning reaction. *Japanese J. Nutr. Diet.* **1986**, *44*, 307–315. [CrossRef]
22. Berman, H.M.; Battistuz, T.; Bhat, T.N.; Bluhm, W.F.; Bourne, P.E.; Burkhardt, K.; Feng, Z.; Gilliland, G.L.; Iype, L.; Jain, S. The protein data bank. *Acta Crystallogr. Sect. D Biol. Crystallogr.* **2002**, *58*, 899–907. [CrossRef]
23. Lenaeus, M.J.; Burdette, D.; Wagner, T.; Focia, P.J.; Gross, A. Structures of KcsA in complex with symmetrical quaternary ammonium compounds reveal a hydrophobic binding site. *Biochemistry* **2014**, *53*, 5365–5373. [CrossRef]
24. Retailleau, P.; Colloc'h, N.; Vivarès, D.; Bonnete, F.; Castro, B.; El Hajji, M.; Mornon, J.-P.; Monard, G.; Prangé, T. Complexed and ligand-free high-resolution structures of urate oxidase (Uox) from Aspergillus flavus: A reassignment of the active-site binding mode. *Acta Crystallogr. Sect. D Biol. Crystallogr.* **2004**, *60*, 453–462. [CrossRef] [PubMed]
25. Nissen, N. Practitioners of Western herbal medicine and their practice in the UK: Beginning to sketch the profession. *Complement. Ther. Clin. Pract.* **2010**, *16*, 181–186. [CrossRef] [PubMed]
26. Fuchs, E.; Flügge, G. Experimental animal models for the simulation of depression and anxiety. *Dialogues Clin. Neurosci.* **2006**, *8*, 323. [PubMed]
27. Lister, R.G. The use of a plus-maze to measure anxiety in the mouse. *Psychopharmacology* **1987**, *92*, 180–185. [CrossRef]
28. Rodgers, R.J.; Cao, B.-J.; Dalvi, A.; Holmes, A. Animal models of anxiety: An ethological perspective. *Brazilian J. Med. Biol. Res.* **1997**, *30*, 289–304. [CrossRef]
29. Sillaber, I.; Panhuysen, M.; Henniger, M.S.H.; Ohl, F.; Kühne, C.; Pütz, B.; Pohl, T.; Deussing, J.M.; Paez-Pereda, M.; Holsboer, F. Profiling of behavioral changes and hippocampal gene expression in mice chronically treated with the SSRI paroxetine. *Psychopharmacology* **2008**, *200*, 557–572. [CrossRef]
30. Colombo, G.; Agabio, R.; Lobina, C.; Reali, R.; Vacca, G.; Gessa, G.L. Stimulation of locomotor activity by voluntarily consumed ethanol in Sardinian alcohol-preferring rats. *Eur. J. Pharmacol.* **1998**, *357*, 109–113. [CrossRef]
31. Prut, L.; Belzung, C. The open field as a paradigm to measure the effects of drugs on anxiety-like behaviors: A review. *Eur. J. Pharmacol.* **2003**, *463*, 3–33. [CrossRef]
32. Mandelli, M.; Tognoni, G.; Garattini, S. Clinical pharmacokinetics of diazepam. *Clin. Pharmacokinet.* **1978**, *3*, 72–91. [CrossRef]
33. Sarris, J.; Panossian, A.; Schweitzer, I.; Stough, C.; Scholey, A. Herbal medicine for depression, anxiety and insomnia: A review of psychopharmacology and clinical evidence. *Eur. Neuropsychopharmacol.* **2011**, *21*, 841–860. [CrossRef]
34. Mennini, T.; Caccia, S.; Garattini, S. Mechanism of action of anxiolytic drugs. In Progress in Drug Research/Fortschritte der Arzneimittelforschung/Progrès des recherches pharmaceutiques. Springer Birkhäuser: Basel, Switzerland, 1987; pp. 315–347.
35. Gadekar, D.H.; Sourabh, J.; Jitender, M.K. Evaluation of anxiolytic activity of Boerhaavia diffusa hydro-alcoholic extract of leaves in rats. *Int Res J Pharm* **2011**, *2*, 90–92.
36. Delattre, J.; Beaudeux, J.-L.; Bonnefont-Rousselot, D. Radicaux Libres et Stress Oxydant(Aspects Biologiques et Pathologiques). Tec & Doc Lavoisier: Paris, France, 2005; pp. 1–547.

37. Rammal, H.; Bouayed, J.; Younos, C.; Soulimani, R. Evidence that oxidative stress is linked to anxiety-related behaviour in mice. *Brain. Behav. Immun.* **2008**, *22*, 1156–1159. [CrossRef] [PubMed]
38. Adnan, M.; Chy, M.N.U.; Rudra, S.; Tahamina, A.; Das, R.; Tanim, M.A.H.; Siddique, T.I.; Hoque, A.; Tasnim, S.M.; Paul, A. Evaluation of Bonamia semidigyna (Roxb.) for antioxidant, antibacterial, anthelmintic and cytotoxic properties with the involvement of polyphenols. *Orient. Pharm. Exp. Med.* **2018**, *9*, 187–199. [CrossRef]
39. Lee, J.; Koo, N.; Min, D.B. Reactive oxygen species, aging, and antioxidative nutraceuticals. *Compr. Rev. food Sci. food Saf.* **2004**, *3*, 21–33. [CrossRef]
40. Hatano, T.; Edamatsu, R.; Hiramatsu, M.; Mori, A.; Fujita, Y.; Yasuhara, T.; Yoshida, T.; Okuda, T. Effects of the interaction of tannins with co-existing substances. VI.: effects of tannins and related polyphenols on superoxide anion radical, and on 1, 1-Diphenyl-2-picrylhydrazyl radical. *Chem. Pharm. Bull.* **1989**, *37*, 2016–2021. [CrossRef]
41. Kähkönen, M.P.; Hopia, A.I.; Vuorela, H.J.; Rauha, J.-P.; Pihlaja, K.; Kujala, T.S.; Heinonen, M. Antioxidant activity of plant extracts containing phenolic compounds. *J. Agric. Food Chem.* **1999**, *47*, 3954–3962. [CrossRef]
42. Phillips, M.A.; Stewart, M.A.; Woodling, D.L.; Xie, Z.-R. Has Molecular Docking Ever Brought us a Medicine? In Molecular Docking. IntechOpen Limited: London, UK, 2018; p. 141.
43. Gilhotra, N.; Dhingra, D. Possible involvement of GABAergic and nitriergic systems for antianxiety-like activity of piperine in unstressed and stressed mice. *Pharmacol. Rep.* **2014**, *66*, 885–891. [CrossRef]
44. Mittal, R.; Gupta, R.L. In vitro antioxidant activity of piperine. *Methods Find. Exp. Clin. Pharmacol.* **2000**, *22*, 271–274. [CrossRef]
45. Karki, K.; Hedrick, E.; Kasiappan, R.; Jin, U.-H.; Safe, S. Piperlongumine induces reactive oxygen species (ROS)-dependent downregulation of specificity protein transcription factors. *Cancer Prev. Res.* **2017**, *10*, 467–477. [CrossRef]
46. Bezerra, D.P.; Pessoa, C.; de Moraes, M.O.; Saker-Neto, N.; Silveira, E.R.; Costa-Lotufo, L. V Overview of the therapeutic potential of piplartine (piperlongumine). *Eur. J. Pharm. Sci.* **2013**, *48*, 453–463. [CrossRef]
47. Gutiérrez, R.M.P.; Gonzalez, A.M.N.; Hoyo-Vadillo, C. Alkaloids from piper: A review of its phytochemistry and pharmacology. *Mini-Reviews Med. Chem.* **2013**, *13*, 163–193.

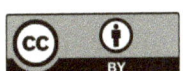

© 2020 by the authors. Licensee MDPI, Basel, Switzerland. This article is an open access article distributed under the terms and conditions of the Creative Commons Attribution (CC BY) license (http://creativecommons.org/licenses/by/4.0/).

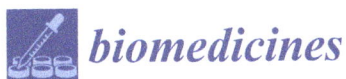

Article

Orthosiphon stamineus Standardized Extract Reverses Streptozotocin-Induced Alzheimer's Disease-Like Condition in a Rat Model

Thaarvena Retinasamy [1], Mohd. Farooq Shaikh [1,*], Yatinesh Kumari [1], Syafiq Asnawi Zainal Abidin [1,2] and Iekhsan Othman [1,2,*]

1. Neuropharmacology Research Strength, Jeffrey Cheah School of Medicine and Health Sciences, Monash University Malaysia, Bandar Sunway, Selangor 47500, Malaysia; thaarvena@gmail.com (T.R.); yatinesh.kumari@monash.edu (Y.K.); syafiq.asnawi@monash.edu (S.A.Z.A.)
2. Liquid Chromatography Mass Spectrometry (LC-MS) Platform, Jeffrey Cheah School of Medicine and Health Sciences, Monash University Malaysia, Bandar Sunway, Selangor 47500, Malaysia
* Correspondence: farooq.shaikh@monash.edu (M.F.S.); iekhsan.othman@monash.edu (I.O.)

Received: 7 April 2020; Accepted: 29 April 2020; Published: 30 April 2020

Abstract: Alzheimer's disease (AD) is a chronic neurodegenerative brain disease that is characterized by impairment in cognitive functioning as well as the presence of intraneuronal neurofibrillary tangles (NFTs) and extracellular senile plaques. There is a growing interest in the potential of phytochemicals to improve memory, learning, and general cognitive abilities. The Malaysian herb *Orthosiphon stamineus* is a traditional remedy that possesses anti-inflammatory, anti-oxidant, and free-radical scavenging abilities, all of which are known to protect against AD. Previous studies have reported that intracerebroventricular (ICV) administration of streptozotocin (STZ) mimics a condition similar to that observed in AD. This experiment thus aimed to explore if an ethanolic leaf extract of *O. stamineus* has the potential to be a novel treatment for AD in a rat model and can reverse the STZ- induced learning and memory dysfunction. The results of this study indicate that *O. stamineus* has the potential to be potentially effective against AD-like condition, as both behavioral models employed in this study was observed to be able to reverse memory impairment. Treatment with the extract was able to decrease the up-regulated expression levels of amyloid precursor protein (APP), microtubule associated protein tau (MAPT), Nuclear factor kappa-light-chain-enhancer of activated B cells (NFκB), glycogen synthase kinase 3 alpha (GSK3α), and glycogen synthase kinase 3 beta (GSK3β) genes indicating the extract's neuroprotective ability. These research findings suggest that the *O. stamineus* ethanolic extract demonstrated an improved effect on memory, and hence, could serve as a potential therapeutic target for the treatment of neurodegenerative diseases such as AD.

Keywords: Alzheimer's disease; cognitive function; streptozotocin; *Orthosiphon stamineus*; oxidative stress

1. Introduction

Alzheimer's disease (AD) is an age-related brain disease and one of the most common types of dementia. AD is characterized by chronic and progressive neurodegeneration that triggers advanced cognitive impairment, ultimately leading to death [1,2]. The pervasiveness of this disease is expected to quadruple from 26.6 million cases (1 in 253 people) to 1 in 85 people living with the disease by 2050 [3]. Those diagnosed with this disease are unable to encode new memories, which in turn damages both declarative and non-declarative memory, thus gradually reducing the ability for reasoning, abstraction, and language [4]. Elderly people are most predisposed to developing AD and the risk increases with age. There are namely two forms of the disease, sporadic (SAD) and familial (FAD). It has been predicted that the pervasiveness of SAD is projected to be increased to 131.5 million in 2050 which in turn could lead to a serious socio-economic burden [5].

AD is largely characterized by the presence of intraneuronal neurofibrillary tangles (NFTs) and extracellular senile plaques together with neurodegeneration in the brain [2,6]. The key etiological component of AD includes a causative protein, amyloid β protein, whereby the aggregation and deposition of the amyloid β protein activate an inflammatory immune reaction that in turn obliterates the brain neurons [7]. The synthesis of amyloid is regulated by the secretase enzyme. Thus, it can be further said that the damage to the amyloid β peptide cerebral clearance causes an abnormal increase in its brain level during the late onset of AD, which in turn accounts for most of the AD cases [8]. Another key hallmark of AD is the decrease in the production of the neurotransmitter acetylcholine, which is vital in controlling various memory-related functions [9]. AD predominantly affects cholinergic neurons in the cerebral cortex of the brain, whereby the neuronal activity is largely controlled by the neurotransmitter "acetylcholine" [10,11]. In AD, memory decline occurs because the enzyme that produces acetylcholine becomes defective resulting in a shortage of this neurotransmitter at the neuronal synapse [11]. Additionally, recent studies have shown that neuronal degeneration linked with AD has been triggered largely by neuroinflammation, oxidative stress, neurotransmitter imbalance, and neurotoxicity [5,12,13].

Streptozotocin (STZ) is a glucosamine-nitrosourea compound that produces a cytotoxic agent that particularly affects the β cells in the pancreatic islet, impairing the brain biochemistry and cholinergic transmission, as well as increasing the generation of free radicals [14–16]. Intracerebroventricular administration of STZ has been shown to resemble the similar neuropathology and biochemical alterations observed during an AD condition thus resulting in STZ-induced models playing a vital role in the pathophysiology of sporadic Alzheimer's.

In recent times, there has been a growing interest in using complementary therapy and phytochemicals from medicinal herbs to enhance the quality of life and prevent therapy-induced side-effects, particularly in using phytochemicals from medicinal herbs, as they possess anti-inflammatory and antioxidant activities that may potentially hinder neurodegeneration and improve memory and cognitive functioning [17]. *Orthosiphon stamineus* Benth. (Lamiaceae) is a medicinal herb that is extensively distributed in South East Asia. Various in vitro and in vivo models have addressed the presence of different types of phytochemicals in this plant-like flavonoids, terpenoids, and essential oils. Earlier studies have demonstrated that *O. stamineus* (OS) leaves extracts to possess strong antioxidant, anti-inflammatory, and anti-bacterial properties, with more than 20 phenolic compounds, two flavonol glycosides, nine lipophilic flavones, and nine caffeic acid derivatives, such as rosmarinic acid and 2,3-di-caffeoyl tartaric acid and nitric oxide inhibitory isopimarane-diterpenes [18–21]. For instance, Rosmarinic acid, a major flavonoid component of *O. stamineus* has been shown to have various pharmacological properties. Flavonoids, which are the principal group of polyphenols, are also reported to be efficacious in decreasing oxidative stress and are said to promote various physiological benefits, particularly in learning and memory, scavenging free radicals and improving cognition [6,22]. Besides that, standardized ethanolic extract of *O. stamineus* was also found to be able to reverse age-related deficits in short-term memory as well as prevent and reduce the rate of neurodegeneration [23]. Moreover, in vitro studies have demonstrated that *O. stamineus* enhanced H_2O_2 induced oxidative stress by antioxidant mechanisms in SH-SY5Y human neuroblastoma cells [24].

Therefore, since the OS extract has been observed to demonstrate strong antioxidant and anti-inflammatory properties, these reports on the OS extract further support its neuroprotective potential in combating neurodegenerative diseases such as AD. Based on the activity profile of OS extract, it can be hypothesized that OS could serve to halt or modify intricate neurodegenerative diseases such as AD. Thus, the aim of this study was to investigate the protective potential of OS against STZ-induced AD-like condition, using two established behavioral paradigms for learning and memory as well as to observe the hippocampal alterations associated. Since preliminary studies have demonstrated a neuroprotective as well as cholinesterase inhibitory effect; hence, it is hypothesized that *O. stamineus* can be established as an effective and safer potential therapeutic agent to combat cognitive alterations in AD.

2. Materials and Methods

2.1. Plant Extract Standardization of Orthosiphon stamineus 50% Ethanolic Extract

The plant material was collected from NatureCeuticals HiTech Plantation, Jalan Kampung Binjai, Kampung Binjai, 11960 Batu Maung, Pulau Pinang, Malaysia (5°16′59.4″ N 100°15′30.3″ E) and the sample was authenticated and deposited at the Herbarium of School of Biology, Universiti Sains Malaysia with voucher #11009. The 50% ethanolic OS extract was procured from NatureCeuticals Sendirian Berhad, Kedah DA, Malaysia. The standardized extract from leaves of Orthosiphon stamineus was prepared under a good manufacturing practice (GMP)-based environment using Digmaz technology by Natureceuticals Sdn. Bhd., Malaysia. The 50% ethanolic *O. stamineus* extract was standardized by Natureceuticals Sdn. Bhd., Malaysia. As per their standardization report, the standardization of the extract was carried out against four bioactive standard markers; rosmarinic acid (RA), sinensetin (SIN), eupatorin (EUP), and 3′hydroxy-5,6,7,4′-tetramethoxyflavone (TMF).

2.2. LC-MS Analysis

The MS analysis was performed on an Agilent UHPLC 1290 Infinity system coupled to Agilent quadrupole-time-of-flight 6520 mass spectrometer with dual ESI source. The sample was loaded on a C18 column (XDB-C18 Agilent Zorbax Eclipse, narrow-bore 2.1 × 150 mm, 3.5 micron, P/N: 930990–902). The thermostat temperature was maintained at 25 °C and the auto-sampler temperature was set at 4 °C. The mobile phases used were 0.1% formic acid in water (A) and 0.1% formic acid in acetonitrile (B). The sample was eluted by increasing the gradient of buffer B from 5–95% over 25 min at a flow rate of 0.5 mL/min. The injection volume was 1.0 µL. MS analysis scan was carried out in a range of m/z 100–1000 employing electrospray ion source in the positive ionization mode. Nitrogen gas flow rate and drying gas were set at 25 L/h and 600 L/h, respectively. Drying gas temperature was set at 350 °C. The fragmentation voltage was optimized to 125 v, while the capillary voltage for analysis was 3500 v.

2.3. Animals

Locally-bred adult male Sprague Dawley (SD) rats weighing between 200–300 g were acquired from the animal facility of Jeffrey Cheah School of Medicine and Health Sciences, Monash University Malaysia. The rats were maintained under standard husbandry conditions (12:12 h light/dark cycle, at controlled room temperature (22 ± 2 °C), stress-free, water ad libitum, standard diet, and sanitary conditions). The experiment protocols were approved and conducted according to the approval of the Animal Ethics Committee Monash University, Animal Research Platform (MARP/2016/028).

2.4. Intracerebroventricular (ICV) Infusion of Streptozotocin

Streptozotocin (STZ) was injected ICV bilaterally at a dose of 3 mg/kg as described previously [15]. Briefly, the rats were firstly anesthetized using a combination of ketamine hydrochloride (75 mg/kg, intraperitoneally (i.p.)) and xylazine (10 mg/kg, i.p.). The head was positioned and fixed on the stereotaxic frame. A midline sagittal incision was done on the scalp and a burr hole was drilled through the skull on both sides over the lateral ventricles. The coordinates employed were: 0.8 mm posterior to bregma, 1.5 mm lateral to the sagittal suture, and 3.6 mm beneath the surface of the brain [25]. An injection cannula was lowered very slowly into the lateral ventricles to deliver STZ (3 mg/kg, 10 µL/injection site) or saline (10 µL/injection site) through the skull holes. STZ was prepared freshly before each injection. The injection cannula was connected to a Hamilton syringe and the injection was done using a micro-injector unit. The cannula was left in situ for a further 5 min following the injection to allow passive diffusion from the cannula tip and to minimize spread into the injection tract. The cannula was then removed slowly from the scalp and the cut skin was closed with sutures.

Following the surgery, postoperative care was made by applying the betadine povidone-iodine solution on the wound. The rats were also placed on thermal sheets to maintain body temperature and were kept under close observation for the next four days.

2.5. Experimental Design

Before the experiment, animals were acclimatized to the surroundings and were handled for one week to reduce the stress. The animals were then randomly divided into five groups (n = 8/group) as described below. The ethanolic extract of OS was dissolved in distilled water before administration.

Group 1: Sham-control (Saline)
Group 2: Negative control (Saline + STZ; 3 mg/kg)
Group 3: STZ (3 mg/kg) + Orthosiphon stamineus Low dose (50 mg/kg OS)
Group 4: STZ (3 mg/kg) + Orthosiphon stamineus Medium dose (100 mg/kg OS)
Group 5: STZ (3 mg/kg) + Orthosiphon stamineus High dose (200 mg/kg OS)

After seven days of acclimatization period, the animals were subjected to ICV injection. Group 1 rats were sham-operated, where only the surgery was done, and the brain was injected with saline, whereas groups 2–5 received STZ (3 mg/kg, single injection bilaterally). One week after the ICV-STZ injection, the rats were treated with OS extract through oral dosing using oral gavage for 10 days before being subjected to a series of behavioral studies. The behavioral parameters were conducted on day 18, where elevated plus maze test was conducted on the day (18 and 19) and a passive avoidance test was conducted on the day (20 and 21). At the end of the study, the animals were sacrificed, and their brains were isolated for gene expression analysis. The treatment schedule is presented in Figure 1.

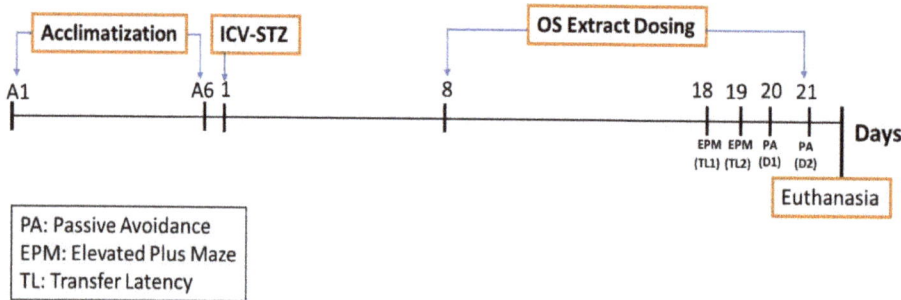

Figure 1. Schematic representation of the experimental flow. ICV-STZ: intracerebroventricular administration of streptozotocin; OS: *Orthosiphon stamineus*.

2.6. Elevated Plus Maze (EPM)

The elevated plus-maze test was employed to evaluate acquisition and retention memory following the procedure previously described [15]. Briefly, after being treated with the OS extract, the rats were put on to the end of the open arm, facing away from the central platform. With the help of the stopwatch, the transfer latency (TL_1) was noted, i.e., the time taken by a rat with all its four legs to move into any one of the enclosed arms. If the rat failed to enter any one of the enclosed arms within 90 s, it was gently pushed into one of the two enclosed arms and the TL was assigned as 90 s. The rat was allowed to explore the maze for the next 10 s and then returned to its home cage. The maze was cleaned with 70% ethanol between runs to minimize scent trails. The retention test phase was carried out 24 h after the training session to assess memory, whereby a decrease in time latency (TL_2) during the test session was deemed as an index of memory improvement. The transfer latency was expressed as an inflexion ratio, calculated using the formula:

$$IR = \frac{(L1 - L0)}{L0} \quad (1)$$

L_0: Initial TL (s) on the 1st day and
L_1: TL (s) on the 2nd day.

2.7. Passive Avoidance (PA)

A step-through passive avoidance (PA) test was carried out to measure memory retention deficit using the Passive Avoidance Box (Panlab, Harvard Apparatus) following the method previously used [26,27]. Briefly, during the acquisition trial, each rat was placed in the light chamber. Following the 60 s of habituation, the guillotine door separating the light and dark chamber was opened and the initial latency time for the rat to enter the dark chamber was recorded. The rats with the initial latency time of more than 60 s were excluded from the study. Once the rat entered the dark chamber, the guillotine door was closed and an electric foot shock (75 V, 0.2 mA, 50 Hz) was delivered to the floor grids for 3 s. Five seconds later, the rat was removed from the dark chamber and returned to its home cage. After 24 h, the retention latency was measured in the same way as the acquisition trial, but the foot shock was not delivered, and the latency time was recorded to a maximum of 300 s.

2.8. Gene Expression

Total RNA from the rat brain's hippocampal and pre-frontal cortical region was extracted following the method employed by [28], with some minor modifications. The single-step method, phenol-chloroform extraction, and Trizol reagent (Invitrogen) were used to isolate the total RNA from both the pre-frontal cortical and hippocampal regions. Briefly, the tissues were homogenized in 200 µL of Trizol solution. The mixture was then extracted using chloroform and centrifuged at 135,000 rpm at 4 °C. The alcohol was removed, and the pellet was washed twice with 70% ethanol and resuspended in 20 µL of RNase free water. RNA concentration was determined by reading absorbance at 260 nm using Nanodrop. A 500 ng amount of total RNA was reverse transcribed to synthesize cDNA using the Quantitect® Reverse Transcription Kit according to the manufacturer's protocol. Then, the mRNA expression of genes encoding amyloid precursor protein (APP), Microtubule Associated Protein Tau (MAPT), Nuclear factor kappa-light-chain-enhancer of activated B (NFκB), Glycogen synthase kinase-3 alpha (GSK3α), Glycogen synthase kinase-3 beta (GSK3β), and IMPDH2 in the hippocampus was measured via real-time PCR using the StepOne Real-Time PCR system. Subsequently, the cDNA from the reverse transcription reaction was subjected to Real-Time PCR using QuantiNova™ SYBR® Green PCR kit according to the manufacturer's protocol. The comparative threshold (C_T) cycle method was used to normalize the content of the cDNA samples, which consists of the normalization of the number of target gene copies versus the endogenous reference gene, IMPDH2.

2.9. Statistical Analysis

All findings were expressed as mean ± standard error of the mean (SEM). The data were analyzed using one-way analysis of variance (ANOVA) followed by Dunnett's tests. All the experimental groups were compared with group 2, the STZ (3 mg/kg) only group, and the *p*-values of * $p < 0.05$, ** $p < 0.01$, and *** $p < 0.001$ were considered to be statistically significant.

3. Results

3.1. Characterization of O. stamineus Ethanolic Extract

The 50% ethanolic extract was found to contain four markers, namely, RA, SIN, EUP, where the amounts of TMF were present in a very low amount as compared to the other markers, while the RA was present in abundance.

3.2. LC-MS Analysis

Identification of small-molecule contents in OS extract were detected using LC-MS analysis. A positive ionization mode was utilized for the tentative identification of the compounds. The total compound chromatogram (TCC) of the extract demonstrated different peaks as shown in Figure 2. The LC-MS analysis of the OS extract identified a total of 87 different compounds (Table 1) belonging to various groups, e.g., phenols, flavonoids, amino acids, coumarins, carboxylic acid, sesquiterpenoid, nucleoside, quinone, and cinnamic acid. Flavonoids were identified as the major compound present in the extract, such as (R)-O-(3,4-Dihydroxycinnamoyl)-3-(3,4-dihydroxy phenyl)lactic acid, Quercetagetin 4'-methyl ether 7-(6-(E)-caffeylglucoside), Luteolin 7-rhamnosyl(1→6)galactoside, Prodelphinidin A1, 6-Hydroxyluteolin 7-rhamnoside, Xanthochymuside, and Iriskumaonin.

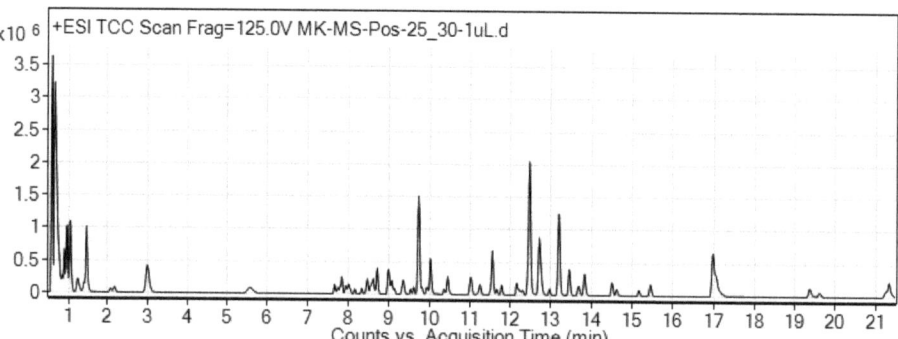

Figure 2. Total Compound Chromatogram (TCC) of *Orthosiphon stamineus* extract..

Table 1. UHPLC-MS small molecules identified in *Orthosiphon Stamineus stamineus* extract.

RT (min)	Mass (m/z)	Compound Identified	DB Formula	Compound Class
0.58	175.9546	Methylselenopyruvate	C4 H6 O3 Se	Oxo carboxylic acid
0.58	150.0317	Piperonal	C8 H6 O3	Benzodioxoles
0.635	103.0993	2-Amino-3-methyl-1-butanol	C5 H13 N O	Valinol
0.648	196.0369	Haematommic Acid	C9 H8 O5	Amides
0.650	360.318	(R)-O-(3,4-Dihydroxycinnamoyl)-3-(3,4- dihydroxyphenyl)lactic acid (Rosmarinic acid)	C18 H16 O8	Flavonoids
0.651	265.1152	D-1-[(3-Carboxypropyl)amino]-1-deoxyfructose	C10 H19 N O7	Carboxylic acid
0.651	404.0875	Asp-Tyr-OH	C18 H16 N2 O9	Amino acid
0.654	309.1058	N-Acetyl-a-neuraminic acid	C11 H19 N O9	Sialic acid (antioxidants)
0.663	117.0789	Valine	C5 H11 N O2	Amino acid
0.673	115.0632	3-Acetamidopropanal	C5 H9 N O2	Monocarboxylic acid amide
0.684	174.0999	Gly Val	C7 H14 N2 O3	Amino acid
0.686	192.0633	Quinic acid	C7 H12 O6	Cyclitol carboxylic acid (plant metabolite)
0.693	232.1057	Asp Val	C9 H16 N2 O5	Amino acid
0.716	125.0477	3-Hydroxyaminophenol	C6 H7 N O2	Phenols
0.717	304.1276	2'-Deoxymugineic acid	C12 H20 N2 O7	Tricarboxylic acid
0.717	135.0546	Adenine	C5 H5 N5	Amino acid
0.753	117.0791	Isoamyl nitrite	C5 H11 N O2	Nitrites
0.758	279.1308	N-(1-Deoxy-1-fructosyl)valine	C11 H21 N O7	Amino acid
0.828	123.0321	Isonicotinic acid	C6 H5 N O2	Carboxylic acid
0.882	208.094	Ethyl beta-D-glucopyranoside	C8 H16 O6	Glucoside
0.883	162.0526	3-Hydroxy-3-methyl-glutaric acid	C6 H10 O5	Carboxylic acid (plant metabolites)
0.886	256.0589	Piscidic Acid	C11 H12 O7	Phenols
0.892	204.0271	Oxaloglutarate	C7 H8 O7	Tricarboxylic acid

Table 1. Cont.

RT (min)	Mass (m/z)	Compound Identified	DB Formula	Compound Class
0.939	271.1054	Deidaclin	C12 H17 N O6	Glycoside
0.947	174.0162	trans-Aconitate	C6 H6 O6	Carboxylic acid anion (metabolite)
0.947	146.0212	Methyloxaloacetate	C5 H6 O5	Dicarboxylic acid
0.948	192.0271	Citric acid	C6 H8 O7	Tricarboxylic acid
0.956	187.048	1-(Malonylamino)cyclopropanecarboxylic acid	C7 H9 N O5	Carboxylic acid
1.024	189.064	L-2-Amino-6-oxoheptanedioate	C7 H11 N O5	Oxo dicarboxylic acid
1.025	171.053	Tetrahydrodipicolinate	C7 H9 N O4	Dicarboxylic acid anion
1.038	293.1473	N-(1-Deoxy-1-fructosyl)isoleucine	C12 H23 N O7	Amino acid
1.074	131.0945	N,N-Diethylglycine	C6 H13 N O2	Amino acid
1.222	100.0164	Succinic anhydride	C4 H4 O3	Tetrahydrofurandione
1.223	118.0263	Erythrono-1,4-lactone	C4 H6 O4	Lactone (butan-4-olide)
1.381	131.0944	L-Leucine	C6 H13 N O2	Amino acid
1.403	283.0918	8-hydroxy-2'-deoxy Guanosine	C10 H13 N5 O5	Nucleoside
1.452	127.0631	Guvacine	C6 H9 N O2	Amino acid
1.453	145.074	Isobutyrylglycine	C6 H11 N O3	Carboxylic acid (N-acylglycine)
2.075	327.1319	N-(1-Deoxy-1-fructosyl)phenylalanine	C15 H21 N O7	Monosaccharide derivative
2.176	165.0784	Gentiatibetine	C9 H11 N O2	Alkaloids
3.004	198.0526	2-Hydroxy-3,4-dimethoxybenzoic Acid	C9 H10 O5	Phenolic acid
3.005	152.0465	p-Anisic acid	C8 H8 O3	Phenolic acid
5.57	162.0313	3-Hydroxycoumarin	C9 H6 O3	Coumarin
7.663	712.2231	Isoliquiritigenin 4'-O-glucoside 4-O-apiofuranosyl-(1'''->2''')-glucoside	C32 H40 O18	Flavonoids
7.742	684.1694	Cosmosiin Hexaacetate	C33 H32 O16	Phenols
7.802	180.0416	4-Hydroxyphenylpyruvic acid	C9 H8 O4	Carboxylic acid (oxo carboxylic acid)
7.923	206.1302	2-Phenylethyl 3-methylbutanoate	C13 H18 O2	Carboxylic ester

Table 1. Cont.

RT (min)	Mass (m/z)	Compound Identified	DB Formula	Compound Class
7.944	656.1391	Quercetagetin 4′-methyl ether 7-(6-(E)-caffeylglucoside)	C31 H28 O16	Flavonoids
7.993	517.1616	Piperacillin	C23 H27 N5 O7S	Penicillin
8.013	594.1598	Luteolin 7-rhamnosyl(1->6)galactoside	C27 H30 O15	Flavonoids
8.442	226.1203	12-hydroxyjasmonic acid	C12 H18 O4	Oxo carboxylic acid
8.467	608.1184	Prodelphinidin A1	C30 H24 O14	Flavonoids
8.538	206.1301	2-Phenylethyl 3-methylbutanoate	C13 H18 O2	Carboxylic ester
8.582	596.1388	Quercetin 3-alpha-arabinopyranosyl-(1->2)-glucoside	C26 H28 O16	Flavonoid glycoside
8.612	448.1012	6-Hydroxyluteolin 7-rhamnoside	C21 H20 O11	Flavonoids
8.702	464.0979	Robinetin 7-glucoside	C21 H20 O12	Flavonoids
8.985	464.096	5,6,7,3′,4′-Pentahydroxy-8-methoxyflavone 7-apioside	C21 H20 O12	Flavonoids
9.062	294.0376	Tricrozarin A	C13 H10 O8	Quinone
9.316	196.1096	4-(2-hydroxypropoxy)-3,5-dimethyl-Phenol	C11 H16 O3	Phenols
9.339	448.1013	6-Hydroxyluteolin 5-rhamnoside	C21 H20 O11	Flavonoids
9.365	720.1688	Xanthochymuside	C36 H32 O16	Flavonoids
9.612	520.1583	5-Hydroxy-7,8,2′,3′-tetramethoxyflavone 5-glucoside	C25 H28 O12	Flavonoids
9.733	342.0744	Iriskumaonin	C18 H14 O7	Flavonoids
9.734	162.0318	3-Hydroxycoumarin	C9 H6 O3	Coumarins
9.734	180.0424	4-Hydroxyphenylpyruvic acid	C9 H8 O4	Phenols
9.823	520.1575	Quercetin 5,7,3′,4′-tetramethyl ether 3-galactoside	C25 H28 O12	Flavonoids
10.028	538.1122	Lithospermic acid	C27 H22 O12	Benzofuran
10.028	718.1537	Salvianolic acid L	C36 H30 O16	Stilbenoids
10.352	506.143	Morin 3,7,4′-trimethyl ether 2′-glucoside	C24 H26 O12	Flavonoids
10.441	520.1012	Melitric acid B	C27 H20 O11	Cinnamic acids
10.444	538.1113	Melitric acid A	C27 H22 O12	Cinnamic acids
10.996	208.0736	2,5-Dimethoxycinnamic acid	C11 H12 O4	Cinnamic acids

Table 1. Cont.

RT (min)	Mass (m/z)	Compound Identified	DB Formula	Compound Class
11.032	330.0741	Hypolaetin 8,3′-diimethyl ether	C17 H14 O7	Flavonoids
11.246	254.1879	Kikkanol A	C15 H26 O3	Sesquiterpenoid
11.55	358.1057	Corymbosin	C19 H18 O7	Flavonoids
11.664	374.1366	(2S)-5,6,7,3′,4′-Pentamethoxyflavanone	C20 H22 O7	Flavonoids
11.783	328.0949	Luteolin 7,3′,4′-trimethyl ether	C18 H16 O6	Flavonoids
12.256	342.1106	5,7-Dihydroxy-3′,4′-dimethoxy-6,8-dimethylflavone	C19 H18 O6	Flavonoids
12.306	272.2345	16-hydroxy hexadecanoic acid	C16 H32 O3	Juniperic acid
12.42	180.1145	3-tert-Butyl-5-methylcatechol	C11 H16 O2	Phenols
12.465	372.1213	7,8,3′,4′,5′-Pentamethoxyflavone	C20 H20 O7	Flavnonoids
12.706	344.09	Wightin	C18 H16 O7	Flavonoids
12.764	314.0793	Luteolin 5,3′-dimethyl ether	C17 H14 O6	Flavonoids
13.198	342.1108	5,7,2′,5′-tetramethoxyflavone	C19 H18 O6	Flavonoids
13.673	310.1784	methyl 8-[2-(2-formyl-vinyl)-3-hydroxy-5-oxo-cyclopentyl]-octanoate	C17 H26 O5	Long chain fatty acid
14.622	328.0942	Luteolin 7,3′,4′-trimethyl ether	C18 H16 O6	Flavonoids
21.342	390.2771	3α,12α-Dihydroxy-5β-chol-8(14)-en-24-oic Acid	C24 H38 O4	Cholanoids

3.3. Effect of OS Extract on Memory Performance in EPM and PA Task in ICV-STZ Infused Rats

Both the EPM and PA task was carried out to assess spatial long-term memory retention. In the EPM task, as observed in Figure 3A, the negative (only STZ-induced) group demonstrated a notable decrease in inflexion ratio whereas the OS treated groups demonstrated a significant increase in inflexion ratio when compared to the negative group. In the PA task, memory performance was assessed by determining the latencies to enter the dark (shock-paired) compartment during the post-24-h retention trial. All the groups did not demonstrate any differences in latency during the learning trial (data not shown), signifying that all rats showed similar responses to the testing environment and electric shocks. On the other hand, the retention test that was performed 24 h following the initial training demonstrated a significant decrease in step-through latency in the negative (only STZ-induced) group as compared to the sham-operated and the other treated groups as depicted in Figure 3B. However, when the STZ-induced rats were treated with all the three doses (50, 100, and 200 mg/kg) of OS extract, a significant increase in step-through latency was observed, indicating improved memory retention. Based on these results obtained, it can be said that OS extract does improve memory retention.

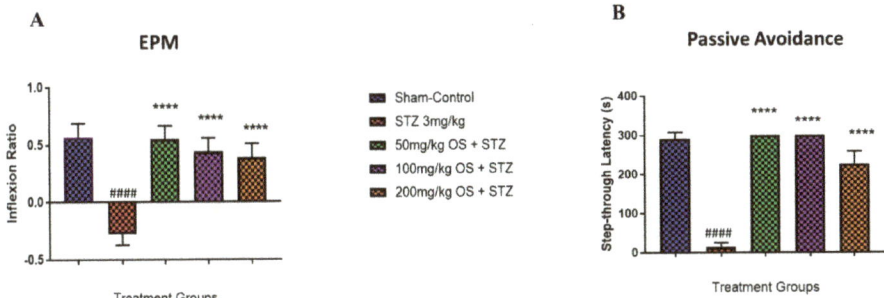

Figure 3. Behavioral analysis for elevated plus maze (EPM) and passive avoidance (PA). (**A**) represents the graph plot for the inflection ratio; (**B**) represents the graph plot for the step-through latency in PA. The behavioral analysis for the treatment groups (**A**,**B**) was compared to the negative group (3 mg/kg STZ) and the negative group (3 mg/kg STZ) was compared to the control group. Data are expressed as Mean ± SEM, $n = 8$ and statistical analysis by one-way ANOVA followed by Dunnett test **** $p < 0.0001$, #### $p < 0.0001$.

3.4. Effect of OS Extract on the Gene Expression in the Rat Hippocampal and Prefrontal Cortical Region

In the hippocampal region, the APP mRNA levels were significantly up-regulated when administered with STZ as compared to the control group, depicted in Figure 4A. Similarly, even the MAPT, NFκB, GSK3α, and GSK3β were observed to be up-regulated when administered with STZ as demonstrated in Figure 4B–E, respectively. This up-regulation was decreased significantly by OS extract treatment as compared with the negative (STZ 3 mg/kg) group. All the five mRNA expression levels, namely APP, MAPT, NFκB, GSK3α, and GSK3β, were observed to be significantly lower when treated with OS extract. The expression of APP mRNA was observed to be down-regulated in all the three doses of OS extract, and similarly, even the expression levels of MAPT, NFκB, GSK3α, and GSK3β mRNA were observed to be decreased in all the three doses of OS extract.

On the other hand, in the pre-frontal cortical region, similar results were also observed, whereby the APP mRNA levels were observed to be significantly augmented when administered with STZ as compared to the control group, as shown in Figure 5A. Likewise, even the MAPT, NFκB, GSK3α, and GSK3β were observed to be increased when administered with STZ as demonstrated in Figure 5B–E, respectively. This up-regulation was decreased significantly by OS extract treatment, whereby all five mRNA expression levels, namely APP, MAPT, NFκB, GSK3α, and GSK3β, were observed to be significantly higher when treated with the OS extract.

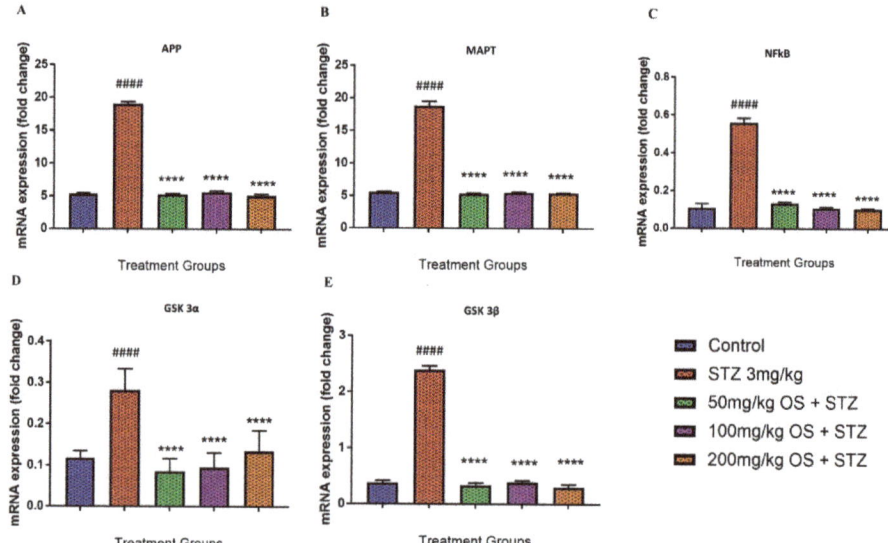

Figure 4. Gene expression in the rat hippocampi determined by real time-PCR. The genes included are (**A**) APP, (**B**) MAPT, (**C**) NFkB, (**D**) GSK 3α, and (**E**) GSK 3β. All changes in the expression levels were compared to the negative control group (STZ 3 mg/kg) and the negative group (3 mg/kg STZ) was compared to the control group. Data are expressed as Mean ± SEM, n = 4 and statistical analysis by one-way ANOVA followed by Dunnett test **** $p < 0.0001$, #### $p < 0.0001$.

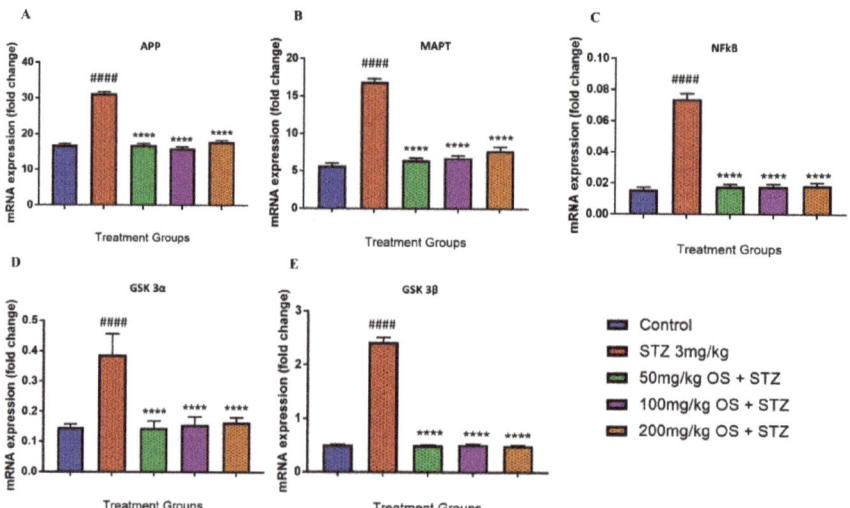

Figure 5. Gene expression in the rat pre-frontal cortical determined by real time-PCR. The genes included are (A) APP, (B) MAPT, (C) NFkB, (D) GSK 3α, and (E) GSK 3β. All changes in the expression levels were compared to the negative control group (STZ 3 mg/kg) and the negative group (3 mg/kg STZ) was compared to the control group. Data are expressed as Mean ± SEM, n = 4 and statistical analysis by one-way ANOVA followed by Dunnett test **** $p < 0.0001$, #### *p < 0.0001*.

4. Discussion

The present work aimed at determining if the ethanolic leaf extract of *O. stamineus* has the potential to be a novel treatment for AD. A preliminary dose deciding study to ascertain the therapeutic dose of OS extract was conducted where the LD50 value was found to be more than 2000 mg/kg, and therefore, the 1/20th, 1/10th, and 1/5th was chosen as therapeutic doses, corresponding to a dose range of 100 mg/kg, 200 mg/kg, and 400 mg/kg, respectively. However, when behavioral studies were conducted using these doses, the 400 mg/kg group were found to be exhibiting a neurobehavioral effect on coordination and motor activity and were not able to demonstrate any reliable results. Thus, for this study, a new range of doses was used. The dose of 200 mg/kg was employed as the highest dose, and 50 mg/kg, as well as 100 mg/kg, were used as the low dose and medium dose, respectively. All three doses did not demonstrate any side effects. *O. stamineus* ethanolic extract was employed in this study as ethanolic extracts of *O. stamineus* were found to possess the highest concentration of phenolic compounds, followed by methanolic and aqueous extracts [29] Therefore, since oxidative stress plays a significant role in AD, particularly the phenols in *O. stamineus* such as rosmarinic acid that exert free radical scavenging, anti-inflammatory and antioxidant effects [21,30], ethanolic extract of *O. stamineus* serves as the ideal choice for this experiment.

ICV injection of STZ has been established to be characterized by a progressive decline in learning and memory [31]. In this present study, a dose of 3 mg/kg STZ was employed, which has been shown to not interfere with the changes in the peripheral blood glucose level but induce a significant cognitive impairment in all animals [15,32,33]. Additionally, central administration of low STZ doses triggers an insulin-resistance brain state that produces similar neuropathology and biochemical alterations observed during AD, enabling the pathophysiology of sporadic Alzheimer's disease (sAD) to be further comprehended. Thus, the expression of increased phosphorylated tau protein in the hippocampus, as well as the accumulation of β amyloid in the meningeal capillaries, suggest that the ICV-STZ model recapitulates most of the sAD pathological feature, and hence, can serve as an apt experimental model of developing the AD hallmarks [13,34].

The performance of animals during the behavioral assessments for spatial memory acquisition and retention using elevated plus maze and passive avoidance test is well documented to estimate the extent of neuronal injury. The present study demonstrated that that treatment with OS extract improved memory retention as evidenced by the improved inflexion ratio observed in the EPM test as well as the increase in the step-through latency observed in the OS treated rats. Previous studies demonstrated significant cognitive impairment in the ICV-STZ treated group [15,35–38]. In our study, similar results were observed, whereby bilateral ICV administration of STZ resulted in spatial memory deficit, as observed by the decrease in step-through latency in the passive avoidance test and decrease in inflexion ratio observed in the elevated plus-maze test indicating memory impairment. However, when the STZ-injected rats were treated with OS extract, improved performances in both tests were observed. The positive effects of OS extract were evident with the rats that were treated with 50 mg/kg and 100 mg/kg OS extract namely where a decrease in transfer latency was observed in which the rats were able to remember and enter the closed arm quickly compared to the training session, which was observable by the improved inflexion ratio. The rats that were treated with 200 mg/kg did show improved memory retention as compared to the STZ treated group, but not as much as that observed in the 50 mg/kg and 100 mg/kg OS treated group. A ceiling effect was observed with higher doses. Therefore, based on the behavioral analyses, we can conclude that the spatial memory was improved. Thus, OS extract might influence spatial memory retention, which needs to be further explored.

The underlying mechanism for the improvement in memory retention observed in the behavioral studies was further explored by evaluating the biochemical parameters, such as the expression of amyloid precursor protein (APP), microtubule-associated protein tau (MAPT), nuclear factor kappa-light-chain-enhancer of activated B (NFκB), glycogen synthase kinase-3 alpha (GSK3-α), and glycogen synthase kinase 3 beta (GSK3-β) genes in rats treated with OS extract and STZ. Beta-amyloid (Aβ) and tau are some of the key aspects of AD and are undeniably crucial in comprehending the pathogenesis of AD. The AD amyloid cascade hypothesis postulates that the up-regulation of Aβ triggers the pathogenic hyperphosphorylation of tau, which in turn leads to the formation of neurofibrillary tangles (NFTs), thus causing neurodegeneration. Furthermore, dysregulation of GSK3 has been implicated in numerous neurodegenerative diseases, including AD [39–41]. Additionally, GSK3 plays a key role in AD as its deregulation accounts for most of the pathological hallmarks of the disease observed in both sporadic and familial AD. Both GSK3β and GSK3α stimulates tau hyper-phosphorylation at both primed and non-primed phosphorylation sites, in both cell culture models, as well as in vitro models of neurodegeneration, further implicating GSK3 as a vital factor in AD [42,43]. GSK3β has been said to influence the abnormal tau hyperphosphorylation, a key component of neurofibrillary tangles observed in the AD brain, which enhances tau aggregation and neurotoxicity [44,45]. On the other hand, GSK3α has been shown to monitor APP cleavage, resulting in the augmented Aβ production [46,47]. Although increased expression of GSK3 is not the main cause of the disease, augmented GSK3 could serve to enhance the production of Aβ, which in turn also trigger tau hyper-phosphorylation and neuronal degeneration in both FAD and sAD, which is in line with the amyloid cascade hypothesis of AD. In the present study, the induction of STZ demonstrated overexpression of all the key genes namely APP, MAPT, GSK3-α, and GSK3-β in both the hippocampus and the prefrontal cortex region. However, when treated with OS extract, the expressions of all these genes were observed to be suppressed indicating maximum protection, and hence, reducing AD pathology.

5. Conclusions

In summary, the present study demonstrated that OS extract is effective in ameliorating ICV streptozotocin-induced behavior alterations. Additionally, we also established that the GSK3α-GSK3β pathway could serve as the potential target for beta-amyloid and tau accumulation characteristically observed in AD condition and OS extract could potentially inactivate this pathway, and hence, serve as a promising treatment for neurodegenerative diseases such as Alzheimer's disease.

Author Contributions: T.R. performed all the experiments and was responsible for the writing of the manuscript in its entirety. Y.K. helped in designing the gene expression study. S.A.Z.A. contributed to the LC-MS analysis. M.F.S. and I.O. were involved in conceptualizing, designing the study, result analysis, and manuscript editing. All authors have read and agreed to the published version of the manuscript.

Funding: This research was funded by the NKEA Research Grant Scheme (NRGS), Ministry of Agriculture and Agro-Based Industry Malaysia (Grant No. NH1014D066).

Conflicts of Interest: The authors declare no conflict of interest.

References

1. Zlokovic, B.V. Vascular disorder in Alzheimer's disease: Role in pathogenesis of dementia and therapeutic targets. *Adv. Drug Deliv. Rev.* **2002**, *54*, 1553–1559. [CrossRef]
2. Zhao, Y.; Gu, J.-H.; Dai, C.-L.; Liu, Q.; Iqbal, K.; Liu, F.; Gong, C.-X. Chronic cerebral hypoperfusion causes decrease of O-GlcNAcylation, hyperphosphorylation of tau and behavioral deficits in mice. *Front. Aging Neurosci.* **2014**, *6*, 10. [CrossRef] [PubMed]
3. Brookmeyer, R.; Johnson, E.; Ziegler-Graham, K.; Arrighi, H.M. Forecasting the global burden of Alzheimer's disease. *Alzheimers Dement* **2014**, *3*, 186–191. [CrossRef] [PubMed]
4. Pluta, R.; Ulamek, M.; Jablonski, M. Alzheimer's mechanisms in ischemic brain degeneration. *Anat. Rec. (Hoboken)* **2009**, *292*, 1863–1881. [CrossRef] [PubMed]
5. Arora, R.; Deshmukh, R. Embelin Attenuates Intracerebroventricular Streptozotocin-Induced Behavioral, Biochemical, and Neurochemical Abnormalities in Rats. *Mol. Neurobiol.* **2017**, *54*, 6670–6680. [CrossRef]
6. Ghumatkar, P.J.; Patil, S.P.; Jain, P.D.; Tambe, R.M.; Sathaye, S. Nootropic, neuroprotective and neurotrophic effects of phloretin in scopolamine induced amnesia in mice. *Pharmacol. Biochem. Behav.* **2015**, *135*, 182–191. [CrossRef]

7. Chen, X.-Q.; Mobley, W.C. Alzheimer Disease Pathogenesis: Insights From Molecular and Cellular Biology Studies of Oligomeric Aβ and Tau Species. *Front. Neurosci.* **2019**, *13*, 659. [CrossRef]
8. Hardy, J.; Selkoe, D.J. The amyloid hypothesis of Alzheimer's disease: Progress and problems on the road to therapeutics. *Science* **2002**, *297*, 353–356. [CrossRef]
9. Muir, J.L. Acetylcholine, aging, and Alzheimer's disease. *Pharmacol. Biochem. Behav.* **1997**, *56*, 687–696. [CrossRef]
10. Contestabile, A. The history of the cholinergic hypothesis. *Behav. Brain Res.* **2011**, *221*, 334–340. [CrossRef]
11. Craig, L.A.; Hong, N.S.; Mcdonald, R.J. Revisiting the cholinergic hypothesis in the development of Alzheimer's disease. *Neurosci. Biobehav. Rev.* **2011**, *35*, 1397–1409. [CrossRef] [PubMed]
12. Salkovic-Petrisic, M.; Osmanovic-Barilar, J.; Brückner, M.K.; Hoyer, S.; Arendt, T.; Riederer, P. Cerebral amyloid angiopathy in streptozotocin rat model of sporadic Alzheimer's disease: A long-term follow up study. *J. Neural Transm.* **2011**, *118*, 765–772. [CrossRef] [PubMed]
13. Salkovic-Petrisic, M.; Knezovic, A.; Hoyer, S.; Riederer, P. What have we learned from the streptozotocin-induced animal model of sporadic Alzheimer's disease, about the therapeutic strategies in Alzheimer's research. *J. Neural. Transm.* **2013**, *120*, 233–252. [CrossRef] [PubMed]
14. Lannert, H.; Hoyer, S. Intracerebroventricular administration of streptozotocin causes long-term diminutions in learning and memory abilities and in cerebral energy metabolism in adult rats. *Behav. Neurosci.* **1998**, *112*, 1199–1208. [CrossRef]
15. Sharma, M.; Gupta, Y.K. Intracerebroventricular injection of streptozotocin in rats produces both oxidative stress in the brain and cognitive impairment. *Life Sci.* **2001**, *68*, 1021–1029. [CrossRef]
16. Singh, H.; Kakalij, R.; Kshirsagar, R.; Kumar, B.; Santhosh, S.; Diwan, P.D. Cognitive effects of vanillic acid against streptozotocin-induced neurodegeneration in mice. *Pharm. Biol.* **2014**, *53*, 1–7. [CrossRef]
17. Essa, M.M.; Vijayan, R.K.; Castellano-Gonzalez, G.; Memon, M.A.; Braidy, N.; Guillemin, G.J. Neuroprotective effect of natural products against Alzheimer's disease. *Neurochem. Res.* **2012**, *37*, 1829–1842. [CrossRef]
18. Sumaryono, W.; Proksch, P.; Wray, V.; Witte, L.; Hartmann, T. Qualitative and Quantitative Analysis of the Phenolic Constituents from Orthosiphon aristatus. *Planta Med.* **1991**, *57*, 176–180. [CrossRef]
19. Awale, S.; Tezuka, Y.; Banskota, A.H.; Adnyana, I.K.; Kadota, S. Nitric Oxide Inhibitory Isopimarane-type Diterpenes from Orthosiphon stamineus of Indonesia. *J. Nat. Prod.* **2003**, *66*, 255–258. [CrossRef]
20. Awale, S.; Tezuka, Y.; Banskota, A.H.; Kadota, S. Inhibition of NO production by highly-oxygenated diterpenes of Orthosiphon stamineus and their structure-activity relationship. *Biol. Pharm. Bull.* **2003**, *26*, 468–473. [CrossRef]
21. Yam, M.F.; Vuanghao, L.; Salman, I.; Ameer, O.; Fung-Ang, L.; Noersal, R.; Albaldawi, M.; Abdullah, G.; Basir, R.; Sadikun, A.; et al. HPLC and Anti-Inflammatory Studies of the Flavonoid Rich Chloroform Extract Fraction of Orthosiphon Stamineus Leaves. *Molecules* **2010**, *15*, 4452–4466. [CrossRef] [PubMed]
22. Bhullar, K.S.; Rupasinghe, H.P. Polyphenols: Multipotent therapeutic agents in neurodegenerative diseases. *Oxid. Med. Cell Longev.* **2013**, *2013*, 891748. [CrossRef] [PubMed]
23. George, A.; Chinnappan, S.; Choudhary, Y.; Choudhary, V.K.; Bommu, P.; Wong, H.J. Effects of a Proprietary Standardized Orthosiphon stamineus Ethanolic Leaf Extract on Enhancing Memory in Sprague Dawley Rats Possibly via Blockade of Adenosine A 2A Receptors. *Evidence-based complementary and alternative medicine. eCAM* **2015**, *2015*, 375837. [PubMed]
24. Sree, N.V.; Sri, P.U.; Ramarao, N. Neuro-protective properties of orthosiphon staminus (benth) leaf methanolic fraction through antioxidant mechanisms on sh-sy5y cells: An in-vitro evaluation. *Int. J. Pharm. Sci. Res.* **2015**, *6*, 1115.
25. Paxinos, G.; Watson, C. *The Rat Brain in Stereotaxic Coordinates*, 5nd ed.; Academic Press: London, UK, 1982; pp. 1–5.
26. Elcioglu, H.K.; Aslan, E.; Ahmad, S.; Alan, S.; Salva, E.; Elcioglu, Ö.H.; Kabasakal, L. Tocilizumab's effect on cognitive deficits induced by intracerebroventricular administration of streptozotocin in Alzheimer's model. *Mol. Cell Biochem.* **2016**, *420*, 21–28. [CrossRef]
27. Nakahara, N.; Iga, Y.; Mizobe, F.; Kawanishi, G. Effects of intracerebroventricular injection of AF64A on learning behaviors in rats. *Jpn. J. Pharm.* **2013**, *48*, 121–130. [CrossRef]
28. Retinasamy, T.; Shaikh, M.F.; Kumari, Y.; Othman, I. Ethanolic Extract of Orthosiphon stamineus Improves Memory in Scopolamine-Induced Amnesia Model. *Front. Pharm.* **2019**, *10*, 1216. [CrossRef]

29. Saidan, N.H.; Hamil, M.S.; Memon, A.H.; Abdelbari, M.M.; Hamdan, M.R.; Mohd, K.S.; Majid, A.M.; Ismail, Z. Selected metabolites profiling of Orthosiphon stamineus Benth leaves extracts combined with chemometrics analysis and correlation with biological activities. *BMC Complement Altern. Med.* **2015**, *15*, 350. [CrossRef]
30. Akowuah, G.A.; Zhari, I.; Norhayati, I.; Sadikun, A.; Khamsah, S.M. Sinensetin, eupatorin, 3′-hydroxy-5, 6, 7, 4′-tetramethoxyflavone and rosmarinic acid contents and antioxidative effect of Orthosiphon stamineus from Malaysia. *Food Chem.* **2004**, *87*, 559–566. [CrossRef]
31. Park, S.A. A Common Pathogenic Mechanism Linking Type-2 Diabetes and Alzheimer's Disease: Evidence from Animal Models. *J. Clin. Neurol.* **2011**, *7*, 10–18. [CrossRef]
32. Arafat, O.M.; Roghani, M.; Khalili, M.; Baluchnejadmojarad, T. Studies on diuretic and hypouricemic effects of Orthosiphon stamineus methanol extracts in rats. *J. Ethnopharmacol.* **2008**, *118*, 354–360. [CrossRef] [PubMed]
33. Balouchnejadmojarad, T. The effect of genistein on intracerebroventricular streptozotocin-induced cognitive deficits in male rat. *Basic Clin. Neurosci. J.* **2009**, *1*, 17–21.
34. Grunblatt, E.; Salkovic-Petrisic, M.; Osmanovic, J.; Riederer, P.; Hoyer, S. Brain insulin system dysfunction in streptozotocin intracerebroventricularly treated rats generates hyperphosphorylated tau protein. *J. Neurochem.* **2007**, *101*, 757–770. [CrossRef] [PubMed]
35. Veerendra Kumar, M.H.; Gupta, Y.K. Effect of Centella asiatica on cognition and oxidative stress in an intracerebroventricular streptozotocin model of Alzheimer's disease in rats. *Clin. Exp. Pharmacol. Physiol.* **2003**, *30*, 336–342. [CrossRef] [PubMed]
36. Tota, S.; Kamat, P.K.; Awasthi, H.; Singh, N.; Raghubir, R.; Nath, C.; Hanif, K. Candesartan improves memory decline in mice: Involvement of AT1 receptors in memory deficit induced by intracerebral streptozotocin. *Behav. Brain. Res.* **2009**, *199*, 235–240. [CrossRef] [PubMed]
37. Agrawal, R.; Mishra, B.; Tyagi, E.; Nath, C.; Shukla, R. Effect of curcumin on brain insulin receptors and memory functions in STZ (ICV) induced dementia model of rat. *Pharm. Res.* **2010**, *61*, 247–252. [CrossRef]
38. Mehla, J.; Mehla, J.; Pahuja, M.; Gupta, P.; Dethe, S.; Agarwal, A.; Gupta, Y.K. Clitoria ternatea ameliorated the intracerebroventricularly injected streptozotocin induced cognitive impairment in rats: Behavioral and biochemical evidence. *Psychopharmacology* **2013**, *230*, 589–605. [CrossRef]
39. Martinez, A.; Perez, D.I. GSK-3 inhibitors: A ray of hope for the treatment of Alzheimer's disease? *J. Alzheimers Dis.* **2008**, *15*, 181–191. [CrossRef]
40. Kremer, A.; Louis, J.V.; Jaworski, T.; VAN Leuven, F. GSK3 and Alzheimer's Disease: Facts and Fiction. *Front. Mol. Neurosci.* **2011**, *4*, 17. [CrossRef]
41. DaRocha-Souto, B.; Coma, M.; Pérez-Nievas, B.G.; Scotton, T.C.; Siao, M.; Sánchez-Ferrer, P.; Hashimoto, T.; Fan, Z.; Hudry, E.; Barroeta, I.; et al. Activation of glycogen synthase kinase-3 beta mediates β-amyloid induced neuritic damage in Alzheimer's disease. *Neurobiol. Dis.* **2012**, *45*, 425–437. [CrossRef]
42. Cho, J.H.; Johnson, G.V. Glycogen synthase kinase 3beta phosphorylates tau at both primed and unprimed sites. Differential impact on microtubule binding. *J. Biol. Chem.* **2003**, *278*, 187–193. [CrossRef] [PubMed]
43. Asuni, A.A.; Hooper, C.; Reynolds, C.H.; Lovestone, S.; Anderton, B.H.; Killick, R. GSK3alpha exhibits beta-catenin and tau directed kinase activities that are modulated by Wnt. *Eur. J. Neurosci.* **2006**, *24*, 3387–3392. [CrossRef] [PubMed]
44. Engel, T.; Goni-Oliver, P.; Lucas, J.J.; Avila, J.; Hernandez, F. Chronic lithium administration to FTDP-17 tau and GSK-3beta overexpressing mice prevents tau hyperphosphorylation and neurofibrillary tangle formation, but pre-formed neurofibrillary tangles do not revert. *J. Neurochem.* **2006**, *99*, 1445–1455. [CrossRef] [PubMed]
45. Lucas, J.J.; Hernández, F.; Gómez-Ramos, P.; Morán, M.A.; Hen, R.; Avila, J. Decreased nuclear beta-catenin, tau hyperphosphorylation and neurodegeneration in GSK-3beta conditional transgenic mice. *Embo J.* **2001**, *20*, 27–39. [CrossRef] [PubMed]
46. Phiel, C.J.; Wilson, C.A.; Lee, V.M.; Klein, P.S. GSK-3alpha regulates production of Alzheimer's disease amyloid-beta peptides. *Nature* **2003**, *423*, 435–439. [CrossRef]
47. Sun, X.; Sato, S.; Murayama, O.; Murayama, M.; Park, J.M.; Yamaguchi, H.; Takashima, A. Lithium inhibits amyloid secretion in COS7 cells transfected with amyloid precursor protein C100. *Neurosci. Lett.* **2002**, *321*, 61–64. [CrossRef]

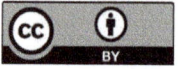

© 2020 by the authors. Licensee MDPI, Basel, Switzerland. This article is an open access article distributed under the terms and conditions of the Creative Commons Attribution (CC BY) license (http://creativecommons.org/licenses/by/4.0/).

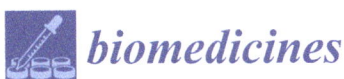

Article

Preparation of Terpenoid-Invasomes with Selective Activity against *S. aureus* and Characterization by Cryo Transmission Electron Microscopy

Bernhard P. Kaltschmidt [1], Inga Ennen [1], Johannes F. W. Greiner [2], Robin Dietsch [3], Anant Patel [3], Barbara Kaltschmidt [2,4], Christian Kaltschmidt [2,†] and Andreas Hütten [1,*,†]

[1] Thin Films & Physics of Nanostructures, Bielefeld University, Universitätsstrasse 25, 33615 Bielefeld, Germany; b.kaltschmidt@uni-bielefeld.de (B.P.K.); ennen@physik.uni-bielefeld.de (I.E.)
[2] Department of Cell Biology, Bielefeld University, Universitätsstrasse 25, 33615 Bielefeld, Germany; johannes.greiner@uni-bielefeld.de (J.F.W.G.); barbara.kaltschmidt@uni-bielefeld.de (B.K.); c.kaltschmidt@uni-bielefeld.de (C.K.)
[3] Fermentation and Formulation of Biologicals and Chemicals, Bielefeld University of Applied Sciences, Interaktion 1, 33619 Bielefeld, Germany; robin.dietsch@fh-bielefeld.de (R.D.); anant.patel@fh-bielefeld.de (A.P.)
[4] Molecular Neurobiology, Bielefeld University, Universitätsstrasse 25, 33615 Bielefeld, Germany
* Correspondence: huetten@physik.uni-bielefeld.de; Tel.: +49-521-106-5418
† These authors contributed equally to this work.

Received: 7 April 2020; Accepted: 30 April 2020; Published: 1 May 2020

Abstract: Terpenoids are natural plant-derived products that are applied to treat a broad range of human diseases, such as airway infections and inflammation. However, pharmaceutical applications of terpenoids against bacterial infection remain challenging due to their poor water solubility. Here, we produce invasomes encapsulating thymol, menthol, camphor and 1,8-cineol, characterize them via cryo transmission electron microscopy and assess their bactericidal properties. While control- and cineol-invasomes are similarly distributed between unilamellar and bilamellar vesicles, a shift towards unilamellar invasomes is observable after encapsulation of thymol, menthol or camphor. Thymol- and camphor-invasomes show a size reduction, whereas menthol-invasomes are enlarged and cineol-invasomes remain unchanged compared to control. While thymol-invasomes lead to the strongest growth inhibition of *S. aureus*, camphor- or cineol-invasomes mediate cell death and *S. aureus* growth is not affected by menthol-invasomes. Flow cytometric analysis validate that invasomes comprising thymol are highly bactericidal to *S. aureus*. Notably, treatment with thymol-invasomes does not affect survival of Gram-negative *E. coli*. In summary, we successfully produce terpenoid-invasomes and demonstrate that particularly thymol-invasomes show a strong selective activity against Gram-positive bacteria. Our findings provide a promising approach to increase the bioavailability of terpenoid-based drugs and may be directly applicable for treating severe bacterial infections such as methicillin-resistant *S. aureus*.

Keywords: terpenoids; invasomes; thymol; menthol; camphor; cineol; *S. aureus*; *E. coli*; bactericidal

1. Introduction

Terpenes are secondary plant metabolides with aromatic characters found in the oil fraction of various plants, where they serve for protection against predators or pathogens [1,2]. Notably, the oxygenated derivatives of terpenes, so-called terpenoids, have strong antioxidant and anti-inflammatory as well as antimicrobial properties [3,4]. For instance, the terpenoid thymol was reported to attenuate allergic airway inflammation in mice [5] and inhibit lipopolysaccharide-stimulated inflammatory responses via down-regulation of the transcription factor NF-κB [6]. Additionally, the terpenoid cineol was shown to inhibit pro-inflammatory signaling mediated by NF-κB [7], while simultaneously potentiating IRF3-mediated antiviral responses [8]. In addition, cineol reduced production of mucus in a human ex vivo model of late rhinosinusitis [9]. Regarding the antimicrobial properties of terpenoids, thymol was reported to have direct bactericidal effects against S. aureus and S. epidermidis [10]. The terpenoids menthol and camphor also showed anti-bacterial activity against different bacterial species such as streptococci or mycobacteria [11,12]. Cineol was also recently demonstrated to display antibacterial activities against pathogenic bacteria present in chronic rhinosinusitis such as S. aureus [13]. Despite these promising anti-inflammatory and anti-bacterial properties, pharmaceutical applications of terpenoids against bacterial infection remain challenging due to their poor water solubility and high volatility.

Here, we address this challenge by utilizing liposomal packaging for drug delivery of terpenoids. Liposomes are spherical vesicles of phospholipid bilayers, which are commonly used for encapsulation of drugs and particularly for increasing or allowing their anti-microbial activity [14]. For instance, Aravevalo and colleagues showed an increase in antibiotic activity of ß-Lactam against resistant S. aureus after encapsulation within coated-nanoliposomes [15]. In addition, Moyá and coworkers recently demonstrated a bactericidal activity of Cefepime encapsulated into cationic liposomes against E. coli [16]. Engel and colleagues assessed the antimicrobial activity of thymol and carvacrol encapsulated into liposomes by thin-film hydration and observed an inhibition of S. aureus and S. enterica growing on stainless steel [17]. As recently reported by Usach and coworkers, pompia essential oil (containing limonene and citral) as well as citral itself were successfully loaded into liposomes via hydration followed by ultrasonic disintegration. The respective encapsulated terpenoids had antimicrobial properties against different bacterial species such as S. aureus or P. aeruginosa [18]. A nanoemulsion comprising eucalyptus oil obtained by ultrasonic emulsification was also shown to have antibacterial activity against S. aureus [19]. Cui and colleagues further observed an antibacterial effect of cinnamon oil (with eugenol being its main compound) encapsulated into liposomes against methicillin-resistant S. aureus (MRSA) alone or cultivated as a biofilm [20]. In addition to increasing the anti-microbial activity of drugs, encapsulation into liposomal structures was already described to enhance the anti-inflammatory capacity of terpenoids. In this regard, nanostructured lipid carriers encapsulating thymol were shown to provide a sustained release of the terpenoid as well as an increase in anti-inflammatory activity within mouse models of skin inflammation [21]. In addition to nanostructured lipid carriers, terpenoids can also be delivered by encapsulation into polymeric nanostructured systems or by molecular complexation [2]. In addition to increasing stability of encapsulated compounds, terpenoid-encapsulation systems are widely accepted to be non-cytotoxic and enhance the antioxidant and anti-inflammatory activities of terpenoids ([18,21–23] reviewed in [2,24]). For instance, Manconi and colleagues reported the liposomal formulation of thymus essential oil to be highly biocompatible and to counteract oxidative stress in keratinocytes [22]. Thymol encapsulated in nanostructured lipid carriers further showed anti-inflammatory activity in different mouse models of skin inflammation in vivo [21].

In the present study, we took advantage of a liposome-based system, the so-called invasomes, for encapsulating the terpenoids thymol, menthol, camphor and cineol (Figure 1). Invasomes are liposomes composed of unsaturated phospholipids, small amounts of ethanol, terpenes and water [25]. In our present approach, terpenoid-invasomes were produced via extrusion of a solution comprising the respective terpenoid solved in ethanol, while soybean lecithin served as a lipid source. We aimed to characterize the produced invasomes in terms of their lamellarity, size and bilayer thickness using cryo transmission electron microscopy (Cryo TEM). Although being commonly utilized for the formulation of invasomes [26,27], terpenoids mostly serve as permeation enhancer for transdermal delivery and bioavailability rather than being bioactive components [2]. In the present study, we focused on the production of invasomes with terpenoids as the bioactive components to inhibit bacterial cell growth. With respect to pharmaceutical applications for treating bacterial infection, we therefore assessed potential bactericidal effects of our produced terpenoid-invasomes against S. aureus and E. coli.

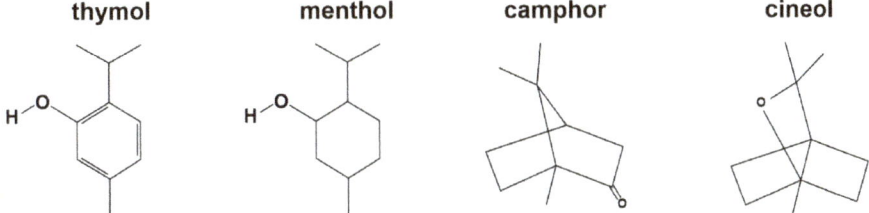

Figure 1. Structural formulas of the terpenoids thymol, menthol, camphor and cineol used for encapsulation into invasomes.

2. Materials and Methods

2.1. Preparation of Invasomes and Encapsulation of Terpeonoids

For production of invasomes, 20 mg of the respective terpenoid thymol, menthol, camphor or cineol (Caesar and Loretz GmbH, Hilden, Germany) was solved in 1.32 mL of 99.6% Ethanol. This mixture was subsequently added to 40 mL of 0.9% saline to reach a final concentration of 0.5 mg terpenoid per mL. A quantity of 100 mg of soybean lecithin (Lipoid S 100, Batch 579000-1160713-01/704, Lipoid GmbH, Ludwigshafen am Rhein, Germany) was added to 2 mL of this solution comprising the terpenoid, ethanol and saline followed by vortexing for 5 min to reach a homogenous solution. For control formulation, a solution without terpenoids was applied. Invasomes were formed by extrusion using the Avanti Mini-Extruder (Avanti Polar Lipids, Alabaster, AL, USA) by passing 1 mL of final solution 10 times back and forth through a polycarbonate membrane with 100 nm pores.

2.2. Cryo Transmission Electron Microscopy (Cryo TEM)

For Cryo TEM analysis, 3 µL of the respective invasome-dispersion produced as described above was placed on a TEM copper grid (Quantifoil Micro Tools GmBH, Großlöbichau, Germany). Plunging into liquid ethane using Leica EM GP (Leica Microsystems, Wetzlar, Germany) with 80% moisture, 10 s pre-blotting time, 3 s blotting time and 20 °C temperature was followed by transporting the samples to the cryo transfer station (Fischione Intruments, Export, PA, USA) in liquid nitrogen. Analysis was done at the OWL Analytic Center using Jeol JEM 2200 FS (JEOL Ltd., Tokyo, Japan) operated at 200 kV.

2.3. Determination of Zeta Potentials

Zeta potentials were measured using Beckmann Coulter Delsa Nano C Particle Analyzer (Beckman Coulter, Brea, CA, USA) in a flow cell after dilution of samples with water from 50 mg/mL to 500 µg/mL. Measurements were repeated ten times.

2.4. Evaluation of Invasome Size and Bilayer Thickness

Area and bilayer thickness of produced invasomes were measured using FIJI [28] by utilizing Cryo TEM images. Briefly, the area of every invasome was marked with the circular selection tool and the measurement function was applied to calculate the area of the selections followed by calculation of the radius. For assessing bilayers thickness, the segmented area selection tool of FIJI was used followed by the straighten function of FIJI to obtain straight selection and calculation of a line profile. Respective line profiles showed a clear dent at the bilayer position and thickness was measured at half maximum. A Gauss distribution was fitted to all histograms.

2.5. Growth-Inhibition Zone Assay

Overnight suspension cultures of *S. aureus* (*Staphylococcus aureus* Rosenbach 1884, DSM 24167, German Collection of Microorganisms and Cell Cultures GmbH (DSMZ), Braunschweig, Germany) were inoculated on Brain Heart Infusion Broth (BHI) agar plates (Sigma-Aldrich Corporation, Merck KGaA, Darmstadt, Germany). Filter plates loaded with 10 µL of respective invasome-dispersion were placed on the BHI agar plates followed by incubation overnight at 37 °C. Diameters of the growth-inhibition zones were measured and calculated using FIJI [28].

2.6. Analysis of Encapsulation Efficiency and Loading Capacity

Encapsulation efficiency (EE %) was analyzed as described in [29]. EE% was calculated by (total drug added − free non-entrapped drug) divided by the total drug added. Loading capacity (LC) was calculated as the amount of drug loaded per unit weight of total invasomes (weight of lipids). Free drug was separated from invasome preparation by ultrafiltration (1000× g for 30 min at 4 °C) using an Amicon Centricon device with a molecular weight cut-off of 30,000. Drug stocks for measurement were prepared in methanol for HPLC (VWR) at a concentration of 1 mg/mL. A linear dilution was prepared in methanol and absorbance was measured at 276 nm using an Ultrasspec 2100 pro photometer (Amersham Biosciences, Little Chalfont, UK). Linearity was proven between 0.0015 mg/mL and 0.025 mg/mL thymol. EE% for thymol was calculated as (0.5 mg/mL−0.0041 mg/mL)/0.5 mg/mL = 0.9918 resulting in 99.18% EE. LC% was calculated as (0.5 mg/mL−0.0041 mg/mL)/(50 + 0.5) mg/mL= 0.01, which equals 1%.

2.7. Flow Cytometric Measurement of Cell Death

For flow cytometric measurement of cell death, *S. aureus* or *E. coli* (*Escherichia coli* DH5-Alpha) were exposed to respective invasome-dispersions (0.5 mg/mL, 1 mg/mL, 2 mg/mL final terpenoid concentration) for 24 h. Cells were fixed with 0.4% PFA for 20 min followed by staining with 1 µL/mL propidium iodide (PI, Sigma Aldrich) for 10 min. PI-stained bacterial cultures were analyzed using a Beckman Coulter Gallios Flow Cytometer (Beckman Coulter) followed by data analysis with Kaluza software (Beckman Coulter).

2.8. Statistical Analysis

For assessment of lamellarity and size of invasomes encapsulating a distinct terpenoid, up to 200 invasomes per Cryo TEM image were measured in 3–4 representative Cryo TEM images. For evaluation of bilayer thickness, up to 30 invasomes were measured in 3–4 representative Cryo TEM images for each of the different terpenoid-invasomes. Examples of small representative sections of original cryo electron micrographs used for measuring invasomes size are included within the respective figures, details of measuring are described above. Statistical analysis was performed using Graph Pad Prism (GraphPad Software, San Diego, CA, USA). The p value is a probability, with a value ranging from zero to one. The first step is to state the null hypothesis, here that the terpenoids do not affect the size of the invasomes and all differences in size are due to random sampling. The p-value is the probability of obtaining results as extreme as the observed results of a statistical hypothesis test, assuming that the null hypothesis is correct. The p-value is used as an alternative to rejection points to provide the smallest level of significance at which the null hypothesis would be rejected. A smaller p-value means that there is stronger evidence in favour of the alternative hypothesis. For analysis of lamellarity, * $p < 0.05$ was considered significant (Mann–Whitney test, one-tailed). For analysis of invasome size, $p < 0.0001$ was considered significant (unpaired t-test, one-tailed). Growth-inhibition zone assay was performed as biological triplicate and Graph Pad Prism served for statistical analysis with * $p < 0.05$ being considered significant (Mann–Whitney test, one-tailed).

3. Results and Discussion

3.1. Succsessfull Preparation of Invasomes Encapsulating the Terpenoids Thymol, Menthol, Camphor and Cineol

To encapsulate terpenoids into invasomes, we aimed to produce liposomes by extrusion of a homogenous solution comprising the respective terpene solved in ethanol, 0.9% saline and soybean lecithin. Extrusion of a solution without terpenoids served as control and resulted in the formation of invasomes, as visualized by cryo transmission electron microscopy (Cryo TEM) (Figure 2A).

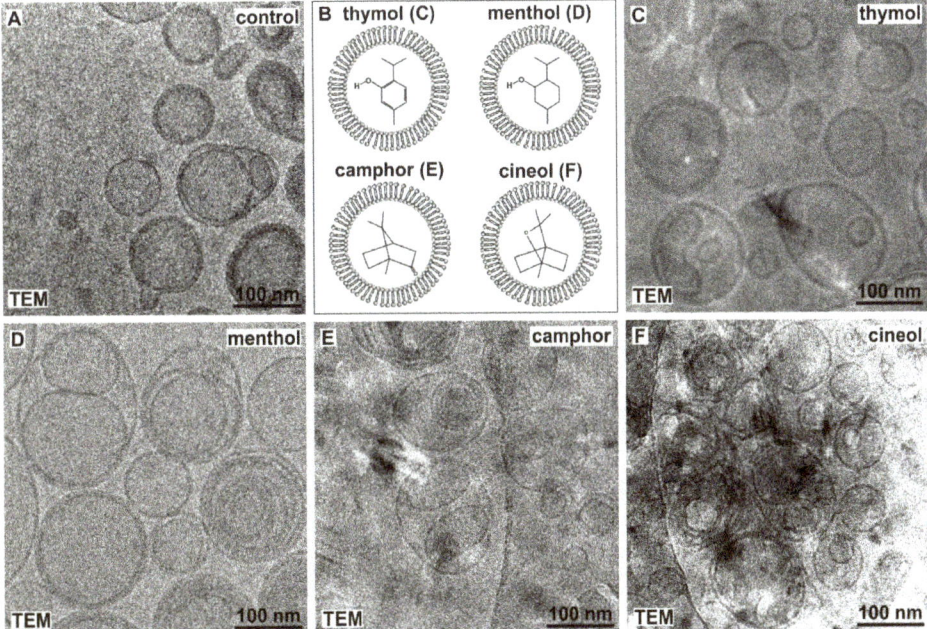

Figure 2. Successful production of invasomes encapsulating thymol, menthol, camphor and cineol by extrusion. (**A**) Cryo transmission electron microscopy (TEM) showing control invasomes without terpenoids (small representative section of original micrograph). (**B**) Schematic view of terpenoids encapsulated by invasomes. Localization of terpenoids within the aqueous phase of the invasome was chosen only for visualization reasons and does not represent their natural localization. (**C–F**) Small representative sections of original cryo electron micrographs revealed invasomes comprising thymol (**C**), menthol (**D**), camphor (**E**) or cineol (**F**) after extrusion. TEM: Cryo transmission electron microscopy.

We next applied the terpenoids thymol, menthol, camphor or cineol for production of invasomes (Figure 2B). Cryo TEM micrographs showed the presence of invasomes comprising thymol (Figure 2C), menthol (Figure 2D), camphor (Figure 2E) or cineol (Figure 2F) after extrusion. Interestingly, Cryo TEM allowed us to observe multilamellar membrane boundaries in all five approaches (Figure 2A,C–F).

During characterization of the newly produced invasomes via Cryo TEM, we observed that encapsulation of thymol and camphor resulted in a significant shift towards unilamellar vesicles. We suggest that terpenoids such as thymol might decrease membrane fluidity and thus lead to more unilamellar liposomes. On the contrary, cineol-invasomes revealed a similar distribution between unilamellar and bilamellar vesicles comparable to control. Furthermore, cineol-invasomes showed a similar size to control-invasomes, while encapsulation of thymol and camphor led to significantly smaller invasomes and menthol-comprising invasomes were significantly enlarged compared control.

We suggest this observation to be based on the elevated water solubility of cineol (3500 mg/L) compared to camphor (1600 mg/L), thymol (900 mg/L) and menthol (420 mg/L).

Analysis of Zeta potentials revealed approximately neutral potentials of control invasomes (−2 ± 5 mV, Figure 3A). We also observed approximately neutral Zeta potentials for invasomes encapsulating the terpenoids thymol (−3 ± 6 mV, Figure 3B), menthol (−1 ± 5 mV, Figure 3C), camphor (−2 ± 5 mV, Figure 3D) or cineol (0 ± 5 mV, Figure 3E).

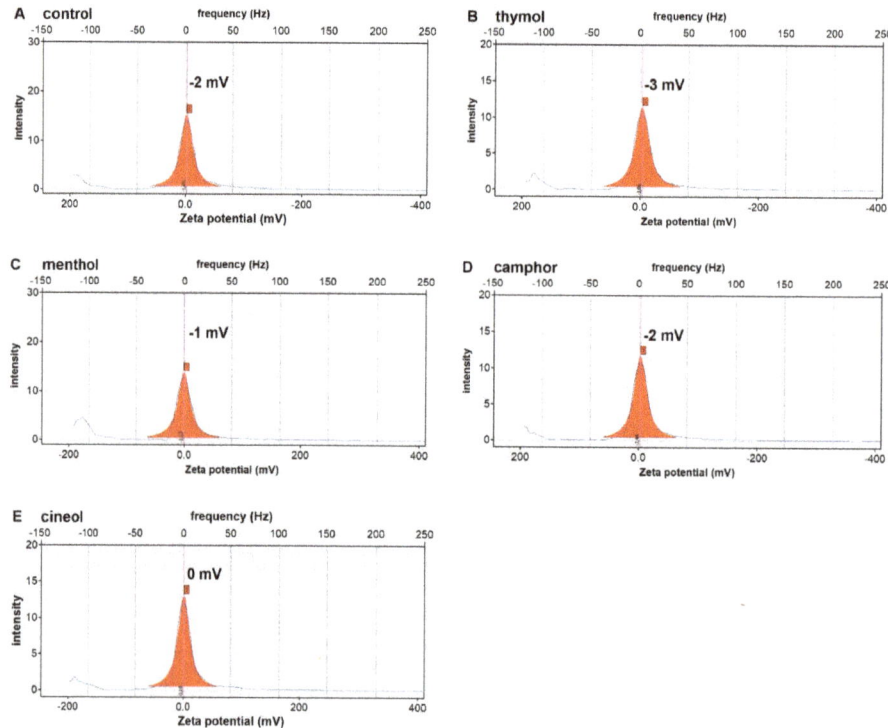

Figure 3. Invasomes without tepenoids (**A**) and encapsulating the terpenoids thymol (**B**) menthol (**C**) camphor (**D**) or cineol (**E**) reveal neutral Zeta potentials.

In terms of invasomal stability, high Zeta potentials of at least ± 20 mV are generally considered as an indicator for electrostatical and steric stabilization of invasomes [30,31]. Although all produced terpenoid-invasomes showed neutral Zeta potentials in the present study, we observed the presence of stable invasomes using Cryo TEM after extrusion. A limitation of our study was that the low values of zeta potential could only be measured with low precision, e.g., 3 mV ± 6 for thymol-containing invasomes. Furthermore, measurements of Zeta potentials in nano carrier systems such as invasomes are hampered by measuring limitations arising in diluted samples. Hence, plenty of parameters which influence zeta potentials such as viscosity, pH, and dielectric constant are not correctly reflected in diluted samples [32]. Cryo TEM, to the best of our knowledge, does not have these limitations, since samples with much higher concentrations of invasomes could be analysed in their native diluent.

In accordance with our findings, Sebaaly and colleagues reported neutral Zeta potentials of −3.9 ± 1.9 mV for eugenol-loaded Lipoid S100-liposomes prepared by ethanol injection method. Although the authors demonstrated an increase in liposome size and size distribution after storage in aqueous suspension at 4 °C for 2 months, encapsulation efficiencies of eugenol (86.6%) were unchanged [33]. We suggest that encapsulation efficiencies of our produced invasomes may not be affected over time, despite their neutral Zeta potentials.

In addition to providing an increased bioavailability and a more controlled drug release, our approach may also facilitate topical administration of thymol-invasomes due to the high permeability rate of invasomes through the skin [2,21,24].

Notably, extrusion of solution without addition of ethanol for solving the terpenoid of interest did not result in the formation of invasomes (data not shown). In summary, we successfully prepared invasomes encapsulating the terpenoids thymol, menthol, camphor and cineol.

3.2. Encapsulation of Terpenoids Significantly Changes Lamellarity and Size of Invasomes without Affecting Bilayer Thickness

We next characterized the produced invasomes in more detail in terms of their lamellarity, size and bilayer thickness. For investigation of lamellarity, we determined individual types of lamellar phase lipid bilayers ranging from one lipid bilayer (MLV1) up to eight lamellar phase lipid bilayers (MLV8) (Figure 4A). Cryo electron micrographs (see also Figure 2) served for determination of the individual types of lamellar phase lipid bilayers, which we present in relation to their distribution. Notably, we observed strong differences in lamellarity of invasomes depending on the added terpenoids and in comparison to control. Without the addition of a terpenoid (control, Figure 4B), mostly unilamellar (37 ± 8%) and bilamellar vesicles (37 ± 13%) were formed (* $p < 0.05$, Figure 4B) and showed almost equal proportions ($p = 0.4$ was not considered significant, Mann–Whitney test, one-tailed).

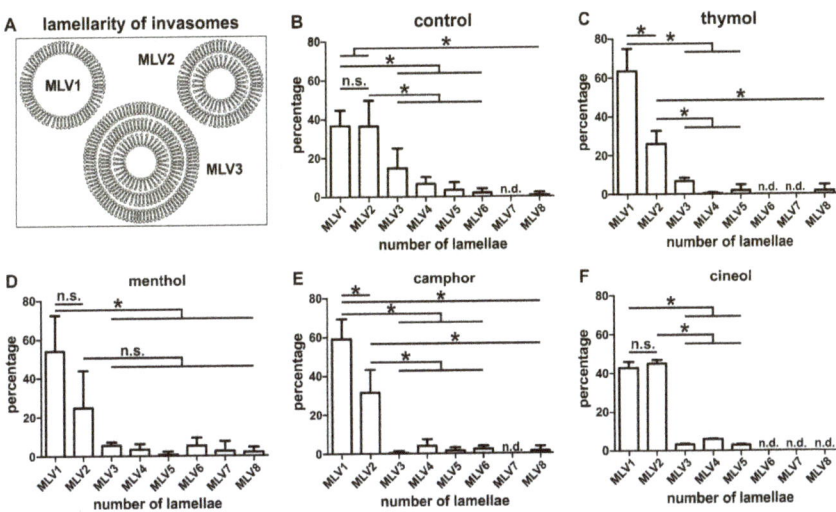

Figure 4. Characterization of lamellarity of the produced terpenoid-comprising invasomes. (**A**) Schematic view of individual types of lamellar phase lipid bilayers. (**B**) Without the addition of a terpenoid (control, **B**), mostly unilamellar and bilamellar vesicles were formed in equal proportions. (**C–E**) Invasomes comprising of thymol or camphor showed mostly unilamellar vesicles and a significantly smaller amount of bilamellar vesicles, while menthol-invasomes revealed no changes between MLV1 and MVL2. (**D**) Cineol-invasomes revealed a similar distribution between unilamellar and bilamellar vesicles. Distribution of the individual vesicle types is depicted in relation to their lamellarity measured from respective cryo electron micrographs. * p 0.05 was considered significant (Mann–Whitney test, one-tailed). MLV: Multilamellar vesicles. (n.s. means not significant)

On the contrary, a shift towards 63 ± 11% unilamellar vesicles (MLV1, Figure 4C) and a significantly decreased amount of 26 ± 7% bilamellar vesicles (MLV2, * $p < 0.05$, Figure 4C) were observed for invasomes comprising of thymol. Production of invasomes with menthol resulted in a significantly increased amount of unilamellar vesicles (54 ± 18%) compared to MLV3–8 (* $p < 0.05$), but no significant changes between the amounts of MLV1 and MLV2 ($p = 0.0571$ was not considered significant, Mann–Whitney test, one-tailed, Figure 4D). Similarly to thymol-invasomes, encapsulation of camphor resulted in mostly unilamellar vesicles (59 ± 10%, * $p < 0.05$) and significantly decreased amounts of bilamellar vesicles (32 ± 12%, * $p < 0.05$, Figure 4E). Interestingly, invasomes containing cineol revealed a similar lamellarity as the control with a similar distribution between unilamellar (43 ± 3%) and bilamellar vesicles (45 ± 2%, $p = 0.2000$ was not considered significant, Mann–Whitney test, one-tailed, Figure 4F). In addition, no MLV6–8 were observable in invasomes encapsulating cineol (Figure 4F).

In addition to their lamellarity, we measured and calculated the size of the produced invasomes (Figure 5A). All invasomes including the control showed a large distribution in size but also specific changes according the encapsulated terpenoid. Compared to control invasomes showing a size distribution from about 20 up to 80 nm radius and a mean of 40 ± 15 nm (Figure 5B), thymol-containing invasomes revealed a significantly smaller radius of 33 ± 18 nm (Figure 5C, *** $p < 0.0001$ was considered significant, unpaired t-test, one-tailed). Preparation of invasomes with camphor also resulted in a significantly smaller invasomes size (30 ± 16 nm radius, Figure 5E) compared to control (*** $p < 0.0001$, unpaired t-test, one-tailed). On the contrary, menthol-comprising invasomes revealed a significantly increased radius of 58 ± 22 nm (Figure 5D) compared to all other terpenoid-encapsulating invasomes and control invasomes (*** $p < 0.0001$, unpaired t-test, one-tailed). Interestingly, although their distribution showed a peak at 35–40 nm radius, the size of invasomes with cineol (43 ± 17 nm radius, Figure 5F) was similar to control (40 ± 15 nm, $p = 0.13$ was not considered significant, unpaired t-test, one-tailed).

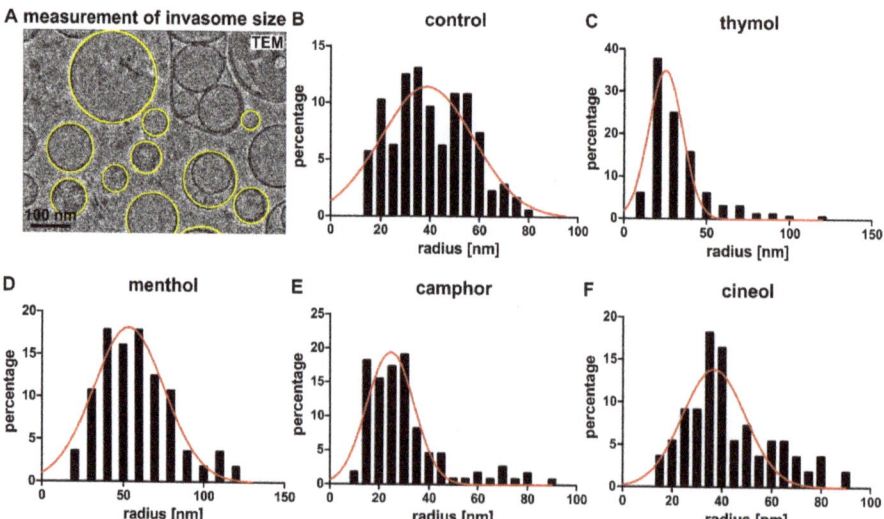

Figure 5. Encapsulation of terpenoids directly affects invasomes size. (**A**) Example of a small representative section of an original cryo-electron micrograph used for measuring invasomes' size. (**B**) Control invasomes without terpenoid showing a mean radius of 40 ± 15 nm. (**C**) Thymol-comprising invasomes revealed a smaller radius of 33 ± 18 nm compared to control. (**D**) Production of invasomes with menthol resulted in an increased invasome radius of 59 ± 22 nm. (**E**) Like thymol, camphor-invasomes also shower a smaller invasome size (30 ± 16 nm radius) compared to control. (**F**) With a mean radius of 43 ± 17 nm, the size of invasomes with cineol was similar to control. Frequency plots of the radius distribution of the invasomes. A fit with the Gaussian function is displayed as a red line.

As a third parameter for characterization of our newly produced invasomes, thickness of the liposomal bilayer was measured by evaluating cryo-electron micrographs (Figure 6A). We observed no significant differences (Mann–Whitney test, one-tailed) in the liposomal bilayer thickness of control invasomes (4 ± 0.5 nm, Figure 6B) compared to menthol-invasomes (4 ± 0.3 nm, $p = 0.2482$, Figure 6D) and invasomes encapsulating camphor (4 ± 0.5 nm, $p = 0.2987$, Figure 6E). Invasomes produced with thymol revealed a slightly but significantly increased bilayer thickness of 5 ± 1 nm (Figure 6C) compared to control (** $p < 0.01$), camphor-invasomes (* $p < 0.05$) and cineol-invasomes (** $p < 0.01$, Mann–Whitney test, one-tailed). In contrast, cineol-comprising invasomes showed a minor decrease in bilayer thickness (4 ± 0.5 nm, Figure 6F) in comparison to the other approaches.

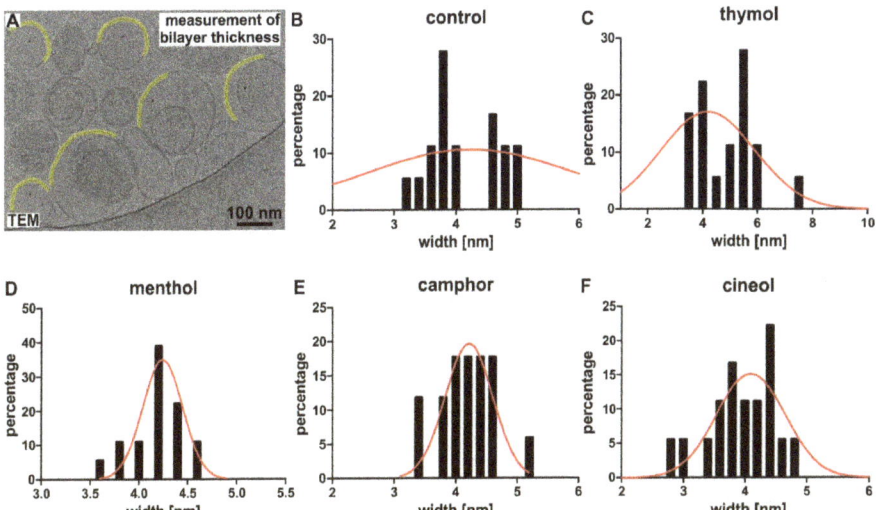

Figure 6. Encapsulation of terpenoids does not affect the bilayer thickness of invasomes. (**A**) Example of a small representative section of an original cryo-electron micrograph used for measurement of the bilayer thickness. (**B–F**) A similar liposomal bilayer thickness was observable for control invasomes (4 ± 0.5 nm), thymol-invasomes (5 ± 1 nm) menthol-invasomes (4 ± 0.3 nm), camphor-invasomes (4 ± 0.5 nm) or cineol-invasomes (4 ± 0.5 nm). Frequency plots of the bilayer thickness distribution of invasomes. A fit with the Gaussian function is displayed as a red line.

Taken together, invasomes with terpenoids showed a shift towards unilamellar vesicles, except for cineol with a similar distribution between unilamellar and bilamellar vesicles comparable to control. While the bilayer thickness of invasomes was comparable in all approaches, preparation of invasomes with thymol and camphor led to significantly smaller invasomes compared control. On the contrary, menthol-comprising invasomes were significantly enlarged and we observed the radius of cineol-invasomes to be comparable to control.

3.3. Invasomes Encapsulating Thymol, Camphor and Cineol Show Bactericidal Activity against S. aureus in a Growth-Inhibition Zone Assay

After successfully producing and characterizing terpenoid-comprising invasomes, we assessed their potential bactericidal activity against *S. aureus* in a growth-inhibition zone assay. After exposure of *S. aureus* to different terpenoid-invasomes overnight, we determined the size of the inhibitory zones. Control invasomes without terpenoids did not result in growth inhibition of *S. aureus* (Figure 7A). Compared to unaffected control, we observed a clearly visible growth inhibition of *S. aureus* exposed to invasomes comprising thymol, camphor or cineol (Figure 7B,D,E). Interestingly, invasomes encapsulating menthol did not affect growth of *S. aureus* (Figure 7C). Statistical evaluation of the measured areas of inhibition validated a strong and significant inhibition of bacterial growth by thymol-containing invasomes compared to all other terpenoid-invasomes and control (Figure 7F). However, invasomes comprising camphor or cineol still caused a significant increase in the zone of inhibition compared to control and menthol-invasomes, which revealed no zone of inhibition (Figure 7F).

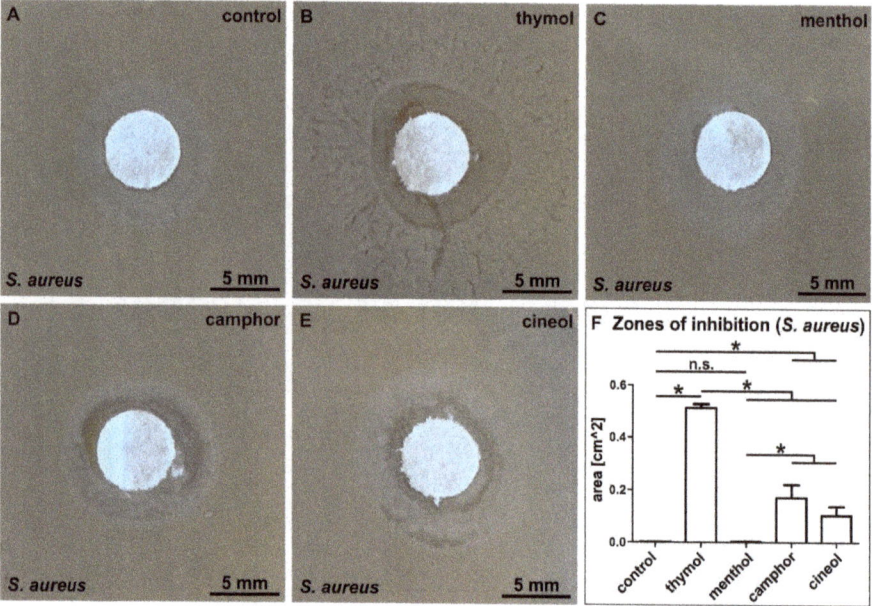

Figure 7. Invasomes encapsulating thymol, camphor and cineol show bactericidal activity against *S. aureus* in a growth-inhibition zone assay. (**A**) Control invasomes without terpenoids did not affect bacterial growth. (**B**) Strong growth inhibition of *S. aureus* exposed to invasomes comprising thymol. (**C**) Invasomes encapsulating menthol did not affect growth of *S. aureus*. (**D–E**) Growth inhibition of *S. aureus* exposed to invasomes comprising camphor and cineol. (**F**) Statistical evaluation of the measured zones of inhibition validated the significant inhibition of *S. aureus* growth by thymol-containing invasomes compared to all other terpenoid-invasomes and control. * p 0.05 was considered significant (Mann–Whitney test, one-tailed). (n.s. means not significant)

In Table 1, the particle size of different terpenoid formulations is depicted as measured in Figure 5. When the formulations are sorted from the highest antibacterial activity (thymol) to the lowest (cineol), as measured in Figure 7, it becomes evident that the terpenoids with the highest antibacterial activity have the highest polydispersity index also (Table 1).

Table 1. Invasome Particle Size and the Polydispersity Index.

Formulation	Particle Size (nm)	Polydispersity Index
Thymol	66 ± 36	0.3 ± 0.05
Camphor	60 ± 32	0.3 ± 0.04
Cineol	86 ± 34	0.2 ± 0.03
Menthol	118 ± 44	0.2 ± 0.03
Control	80 ± 30	0.1 ± 0.02

3.4. Flow Cytometric Analysis of Cell Death Validate High Bactericidal Activity of Thymol-Loaded Invasomes against Gram-Positive S. aureus

To validate the strong bactericidal activity of thymol-invasomes against *S. aureus* in the growth-inhibition zone assay, we also assessed the anti-bacterial activity of thymol-invasomes quantitatively using flow cytometry. Bacterial cell death was measured by the DNA-intercalating dye Propidum Iodide (PI), which is incorporated only by dead cells. Prior to this analysis, we determined the encapsulation efficiency and loading capacity of thymol-invasomes to ensure proper encapsulation of the terpenoid. Here, we observed an encapsulation efficiency of 47 ± 13% as well as a loading capacity of 0.5 ± 0.1% for invasomes encapsulating thymol. Compared to untreated negative control (4–9% cell death), 0.5 mg/mL thymol packaged in invasomes resulted in a profound cell death of 70% (Figure 8A). Exposure of 1 mg/mL invasome-encapsulated thymol even resulted in 75% bacterial cell death (Figure 8B). Since 2 mg/mL thymol packaged in invasomes resulted in only 9% PI-stained *S. aureus* (Figure 8C), we additionally assessed the cell count per second during the flow cytometric measurement. Here, only around 1000 cells/second were observed in the *S. aureus* population treated with 2 mg/mL thymol-comprising invasomes, whereas the cell count for control conditions ranged around 40,000 cells/second (Figure 8D). Treatment of *S. aureus* with 0.5 mg/mL or 1 mg/mL invasome-encapsulated thymol resulted in cell flow of around 33,000 cells/second (Figure 8D). Thus, we suggest that 2 mg/mL thymol packaged in invasomes already resulted in a nearly complete cell death of *S. aureus* prior to PI-staining and following flow cytometric measurements. We conclude invasomes encapsulating thymol to be strongly bactericidal against Gram-positive bacteria such as *S. aureus*.

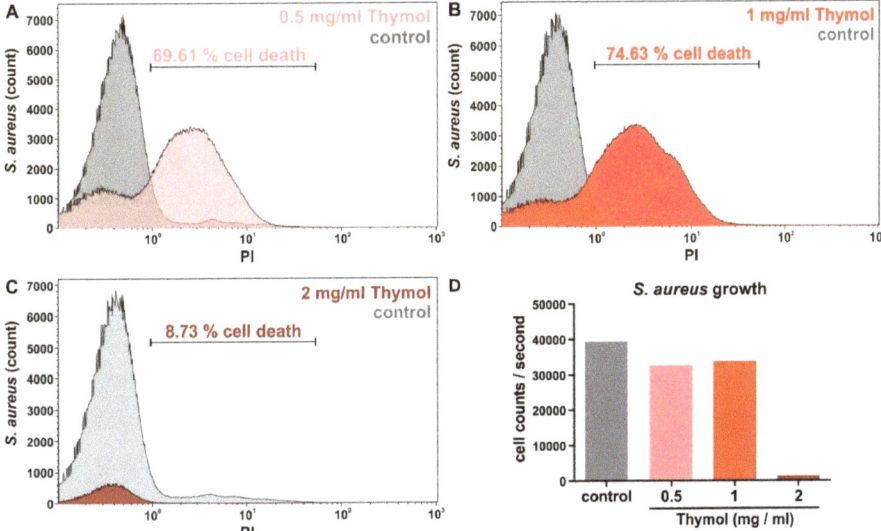

Figure 8. Flow cytometric analysis of cell death validate invasomes encapsulating thymol to be strongly bactericidal against Gram-positive bacteria like *S. aureus*. (**A,B**) Compared to untreated negative control, 0.5 mg/mL or 1 mg/mL thymol packaged in invasomes resulted in a profound cell death depicted by PI-staining. (**C**) 2 mg/mL thymol packaged in invasomes resulted in only 9% PI-stained *S. aureus*. (**D**) Assessment of cell flow revealed only around 1000 cells/second in the *S. aureus* population treated with 2 mg/mL thymol-comprising invasomes, suggesting a nearly complete cell death prior to following flow cytometric analysis. PI: Propidium iodide.

3.5. Thymol-Loaded Invasomes Do Not Affect Survival of Gram-Negative E. coli

Next to Gram-positive bacteria such as *S. aureus,* we assessed the potential anti-bacterial activity of thymol-invasomes against Gram-negative species such as *E. coli.* Notably, 0.5 mg/mL thymol packaged in invasomes resulted in only 0.2% PI-stained dead cells (Figure 9A). Treatment of *E. coli* with 1 mg/mL or 2 mg/mL invasome-encapsulated thymol only led to 6% or 5% cell death (Figure 9B,C). With regards to the low amount of PI-stained cells, we also assessed the cell count per second during the flow cytometric measurement. Here, we observed no relevant effects of the different concentrations of invasome-encapsulated thymol on the growth of *E. coli* (cell count per second, Figure 9D). In summary, the invasomes comprising thymol produced in this study are highly bactericidal to Gram-positive *S. aureus,* but do not affect survival of Gram-negative *E. coli.*

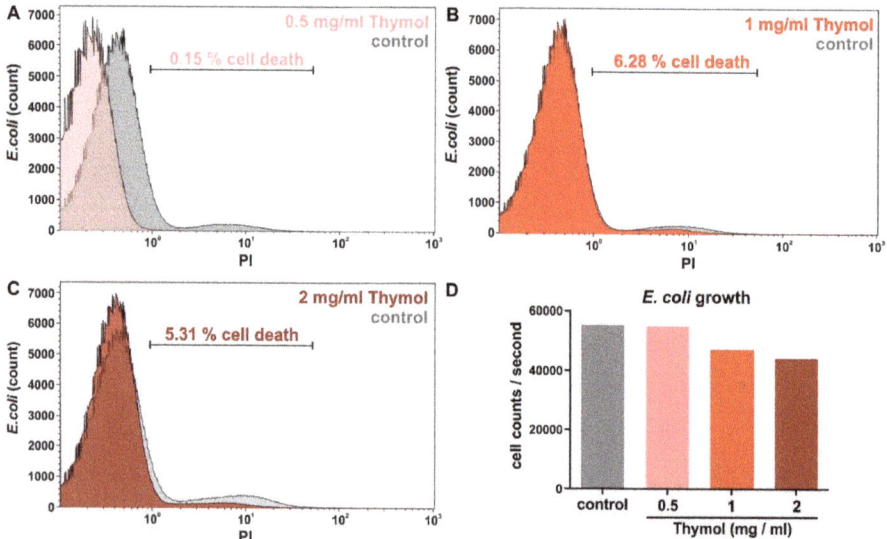

Figure 9. Invasomes encapsulating thymol are not bactericidal against Gram-negative bacteria such as *E. coli.* (**A–C**) Compared to untreated negative control, treatment of *E. coli.* with 0.5 mg/mL, 1 mg/mL or 2 mg/mL thymol packaged in invasomes did not result in elevated amounts of cell death. (**D**) Assessment of cell flow revealed no relevant effects of the different concentrations of invasome-encapsulated thymol on the growth of *E. coli.*

3.6. Growth-Inhibition Zone Assay Shows Strong Bactericidal Activity of Cineol Invasomes against E. coli

In addition to thymol-invasomes, we assessed the potential bactericidal activity of invasomes encapsulating menthol, camphor and cineol against *E. coli.* In line with our flow cytometric analysis of cell death, thymol-invasomes revealed no elevated growth inhibition of *E. coli,* similarly to control-invasomes without encapsulated terpenoids (Figure 10A,B). While menthol-invasomes led to a slight growth inhibition of *E. coli* (Figure 10C), invasomes encapsulating camphor showed no bactericidal activity against *E. coli* (Figure 10D). Notably, exposure of *E. coli* to invasomes loaded with cineol resulted in a strong and significant growth inhibition (Figure 10E,F).

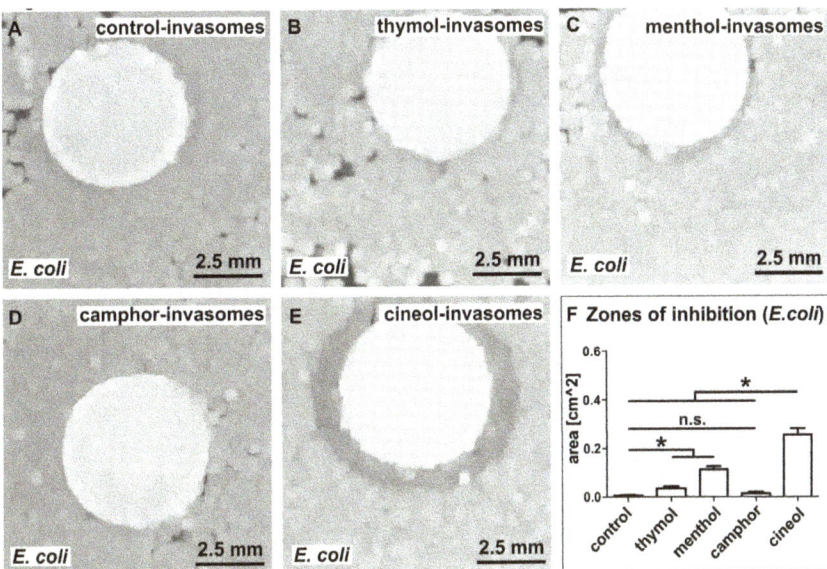

Figure 10. Invasomes encapsulating cineol reveal bactericidal activity against *E. coli* in a growth-inhibition zone assay. (**A,B**) Control invasomes without terpenoids or thymol invasomes did not affect bacterial growth. (**C,D**) While menthol-invasomes led to a slight inhibition of *E. coli* growth, camphor-invasomes did not affect growth of *S. aureus*. (**E**) Strong growth inhibition of *E. coli* exposed to invasomes comprising cineol. (**F**) Statistical evaluation of the measured zones of inhibition validated the significant inhibition of *E. coli* growth by cineol-containing invasomes compared to all other terpenoid-invasomes and control. * p 0.05 was considered significant (Mann–Whitney test, one-tailed). (n.s. means not significant)

We next determined the potential bactericidal activity of non-extruded terpenoids as a control to our encapsulation approach. In contrast to terpenoids encapsulated in invasomes (Figures 7–10), application of non-extruded terpenoids did not result in growth inhibition of *E. coli* or *S. aureus* (data not shown). In summary, the invasomes comprising thymol produced here are highly bactericidal to Gram-positive *S. aureus*, while cineol-invasomes affect the survival of Gram-negative *E. coli* (Figures 7–10).

Potential antibacterial mechanisms of invasome formulations with terpenoids are depicted in Figure 11.

Although terpenoids such as limonene, cineole or beta-citronellene have been widely used for formulation of invasomes [26,27], they were mostly applied as permeation enhancer for transdermal delivery and bioavailability and not as bioactive components [2]. In the present study, we focused on the production of invasomes with terpenoids as the bioactive components to inhibit bacterial cell growth. We found our terpenoids-invasomes to be bactericidal against Gram-positive *S. aureus*, with increasing efficiency from cineol- and camphor-invasomes (moderate bactericidal activity) to thymol-invasomes showing the strongest bactericidal effects. These findings are in line with the commonly reported bactericidal activity of thymol, camphor and cineol [10,12,13]. Interestingly, Mulyaningsih and colleagues reported that exposure of MRSA even to high concentrations of cineol does not inhibit multi-resistant *S. aureus*. However, a combination of the terpene aromadendrene with cineol resulted in reduced bacterial cell growth [34]. Extending these findings, we show that encapsulation of cineol into invasomes alone is sufficient for inhibiting growth of *S. aureus* without the application of additional terpenes. In accordance to the strong bactericidal effects of thymol-invasomes observed here, encapsulation of thymol into other nanocarriers such as ethylcellulose/methylcellulose nanospheres was also reported to preserve its anti-bacterial activity against *S. aureus* [35]. In contrast to invasomes encapsulating thymol, camphor and cineol, we observed no anti-bacterial effects for menthol-invasomes against *S. aureus*, which is contrary to the already described bactericidal activity of menthol [11,12]. With regard to the very low water-solubility of menthol, we suggest the invasomal packaging of menthol to be challenging, in turn, affecting its bactericidal activity. In this line, we observed an increased average size of menthol-invasomes compared to all other terpenoid-invasome preparations and control-invasomes lacking terpenoids. In addition polydispersity index as a measurement of the uniformity of invasome size distribution, with a higher value resulting in a broader distribution, was highest with thymol (0.3) and camphor (0.3), suggesting a correlation to antibacterial activity.

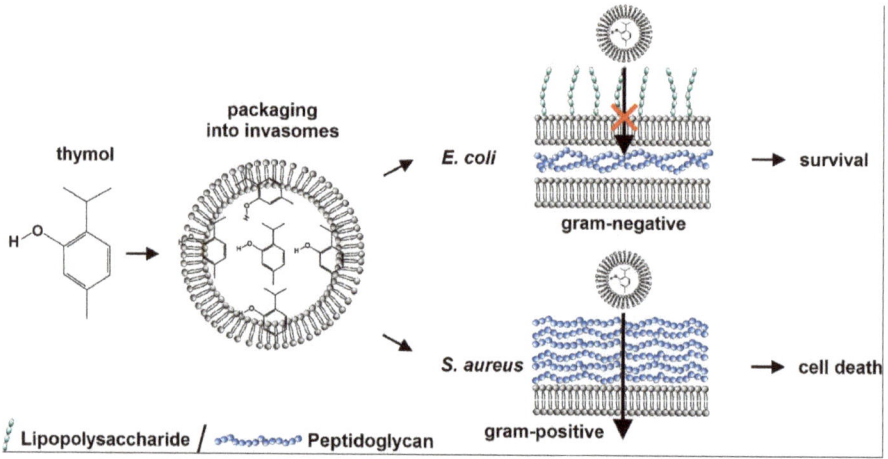

Figure 11. Schematic view on invasomal packaging of thymol and its selective bactericidal activity against Gram-positive *S. aureus*.

Next to Gram-positive bacterial species such as *S. aureus*, we also investigated potential anti-bacterial properties of our invasomes and particularly, thymol-invasomes on Gram-negative *E. coli*. Here, cineol-comprising invasomes led to a strong inhibition of *E. coli* growth, which is in line with our previous observations [13]. In contrast to the strong bactericidal effects against *S. aureus*, cell growth of Gram-negative *E. coli* was not affected by thymol-invasomes. These observations are contrary to the findings by Salvia-Trujillo and colleagues reporting a bactericidal activity of essential oils of thyme (containing thymol) after incorporation into nano-emulsions [35]. In particular, nano-emulsions comprising essential oils of thyme with heterogeneous droplets sizes between 10 nm to 500 nm were shown to reduce growth of *E. coli* [36]. However, the authors applied unfractionated essential oils, suggesting a synergistic action of many terpenes to be necessary for bactericidal activity against Gram-negative species. Interestingly, Trombetta and coworkers demonstrated that *S. aureus* appears to be far more sensitive to thymol than *E. coli* [37], which is in line with our present data. The authors reported a minimal inhibiting concentration of 5.00 mg/mL thymol for *E. coli* [37], suggesting the concentration of up to 2 mg/mL thymol in the invasomes applied here to be not sufficient for inhibition of *E. coli* growth. Furthermore, *S. aureus* is known to secrete pore-forming toxins (PFTs), which were shown to mediate the release of encapsulated clove oil from liposomes. In particular, Cui and coworkers reported that PFTs form pores within the liposome membranes, allowing release of the encapsulated clove oil and facilitating its antibacterial activity. On the contrary, liposomal packaged clove oil had no bactericidal effects on *E. coli*, which does not secrete PFTs and thus prevents the release of antibacterial essential oil from the invasome [38]. Our present observations may suggest a similar mechanism for thymol-invasomes leading to its selective activity against *S. aureus* (Figure 11).

In addition, electrophoretic mobility measurement revealed a harder surface of *E. coli* compared to *S. aureus* [39]. The softer surface of *S. aureus* mainly comprising peptidoglycan may facilitate entry of thymol-invasomes into the bacterial cells more easily compared to Gram-negative *E. coli* (Figure 11). Accordingly, we achieved a highly efficient killing of *S. aureus* with only 0.5 mg/mL thymol encapsulated in invasomes in the present study (Figure 11).

In summary, we demonstrate the successful production of invasomes encapsulating thymol, menthol, camphor or cineol and show a strong selective activity of thymol-invasomes against Gram-positive *S. aureus*. As a further benefit of our approach, encapsulation of terpenoids into nanocarrier systems such as invasomes is suggested to increase stability and protect against environmental factors causing degradation [2,33,40]. Here, liposomes composed of lipid S100 and cholesterol were reported to retain considerable concentrations of isoeugenol, pulegone, terpineol, and thymol liposomes even after 10 months [29]. The application of soy lecithin liposomes comprising cinnamon oil was further shown to improve stability of the essential oil and extend the bactericidal action time [20]. In addition, the application of invasomes was particularly found to elevate the stability of the encapsulated compounds (reviewed in [24]).

There are several nanocarrier systems, encapsulating terpenoids, which are systematically reviewed in [2]. The formulation systems encapsulating terpenoids include polymer-based systems such as nano-capsules, nano-particles, nano-fibers and nano-gels. Furthermore, lipid-based systems are frequently used (67% of the formulations), presumably due to the low toxicity. A subgroup of lipid systems are the vesicular systems, which include invasomes. The most investigated biological activity of terpenoids in nano carrier systems is the anti-inflammatory action. Invasomes were used as anti-acne treatments, hypertension treatment and photosensation therapy [2].

Antimicrobial activity was reported with nano capsules with essential oils from lemon grass, nano emulsions with tea tree oil and penetration-enhancing vehicles with essential oil from Santolina insularis. Here, we report a novel antimicrobial application of invasome formulations with terpenoids.

We conclude that our findings might provide a promising approach to increase the bioavailability of terpenoid-based drugs and might be applicable for treating severe bacterial infections such as MRSA in the future. In this regard, the major treatment aims of our formulations include a broad spectrum of applications, ranging from mucosal infections in airway diseases to systemic infections such as sepsis. In this direction, we have previously shown that patients with chronic rhinosinusitis have increased levels of S. aureus-containing biofilms in the nose [13]. Growth of *S. aureus* biofilms on the nasal mucosa could be inhibited by 1,8-cineol. Here, we extend these findings to thymol-containing invasomes, which have superior antibacterial activity than formulations with 1,8-cineol (see Figure 7). Taken together, an invasome formulation as described here, containing thymol might be useful as an aerosol spray for pre-operative nose cleaning and might have fewer side effects in comparison to disinfectants directly applied on the mucosa. As a general use, it might be envisaged that invasomes containing thymol or other terpenoids could be employed to treat infected surfaces as in nose, lung and skin wounds. Finally, invasomes containing terpenoids might be used in addition or as an alternative to antibiotics.

Author Contributions: Conceptualization, A.H., C.K. and B.K.; validation, A.H., C.K. and B.K.; formal analysis, B.P.K., J.F.W.G., I.E. and A.H.; investigation, B.P.K., I.E., J.F.W.G. and R.D.; resources, A.H., C.K., B.K. and A.P.; data curation, A.H., C.K., B.K. and J.F.W.G.; writing—original draft preparation, B.P.K. and J.F.W.G.; writing—review and editing, A.H., C.K., B.K., I.E., R.D. and A.P.; visualization, B.P.K. and J.F.W.G.; supervision, A.H., C.K. and B.K.; project administration, A.H., C.K. and B.K.; funding acquisition, A.H., C.K., B.K. and A.P. All authors have read and agreed to the published version of the manuscript.

Funding: This research was funded by the University of Bielefeld and received no external funding.

Acknowledgments: The excellent technical help of Angela Kralemann-Köhler is gratefully acknowledged.

Conflicts of Interest: The authors declare no conflict of interest. The funders had no role in the design of the study; in the collection, analyses, or interpretation of data; in the writing of the manuscript, or in the decision to publish the results.

References

1. Gershenzon, J.; Dudareva, N. The function of terpene natural products in the natural world. *Nat. Chem. Biol.* **2007**, *3*, 408–414. [CrossRef] [PubMed]
2. de Matos, S.P.; Teixeira, H.F.; de Lima, A.A.N.; Veiga-Junior, V.F.; Koester, L.S. Essential Oils and Isolated Terpenes in Nanosystems Designed for Topical Administration: A Review. *Biomolecules* **2019**, *9*, 138. [CrossRef] [PubMed]
3. Zengin, H.; Baysal, A.H. Antibacterial and antioxidant activity of essential oil terpenes against pathogenic and spoilage-forming bacteria and cell structure-activity relationships evaluated by SEM microscopy. *Molecules* **2014**, *19*, 17773–17798. [CrossRef] [PubMed]
4. Salminen, A.; Lehtonen, M.; Suuronen, T.; Kaarniranta, K.; Huuskonen, J. Terpenoids: Natural inhibitors of NF-kappaB signaling with anti-inflammatory and anticancer potential. *Cell Mol. Life Sci.* **2008**, *65*, 2979–2999. [CrossRef] [PubMed]
5. Zhou, E.; Fu, Y.; Wei, Z.; Yu, Y.; Zhang, X.; Yang, Z. Thymol attenuates allergic airway inflammation in ovalbumin (OVA)-induced mouse asthma. *Fitoterapia* **2014**, *96*, 131–137. [CrossRef]
6. Liang, D.; Li, F.; Fu, Y.; Cao, Y.; Song, X.; Wang, T.; Wang, W.; Guo, M.; Zhou, E.; Li, D.; et al. Thymol inhibits LPS-stimulated inflammatory response via down-regulation of NF-kappaB and MAPK signaling pathways in mouse mammary epithelial cells. *Inflammation* **2014**, *37*, 214–222. [CrossRef]
7. Greiner, J.F.; Muller, J.; Zeuner, M.T.; Hauser, S.; Seidel, T.; Klenke, C.; Grunwald, L.M.; Schomann, T.; Widera, D.; Sudhoff, H.; et al. 1,8-Cineol inhibits nuclear translocation of NF-kappaB p65 and NF-kappaB-dependent transcriptional activity. *Biochim. Biophys. Acta* **2013**, *1833*, 2866–2878. [CrossRef]
8. Müller, J.; Greiner, J.F.; Zeuner, M.; Brotzmann, V.; Schafermann, J.; Wieters, F.; Widera, D.; Sudhoff, H.; Kaltschmidt, B.; Kaltschmidt, C. 1,8-Cineole potentiates IRF3-mediated antiviral response in human stem cells and in an ex vivo model of rhinosinusitis. *Clin. Sci. (Lond.)* **2016**, *130*, 1339–1352. [CrossRef]
9. Sudhoff, H.; Klenke, C.; Greiner, J.F.; Muller, J.; Brotzmann, V.; Ebmeyer, J.; Kaltschmidt, B.; Kaltschmidt, C. 1,8-Cineol Reduces Mucus-Production in a Novel Human Ex Vivo Model of Late Rhinosinusitis. *PLoS ONE* **2015**, *10*, e0133040. [CrossRef]
10. Nostro, A.; Sudano Roccaro, A.; Bisignano, G.; Marino, A.; Cannatelli, M.A.; Pizzimenti, F.C.; Cioni, P.L.; Procopio, F.; Blanco, A.R. Effects of oregano, carvacrol and thymol on Staphylococcus aureus and Staphylococcus epidermidis biofilms. *J. Med. Microbiol.* **2007**, *56*, 519–523. [CrossRef]
11. Pattnaik, S.; Subramanyam, V.R.; Bapaji, M.; Kole, C.R. Antibacterial and antifungal activity of aromatic constituents of essential oils. *Microbios* **1997**, *89*, 39–46. [PubMed]
12. Freires, I.A.; Denny, C.; Benso, B.; de Alencar, S.M.; Rosalen, P.L. Antibacterial Activity of Essential Oils and Their Isolated Constituents against Cariogenic Bacteria: A Systematic Review. *Molecules* **2015**, *20*, 7329–7358. [CrossRef] [PubMed]
13. Schurmann, M.; Oppel, F.; Gottschalk, M.; Buker, B.; Jantos, C.A.; Knabbe, C.; Hutten, A.; Kaltschmidt, B.; Kaltschmidt, C.; Sudhoff, H. The Therapeutic Effect of 1,8-Cineol on Pathogenic Bacteria Species Present in Chronic Rhinosinusitis. *Front. Microbiol.* **2019**, *10*, 2325. [CrossRef] [PubMed]
14. Rukavina, Z.; Vanic, Z. Current Trends in Development of Liposomes for Targeting Bacterial Biofilms. *Pharmaceutics* **2016**, *8*, 18. [CrossRef]
15. Arevalo, L.M.; Yarce, C.J.; Onate-Garzon, J.; Salamanca, C.H. Decrease of Antimicrobial Resistance through Polyelectrolyte-Coated Nanoliposomes Loaded with beta-Lactam Drug. *Pharmaceuticals* **2018**, *12*, 1. [CrossRef]
16. Moya, M.L.; Lopez-Lopez, M.; Lebron, J.A.; Ostos, F.J.; Perez, D.; Camacho, V.; Beck, I.; Merino-Bohorquez, V.; Camean, M.; Madinabeitia, N.; et al. Preparation and Characterization of New Liposomes. Bactericidal Activity of Cefepime Encapsulated into Cationic Liposomes. *Pharmaceutics* **2019**, *11*, 69. [CrossRef]
17. Engel, J.B.; Heckler, C.; Tondo, E.C.; Daroit, D.J.; da Silva Malheiros, P. Antimicrobial activity of free and liposome-encapsulated thymol and carvacrol against Salmonella and Staphylococcus aureus adhered to stainless steel. *Int. J. Food Microbiol.* **2017**, *252*, 18–23. [CrossRef]
18. Usach, I.; Margarucci, E.; Manca, M.L.; Caddeo, C.; Aroffu, M.; Petretto, G.L.; Manconi, M.; Peris, J.E. Comparison between Citral and Pompia Essential Oil Loaded in Phospholipid Vesicles for the Treatment of Skin and Mucosal Infections. *Nanomaterials* **2020**, *10*, 286. [CrossRef]

19. Sugumar, S.; Ghosh, V.; Nirmala, M.J.; Mukherjee, A.; Chandrasekaran, N. Ultrasonic emulsification of eucalyptus oil nanoemulsion: Antibacterial activity against Staphylococcus aureus and wound healing activity in Wistar rats. *Ultrason Sonochem.* **2014**, *21*, 1044–1049. [CrossRef]
20. Cui, H.; Li, W.; Li, C.; Vittayapadung, S.; Lin, L. Liposome containing cinnamon oil with antibacterial activity against methicillin-resistant Staphylococcus aureus biofilm. *Biofouling* **2016**, *32*, 215–225. [CrossRef]
21. Pivetta, T.P.; Simoes, S.; Araujo, M.M.; Carvalho, T.; Arruda, C.; Marcato, P.D. Development of nanoparticles from natural lipids for topical delivery of thymol: Investigation of its anti-inflammatory properties. *Colloids Surf. B Biointerfaces* **2018**, *164*, 281–290. [CrossRef] [PubMed]
22. Manconi, M.; Petretto, G.; D'Hallewin, G.; Escribano, E.; Milia, E.; Pinna, R.; Palmieri, A.; Firoznezhad, M.; Peris, J.E.; Usach, I.; et al. Thymus essential oil extraction, characterization and incorporation in phospholipid vesicles for the antioxidant/antibacterial treatment of oral cavity diseases. *Colloids Surf. B Biointerfaces* **2018**, *171*, 115–122. [CrossRef] [PubMed]
23. Zhang, K.; Zhang, Y.; Li, Z.; Li, N.; Feng, N. Essential oil-mediated glycerosomes increase transdermal paeoniflorin delivery: Optimization, characterization, and evaluation in vitro and in vivo. *Int. J. Nanomed.* **2017**, *12*, 3521–3532. [CrossRef] [PubMed]
24. Babaie, S.; Bakhshayesh, A.R.D.; Ha, J.W.; Hamishehkar, H.; Kim, K.H. Invasome: A Novel Nanocarrier for Transdermal Drug Delivery. *Nanomaterials* **2020**, *10*, 341. [CrossRef] [PubMed]
25. Dragicevic, N.; Verma, D.D.; Fahr, A. Invasomes: Vesicles for Enhanced Skin Delivery of Drugs. In *Percutaneous Penetration Enhancers Chemical Methods in Penetration Enhancement: Nanocarrier*; Dragicevic, N., Maibach, H.I., Eds.; Springer: Heidelberg, Germany, 2016; pp. 77–92.
26. Charoenputtakun, P.; Pamornpathomkul, B.; Opanasopit, P.; Rojanarata, T.; Ngawhirunpat, T. Terpene composited lipid nanoparticles for enhanced dermal delivery of all-trans-retinoic acids. *Biol. Pharm. Bull.* **2014**, *37*, 1139–1148. [CrossRef] [PubMed]
27. Kamran, M.; Ahad, A.; Aqil, M.; Imam, S.S.; Sultana, Y.; Ali, A. Design, formulation and optimization of novel soft nano-carriers for transdermal olmesartan medoxomil delivery: In vitro characterization and in vivo pharmacokinetic assessment. *Int. J. Pharm.* **2016**, *505*, 147–158. [CrossRef]
28. Schindelin, J.; Arganda-Carreras, I.; Frise, E.; Kaynig, V.; Longair, M.; Pietzsch, T.; Preibisch, S.; Rueden, C.; Saalfeld, S.; Schmid, B.; et al. Fiji: An open-source platform for biological-image analysis. *Nat. Methods* **2012**, *9*, 676–682. [CrossRef]
29. Hammoud, Z.; Gharib, R.; Fourmentin, S.; Elaissari, A.; Greige-Gerges, H. New findings on the incorporation of essential oil components into liposomes composed of lipoid S100 and cholesterol. *Int. J. Pharm.* **2019**, *561*, 161–170. [CrossRef]
30. Patel, V.R.; Agrawal, Y.K. Nanosuspension: An approach to enhance solubility of drugs. *J. Adv. Pharm. Technol. Res.* **2011**, *2*, 81–87. [CrossRef]
31. Yang, J.Z.; Young, A.L.; Chiang, P.C.; Thurston, A.; Pretzer, D.K. Fluticasone and budesonide nanosuspensions for pulmonary delivery: Preparation, characterization, and pharmacokinetic studies. *J. Pharm. Sci.* **2008**, *97*, 4869–4878. [CrossRef]
32. Bhattacharjee, S. DLS and zeta potential-What they are and what they are not? *J. Control Release* **2016**, *235*, 337–351. [CrossRef] [PubMed]
33. Sebaaly, C.; Greige-Gerges, H.; Stainmesse, S.; Fessi, H.; Charcosset, C. Effect of composition, hydrogenation of phospholipids and lyophilization on the characteristics of eugenol-loaded liposomes prepared by ethanol injection method. *Food Biosci.* **2016**, *15*, 1–10. [CrossRef]
34. Mulyaningsih, S.; Sporer, F.; Zimmermann, S.; Reichling, J.; Wink, M. Synergistic properties of the terpenoids aromadendrene and 1,8-cineole from the essential oil of Eucalyptus globulus against antibiotic-susceptible and antibiotic-resistant pathogens. *Phytomedicine* **2010**, *17*, 1061–1066. [CrossRef] [PubMed]
35. Wattanasatcha, A.; Rengpipat, S.; Wanichwecharungruang, S. Thymol nanospheres as an effective anti-bacterial agent. *Int. J. Pharm.* **2012**, *434*, 360–365. [CrossRef] [PubMed]
36. Salvia-Trujillo, L.; Rojas-Graü, A.; Soliva-Fortuny, R.; Martín-Belloso, O. Physicochemical characterization and antimicrobial activity of food-grade emulsions and nanoemulsions incorporating essential oils. *Food Hydrocoll.* **2015**, *43*, 547–556. [CrossRef]
37. Trombetta, D.; Castelli, F.; Sarpietro, M.G.; Venuti, V.; Cristani, M.; Daniele, C.; Saija, A.; Mazzanti, G.; Bisignano, G. Mechanisms of antibacterial action of three monoterpenes. *Antimicrob. Agents Chemother.* **2005**, *49*, 2474–2478. [CrossRef]

38. Cui, H.; Zhao, C.; Lin, L. The specific antibacterial activity of liposome-encapsulated Clove oil and its application in tofu. *Food Control* **2015**, *56*, 128–134. [CrossRef]
39. Sonohara, R.; Muramatsu, N.; Ohshima, H.; Kondo, T. Difference in surface properties between Escherichia coli and Staphylococcus aureus as revealed by electrophoretic mobility measurements. *Biophys. Chem.* **1995**, *55*, 273–277. [CrossRef]
40. Bilia, A.R.; Guccione, C.; Isacchi, B.; Righeschi, C.; Firenzuoli, F.; Bergonzi, M.C. Essential oils loaded in nanosystems: A developing strategy for a successful therapeutic approach. *Evid.-Based Complement. Altern. Med.* **2014**, *2014*, 651593. [CrossRef]

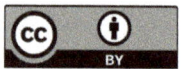

© 2020 by the authors. Licensee MDPI, Basel, Switzerland. This article is an open access article distributed under the terms and conditions of the Creative Commons Attribution (CC BY) license (http://creativecommons.org/licenses/by/4.0/).

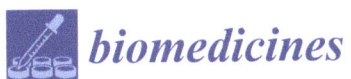

Article

Aristolochia trilobata: Identification of the Anti-Inflammatory and Antinociceptive Effects

Dayana da Costa Salomé [1], Natália de Morais Cordeiro [1], Tayná Sequeira Valério [1], Darlisson de Alexandria Santos [2,3], Péricles Barreto Alves [2], Celuta Sales Alviano [4], Daniela Sales Alviano Moreno [4] and Patricia Dias Fernandes [1,*]

1. Laboratório de Farmacologia da Dor e da Inflamação, Instituto de Ciências Biomédicas, Universidade Federal do Rio de Janeiro, Rio de Janeiro 21941-902, Brazil; daycsalome@gmail.com (D.d.C.S.); natmoraiss@gmail.com (N.d.M.C.); tayna.sequeira@gmail.com (T.S.V.)
2. Departamento de Química, Universidade Federal de Sergipe, Sergipe 49100-000, Brazil; darlisson@unifesspa.edu.br (D.d.A.S.); pericles@ufs.br (P.B.A.)
3. Instituto de Ciências Exatas, Faculdade de Química, Universidade Federal do Sul e Sudeste do Pará, Marabá 68507-590, Brazil
4. Laboratório de Superfície de Fungos, Instituto de Microbiologia Professor Paulo de Góes, Universidade Federal do Rio de Janeiro, Rio de Janeiro 21941-902, Brazil; alviano@micro.ufrj.br (C.S.A.); danialviano@micro.ufrj.br (D.S.A.M.)
* Correspondence: patricia.dias@icb.ufrj.br; Tel.: +55-21-39386442

Received: 30 March 2020; Accepted: 21 April 2020; Published: 6 May 2020

Abstract: *Aristolochia trilobata*, popularly known as "mil-homens," is widely used for treatment of stomach aches, colic, asthma, pulmonary diseases, diabetes, and skin affection. We evaluated the antinociceptive and anti-inflammatory activities of the essential oil (EO) and the main constituent, 6-methyl-5-hepten-2-yl acetate (sulcatyl acetate, SA). EO and SA (1, 10, and 100 mg/kg, p.o.) were evaluated using chemical (formalin-induced licking) and thermal (hot-plate) models of nociception or inflammation (carrageenan-induced cell migration into the subcutaneous air pouch, SAP). The mechanism of antinociceptive activity was evaluated using opioid, cholinergic receptor antagonists (naloxone and atropine), or nitric oxide synthase inhibitor (L-NAME). EO and SA presented a central antinociceptive effect (the hot-plate model). In formalin-induced licking response, higher doses of EO and SA also reduced 1st and 2nd phases. None of the antagonists and enzyme inhibitor reversed antinociceptive effects. EO and SA reduced the leukocyte migration into the SAP, and the cytokines tumor necrosis factor and interleukin-1 (TNF-α and IL-1β, respectively) produced in the exudate. Our results are indicative that EO and SA present peripheral and central antinociceptive and anti-inflammatory effects.

Keywords: *Aristolochia trilobata*; sulcatyl acetate; antinociceptive effect; anti-inflammatory activity

1. Introduction

Inflammation and pain continue to be major problems in individuals. Both of them are a normal response of the body against invasion and/or damage. Inflammation can develop in response to an invasion by a microorganism or by physical damage and is a critical protective action to injury or infection. This phenomenon presents the five cardinal signs (i.e., redness, heat, swelling, pain, and loss of function) [1]. Pain, one sign of inflammation, is an international health problem, affecting about one in five individuals. Both situations affect almost 20% of worldwide population. Drugs used to treat the symptoms can be the non-steroidal anti-inflammatory drugs (NSAIDs) and/or opioids (specifically to pain treatment). However, both groups present a large variety of side effects. For example, opioid drugs are responsible for abuse and dependence affecting 2.1 million people, and NSAIDs also increase the risk of gastrointestinal bleeding and cardiac events [2].

In Central and South America, *Aristolochia trilobata* L. (Aristolochiaceae), popularly known as "mil-homens", is widely used in folk medicine and is an important medicinal plant [3,4]. Conditions such as stomach ache, colic, poisoning, asthma, pulmonary diseases, diabetes, and skin affections have been treated with different species from *Aristolochia* genus [5,6]. Previous studies have shown that a chloroform extract of *A. trilobata* leaves had antiphlogistic potency similar to that of indomethacin (a non-steroidal anti-inflammatory drug) [7].

The present work aims to demonstrate the traditional use of *A. trilobata* for treatment of inflammation and pain. For these purposes, we decided to obtain the essential oil of *A. trilobata* stems from enriching volatile substances, enabling a scientific study to evaluate their possible involvement in the anti-inflammatory and antinociceptive effects testing it in a well-known thermal (hot-plate) model of nociception and carrageenan-induced cell migration as a model of inflammation. We also tried to identify the mechanism by which *A. trilobata* presents its effect.

2. Experimental Section

2.1. Animals

All protocols used Swiss Webster mice (male, 20–25 g, 8–10 weeks) donated by the Instituto Vital Brazil (Niterói, Rio de Janeiro, Brazil). National Council for the Control of Animal Experimentation (CONCEA), the Biomedical Science Institute/UFRJ, and Ethical Committee for Animal Research approved the protocols used (DFBCICB015–04/16). The animals were maintained under standard conditions (a room with a 12 h light–dark cycle at 22 ± 2 °C, 60% to 80% humidity, and with food and water provided ad libitum).

2.2. Plant Material

Stems of *Aristolochia trilobata* were collected in Estância/SE, Brazil, in October/2011 (Geographic coordinates: S 11° 14′ 22.4″ and W 037° 25′ 00.5″) and received a voucher # ASE 23.161 deposited in the Herbarium of the Federal University of Sergipe. Stems of *A. trilobata* were cut in small pieces and crushed in a fourknife mill (Marconi, model MA680). The essential oil (EO) was obtained after hydrodistillation of 200 g of stem (in 1500 mL of distilled water) along 3 h and with help of a Clevenger-type apparatus. After physically separating oil and water, the first one was dried over anhydrous sodium sulfate and filtered. EO was stored in a freezer until further analyses and assays. Identification of constituents of EO was performed as Santos and collaborators [8].

2.3. Drugs and Treatments

Acetylsalicylic acid (ASA), atropine sulfate monohydrate, dexamethasone, and L-nitro arginine methyl ester (L-NAME) were purchased from Sigma-Aldrich (St. Louis, MO, USA). Morphine sulfate and naloxone hydrochloride were kindly provided by Cristália (São Paulo, Brazil) and formalin was purchased from Isofar (Rio de Janeiro, Brazil). EO was dissolved in pure oil in order to prepare a stock solution (100 mg/mL). From this stock solution, intermediate solutions were prepared and administered by oral gavage at doses varying from 1 to 100 mg/kg, in a final volume of 0.1 mL of pure oil per animal. Essential oil, as well as all drugs, were diluted just before use and the pure oil used as vehicle did not present any effect per se.

2.4. Formalin-Induced Licking Behavior

Formalin (2.5%, μL v/v) was injected into the dorsal surface of the left hind paw of mice. The time in which animals remained licking the formalin-injected paw was recorded according to Reference [9] with some adaptations done by Matheus et al. [10]. The response was divided into two phases: the first one (neurogenic phase) occurs in the first 5 min post-formalin injection and the second one (inflammatory phase) occurs between 15 and 30 min post-formalin injection.

2.5. Thermal Nociception Model (Hot-Plate)

The reaction time (licked fore and hind paws) that mice remained on a hot plate (Insight Equipment, Brazil) set at 55 ± 1 °C was recorded at several intervals of 30 min post-oral administration of EO or sulcatyl acetate (1, 10, or 100 mg/kg), vehicle, morphine, or antagonists. Baseline was calculated by the mean of two reaction time measurements at 60 and 30 min before oral administration [9] adapted by Matheus et al. [10]. Area under the curve (AUC) graphs were calculated from time–course graphs. The following formula, which is based on the trapezoid rule, was used to calculate the AUC: AUC = 30 × IB [(min 30) + (min 60) + ... + (min 180)]/2, where IB is the increase from the baseline (in %).

2.6. Evaluation of the Possible Mechanisms of Antinociception of A. Trilobata EO and Sulcatyl Acetate

The participation of nitrergic, opioid, and cholinergic pathways in the antinociception caused by EO and sulcatyl acetate was evaluated 15 min after intraperitoneal injection of antagonists and prior to oral administration of EO or sulcatyl acetate (at 100 mg/kg dose each). In assays conducted in our laboratory, dose–response curves for each antagonist against the respective agonist were previously constructed and the dose that reduced the agonist effect by 50% was chosen for the assays. Based on these data the doses used were: naloxone (opioid receptor antagonist) 1 mg/kg, atropine (cholinergic receptor antagonist) 1 mg/kg, L-NAME (nitric oxide synthase inhibitor) 3 mg/kg. The antinociceptive effect was evaluated via the hot plate test as described above.

2.7. Carrageenan-Induced Leukocyte Migration into the Subcutaneous Air Pouch (SAP)

Mice back received a subcutaneous injection of sterile air (10 mL) with a replacement of another 7 mL after 3 days. Twenty-four hours after the last injection of air, a solution of carrageenan (1%, 0.5 mL) was injected in subcutaneous air pouches [11,12] with modifications described in Raymundo et al. [13]. Treated groups were composed of mice that received oral administration of vehicle, EO (1, 10, or 100 mg/kg), sulcatyl acetate (1, 10, or 100 mg/kg), or dexamethasone (0.3 mg/kg, i.p.) 1 h before carrageenan injection in the SAP. The negative control group was composed of animals that received oral administration of pure oil and phosphate buffer saline (PBS, 1 mL) in SAP. After 24 h, animals were euthanized, the pouches were washed with 1 mL of sterile PBS, and exudates were collected. The total number of leukocytes was determined using a CellPocH-100Iv Diff (Sysmex) hematology analyzer. Exudates were centrifuged at 170× g for 10 min at 4 °C, and the supernatants were collected and stored at −20 °C until use.

To rule out a possible toxic effect of EO and sulcatyl acetate, mice treated with the highest dose of each one had their bone marrow cells collected through flushing the femur with 1 mL of PBS. Peripheral blood was also collected in heparinized tubes. The counting of the cells in the femoral lavage or in the blood was performed with the aid of a CellPocH-100Iv Diff (Sysmex) hematology analyzer.

2.8. Cell Culture

All cell culture reagents were purchased from Sigma-Aldrich (USA). RAW 264.7 (TIB-71) was obtained from the American Type Culture Collection. Cells were routinely grown in Roswell Park Memorial Institute (RPMI) medium containing 10% fetal bovine serum, 1% L-glutamine, and 1% penicillin-streptomycin (henceforth called RPMI) in a humidified 5% CO_2 atmosphere at 37 °C. Cells were cultured up to confluence and used in the assays.

2.9. Cell Viability Assay

Cell viability was determined using 3-(4,5-dimethyl-2-thiazyl)-2,5-diphenyl-2*H*-tetrazolium bromide (MTT) reagent (Sigma-Aldrich, USA) using method described by Denizot and Lang [14]. Briefly, cells were plated at an initial density of 5×10^4 cells per well in 96-well plates and incubated for 24 h at 37 °C and 5% CO_2. After 24 h, cultures were treated with EO or SA at a final concentration of 10, 30, or 100 µg/mL and further incubated for 24 h. The supernatants were removed and then 10 µL of MTT solution (5 mg/mL in RPMI)/100 µL of medium were added to each well and incubated for 4 h at 37 °C, 5% CO_2. The resultant formazan crystals were dissolved in dimethylsulfoxide (100 µL) and absorbance was measured in a microplate reader (FlexStation Reader, Molecular Devices, San Jose, CA, USA) at 570 nm. All experiments were performed in triplicate, and cell viability was expressed as a percentage relative to the untreated control cells.

2.10. Quantification of TNF-α and IL-1β

Supernatants from the exudates collected from the SAP were used to measure the levels of the cytokines tumor necrosis factor-α (TNF-α) and interleukin 1β (IL-1β) by enzyme-linked immunosorbent assay (ELISA) using the protocol supplied by the manufacturer (B&D, Franklin Lakes, NJ, USA).

2.11. Nitrate and Nitrite Measurement

To evaluate the nitrate accumulated in SAP, exudates were measured according to the method described by Bartholomew [15] and adapted by Raymundo et al. [13], followed by measurement of nitrite according to the Griess reaction [16].

2.12. Detection of Enzymes Expression

Immunoblots were carried out as described previously [17]. Briefly, RAW 264.7 cells (4 × 106/mL) were plated in 12-well plate, incubated for 1 h with EO or SA, activated with lipopolysaccharide (LPS) (1 µg/mL), and further incubated for 10 min, 1 h, or 8 h. Cells were lysed with cold lysis buffer (10% NP40, 150 Mm NaCl, 10 Mm Tris HCl pH 7.6, 2 Mm PMSF, and 5 µM leupeptin). After determination of the protein concentration in the suspensions by the BCA method (BCA™ Protein Assay Kit, Pierce, Waltham, MA, USA), the suspensions were boiled in application buffer (DTT 100 Mm, Bromophenol Blue 0.1%). Aliquots of 30 µg of protein were submitted to electrophoresis in 10% polyacrylamide gel. Proteins were electrophoretically transferred onto nitrocellulose membranes. Membranes were incubated with primary antibodies (Cell Signaling, Danvers, MA, USA) and further with secondary antibodies (anti-mouse IgG antibody conjugated to horseradish peroxidase). Proteins were detected using enhanced chemiluminescence (ECL) reagents and quantified using a ChemiDoc system (BioRad, Hercules, CA, USA).

2.13. Statistical Analysis

Each experimental group consisted of 6 to 8 mice, and the results are expressed as the mean ± S.D. The area under the curve (AUC) was calculated using Prism Software 5.0 (GraphPad Software, La Jolla, CA, USA). Significant differences between the groups were established using Bonferroni's test for multiple comparisons after analysis of variance (ANOVA) testing. p values less than 0.05 were considered significant.

3. Results

3.1. Antinociceptive Effect

3.1.1. Formalin-Induced Licking Behavior

We further decided to evaluate a possible antinociceptive activity from the EO and its major component, sulcatyl acetate. Doses of 1, 10, or 100 mg/kg given orally significantly reduced both phases of formalin-induced licking behavior (1st and 2nd). While first phase was inhibited by 10 and 100 mg/kg, the second phase was only inhibited by the highest dose (of 100 mg/kg) of EO. When studying sulcatyl acetate it could be observed that even 1 mg/kg dose significantly reduced the first phase, while only the highest dose reduced the second phase (Figure 1).

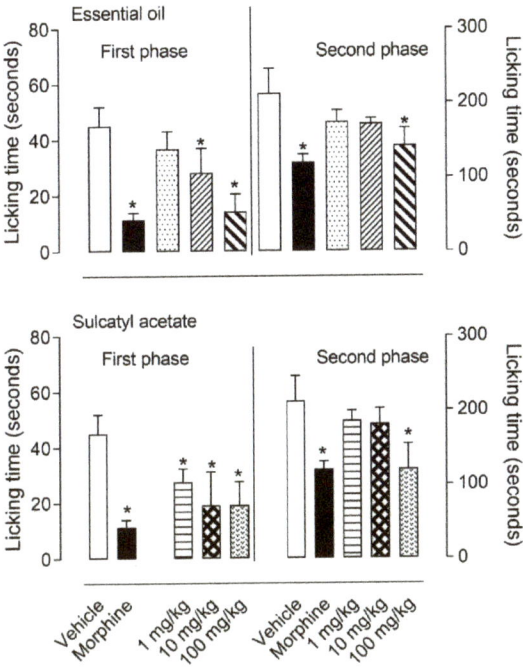

Figure 1. Effect of essential oil from *Aristolochia trilobata* and sulcatyl acetate on formalin-induced licking response in mice. Animals were orally pretreated with essential oil of sulcatyl acetate (1, 10, or 100 mg/kg), acetylsalicylic acid (ASA, 200 mg/kg), morphine (2.5 mg/kg), or vehicle (DMSO + phosphate buffer saline (PBS) 60 min before intraplantar injection of formalin (2.5%). The results are expressed as the mean ± S.D. ($n = 6$) of the time the animals spent licking the formalin-injected paw. Statistical significance was calculated by one-way ANOVA with Bonferroni's as post-test. * indicates $p < 0.05$ when compared to the vehicle-treated mice.

3.1.2. Hot-Plate Model

The significant effect observed in the first phase of the formalin-induced licking behavior is suggestive of an antinociceptive activity. Previous data from literature had shown that EO from *A. trilobata* presented antinociceptive effect in models of chemical nociception (acetic acid-induced writhings and formalin-induced licking response). However, in such paper, authors used high doses (25, 50, and 100 mg/kg) [6]. We further decided to evaluate if lower doses of EO and its majority component (sulcatyl acetate) present antinociceptive effect in thermal model of nociception (the hot plate). We also tried to evaluate the possible mechanism of action.

Data showed in Figure 2 indicate that both EO and sulcatyl acetate presented central antinociceptive effect. Even 30 min after oral administration of EO a significant effect was observed with all three doses tested (1, 10, and 100 mg/kg). This effect was maintained until 90 min post-oral administration and being gradually reduced in later times. The conversion of data from line graphs to area under the curve graph demonstrated that all three doses tested developed a significant central antinociceptive effect when comparing to the vehicle-treated group.

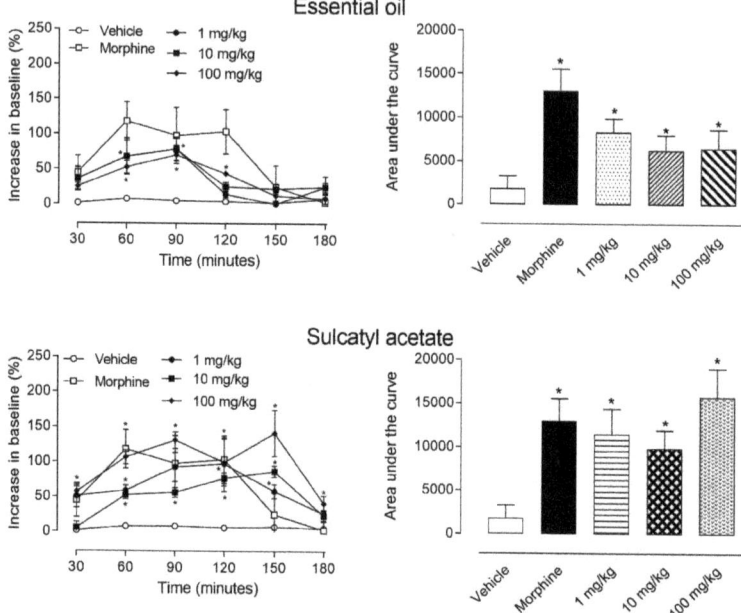

Figure 2. Effect of essential oil from *A. trilobata* and sulcatyl acetate on thermal nociception model (the hot plate) in mice. Animals were orally pretreated with essential oil of sulcatyl acetate (1, 10, or 100 mg/kg), morphine (2.5 mg/kg), or vehicle (DMSO + PBS). The results are presented as the mean ± S.D. ($n = 6–8$) of the increase in the response time relative to baseline levels (left graphs) or area under the curve (right graphs) calculated with the Prism Software 5.0. Statistical significance was calculated by one-way ANOVA with Bonferroni's as post-test. * indicates $p < 0.05$ when compared to the vehicle-treated mice. Where no error bars are shown is because they are smaller than the symbol.

When mice were orally treated with sulcatyl acetate, we could observe a significant effect after 30 min of administration. Differently to that observed with EO, sulcatyl acetate antinociception was maintained until 150 min. At this time point, antinociceptive effect was even higher than morphine-treated mice. The graph of the area under the curve demonstrated that all 3 doses presented a significant antinociceptive effect.

3.1.3. Mechanism of Antinociceptive Action

In the next step, we decided to investigate which pathways could be involved in the central antinociceptive effect of EO and sulcatyl acetate. Mice were pretreated with an opioid antagonist (naloxone), a cholinergic antagonist (atropine), or with an inhibitor of nitric oxide synthase enzyme (L-NAME). Data obtained showed that none of the antagonists of inhibitor significantly reversed the antinociceptive effect of either EO or sulcatyl acetate (Figure 3).

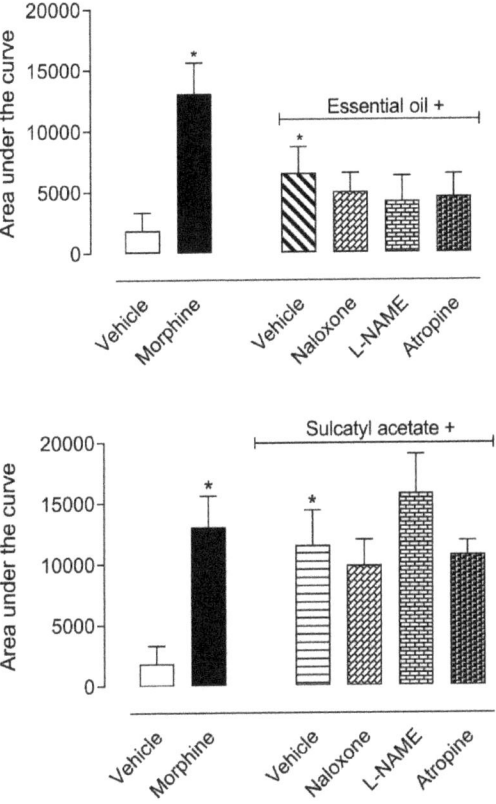

Figure 3. Effect of the different antagonists on the antinociceptive activity of essential oil from *A. trilobata* and sulcatyl acetate in the hot-plate model. The animals were pretreated with naloxone (1 mg/kg, i.p.), atropine (1 mg/kg, i.p.), or L-NAME (3 mg/kg, i.p.) 15 min before oral administration of essential oil or sulcatyl acetate (100 mg/kg) or vehicle. The results are expressed as the mean ± S.D. of the area under the curve calculated with Prism Software 5.0 ($n = 6-8$). One-way ANOVA followed by Bonferroni's test was used to calculate the statistical significance. * indicates $p < 0.05$ when compared to the vehicle-treated group.

3.2. Anti-Inflammatory Effect

The observation that EO and sulcatyl acetate inhibited the second phase of formalin-induced licking, a well-known inflammatory phase, led us to investigate if both substances could present an anti-inflammatory effect. In this regard, EO and sulcatyl acetate were evaluated in their abilities in reducing carrageenan-induced leukocyte migration into a subcutaneous air pouch (SAP) and cytokines production.

3.2.1. Leukocyte Migration

Injection of carrageenan into the SAP led to a 76-fold increase in leukocyte number ($2.14 \pm 1.65 \times 10^6$ cells/mL in the group that received saline in SAP versus $162.6 \pm 31.17 \times 10^6$ cells/mL in the group that received carrageenan in SAP). Pretreatment of mice with the steroidal anti-inflammatory drug (SAID), dexamethasone (Dex) resulted in a reduction of 50% in leukocyte number present in SAP. The crescent doses of EO (1, 10, and 100 mg/kg) significantly reduced the cell migration with values similar to the SAID. Sulcatyl acetate also reduced the number of cells that migrated to the pouch. However, this effect was less prominent when compared with that obtained with EO (Figure 4).

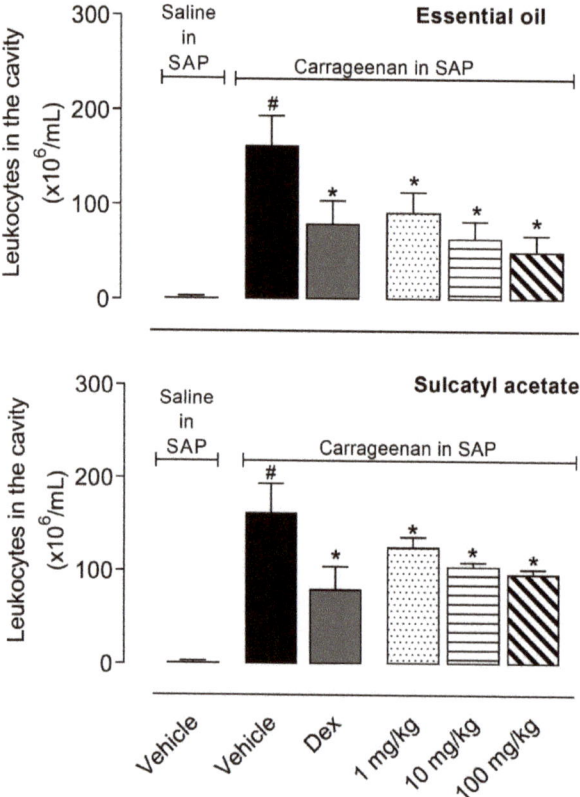

Figure 4. Effect of essential oil from *A. trilobata* and sulcatyl acetate in leukocyte migration into the subcutaneous air pouch (SAP). The animals were pretreated with dexamethasone (Dex, 1 mg/kg, i.p.), essential oil, or sulcatyl acetate (1, 10, or 100 mg/kg) or vehicle, 1 h before carrageenan injection into the SAP. The results are expressed as the mean ± S.D. calculated with Prism Software 5.0 ($n = 6$–8). One-way ANOVA followed by Bonferroni's test was used to calculate the statistical significance. * indicates $p < 0.05$ when compared to the vehicle-treated group (animals that received carrageenan in the SAP) and # indicates $p < 0.05$ when compared to the vehicle-treated group (animals that received saline in the SAP).

3.2.2. Protein Extravasation

As EO and SA presented a significative effect in reducing leukocyte migration into SAP similarly to that observed with the positive control group (SAID), we decided to further investigate if they could reduce other parameters of the inflammatory process in a tentative to investigate the possible mechanism of anti-inflammatory action. The exudate collected in the SAP protein was measured and results demonstrated that pretreatment of mice with 10 or 100 mg/kg doses of EO significantly reduced the amount of protein in exudate. It is interesting to note that none of the doses of SA inhibit protein extravasation even at a higher dose (100 mg/kg) (Figure 5).

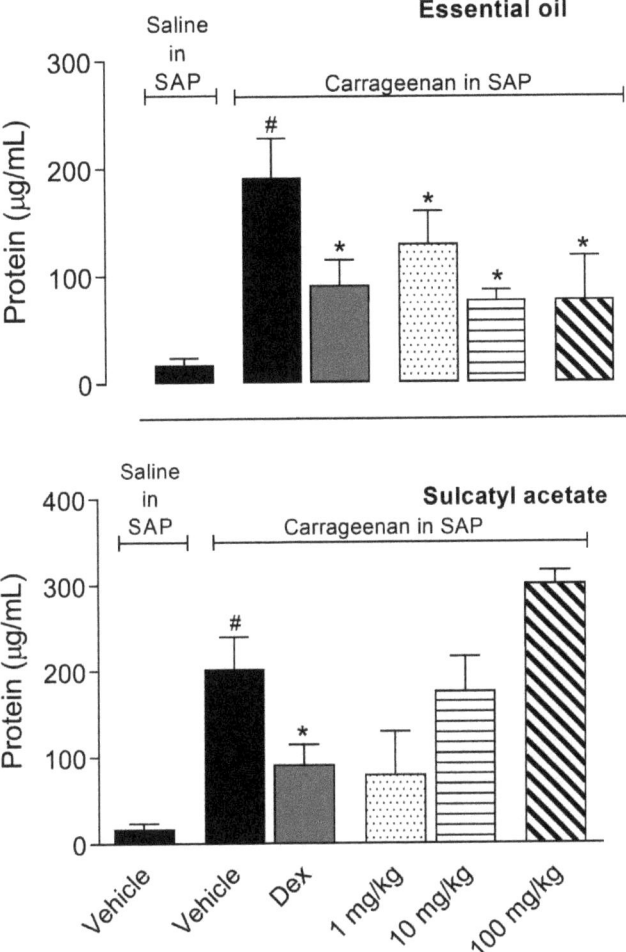

Figure 5. Effect of essential oil from *A. trilobata* and sulcatyl acetate in protein extravasation into the subcutaneous air pouch (SAP). The animals were pretreated with dexamethasone (Dex, 1 mg/kg, i.p.), essential oil, or sulcatyl acetate (1, 10, or 100 mg/kg) or vehicle 1 h before carrageenan injection into the SAP. The results are expressed as the mean ± S.D. calculated with Prism Software 5.0 (n = 6–8). One-way ANOVA followed by Bonferroni's test was used to calculate the statistical significance. * indicates $p < 0.05$ when compared to the vehicle-treated group (animals that received carrageenan in the SAP) and # indicates $p < 0.05$ when compared to the vehicle-treated group (animals that received saline in the SAP).

3.2.3. Nitric Oxide Production

We also decided to quantify the amount of nitric oxide (NO) produced in the exudate. When NO is produced in biological fluids it decays to the stable metabolite nitrate. Figure 6 shows that injection of carrageenan in the SAP lead to an increase in the amount of NO accumulated in the pouch when compared with mice that received saline. EO almost completely abolished NO production resulting in NO levels similar to those observed in saline-treated mice. Although SA did not completely inhibit the NO production, the reduction observed vary between 50% and 80% (Figure 6).

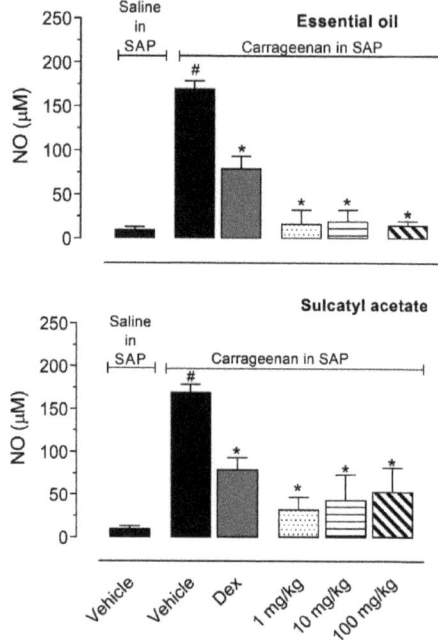

Figure 6. Effect of essential oil from *A. trilobata* and sulcatyl acetate in nitric oxide production into the subcutaneous air pouch (SAP). The animals were pretreated with dexamethasone (Dex, 1 mg/kg, i.p.), essential oil, or sulcatyl acetate (1, 10, or 100 mg/kg) or vehicle 1 h before carrageenan injection into the SAP. The results are expressed as the mean ± S.D. calculated with Prism Software 5.0 (n = 6–8). One-way ANOVA followed by Bonferroni's test was used to calculate the statistical significance. * indicates $p < 0.05$ when compared to the vehicle-treated group (animals that received carrageenan in the SAP) and # indicates $p < 0.05$ when compared to the vehicle-treated group (animals that received saline in the SAP).

3.2.4. Cytokine Production

The measurement of cytokines TNF-α and IL-1β accumulated in the exudate obtained from SAP showed that highest doses of EO (10 and 100 mg/kg) significantly reduced levels of both cytokines. However, pretreatment of mice with the majority component of the EO, sulcatyl acetate, led to an almost 50% reduction in cytokines production even with 1 mg/kg dose (Figure 7).

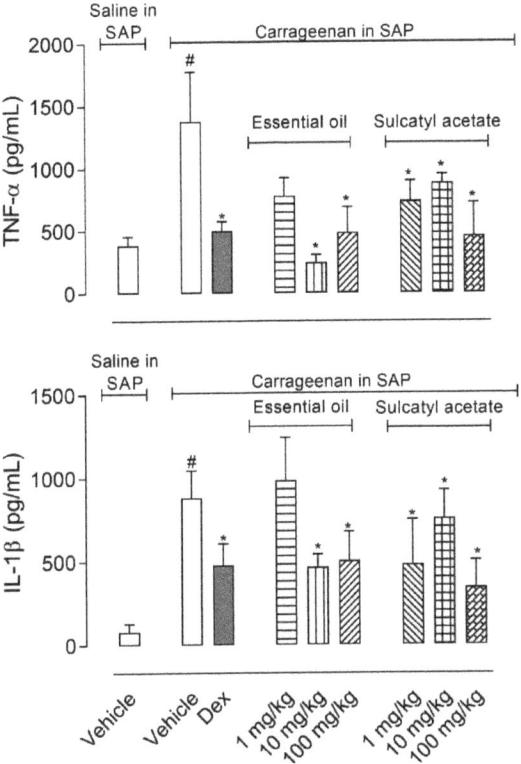

Figure 7. Effect of essential oil from *A. trilobata* and sulcatyl acetate in TNF-α and IL-1β production in the subcutaneous air pouch (SAP). The animals were pretreated with dexamethasone (1 mg/kg, i.p.), essential oil, or sulcatyl acetate (1, 10 or 100 mg/kg) or vehicle 1 h before carrageenan injection into the SAP. The results are expressed as the mean ± S.D. calculated with Prism Software 5.0 ($n = 6$–8). One-way ANOVA followed by Bonferroni's test was used to calculate the statistical significance. * indicates $p < 0.05$ when compared to the vehicle-treated group (animals that received carrageenan in the SAP) and # indicates $p < 0.05$ when compared to the vehicle-treated group (animals that received saline in the SAP).

3.2.5. In Vitro Cell Viability and Nitric Oxide Production

To further evaluate the possible anti-inflammatory mechanism of action, we decided to study the effects of EO and SA in vitro using macrophage cell line RAW 264.7. Data obtained showed that none of the concentrations used (1, 10, or 30 µg/mL) significantly affected the cell viability (data not shown). We next measure NO production by LPS-activated cells incubated or not with the three concentrations of EO and SA. Neither EO nor SA did induce NO production *per se* (data not shown). Figure 8 shows that there is an inhibitory effect on NO production when LPS-activated cells were pre-incubated with SA for 1 h (Figure 8D). In another set of experiments, cells were activated with LPS and after 8 h different concentrations of OE or SA were added to each group. As can be observed in Figure 8C,D, we do not observe inhibitory effect in NO production when EO or SA was added 8 h post-LPS.

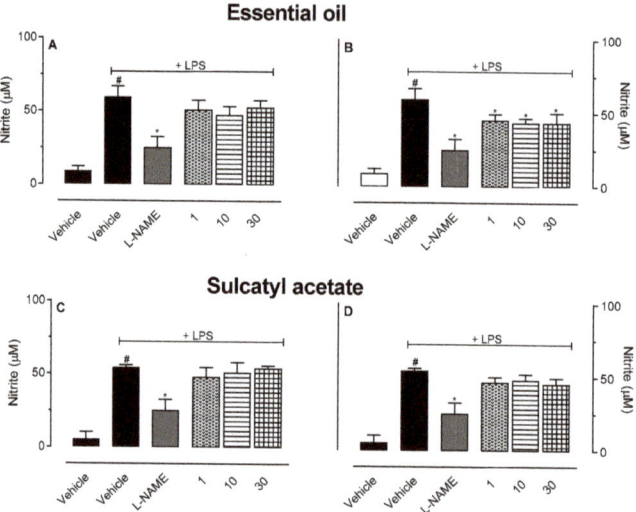

Figure 8. Effect of essential oil from *A. trilobata* (EO) and sulcatyl acetate (SA) in nitric oxide production by RAW 264.7 macrophage. Cells (2×10^6/mL) were incubated with lipopolysaccharide (LPS, 1 µg/mL) and EO or SA (1, 10, or 30 µg/mL). Graphs **A** and **B** show the results of pre-incubation of cells for 1 h before LPS addition to cells. Graphs **C** and **D** show the results of NO production when EO or SA was added 8 h post-LPS activation. The results are expressed as the mean ± S.D. calculated with Prism Software 5.0 ($n = 6$). One-way ANOVA followed by Bonferroni's test was used to calculate the statistical significance. # indicates $p < 0.05$ when compared to the vehicle (non-LPS group). * indicates $p < 0.05$ when compared to the group that was activated with LPS and received vehicle.

In a tentative to demonstrate the possible mechanism of anti-inflammatory effect of EO and SA, we decided to evaluate their effects on some inflammatory pathways. For this purpose, expression of inducible nitric oxide synthase (iNOS), p38 mitogen-activated protein kinase (p38 MAPK), its activated form (the phosphorylated p38), and spleen tyrosine kinase (Syk) was evaluated after incubation of RAW 264.7 cells with EO or SA (30 µg/mL) and LPS. As expected, non-activated cells did not express those inflammatory enzymes, while LPS incubation induced an increase in levels of all of them. As illustrated in Figure 9, preincubation with EO significantly reduced the expression of iNOS. To ascertain whether the mechanism by which both substances were reducing the expression of the enzyme, we evaluated the involvement of enzymes present in the early stages of the activation pathways triggered by LPS in the toll receptor 4. In this regard, we evaluated expression of p38 MAPK and Syk and the corresponding increase in levels of phosphorylated p38, a consequence of cell activation and p38 activation. It can be observed that EO reduced expression of Syk enzyme. After an activation induced by LPS we can observe the activation/phosphorylation of p38 MAPK. In this context, it could be noted an increase in levels of this enzyme (p-p38). However, preincubation of activated cells with EO or SA did not affect phosphorylation levels of p38 MAPK. In summary, EO and SA did not affect the levels of p-p38 expressed in cells after activation with LPS (Figure 9).

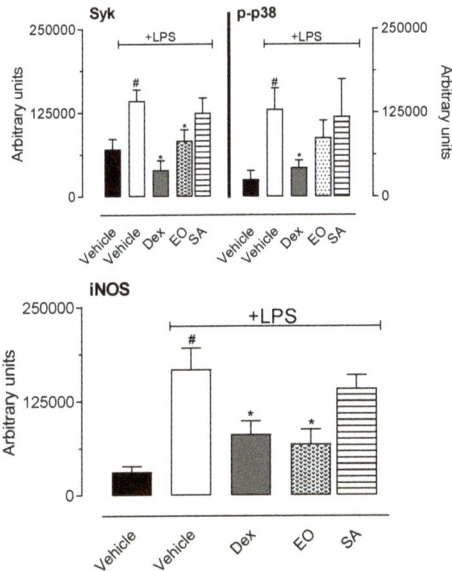

Figure 9. Effect of essential oil from *A. trilobata* (EO) and sulcatyl acetate (SA) in expression of Syk, p38 MAPK, or inducible nitric oxide synthase (iNOS) by RAW 264.7 cells. Cells ($2 \times 10^{6/mL}$) were incubated with dexamethasone (350 µg/mL), EO, or SA (30 µg/mL) 1 h before lipopolysaccharide (LPS, 1 µg/mL). After 10 min (for Syk and p38 MAPK) or 8 h (for iNOS), cell lysates were collected for Western blot analyses. The results are expressed as the mean ± S.D. calculated with Prism Software 5.0 ($n = 3$). One-way ANOVA followed by Newman's test was used to calculate the statistical significance. # indicates $p < 0.05$ when compared to the vehicle (non-LPS group). * indicates $p < 0.05$ when compared to the group that was activated with LPS and received vehicle.

4. Discussion

The present work demonstrated that the essential oil (EO) of *A. trilobata* and its majoritarian substance, sulcatyl acetate (SA), present significant anti-inflammatory and antinociceptive effects. We also demonstrated that opioidergic, nitrergic, and cholinergic pathways do not participate in the antinociceptive effect. Contributing to the knowledge about this species, we also demonstrated that both EO and SA presented anti-inflammatory effect reducing leukocyte migration, production of cytokines, nitric oxide (NO), and protein extravasation.

The evaluation of *A. trilobata* EO chemical constituents highlighted the presence of SA as the major substance. This characteristic is not usual in essential oils in general. However, this finding confirms previous works, which states *A. trilobata* EO as a rich source of SA [4,7].

Quintas et al. [7] demonstrated that EO from *A. trilobata* and SA presented antinociceptive effect in two models of chemical nociception (i.e., acetic acid-induced writhing and formalin-induced paw licking). Although the essential oil tested in that work was very similar to that used by us, there are several differences among assays and results. In that work, authors used doses varying from 25 to 100 mg/kg, administered by intraperitoneal route. EO and SA were evaluated only in two models of chemical nociception. Differently, in the present work, we evaluated EO and SA administered by oral route and doses of 1, 10, and 100 mg/kg. The effect observed in this model could be explained, at least in part, due to the presence of other substances with antinociceptive activity. It was demonstrated by Amaral and collaborators [18] that the monoterpene limonene presented antinociceptive activity more related to peripheral analgesia. Kaiamoto and collaborators [19] also suggested that limonene may act as a transient receptor potential cation channel 1 (TRPA1) agonist when applied topically. However, when systemically administered, it presents an antinociceptive effect. In our work, we did not test isolated limonene. We used only the majoritarian substance (SA). It is also important to note that formalin-induced licking is a multicomplex phenomenon with the involvement and activation of nuclear factor erythroid 2-related factor 2 (Nrf2) pathway. Nrf2 is a transcriptional factor related to activation of heme-oxygenase 1 (HO-1) [20], leading to an antinociceptive effect in formalin-induced licking [21]. It may be that in such a way, by oral administration, all the substances presented in the EO may acting together to present an anti-inflammatory effect.

Considering the *A. trilobata* EO results and its major substances, a synergistic effect of SA and limonene can be occurring, especially in the second phase of formalin-induced licking response. Besides evaluating the effects in the formalin-induced paw licking, we also used the thermal model of nociception, the hot-plate, and searched the mechanism of action of EO and SA using three different antagonists.

In another group of assays, we also studied the anti-inflammatory effect of EO and SA in their capacity to inhibit the leukocyte migration into the subcutaneous air pouch induced by carrageenan and production of some inflammatory mediators. Our data complement those obtained by the other group and identify the possible mechanism of action. We also demonstrated that EO and SA presented significant effects even when used by oral route at a dose as low as 1 mg/kg.

In the present study, we attempted to further characterize some of the mechanisms through which EO from *A. trilobata* and SA exerts its antinociceptive effect. The sensation of pain can be divided into four components, i.e., transduction, transmission, modulation, and perception. Several systems, such as oxidonitrergic, gamma aminobutyric acid GABAergic, glutamatergic, opioidergic, cholinergic, serotonergic, adrenergic, and others, may act in different steps of the pain turning it a complex phenomenon in such a way that alterations in one of the system cited above can alter the response in all the other systems [22]. A substance, whether natural or synthetic, can then act in one of four components to produce analgesia. Our data are suggestive that nor opioidergic, nitrergic, or cholinergic pathways appear to be involved in the antinociceptive effect of EO and SA since none of the antagonists used (naloxone, L-NAME, or atropine) reversed the effects of EO and SA. Despite the opioid system is one of the most important in pain perception and modulation, the activation of naloxone-sensitive pathway is probably not involved in the antinociception produced by EO and SA because naloxone significantly reversed morphine (data not shown) but not EO and SA antinociception.

We also demonstrated that doses as low as 1 mg/kg significantly reduced the licking response induced by formalin injection in mice paw. Nociception induced by formalin develops a biphasic pattern with an initial phase (5 to 15 min post-injection) followed by a second phase (15 to 30 min post-injection) [23–26]. First phase is due to direct activation of nociceptors, whereas the second one is due to the release of inflammatory mediators acting together in nociceptors and their own local receptors [27–29]. The involvement of serotonin and bradykinin in both phases was also described [30].

As mediators previously cited are also involved in inflammatory processes, we further decided to study if EO and SA could present an anti-inflammatory effect. In this regard, we used the leukocyte migration induced by injection of carrageenan into the subcutaneous air pouch (SAP). Carrageenan-induced inflammation is a multicomplex phenomenon with the involvement of synthesis and/or liberation of a range of mediators such as prostaglandins, histamine, bradykinin, serotonin, nitric oxide, and leukotrienes and chemotaxis of neutrophils and macrophages [31]. After 24 h of carrageenan injection, there is an intense migration of leukocytes and an increase in levels of NO and cytokines [32–36].

Results obtained in the SAP model complement those obtained in the second phase of formalin-induced licking since both models present an inflammatory profile with involvement in a diversity of inflammatory mediators. One hypothesis for the reduction observed in this model could be related to reduction in production and/or liberation of inflammatory substances involved in leukocyte chemotaxis. In this context, we can infer that the reduction in cell migration into the SAP could be due to a reduction in the levels of these cytokines. Our data are in accordance with those obtained in Reference [37], which observed that tacrolimus (an immunosuppressor) reduced neutrophil infiltration in the pancreatitis model due to a reduction in expression of mRNA of TNF-α and IL-1β. In an inflammatory event, inducible nitric oxide synthase is expressed in different cells and culminating with NO production. NO plays multiple roles in the inflammatory response, vasodilation, and regulation of leukocytes rolling, migration, cytokines production, and proliferation. It has been shown that some iNOS inhibitors demonstrated an important effect in several inflammatory models, such as the air pouch model [38,39]. The fact that EO and SA reduced NO levels in exudate also contribute to their anti-inflammatory effect. It is also interesting to note that EO reduced NO levels similar to the positive control group, dexamethasone, a well-known steroidal anti-inflammatory drug.

Data obtained using the in vivo model of SAP was corroborated by in vitro assays. Reduction in nitric oxide production in vitro and in vivo was not due to a direct effect in iNOS enzyme activity. It is well known that iNOS synthesis occurs until 6–8 h after LPS activation. After this time point, nucleus synthesis is finished and enzymes synthesized initiate NO production [39]. Since addition of EO or SA 8 h after LPS activation did not affect NO production, it can be suggested that the inhibitory effect observed was not due to reduced enzyme activity.

As a final step in our effort to delineate the inhibitory effects of EO and SA, we quantified Syk and p38 MAPK enzymes expression. Several intracellular signaling molecules are involved and activated during the inflammatory responses in macrophages. Tyrosine kinase families have been considered as the major effector molecule. Spleen tyrosine kinase (Syk) binds with Toll-like receptor-4 (TLR4) and is activated, resulting in the transduction of stimulatory signals through the activation of various downstream signaling molecules. Since Syk is one of the upstream signaling molecules, it orchestrates many downstream signaling molecules and amplifies inflammatory signals. Therefore, Syk has been considered to play critical roles in inflammatory responses [40–42]. The observation that EO partially reduced expression of Syk can explain the inhibition of expression of iNOS and justify the inhibition observed in NO production.

p38 MAPK was first recognized for its role in inflammation in regulating the biosynthesis of pro-inflammatory cytokines (i.e., IL-1 and TNFα) in LPS-stimulated cells [41] and expression of cycloxigenase-2 (COX2) [42–44]. It can be suggested that EO and SA mechanism of action do not seem to affect p38 MAPK activation into the phosphorylated form (the p-p38). We could speculate that EO effect may act through Syk pathway do not interfere with p38 MAPK since both are independent systems that may act without cross-interference with each other.

Our data also demonstrated that SA did not affect *per se* any of enzymes evaluated (Syk, p38 MAPK, and iNOS). It is important to note that as part of a complex mixture of substances it is reasonable that EO can present effect and one isolated substance cannot present the same effect and mechanism of action.

5. Conclusions

In the present work, we demonstrated that *A. trilobata* essential oil as well as the majority component, sulcatyl acetate, present antinociceptive and anti-inflammatory effects. This activity is accompanied by reduction in cell migration and production of NO and cytokines. It seems that at least part of this effect is mediated by inhibition of Syk and iNOS enzymes expression. Together, we can suggest *A. trilobata* as an anti-inflammatory and antinociceptive species.

Author Contributions: Data curation, P.D.F.; formal analysis, D.d.C.S. and P.D.F.; funding acquisition, P.D.F.; investigation, D.d.C.S., N.d.M.C., P.D.F., and P.D.F.; methodology, D.d.C.S., T.S.V., D.d.A.S., P.B.A., D.S.A.M., and P.D.F.; project administration, P.D.F.; resources, C.S.A. and P.D.F.; supervision, P.B.A. and P.D.F.; writing—original draft, P.D.F.; writing—review and editing, P.D.F. All authors have read and agreed to the published version of the manuscript.

Funding: This research was funded by Conselho Nacional de Pesquisa (CNPq, fellowship and grants for P.D.F. and C.S.A.), Fundação Carlos Chagas Filho de Apoio à Pesquisa (FAPERJ, fellowship and grants for P.D.F., C.S.A., D.S.A.M.), and Coordenação de Aperfeiçoamento de Pessoal (CAPES, for fellowship to NMC, D.d.C.S.).

Acknowledgments: We would like to thank Alan Minho for technical assistance and Instituto Vital Brazil (Niterói, Brazil) for donating the mice.

Conflicts of Interest: The authors declare no conflict of interest.

References

1. Levine, J.D.; Reichling, D.B. Peripheral mechanisms of inflammatory pain. In *Textbook of Pain*, 4th ed.; Will, P.A., Melzack, R., Eds.; Churchil Livingstone: London, UK, 1999; pp. 59–84.
2. Harirforoosh, S.; Asghar, W.; Jamali, F. Adverse effects of nonsteroidal anti-inflammatory drugs: An update of gastrointestinal, cardiovascular and renal complications. *J. Pharm. Pharm. Sci.* **2013**, *16*, 821–847. [CrossRef] [PubMed]
3. Heinrich, M.; Chan, J.; Wanke, S.; Neinhuis, C.; Simmonds, M. Local uses of Aristolochia species and content of nephrotoxic aristolochic acid 1 and 2 a global assessment based on bibliographic sources. *J. Ethnopharmacol.* **2008**, *17*, 108–144. [CrossRef] [PubMed]
4. de Oliveira, B.M.S.; Melo, C.R.; Alves, P.B.; Abraão, A.S.; Santos, A.C.C.; Santana, A.S.; Araújo, A.P.A.; Nascimento, P.E.S.; Blank, A.F.; Bacci, L. Essential oil of *Aristolochia trilobata*: Synthesis, routes of exposure, acute toxicity, binary mixtures and behavioral effects on leaf-cutting ants. *Molecules* **2017**, *22*, 335. [CrossRef] [PubMed]
5. Lans, C. Comparison of plants used for skin and stomach problems in Trinidad and Tobago with Asian ethnomedicine. *J. Ethnobiol. Ethnomed.* **2007**, *3*, 3. [CrossRef] [PubMed]
6. Sosa, S.; Balick, M.J.; Arvigo, R.; Esposito, R.G.; Pizza, C.; Altinier, G. Screening of the topical anti-inflammatory activity of some Central American plants. *J. Ethnopharmacol.* **2002**, *81*, 211–215. [CrossRef]
7. Quintans, J.S.S.; Alves, R.S.; Santos, D.A.; Serafini, M.R.; Alves, P.B.; Costa, E.V.; Zengin, G.; Quintans-Júnior, L.J.; Guimarães, A.G. Antinociceptive effect of *Aristolochia trilobata* stem essential oil and 6-methyl-5-hepten-2yl acetate, its main compound, in rodents. *Zeitschrift Für Naturforschung C* **2017**, *72*, 93–97. [CrossRef]
8. Santos, D.A. Volatile constituents of *Aristolochia trilobata* L. (Aristolochiaceae): A rich source of sulcatyl acetate. *Quim. Nova* **2014**, *37*, 977–981.
9. Sahley, T.L.; Berntson, G.G. Antinociceptive effects of central and systemic administration of nicotine in the rat. *Psychopharmacology* **1979**, *65*, 279–283. [CrossRef]
10. Matheus, M.E.; Berrondo, L.F.; Vieitas, E.C.; Menezes, S.F.; Fernandes, P.D. Evaluation of the antinociceptive properties from *Brillantaisia palisotii* Lindau stems extracts. *J. Ethnopharmacol.* **2005**, *102*, 377–381. [CrossRef]
11. Fernandes, P.D.; Zardo, P.D.; Figueiredo, G.S.M.; Silva, B.A.; Pinto, A.C. Anti-inflammatory properties of convolutamydine A and two structural analogues. *Life Sci.* **2014**, *116*, 16–24. [CrossRef]
12. Sedgwick, A.D.; Lees, P. Studies of eicosanoid production in the air pouch model of synovial inflammation. *Agents Actions* **1986**, *18*, 439–446. [CrossRef] [PubMed]
13. Raymundo, L.J.R.P.; Guilhon, C.C.; Alviano, D.S.; Matheus, M.E.; Antoniolli, A.R.; Cavalcanti, S.C.H.; Alves, P.B.; Alviano, C.S.; Fernandes, P.D. Characterization of the anti-inflammatory and antinociceptive activities of the *Hyptis pectinata* (L.) Poit essential oil. *J. Ethnopharmacol.* **2011**, *134*, 725–732. [CrossRef] [PubMed]
14. Denizot, F.; Lang, R. Rapid colorimetric assay for cell growth and survival. Modifications to the tetrazolium dye procedure giving improved sensitivity and reliability. *J. Immunol. Meth.* **1986**, *89*, 271–277. [CrossRef]
15. Bartholomew, B. A rapid method for the assay of nitrate in urine using the nitrate reductase enzyme of Escherichia coli. *Food Chem. Toxicol.* **1984**, *22*, 541–543. [CrossRef]
16. Green, L.C.; Wagner, D.A.; Glogowski, J.; Skipper, P.L.; Wisnok, J.S.; Tannenbaum, S.R. Analysis of nitrate, nitrite, and [5N] nitrate in biological fluids. *Anal. Biochem.* **1982**, *126*, 131–138. [CrossRef]
17. Fernandes, P.D.; Araujo, H.M.; Riveros-Moreno, V.; Assreuy, J. Depolymerization of macrophage microfilaments prevents induction and inhibits activity of nitric oxide synthase. *Eur. J. Cell Biol.* **1996**, *71*, 356–362.
18. do Amaral, J.F.; Silva, M.I.; Neto, M.R.; Neto, P.F.; Moura, B.A.; de Melo, C.T.; de Araújo, F.L.; de Sousa, D.P.; de Vasconcelos, P.F.; de Vasconcelos, S.M.; et al. Antinociceptive effect of the monoterpene R-(+)-limonene in mice. *Biol. Pharm. Bull.* **2007**, *30*, 1217–1220. [CrossRef]
19. Kaiamoto, T.; Hatakeyama, Y.; Takahashi, K.; Imagawa, T.; Tominaga, M.; Ohta, T. Involvement of transient receptor potential A1 channel in algesic and analgesic actions of the organic compound limonene. *Eur. J. Pain* **2016**, *20*, 1155–1165. [CrossRef]

20. Egea, J.; Rosa, A.O.; Lorrio, S.; Barrio, L.; Cuadrado, A.; López, M.G. Haeme oxygenase-1 overexpression via nAChRs and the transcription factor Nrf2 has antinociceptive effects in the formalin test. *Pain* **2009**, *146*, 75–83. [CrossRef]
21. Rosa, O.A.; Egea, J.; Lorrio, S.; Rojo, A.I.; Cuadrado, A.; Lopez, M.G. Nrf2-mediated haeme oxygenase-1 up-regulation induced by cobalt protoporphyrin has antinociceptive effects against inflammatory pain in the formalin test in mice. *Pain* **2008**, *132*, 332–339. [CrossRef]
22. Xie, Y.F.; Huo, F.Q.; Tang, J.S. Cerebral cortex modulation of pain. *Acta Pharmacol. Sin.* **2009**, *30*, 31–41. [CrossRef] [PubMed]
23. Malmberg, A.B.; Yaksh, T.L. Cyclooxygenase inhibition and the spinal release of prostaglandin E2 nd amino acids evoked by paw formalin injection: A microdialysis study in unanesthetized rats. *J. Neurosci.* **1995**, *15*, 2768–2776. [CrossRef] [PubMed]
24. Shibata, M.; Ohkubo, T.; Takahashi, H.; Inoki, R. Modified formalin test: Characteristic biphasic pain response. *Pain* **1989**, *38*, 347–352. [CrossRef]
25. Teng, C.J.; Abbott, F.V. The formalin test: A dose-response analysis at three developmental stages. *Pain* **1998**, *76*, 337–347. [CrossRef]
26. Ward, L.; Wright, E.; McMahon, S.B. A comparison of the effects of noxious and innocuous counter stimuli on experimentally induced itch and pain. *Pain* **1996**, *64*, 129–138. [CrossRef]
27. Wheeler-Aceto, H.; Porreca, F.; Cowan, A. The rat paw formalin test: Comparison of noxious agents. *Pain* **1990**, *40*, 229–238. [CrossRef]
28. Hunskaar, S.; Hole, K. The formalin test in mice: Dissociation between inflammatory and non-inflammatory pain. *Pain* **1987**, *30*, 103–114. [CrossRef]
29. Jaffery, G.; Coleman, J.W.; Huntley, J.; Bell, E.B. Mast cell recovery following chronic treatment with compound 48/80. *Int. Arch. Allergy Immunol.* **1994**, *105*, 274–280. [CrossRef]
30. Parada, C.A.; Tambeli, C.H.; Cunha, F.Q.; Ferreira, S.H. The major role of peripheral release of histamine and 5-hydroxytryptamine in formalin-induced nociception. *Neuroscience* **2001**, *102*, 937–944. [CrossRef]
31. Di Rosa, M.; Sorrentino, L.; Parente, L. Non-steroidal anti-inflammatory drugs and leucocyte emigration. *J. Pharm. Pharmacol.* **1972**, *24*, 575–577. [CrossRef]
32. Ferrandiz, M.L.; Gil, B.; Sanz, M.L.; Ubeda, A.; Gonzalez, E.; Negrete, R.; Pacheco, S.; Paya, M.; Alcarz, M.L. Effect of bakuchiol on leukocytes function and some inflammatory responses in mice. *J. Pharm. Pharmacol.* **1996**, *48*, 975–980. [CrossRef] [PubMed]
33. Saleh, T.S.; Calixto, J.B.; Medeiros, Y.S. Anti-inflammatory effects of theophylline, cromolyn and salbutamol in a murine model of pleurisy. *Br. J. Pharmacol.* **1996**, *118*, 811–819. [CrossRef] [PubMed]
34. Fröde, T.S.; Medeiros, Y.S. Myeloperoxidase and adenosine-deaminase levels in the pleural fluid leakage induced by carrageenan in the mouse model of pleurisy. *Mediat. Inflamm.* **2001**, *10*, 223–227. [CrossRef] [PubMed]
35. Da Silva, M.B.; Farges, R.C.; Fröde, T.S. Involvement of steroids in anti-inflammatory effects of PK11195 in a murine model of pleurisy. *Mediat. Inflamm.* **2004**, *13*, 93–103. [CrossRef]
36. Koo, H.J.; Lim, K.H.; Jung, H.J.; Park, E.H. Anti-inflammatory evaluation of gardenioa extract, geniposide and genipin. *J. Ethnopharmacol.* **2005**, *103*, 496–500. [CrossRef]
37. Rau, B.M.; Kruger, C.M.; Hasel, C.; Oliveira, V.; Rubie, C.; Beger, H.G.; Schilling, M.K. Effects of immunosuppressive and immunostimulative treatment on pancreatic injury and mortality in severe acute experimental pancreatitis. *Pancreas* **2006**, *33*, 174–183. [CrossRef]
38. Gurik, T.J.; Korbut, R.; Adamek-Gurik, T. Nitric oxide and superoxide in inflammation and immune regulation. *J. Physiol. Pharmacol.* **2003**, *54*, 469–487.
39. Paya, M.; Pastor, P.G.; Coloma, J.; Alcaraz, M.J. Nitric oxide synthase and cyclo-oxygenase pathways in the inflammatory response induced by zymosan in the rat air pouch. *Br. J. Pharmacol.* **1997**, *120*, 1445–1452. [CrossRef]
40. Yi, Y.S.; Son, Y.J.; Ryou, C.; Sung, G.H.; Kim, J.H.; Chol, J.Y. Functional roles of Syk in macrophage-mediated inflammatory responses. *Mediat. Inflamm.* **2014**, 270302. [CrossRef]
41. Lee, J.C.; Laydon, J.T.; McDonnell, P.C.; Gallagher, T.F.; Kumar, S.; Green, D.; McNulty, D.; Blumenthal, M.J.; Heys, J.R.; Landvatter, S.W. A protein kinase involved in the regulation of inflammatory cytokine biosynthesis. *Nature* **1994**, *372*, 739–746. [CrossRef]

42. Hwang, D.; Jang, B.C.; Yu, G.; Boudreau, M. Expression of mitogen inducible cyclooxygenase induced by lipopolysaccharide: Mediation through both mitogen-activated protein kinase and NF-kappaB signaling pathways in macrophages. *Biochem. Pharmacol.* **1997**, *54*, 87–96. [CrossRef]
43. Paul, A.; Cuenda, A.; Bryant, C.E.; Murray, J.; Chilvers, E.R.; Cohen, P.; Gould, G.W.; Plevin, R. Involvement of mitogen-activated protein kinase homologues in the regulation of lipopolysaccharide-mediated induction of cyclo-oxygenase-2 but not nitric oxide synthase in RAW 264.7 macrophages. *Cell. Signal.* **1999**, *11*, 491–497. [CrossRef]
44. Ridley, S.H.; Dean, J.L.; Sarsfield, S.J.; Brook, M.; Clark, A.R.; Saklatvala, J. A p38 MAP kinase inhibitor regulates stability of interleukin-1-induced cyclooxygenase-2 Mrna. *FEBS Lett.* **1998**, *439*, 75–80. [CrossRef]

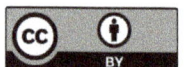 © 2020 by the authors. Licensee MDPI, Basel, Switzerland. This article is an open access article distributed under the terms and conditions of the Creative Commons Attribution (CC BY) license (http://creativecommons.org/licenses/by/4.0/).

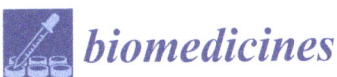

Article

Phytogenic Synthesis of Nickel Oxide Nanoparticles (NiO) Using Fresh Leaves Extract of *Rhamnus triquetra* (Wall.) and Investigation of Its Multiple In Vitro Biological Potentials

Javed Iqbal [1,*,†], Banzeer Ahsan Abbasi [1,†], Riaz Ahmad [2], Mahboobeh Mahmoodi [3], Akhtar Munir [4], Syeda Anber Zahra [1], Amir Shahbaz [1], Muzzafar Shaukat [1], Sobia Kanwal [5], Siraj Uddin [1,6], Tariq Mahmood [1] and Raffaele Capasso [7,*]

1. Department of Plant Sciences, Quaid-i-Azam University, Islamabad 45320, Pakistan; benazirahsanabbasi786@gmail.com (B.A.A.); s.a.zahra786@gmail.com (S.A.Z.); amirqaisrani@gmail.com (A.S.); m.muzaffar.shoukat@gmail.com (M.S.); usiraj85@gmail.com (S.U.); tmahmood.qau@gmail.com (T.M.)
2. College of Life Sciences, Shaanxi Normal University, Xi'an 710119, China; riaz17qau@gmail.com
3. Department of Biomedical Engineering, Yazd Branch, Islamic Azad University, Yazd 8915813135, Iran; m.mahmoodi@iauyazd.ac.ir
4. Department of Chemistry and Chemical Engineering, SBA School of Science and Engineering, Lahore University of Management Sciences (LUMS), DHA, Lahore 54792, Pakistan; 16130031@lums.edu.pk
5. Department of Zoology, University of Gujrat, Sub-Campus Rawalpindi 46000, Pakistan; sobiakanwal16@gmail.com
6. Plant Breeding Institute, Faculty of Agriculture & Environment, University of Sydney, Cobbitty, NSW 2570, Australia
7. Department of Agricultural Sciences, University of Naples Federico II, 80055 Portici, Italy
* Correspondence: javed89qau@gmail.com (J.I.); rafcapas@unina.it (R.C.)
† These authors contributed equally to this work.

Received: 7 April 2020; Accepted: 3 May 2020; Published: 12 May 2020

Abstract: Chemically nickel oxide nanoparticles (NiONPs) involve the synthesis of toxic products, which restrict their biological applications. Hence, we developed a simple, eco-friendly, and cost-efficient green chemistry method for the fabrication of NiONPs using fresh leaf broth of *Rhamnus triquetra* (RT). The RT leaves broth was used as a strong reducing, capping, and stabilizing agent in the formation of RT-NiONPs. The color change in solution from brown to greenish black suggests the fabrication of RT-NiONPs which was further confirmed by absorption band at 333 nm. The synthesis and different physicochemical properties of RT-NiONPs were investigated using different analytical techniques such as UV-Vis (ultraviolet–visible) spectroscopy, XRD (X-ray powder diffraction), FT-IR (Fourier-transform infrared spectroscopy), SEM (scanning electron microscopy), TEM (transmission electron microscopy), EDS (energy-dispersive X-ray spectroscopy), DLS (dynamic light scattering) and Raman. Further, RT-NiONPs were subjected to different in vitro biological activities and revealed distinctive biosafe and biocompatibility potentials using erythrocytes and macrophages. RT-NiONPs exhibited potential anticancer activity against liver cancer cell lines HUH7 (IC_{50}: 11.3 µg/mL) and HepG2 (IC_{50}: 20.73 µg/mL). Cytotoxicity potential was confirmed using Leishmanial parasites promastigotes (IC_{50}: 27.32 µg/mL) and amastigotes (IC_{50}: 37.4 µg/mL). RT-NiONPs are capable of rendering significant antimicrobial efficacy using various bacterial and fungal strains. NiONPs determined potent radical scavenging and moderate enzyme inhibition potencies. Overall, this study suggested that RT-NiONPs can be an attractive and eco-friendly candidate. In conclusion, current study showed potential in vitro biological activities and further necessitate different in vivo studies in various animal models to develop leads for new drugs to treat several chronic diseases.

Keywords: *Rhamnus triquetra*; NiONPs; cytotoxicity; biocompatibility; antimicrobial; enzyme inhibition

1. Introduction

Nanotechnology deals with different approaches to synthesize materials ranging from 1 to 100 nm, at least in one dimension, and have unique properties, such as small size, surface charge, porosity, high surface energy, and high surface area/volume (S/V) ratio, which enhance their catalytic properties and interaction with other molecules. The main reason why metal nanoparticles (MNPs) have gained the specific attention of researchers is due to their unique properties, namely particle size, shape, crystal structure, surface effect, magnetic, catalytic, optical, as well as chemical and mechanical characteristics from their bulk counterpart [1,2]. Until now, different multifunctional metals and metal-oxide nanoparticles have been synthesized [3,4]. Among the different nanoparticles(NPs), NiONPs have gained the specific attention of biologists and chemists due to their numerous applications in battery electrodes, magnetic materials, heterogeneous catalysts, gas sensors, electrochromic films, and solid-oxide fuel cells and help in the adsorption of inorganic pollutants and dyes [5,6]. Further, NiONPs have shown significant antibacterial, antifungal, antioxidants, anti-inflammatory, anticancer, and enzyme inhibition potentials [6,7]. NiONPs have shown toxicity towards different microbial agents and microalgae by producing ROS, inducing oxidative stress and releasing (Ni^{2+}) inside the cell [8].

Currently, NiONPs are fabricated via different physical and chemical approaches. However, these synthesis routes face several challenges as they utilize costly metal salts, organic solvents, toxic reducing agents (sodium borohydrides, hydrazine hydrate, sodium citrate and Gallic acid), stabilizing and capping agents (thiols, amines, sodium citrate), and demand expensive equipment. These approaches are not only expensive at the industrial scale, but also cause some undesired effects on human life and the surrounding environment, and may result in cytotoxicity, carcinogenicity, and genotoxicity, thus restricting their utilization in biomedical purposes [9]. Hence, these problems must be solved, and actions are required to develop an alternative solution for the fabrication of NPs.

Therefore, scientists have developed green chemistry methods which are more sustainable, cleaner and eco-friendly. Presently, new developments have been made in the synthesis of nanomaterials using different biological sources (microbes, algae, fungi, various lower and higher plants). This method is relatively simple, ecofriendly, energy-efficient, nontoxic, eliminates the need for high energy, temperature, and pressure and needs no reducing, stabilizing, and capping agents from outside. The major disadvantages associated with microbial synthesis is the maintenance of an aseptic environment, culturing in media, high isolation cost, high incubation time, difficulty in handling, pathogenicity in nature, and the requirement of comprehensive biological knowledge [10].

Phytofabrication has flourished for the formation of several nanomaterials and has attracted the attention of the nano task force due to its sample, environmentally benign, and cost-effective nature [11–14]. In green synthesis, phytoconstituents (alkaloids, terpenoids, polyphenols, glycosides, flavanoids, proteins, vitamins, polysaccharides) function as a capping and reducing agent like different chemical substitutes used in the chemical synthesis of nanoparticles [15,16]. There are multiple factors that influences green synthesis of nanoparticles, such as nature of plant extracts, concentration of extracts, metal salt, pH, and synthesis protocol used. Thus, for the green synthesis of MNPs, 12 basic principles of green chemistry are now becoming a reference guideline for researchers, chemical technologists, and chemists worldwide to develop less dangerous chemical products and byproducts [17–19]. Therefore, green nanotechnology is an alternate route for the formation of safe and stable materials using different medicinal plants and thus has experienced for rapid rise [20–23].

In the present study, fresh leaves extract of *R. triquetra* were used to synthesize NiONPs. The plant is found in abundance in Pakistan (Kashmir, Margalla Hills), Nepal, and India during the summer season between July and August. The bark, leaves, and fruits of *R. triquetra* are used to treat hemorrhagic septicemia in livestock, intestinal worms, and malarial fevers, possessing significant antimicrobial, deobstruent, anti-inflammatory, astringent, and antioxidant properties. This plant contains several ecofriendly phytoconstituents such as emodin, Kaempferol-7-O-CH$_3$ ether, Kaempferol-4-O-CH$_3$ ether, gluside, quercetins, and physcion [24,25] which help in the phytofabrication of NiONPs. As per the available literature and knowledge, this is perhaps the first study reported on the green synthesis of NiONPs employing *R. triquetra* leaves broth. NiONPs were characterized using different characterization techniques. Further, considering biological and therapeutic potential of *R. triquetra*-NiONPs, different biological activities; anticancer, antimicrobial, antileishmanial, antioxidant, and enzyme inhibitory assays were performed.

2. Material and Methods

2.1. Preparation of R. Triquetra Leaf Extract

The preparation of *R. triquetra* leaves extract was achieved using previously optimized protocol [26]. Precisely, *R. triquetra* leaves were collected from Pir Suhawa Margalla hills Pakistan (33.7870° N, 73.1084° E). The sample was identified by senior taxonomist Dr. Syed Afzal Shah, Department of Plant Sciences, QAU Islamabad, Pakistan. The leaves were thoroughly washed with running tap water followed by washing with distill water. The leaves were shade dried and crushed into fine powder. Then, twenty gram leaves powder was added into 100 mL distill water and heated at 80 °C for 1 h. The resultant extract was filtered three time using Whattman filter paper No.1 (cone shaped), centrifuged at 5000 rpm for 20 min to remove all unwanted aggregates. Finally, the plant extract was stored at 4 °C till further use.

2.2. Green Fabrication of NiONPs

Synthesis of NiONPs was performed by reducing nickel nitrate using *R. triquetra* leaf extract. To achieve this purpose, 100 mL filtered RT leaves extract was steadily mixed with 1 gm NiNO$_3$ salt followed by continuous heating (70 °C) and stirring at 500 rpm for 2 h to achieve homogeneous solution. Further, obtained solution was centrifuged at 4000 rpm/20 min. Supernatant was discarded and pellet containing NiONPs was carefully washed 3 times with distilled water to remove uncoordinated materials. The obtained powder assumed as NiONPs was incubated at ~100 °C until the water evaporated completely, followed by annealing. Further, NiONPs were stored in cool, dry, and dark place. Finally, NiONPs were thoroughly characterized. Figure 1 shows a schematic representation of the synthesis, characterization, and biological application of NiONPs.

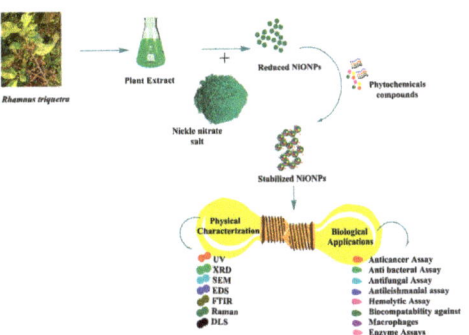

Figure 1. General overview of the study plan.

2.3. Physical Characterizations of NiONPs

The physicochemical properties of RT-NiONPs were investigated using different analytical techniques. The optical properties and bioreduction of nickel ions to NiONPs was confirmed by measuring the absorption spectra of reaction solution using a UV-spectrophotometer, and the solution was scanned between 200 and 600 nm. DLS analyses has provided further insight into the average hydro-dynamic particles diameter (d. nm), ζ-potential and PDI of NiONPs using Malvern Zetasizer Nano (Malvern instrument). RT-NiONPs were analyzed by Fourier transform infrared (FT-IR) spectroscopy to detect different bioactive functional groups responsible for the synthesis and stabilizing NiONPs using various modes of vibrations. FT-IR measurement of the sample was scanned in the wavenumber region 500 cm^{-1} to 4000 cm^{-1}. The structural analysis and crystalline nature of biogenic NiONPs was carried out using XRD analysis (PANalytical XRD (Netherland). The nano-crystallite size was calculated from the width of the XRD peaks using Debye-Scherrer's equation. The vibrational characteristics of RT-NiONPs were studied using Raman spectroscopy. The elements of NiONPs were detected by EDX (energy dispersive X-ray). The morphological features (surface topology) of R. triquetra-NiONPs was studied using SEM (EM (NOVA FEISEM-450 applied with EDX detectors). In addition, the morphological structure and actual particle size was studied under TEM (transmission electron microscopy).

2.4. Antileishmanial Potentials (ALP)

The in vitro antileishmanial potential of NiONPs was investigated using MTT cytotoxicity assay [7]. To confirm the antileishmanicidal potential, *Leishmania tropica* "KWH23 strain" (promastigote and amastigotes parasites) was cultured in MI-99 media containing 10% FBS. The 200 µL reaction mixture is comprised of 100 µL of standardized culture, fresh media (50 µL) and colloidal nanoparticles (50 µL) suspension. Amphoterecin B served as positive while DMSO function as negative control. The leishmanial parasites *L. tropica* were kept in 96-well plate and were treated with different concentration of NiONPs (1100–8.595 µg/mL) to determine their antileishmanial potency. The test sample (NiONPs) was incubated in 5% CO2 incubator at 24 °C/72 h. After treatment and incubation with NiONPs, the reaction mixture was scanned at 540nm using micro-plate analyzer and readings were taken. Both parasites were counted and IC_{50} values were calculated to determine intensity/degree of antileishmanicidal potential using formula below:

$$\%\text{inhibition} = \frac{1 - \text{sample absorbance}}{\text{absorbance of control}} \times 100 \qquad (1)$$

2.5. Anticancer Activity

The in vitro anticancer potential of *R. triquetra* mediated NiONPs was investigated using HepG2 and HuH7 cancer cell lines using an MTT assay [27]. The cancer cells were cultured in flasks containing DMEM media supplemented with 10% FBS, Pen-Strep and kept in 5% CO2 incubator for 24 h/37 °C. The confluent HepG2 and HuH7 cancer cells (4000 cells/well) were carefully seeded in 96-well plate. Further, cells were treated with varying doses of RT-NiONPs (1100–8.595 µg/mL) for 48 h. DMEM media was removed and MTT solution (100 µL) was added in each well followed by further incubation (3 h in 5% CO2 incubator/37 °C). The DMEM media containing other components (FBS, Pen-Strep) was removed and DMSO (100 µL) was loaded in each well followed by incubation for ~20–30 min. The conversion of MTT solution to formazan by living cells was measured using micro plate analyzer 570 nm wavelength. The untreated cancer cells were considered as control and % inhibition of HepG2 and HuH7 cell lines exposed to different concentration of NiONPs was calculated:

$$\%\text{inhibition} = \frac{1 - \text{OD of sample}}{\text{OD of control}} \times 100 \qquad (2)$$

2.6. Biocompatibility with Human Erythrocytes (RBCs) and Macrophages

To determine the non-toxic nature of NiONPs, hemolysis assay was done using erythrocytes cells as discussed in the previously published article [28]. To achieve this purpose, 1 mL freshly isolated human red cells was placed in an Ethylenediaminetetraacetic Acid (EDTA) tube to avoid blood coagulation. Further, erythrocytes were centrifuged at 12,000 rpm/10 min. After centrifugation, supernatant was discarded, and pellet was rinsed three times with PBS. Erythrocytes suspension was made adding 200 µL erythrocytes into 9.8 mL PBS. Further, erythrocytes suspension (100 µL) was treated with various concentration of NiONPs and reaction mixture was incubated at 36 °C for 1 h followed by centrifugation (12,000 rpm/15 min). Supernatant was transferred into 96-well-plate and release of hemoglobin was studied at wavelength (540 nm) using micro-plate analyzer. Triton X-100 was used as positive and DMSO as negative control respectively. The data obtained was calculated as % hemolysis caused by different doses of NiONPs using formula below:

$$\% \text{ hemolysis} = \frac{\text{Sample abs} - \text{Negative control abs}}{\text{Positive control abs} - \text{Negative control abs}} \times 100 \quad (3)$$

The biosafe nature of RT-NiONPs was further confirmed using human macrophages (HM) following previously used protocol [14]. To confirm the biosafe nature, HM cells were culture in flasks containing RPMI media provided with 10% FBS, Hepes, Pen-Strep (antibiotic). For the proper growth and attachment of cells, flasks containing macrophages were transferred in 5% CO_2 incubator for 24 h. After culturing, macrophages (4000 cells/well) were loaded into 96-well-plate. After incubation, macrophages were treated with varying doses of NiONPs (1100–8.595 µg/mL). Finally, the % inhibition of HM cells treated with different doses of RT-NiONPs was calculated using the formula below:

$$\% \text{ inhibition} = \frac{1 - \text{Absorbance of sample}}{\text{Absorbance of control}} \times 100 \quad (4)$$

2.7. Antioxidant Activities

Spectrophotometric procedures were used to confirm the antiradical potentials of RT-NiONPs using Total antioxidant capacity (TAC), CUPARAC, DPPH, and total reducing power (TRP). Total antioxidant capacity (TAC) was determined through the phosphomollybdenum method [29]. The incubation of RT-NiONPs with Molybdenum (VI) demonstrated the presence of antioxidants which were assessed by measuring absorbance at 695 nm. For this purpose, ascorbic acid was used as a positive control and DMSO was taken as negative control. Further, the cupric-ion assay (CUPRAC) was investigated for greenly orchestrated NiONPs [30] and the absorbance of solutions was taken at 515 nm using spectrophotometer. Moreover, the total reducing power (TRP) of greenly prepared NiONPs was studied using potassium ferricyanide method [31]. This method is based on the principle that reductones having reduction potential will reduce potassium ferricyanide (Fe^{3+}) to form potassium ferrocyanide (Fe^{2+}). When potassium ferrocyanide (Fe^{2+}) reacts with $FeCl_3$, it forms Fe^{+2}-Fe^{+3} complex that has maximum absorption at 700 nm. The reducing power of RT-NiONPs was recorded as AAEq/mg. Further, the antioxidant scavenging potential of RT-NiONPs was evaluated. To investigate this potential, 2.4 mg DPPH was mixed with methanol (25 mL) to create a free radical environment. Further, various concentrations (1100–8.595 µg/mL) of NiONPs were prepared in DMSO and studied for their DPPH free-radical scavenging potential. The existence of reductones were determined by measuring maximum absorbance of reaction mixture at 517 nm using microplate analyzer.

$$\% \text{ DPPH scavenging} = 1 - \left(\frac{\text{Absorbance of sample}}{\text{Absorbance of control}}\right) \times 100 \quad (5)$$

2.8. Enzymes Inhibition Potentials

Proteins kinase (PK) inhibition potential of *R. triquetra* synthesized NiONPs was demonstrated using actinobacterium (*Streptomyces* 85E) [32]. To confirm the PK inhibition potential, SP4 minimal media was used to acquire uniform bacterial lawns. Briefly, 100 µL inoculum was taken from standard culture and was equally spread on petri plate to achieve uniform lawns. A sterilized filter disc (6 mm) loaded with various doses of RT-NiONPs were placed on *Streptomyces* 85E painted plate. The surfactin was used as positive and DMSO as negative control. Further, petri plates were incubated (30 °C/72 h) to determine the PK inhibition potential against *Streptomyces* 85E. After incubation, different clear and bald zones were appeared. These different zones determined inhibition potentials of spores/mycelia formation in *Streptomyces* 85E strain. Finally, ZIs were measured in millimeter to determine the PK inhibition potential of RT-NiONPs.

Further, antidiabetic potency of greenly orchestrated RT-NiONPs was studied using alpha amylase (AA) inhibition assay [33]. The reaction mixture was prepared by adding starch solution (45 µL), NiONPs (15 µL), AA enzyme (30 µL), and FBS (20 µL). Further, HCL (25 µL) and iodine solutions (95 µL) were added and incubated at 50 °C for 30 min. Acarbose was used as positive and distill water as negative control respectively. The micro-plate analyzer was used to calculate the optical density at 540 nm and IC_{50} value was recorded. The % inhibition was recorded utilizing below formula:

$$\% \text{ inhibition} = \frac{S(ab) - NC(ab)}{Blank\ (ab) - NC(ab)} \times 100 \qquad (6)$$

2.9. Antifungal Activity

The disc-diffusion method (DDM) was used to study the antifungal potencies of RT-NiONPs using various fungal strains (*A. flavus, M. racemosus, C. albicans, A. niger, F. solani*). Fungal strains were cultured in flasks holding fungal growth media (sabouraud dextrose liquid media) (SDL) and kept in shaking incubator (37 °C/24 h). The SDL media were prepared, autoclaved, and poured in autoclaved petri plates to achieve antifungal activity. Further, 50 µL broth culture was spread on petri plate using autoclaved cotton swab to achieve uniform lawns. Filter discs (~6 mm) loaded with different concentrations (1100–34.38 µg/mL) of RT-NiONPs were kept on media plates. To compare the antifungal potential of RT-NiONPs, Amp B was taken as positive, and DMSO as negative control. Further, fungal plates were placed in an incubator for (24 h/37 °C) and zones of inhibition (ZIs) were observed with time intervals and MICs values were calculated.

2.10. Antibacterial Activity

To further evaluate the antimicrobial potential of RT-NiONPs, in vitro antibacterial potency was investigated using different bacterial strains, namely *P. aeruginosa, B. subtilis, S. aureus, K. pneumoniae,* and *E. coli*. Before antibacterial activity was investigated, bacterial cultures were refreshed in nutrient media and kept in shaking incubator at 37 °C (200 rpm /24 h). Further, bacterial strains were spread on media plates using sterilized cotton swabs. The DDM method was used to confirm the bactericidal potentials. For this purpose, 6 mm (filter disc) loaded with different concentration of RT-NiONPs (1100–34.38 µg/mL) were kept on bacterial lawns. Further, 10 µL of oxytetracycline loaded filter discs were used as positive control for five different bacterial strains. After loading test samples and positive control, petri plates were kept in incubator at 37 °C/24 h and observed after time intervals for ZIs. Finally, MICs were calculated to study the bactericidal potentials of RT-NiONPs.

3. Results and Discussion

The earlier research studies have confirmed the presence of different functional biomolecules such as emodin, Kaempferols-7-O-CH$_3$ ether, Kaempferols-4-O-CH$_3$ ether), gluside, quercetins, and physcion [24,25]. These biomolecules can act as a base source, bioreductant, stabilizers, and capping agents for the convenient synthesis of NiONPs. Previously, NiONPs have been fabricated using a variety of natural plants with potential medicinal values [26]. In the current study, NiONPs has been orchestrated using *R. triquetra* leaf extract via green method. The visual colour change from brown to greenish black revealed the formation of NiONPs. The photo-spectrometric analyses of NiONPs showed broad spectra at 333 nm (λmax), indicating the formation of NiONPs and validating optical observation. The UV visible spectra of green NiONPs are illustrated in Figure 2A. Elemental mapping and atomic content were confirmed using EDS analyses. Figure 2B shows EDS peak indicating strong signals at 0.94, 7.08, an 8.12 KeV for the presence of both nickel and oxygen. The presence of carbon in the spectra is ascribed to grid support. Moreover, no other peak for any elements apart from nickel 'Ni' and oxygen 'O' have been found, indicating the phase purity of greenly synthesized NiONPs.

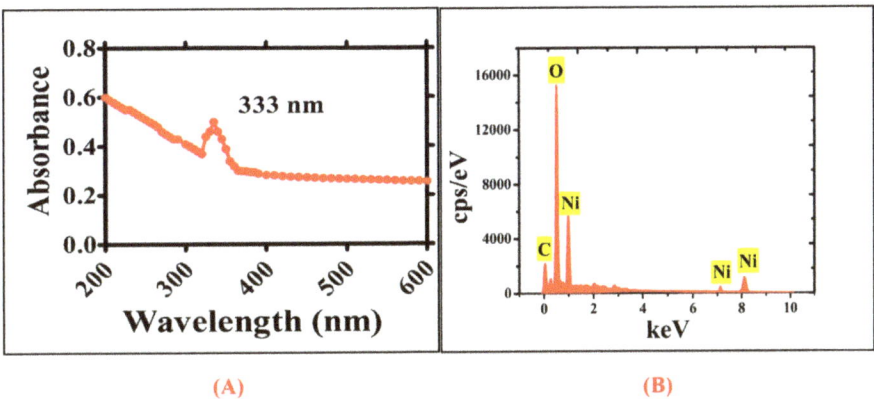

Figure 2. UV visible spectra and EDS analysis for RT. NiONPs (**A**) UV visible spectra for NiONPs (**B**) Elemental composition of NiONPs using EDS analysis.

The hydrodynamic size and stability of RT-NiONPs were demonstrated by DLS and Zeta potential analysis. Zeta-potential or electro-kinetic potential refers to the measure of an effective surface functionality and surface charge on nanoparticle. The magnitude of zeta potential confers to particle stability. Nanoparticles with a high zeta potential exhibit increased stability, i.e., the dispersion or solution will resist the aggregation and agglomeration of nanoparticles. In our research study, data revealed a particle size of 65 nm, zeta-potential of −11 mV, and PDI of 1.000 (Figure 3A,B). Our DLS results are in agreement with previous studies using *Rhamnus virgata* mediated NiONPs [26]. DLS is mostly investigated to confirm the size of nanoscale particles in different suspensions. The mean hydro-dynamic particles diameter (d. nm) in aqueous medium show particles aggregation [11,20,34].

Raman spectral study was further used to analyze the vibrational modes of *R. triquetra* mediated NiONPs. Raman spectra in Figure 4A revealed the positioning of major modes at 358.38 (1 Phonon), 559.57 (1 Phonon), 697.34 (2 Phonon), 1106.18 (2 Phonon), and 1646.51 cm^{-1} (2 Magnon). The intense peaks concluded that the greenly orchestrated nanoparticles are defect rich. The broad peak attributes to the antiferromagnetic behaviour and is related to the spin of individual Ni++. This antiparallel spin behaviour of 'Ni++' also signifies that NiONPs are nano-size in nature (crystal size: ~25 nm). Raman shifts revealed purity and correspond to earlier research studies using *S. thea* and *G. wallichianum* orchestrated NiONPs [7,35]. The difference in Raman scattering peaks might be due to the relative positions, size, intensity and effects of stress and strain [36]. Further, FT-IR analysis was performed to determine the qualitative distribution of functional groups adsorbed on the surface of NiONPs. The infrared absorption bands in Figure 4B revealed significant vibrations at 545.17 cm^{-1} and 657.43 cm^{-1} (Ni-O vibrations in stretching mode), 1025.26 cm^{-1} (Ethers = C-O-C symmetric stretching), 1729.59 cm^{-1} (Aldehyde group of carbonyl '-CHO'), and 3579.43 cm^{-1} (alcohols and phenols of OH stretching). According to previously reported research work, IR bands between 470 and 800 cm^{-1} indicate Ni-O vibrations in the stretching mode [37,38].

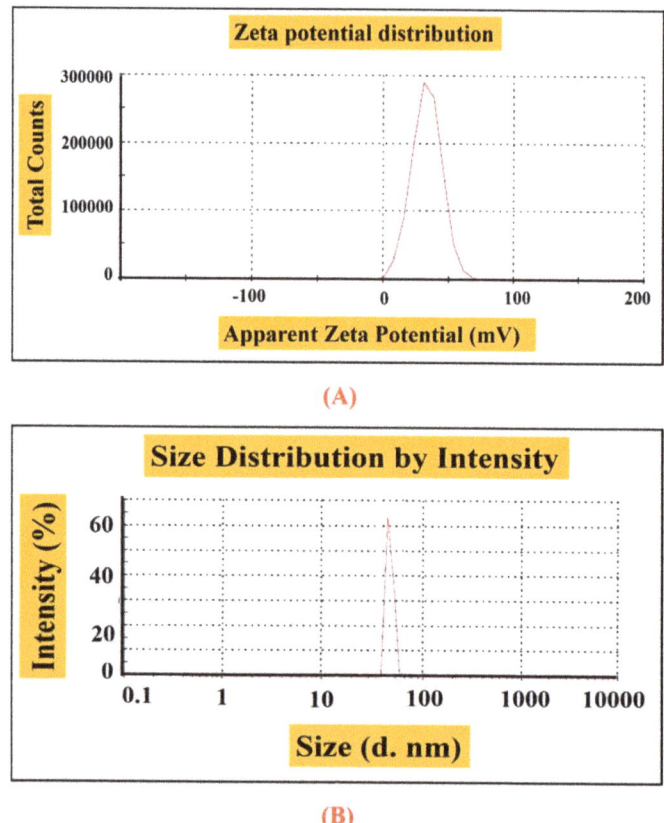

Figure 3. (**A**) Zeta potential of NiONPs (**B**) Size distribution of RT-NiONPs.

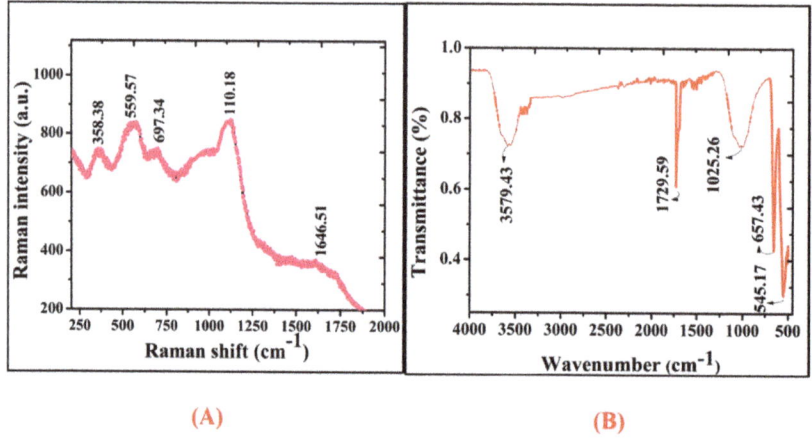

Figure 4. (**A**) Raman spectra of NiONPs (**B**) FT-IR spectra of biogenic NiONPs.

In addition, SEM analysis was performed to know the shape and surface morphology of greenly fabricated NiONPs. Figure 5A,B depicts SEM images of NiONPs confirming the spherical/agglomerated shape of NiONPs. The crystallographic structure and accurate particle size of the biogenic NiONPs were studied by TEM analysis (Figure 5C).

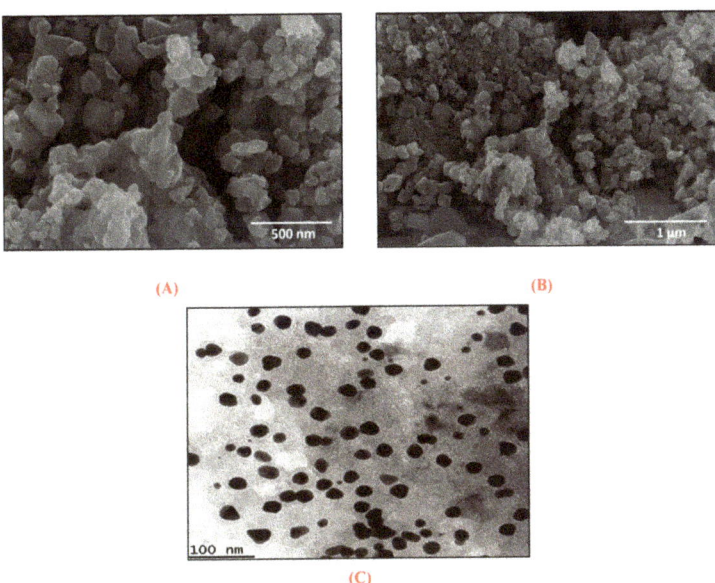

Figure 5. (**A**,**B**) Various SEM images of RT-NiONPs using nickel nitrate salt as a precursor (**C**) TEM images of RT- NiONPs.

Moreover, phase structure of NiONPs was assessed by XRD analyses. The XRD pattern of the synthesized NiONPs and miller indexation have been illustrated in Figure 6A,B, which indicates the diffraction bands at 36.52 (101), 43.44 (012), 63.11 (110), 76.28 (113), and 79.2 (202), corresponding to fcc symmetry in NiONPs crystalline lattice. Previously, Khalil et al. [35] and Iqbal et al. [26] have synthesized biogenic NiONPs from *Sageretia thea* and *Rhamnus virgata* leaf extracts and reported similar results.

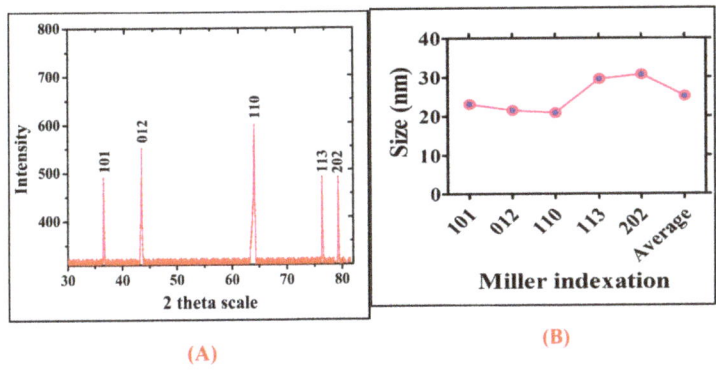

Figure 6. (**A**) XRD Spectra of the RT-NiONPs (**B**) Size calculation and Miller indexation.

3.1. Antimicrobial Potentials

The antibacterial activities of NiONPs were demonstrated against different bacterial strains (*E. coli, P. aeruginosa, B. subtilis, K. pneumoniae, S. aureus*) in concentrations ranging from 34.38 to 1100 µg/mL. Most of the BSs were found susceptible using NiONPs and have shown significant antibacterial activities. Different MIC values were calculated for different bacterial strains *P. aeruginosa* (275 µg/mL), *K. pneumoniae* (137.5 µg/mL), *E. coli* (68.75 µg/mL), and *S. aureus* and *B. subtilis* (34.38 µg/mL). *S. aureus* and *B. subtilis* were found to be the most susceptible strains with MIC: 34.38 µg/mL while *P. aeruginosa* was found to be the least susceptible strain (MIC: 275 µg/mL), as shown in Figure 7A. Oxytetracyclines was taken as positive control and no single concentration of NiONPs determined a stronger potential than Oxytetracyclines. Overall, NiONPs have determined significant antibacterial activities which are in agreement with previous studies of greenly orchestrated NiONPs using *G. wallichianum* and *R. virgata* [7,26]. The strong bactericidal potency of NiONPs might be due to biomolecules adsorbed on NPs surface. In conclusion, RT-NiONPs have shown dose-dependent results. Some studies have explained that the bactericidal potential of NPs is due to ROS generation. Further, NPs damage membrane (membrane proteins) and result in bacterial cell death. Similarly, surface defects in the symmetry of NPs is responsible for the inhibition of bacteria and result in cell damage [39].

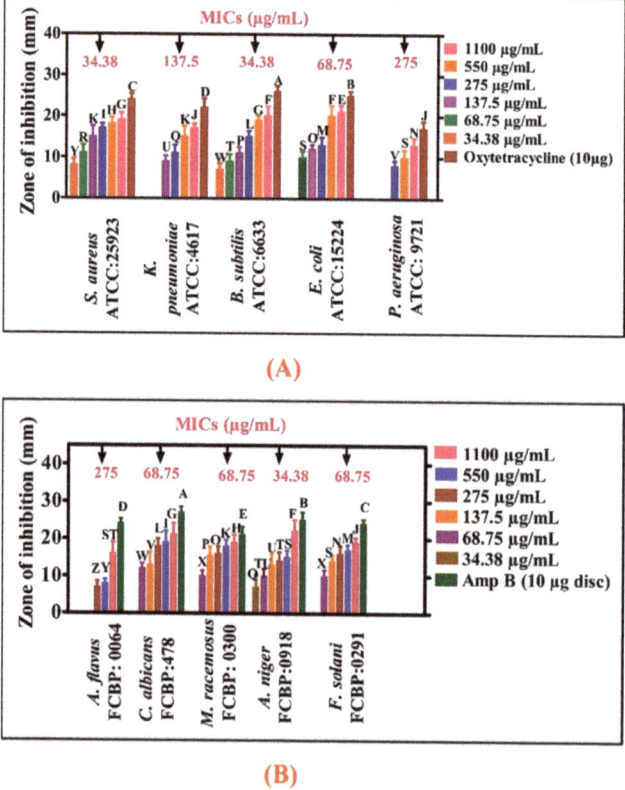

Figure 7. (**A**) Various antimicrobial activities of RT mediated NiONPs. Data represents the mean of three replicates and each alphabet indicates significance at $p < 0.05$ (**A**) MICs values of RT-NiONPs against various pathogenic bacterial strains (**B**) Antifungal potencies of RT-NiONPs against different fungal strains.

Numerous research studies have been conducted on the bactericidal potential of NiONPs while only limited research work has been published on fungicidal activities of NPs. In the present study, the fungicidal potency of RT-NiONPs was investigated using different fungal strains (FS). The different FS such as *F. solani, M. racemosus, A. niger, A. flavus* and *C. albicans* were exposed to different concentration of RT-NiONPs (34.38–1100 μg/mL) (Figure 7B). Amp-B was taken as positive control to confirm the inhibition potential of RT-NiONPs. According to our literature review, the current study, for the first time, reported the antifungal potential of RT-NiONPs. Our *R. triquetra*-NiONPs revealed a concentration-dependent inhibition response against different fungal strains where *A. flavus* was the least susceptible fungal strain (MIC: 275 μg/mL while *A. niger* was the most susceptible strain (MIC: 34.38 μg/mL). Previously, concentration mediated fungicidal activities were reported using different fungal strains [7] and are in line with our presently synthesized RT-NiONPs. The MIC values for different pathogenic bacterial and fungal strains are provided in Figure 7.

3.2. Antileishmanial Potentials

Leishmaniasis is a widespread tropical disease caused by leishmanial parasites [27]. The drug antimonial was developed as a potential candidate to cure leishmaniasis but has lost its therapeutic potential as they have developed resistance. Thus, scientists are involved in designing alternative routes to fight and manage this global disease. Therefore, extensive research studies are needed to design some novel and effective nanomaterials. Various nanomaterials are being used to study their antileishmanial potential [11,14]. However, greenly orchestrated NiONPs are rarely studied to investigate their cytotoxic potential. In current study, antileishmanial potentials of *R. triquetra* orchestrated NiONPs was investigated against *L. tropica*. The parasites were treated with different doses of RT-NiONPs (8.595–1100 μg/mL) (Figure 8A). The antileishmanial potential increased with RT-NiONPs, thus indicating a dose-dependent response. The RT-NiONPs displayed significant potential against *L. tropica* promastigote (IC$_{50}$: 27.32 μg/mL). Similarly, the antileishmanial potential of RT-NiONPs was reported against *L. tropica* amastigotes (IC$_{50}$: 37.4 μg/mL). Our results of RT-NiONPs are in agreement with the previous reports of *Sageretia thea* mediated NiONPs [35].

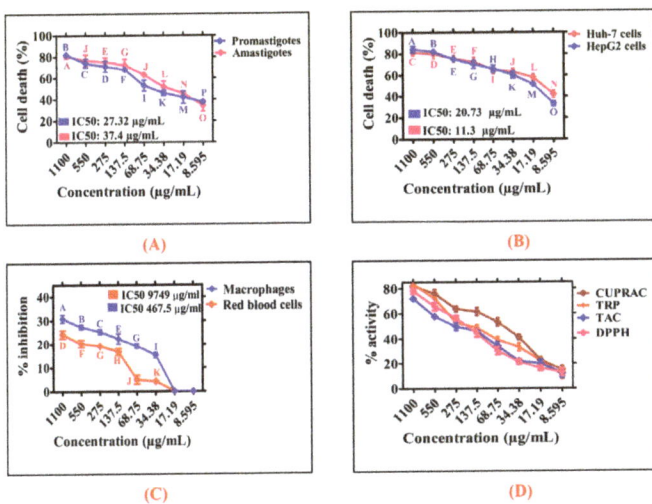

Figure 8. Biocompatibility, cytotoxic and antioxidant properties of NiONPs. Data represents the mean of three replicates and each alphabet indicates significance at $p < 0.05$ (**A**) Antileishmanial activities against Leishmanial parasites (**B**) Anticancer potentials of RT-NiONPs against HUH-7 and HepG2 cell lines (**C**) Biocompatibility of NiONPs against RBCs and Macrophages (**D**) Antioxidant activities of RT-NiONPs.

3.3. Anticancer Potential of NiONPs

Among the different types of cancer, liver cancer is the second deadliest cancer in males and sixth deadliest in females [15,40,41]. Different risk factors are involved in regulating the rate of cancer such as viral infections, heavy consumption of alcohol and toxin exposures (aflatoxin). In the current study, the anticancer potential of greenly orchestrated RT-NiONPs was investigated against HUH-7 and HepG2 liver cancer cell lines using an MTT assay [28]. To achieve this purpose, HUH-7 and HepG2 cancer cells were exposed to different concentrations of RT-NiONPs (1100–8.595 µg/mL) as summarized in Figure 8B. The NiONPs have determined strong reduction in metabolic activities of both HUH-7 and HepG2 cancer cells using different doses of NiONPs. The metabolic activities were decreasing while increasing RT-NiONPs concentration. The highest anticancer activity recorded was 81.41% for HuH-7 and 84.41% for HepG2 at 1100 µg/mL and anticancer activity decreased with NiONPs concentration. Further, IC_{50} values were recorded for RT-NiONPs which are 11.3 µg/mL for (HuH-7) and 20.73 µg/mL (HepG2) cell lines respectively. The anticancer potential induced by RT-NiONPs even at low concentration (8.595 µg/mL) could be due to different functional molecules adsorbed from leaves broth on the surface of NiONPs. The reduction in the metabolic activities have determined that RT-NiONPs have strong anticancer activities. The results of RT-NiONPs using HUH-7 and HepG2 are in correspondence with the previously published reports using *G. wallichianum* and *Euphorbia heterophylla* [7,42].

3.4. Biocompatibility Assays with Human Red Cells and Macrophages

Considering the interest in biomedical applications, the biosafety and biocompatible nature of RT-NiONPs were investigated using previously optimized protocol [7]. According to biosafety principle guidelines, biological and chemical substances having hemolysis >5% are hemolytic, 2–5% are slightly hemolytic, while <2% is non-hemolytic [43]. If the tested NPs are hemolytic, it will damage erythrocytes and result in hemoglobin release from RBCs. To confirm the hemolytic potential, red cells were treated with different doses of RT-NiONPs (1100–8.595 µg/mL) and revealed dose dependent response. The hemoglobin release was 24.23% at highest concentrations of 1100 µg/mL (Figure 8C). Research studies concluded that RT-NiONPs are non-hemolytic at 17.19 µg/mL, slightly hemolytic at 68.75 µg/mL, and hemolytic at >68.75 µg/mL. On the whole, RT-NiONPs are non-toxic and biocompatible at low concentration against red cells. Our biocompatibility results of RT-NiONPs are in line with the previously synthesized *S. thea* and *G. wallichianum* mediated NiONPs [7,35].

The biosafe and biocompatible nature of RT-NiONPs was further determine using normal human macrophages (HM). For this purpose, confluent HM cells were seeded in sterilized 96-well plate containing RPMI media and were cultured for 24 h. Further, the seeded cells were exposed to different doses of RT-NiONPs (1100–8.595 µg/mL). Further, an MTT cell viability assay was performed to confirm the biosafe nature of RT-NiONPs. The results shown in Figure 8C indicate that biosynthesized RT-NiONPs at 1100 µg/mL inhibited the growth of HM cells by ~30.89% confirming its biosafe nature, thus indicating a dose-dependent response. Normally, HM cells have developed a natural strategy to neutralize ROS produced from external sources. Previous research studies reported that ROS are non-toxic to both red cells and HM cells at low concentrations unless concentrations increase beyond the limit, which will result in toxicity to both erythrocytes and macrophages [44]. Previously, Iqbal et al. [26] reported the biocompatibility potential of greenly fabricated NiONPs against HM cells using *Rhamnus virgata*.

3.5. Antioxidant Activities

The antioxidant potential of phytogenic NiONPs was evaluated (Figure 8D). The maximum value for TAC of *R. triquetra* mediated NiONPs in terms of AA Emg^{-1} was reported as 71.93% at 1100 µg/mL. Generally, a TAC assay is performed to evaluate the scavenging potential of reductones/antioxidants present in the test sample towards ROS species. Our TAC results are in correspondence to

Abbasi et al. [7] using *Geranium wallichianum* mediated NiONPs. Further, a cupric-ion assay was investigated to assess the scavenging potentials of antioxidants species adsorbed on the surface of RT-NiONPs. The maximum score for cupric ion assay of green RT-NiONPs was obtained as 81.83%. According to our literature review, a cupric-ion assay was demonstrated for the first time on RT-NiONPs. Moreover, greenly orchestrated NiONPs were further explored to determine the surface adsorbed antioxidant molecules. To achieve this goal, TRP assay was performed. The maximum value for TRP was recorded as 83.41% at 1100 µg/mL which is corroborated with the earlier research report using *Rhamnus virgata* mediated NiONPs [26]. Further, DPPH free radical scavenging assay was demonstrated to assess the presence of radical scavengers (antioxidants) adsorbed on the surface of greenly fabricated NiONPs. The highest DPPH value reported is 77.91% and our DPPH data are in agreement with the previous studies using *Sageretia thea* mediated NiONPs [35]. Together, the antioxidant potential confirmed the presence of radical scavengers on RT-NiONPs which play a potential role in the stabilization, reduction, and capping of nano nickel oxide particles [7].

3.6. Enzymes Inhibition Potentials

Greenly orchestrated RT-NiONPs were examined for their protein kinase (PKs) inhibition activity. Figure 9A shows the significant PK inhibition potential of *R. triquetra* mediated NiONPs using different doses of NiONPs (34.38–1100 µg/mL). Moderate PK inhibition potential was revealed for RT-NiONPs. The maximum value for ZIs was 15.5 mm with $IC_{50} > 1000$ µg/mL. On the whole, ZIs obtained for greenly orchestrated NiONPs were smaller as obtained from surfactin (positive control). These results suggested cell viability at lower concentrations of NiONPs, consistent with a previous research report using *G. wallichianum*–NiONPs [7]. Further, A-amylase assay was demonstrated to evaluate the inhibition potentials of *R. triquetra*-NiONPs using different concentrations (1100–34.38 µg/mL). The biogenic NiONPs were observed to cause increased % inhibition (39.31%) at 1100 µg/mL (Figure 9B). However, the percent inhibition significantly decreased with a decrease in concentration. Overall, a moderate inhibition potential is reported. The results of our current report are in agreement with a previous research study using *S. thea* mediated NiONPs [35].

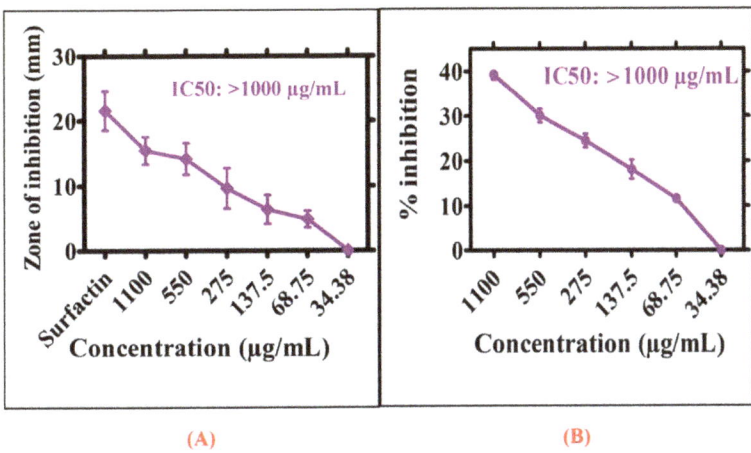

Figure 9. (A) Inhibition potential against protein kinase of RT orchestrated NiONPs (B) Inhibition potential against alpha amylase.

4. Conclusions and Future Directions

This study has established a simple, eco-friendly, and economically viable method to synthesize NiONPs simply by mixing NiNO3 with aqueous broth of *R. triquetra* leaves which are free of toxicants and rich in functional biomolecules. The actions of different functional biomolecules in the leaves extract may result in the reduction, stabilization, and capping of NiONPs. The microscopic analyses from SEM and TEM confirmed the predominant spherical shape and small size of NiONPs (~25 nm). Further, spectroscopic studies from UV–vis, Raman, FT-IR, EDX, zeta potential, and DLS supported the fabrication and stability of NiONPs. Significant anticancer potentials were revealed against different cancer cell lines (HepG2: IC$_{50}$: 20.73 and HuH-7: IC$_{50}$: 11.3 µg/mL). Further, antileishmanial potential was investigated against leishmanial parasites (promastigotes; IC$_{50}$: 27.32, amastigotes: IC$_{50}$: 37.4 µg/mL). The outcomes of a biocompatibility assay revealed that NiONPs are non-toxic and biocompatible. NiONPs determined significant free radical scavenging and moderate enzyme inhibition activities. Further, NiONPs determined significant antimicrobial studies against different bacterial and fungal strains. In conclusion, our results unequivocally indicate that RT-NiONPs may be used as a safer alternative in biotechnological, biomedical, and pharmaceutical industries. Further, more in vitro and in vivo studies are recommended in different animal models before bringing NiONPs into clinical trials.

Author Contributions: J.I., B.A.A., designed and performed the experiments at Quaid-i-Azam University Islamabad, Pakistan. R.A., and M.M., analyzed the data. A.M., S.A.Z., A.S., M.S., S.K., S.U. draft, revised and improved the manuscript. T.M., and R.C. supervised the study. All authors have read and agreed to the published version of the manuscript.

Funding: This research received no external funding.

Conflicts of Interest: The authors declare no conflict of interest.

References

1. Rashmi, B.; Harlapur, S.F.; Avinash, B.; Ravikumar, C.R.; Nagaswarupa, H.; Kumar, M.A.; Gurushantha, K.; Santosh, M.S. Facile green synthesis of silver oxide nanoparticles and their electrochemical, photocatalytic and biological studies. *Inorg. Chem. Commun.* **2020**, *111*, 107580. [CrossRef]
2. Munir, A.; Haq, T.U.; Hussain, I.; Qurashi, A.; Ullah, U.; Iqbal, M.J.; Hussain, I. Ultrasmall Co@Co(OH)2 Nanoclusters Embedded in N-Enriched Mesoporous Carbon Networks as Efficient Electrocatalysts for Water Oxidation. *ChemSusChem* **2019**, *12*, 5117–5125. [CrossRef] [PubMed]
3. Iqbal, J.; Abbasi, B.A.; Ahmad, R.; Mahmood, T.; Ali, B.; Khalil, A.T.; Kanwal, S.; Shah, A.; Alam, M.M.; Badshah, H.; et al. Nanomedicines for developing cancer nanotherapeutics: From benchtop to bedside and beyond. *Appl. Microbiol. Biotechnol.* **2018**, *102*, 9449–9470. [CrossRef] [PubMed]
4. Hameed, S.; Iqbal, J.; Ali, M.; Khalil, A.T.; Abbasi, B.A.; Numan, M.; Shinwari, Z.K. Green synthesis of zinc nanoparticles through plant extracts: Establishing a novel era in cancer theranostics. *Mater. Res. Express* **2019**, *6*, 102005. [CrossRef]
5. Pandian, C.J.; Palanivel, R.; Dhananasekaran, S. Green synthesis of nickel nanoparticles using Ocimum sanctum and their application in dye and pollutant adsorption. *Chin. J. Chem. Eng.* **2015**, *23*, 1307–1315. [CrossRef]
6. Ezhilarasi, A.A.; Vijaya, J.J.; Kaviyarasu, K.; Maaza, M.; Ayeshamariam, A.; Kennedy, L.J. Green synthesis of NiO nanoparticles using Moringa oleifera extract and their biomedical applications: Cytotoxicity effect of nanoparticles against HT-29 cancer cells. *J. Photochem. Photobiol. B Boil.* **2016**, *164*, 352–360. [CrossRef]
7. Abbasi, B.A.; Iqbal, J.; Mahmood, T.; Ahmad, R.; Kanwal, S.; Afridi, S. Plant-mediated synthesis of nickel oxide nanoparticles (NiO) via Geranium wallichianum: Characterization and different biological applications. *Mater. Res. Express* **2019**, *6*, 0850a7. [CrossRef]
8. Gong, N.; Shao, K.; Feng, W.; Lin, Z.; Liang, C.; Sun, Y. Biotoxicity of nickel oxide nanoparticles and bio-remediation by microalgae Chlorella vulgaris. *Chemosphere* **2011**, *83*, 510–516. [CrossRef]
9. Anastas, P.T.; Eghbali, N. Green Chemistry: Principles and Practice. *Chem. Soc. Rev.* **2010**, *39*, 301–312. [CrossRef]
10. Mohamed, H.E.A.; Afridi, S.; Khalil, A.T.; Zia, D.; Iqbal, J.; Ullah, I.; Shinwari, Z.K.; Maaza, M. Biosynthesis of silver nanoparticles from Hyphaene thebaica fruits and their in vitro pharmacognostic potential. *Mater. Res. Express* **2019**, *6*, 1050c9. [CrossRef]

11. Abbasi, B.A.; Iqbal, J.; Mahmood, T.; Qyyum, A.; Kanwal, S. Biofabrication of iron oxide nanoparticles by leaf extract of Rhamnus virgata: Characterization and evaluation of cytotoxic, antimicrobial and antioxidant potentials. *Appl. Organomet. Chem.* **2019**, *33*, e4947. [CrossRef]
12. Abbasi, B.A.; Iqbal, J.; Ahmad, R.; Zia, L.; Kanwal, S.; Mahmood, T.; Wang, C.; Chen, J.-T. Bioactivities of Geranium wallichianum Leaf Extracts Conjugated with Zinc Oxide Nanoparticles. *Biomolecules* **2019**, *10*, 38. [CrossRef] [PubMed]
13. Hameed, S.; Khalil, A.T.; Ali, M.; Numan, M.; Khamlich, S.; Shinwari, Z.K.; Maaza, M. Greener synthesis of ZnO and Ag–ZnO nanoparticles using Silybum marianum for diverse biomedical applications. *Nanomedicine* **2019**, *14*, 655–673. [CrossRef] [PubMed]
14. Lingamdinne, L.P.; Chang, Y.-Y.; Yang, J.-K.; Singh, J.; Choi, E.H.; Shiratani, M.; Koduru, J.R.; Attri, P. Biogenic reductive preparation of magnetic inverse spinel iron oxide nanoparticles for the adsorption removal of heavy metals. *Chem. Eng. J.* **2017**, *307*, 74–84. [CrossRef]
15. Iqbal, J.; Abbasi, B.A.; Batool, R.; Khalil, A.T.; Hameed, S.; Kanwal, S.; Ullah, I.; Mahmood, T. Biogenic synthesis of green and cost effective cobalt oxide nanoparticles using Geranium wallichianum leaves extract and evaluation of in vitro antioxidant, antimicrobial, cytotoxic and enzyme inhibition properties. *Mater. Res. Express* **2019**, *6*, 115407. [CrossRef]
16. Hussain, I.; Singh, N.B.; Singh, A.; Singh, N.B.; Singh, S.C. Green synthesis of nanoparticles and its potential application. *Biotechnol. Lett.* **2015**, *38*, 545–560. [CrossRef]
17. Gupta, M.; Paul, S.; Gupta, R. General aspects of 12 basic principles of green chemistry with applications. *Curr. Sci.* **2010**, *1*, 1341–1360.
18. Kharissova, O.V.; Dias, H.V.R.; Kharisov, B.I.; Pérez, B.O.; Jiménez-Pérez, V.M. The greener synthesis of nanoparticles. *Trends Biotechnol.* **2013**, *31*, 240–248. [CrossRef] [PubMed]
19. Narayanan, K.B.; Sakthivel, N. Synthesis and characterization of nano-gold composite using Cylindrocladium floridanum and its heterogeneous catalysis in the degradation of 4-nitrophenol. *J. Hazard. Mater.* **2011**, *189*, 519–525. [CrossRef]
20. Iqbal, J.; Abbasi, B.A.; Mahmood, T.; Kanwal, S.; Ahmad, R.; Ashraf, M. Plant-extract mediated green approach for the synthesis of ZnONPs: Characterization and evaluation of cytotoxic, antimicrobial and antioxidant potentials. *J. Mol. Struct.* **2019**, *1189*, 315–327. [CrossRef]
21. Wardani, M.; Yulizar, Y.; Abdullah, I.; Apriandanu, D.O.B. Synthesis of NiO nanoparticles via green route using Ageratum conyzoides L. leaf extract and their catalytic activity. *IOP Conf. Ser. Mater. Sci. Eng.* **2019**, *509*, 012077. [CrossRef]
22. Sharma, J.; Srivastava, P.; Singh, G.; Akhtar, M.S.; Ameen, S. Biosynthesized NiO nanoparticles: Potential catalyst for ammonium perchlorate and composite solid propellants. *Ceram. Int.* **2015**, *41*, 1573–1578. [CrossRef]
23. Sulaiman, N.; Yulizar, Y. Spectroscopic, Structural, and Morphology of Nickel Oxide Nanoparticles Prepared Using Physalis angulata Leaf Extract. *Mater. Sci. Forum* **2018**, *917*, 167–171. [CrossRef]
24. Ram, S.N.; Pandey, V.B.; Dwivedi, S.P.D.; Goel, R.K. Further constituents of Rhamnus triquetra and CNS activity of emodin. *Fitoterapia* **1994**, *65*, 275–278.
25. Mazhar, F.; Jahangir, M.; Abbasi, M.A.; Rehman, A.-U.; Ilyas, S.A.; Khalid, F.; Khanum, R.; Jamil, S.; Kausar, S.; Ajaib, M. Rhamnus triquetra: A Valuable Source of Natural Antioxidants to Shield from Oxidative Stress. *Asian J. Chem.* **2013**, *25*, 8569–8573. [CrossRef]
26. Iqbal, J.; Abbasi, B.A.; Mahmood, T.; Hameed, S.; Munir, A.; Kanwal, S. Green synthesis and characterizations of Nickel oxide nanoparticles using leaf extract of Rhamnus virgata and their potential biological applications. *Appl. Organomet. Chem.* **2019**, *33*, e4950. [CrossRef]
27. Iqbal, J.; Abbasi, B.A.; Ahmad, R.; Shahbaz, A.; Zahra, S.A.; Kanwal, S.; Munir, A.; Rabbani, A.; Mahmood, T. Biogenic synthesis of green and cost effective iron nanoparticles and evaluation of their potential biomedical properties. *J. Mol. Struct.* **2020**, *1199*, 126979. [CrossRef]
28. Iqbal, J.; Abbasi, B.A.; Munir, A.; Uddin, S.; Kanwal, S.; Mahmood, T. Facile green synthesis approach for the production of chromium oxide nanoparticles and their different in vitro biological activities. *Microsc. Res. Tech.* **2020**, 1–30. [CrossRef]
29. Özyürek, M.; Güngör, N.; Baki, S.; Güçlü, K.; Apak, R. Development of a Silver Nanoparticle-Based Method for the Antioxidant Capacity Measurement of Polyphenols. *Anal. Chem.* **2012**, *84*, 8052–8059. [CrossRef]

30. Apak, R.; Güçlü, K.; Özyürek, M.; Karademir, S.E. Novel Total Antioxidant Capacity Index for Dietary Polyphenols and Vitamins C and E, Using Their Cupric Ion Reducing Capability in the Presence of Neocuproine: CUPRAC Method. *J. Agric. Food Chem.* **2004**, *52*, 7970–7981. [CrossRef]
31. Ul-Haq, I.; Ullah, N.; Bibi, G.; Kanwal, S.; Ahmad, M.S.; Mirza, B. Antioxidant and Cytotoxic Activities and Phytochemical Analysis of Euphorbia wallichii Root Extract and its Fractions. *Iran. J. Pharm. Res. IJPR* **2012**, *11*, 241–249. [PubMed]
32. Zia, M.; Gul, S.; Akhtar, J.; Ul Haq, I.; Abbasi, B.H.; Hussain, A.; Naz, S.; Chaudhary, M.F. Green synthesis of silver nanoparticles from grape and tomato juices and evaluation of biological activities. *IET Nanobiotechnol.* **2017**, *11*, 193–199. [CrossRef] [PubMed]
33. Nithiya, S.; Sangeetha, R. Amylase inhibitory potential of silver nanoparticles biosynthesized using Breynia retusa leaf extract. *World J. Pharm. Res.* **2014**, *3*, 1055–1066.
34. Sudhasree, S.; Banu, A.S.; Brindha, P.; Kurian, G.A. Synthesis of nickel nanoparticles by chemical and green route and their comparison in respect to biological effect and toxicity. *Toxicol. Environ. Chem.* **2014**, *96*, 743–754. [CrossRef]
35. Khalil, A.T.; Ovais‡, M.; Ullah, I.; Ali, M.; Shinwari, Z.K.; Hassan, D.; Maaza, M. Sageretia thea (Osbeck.) modulated biosynthesis of NiO nanoparticles and their in vitro pharmacognostic, antioxidant and cytotoxic potential. *Artif. Cells Nanomed. Biotechnol.* **2017**, *46*, 838–852. [CrossRef]
36. Burmistrov, I.; Agarkov, D.; Tartakovskii, I.; Kharton, V.; Bredikhin, S. Performance Optimization of Cermet SOFC Anodes: An Evaluation of Nanostructured NiO. *ECS Meet. Abstr.* **2015**, *68*, 1265–1274. [CrossRef]
37. Rahdar, A.; Aliahmad, M.; Azizi, Y. NiO nanoparticles: Synthesis and Characterization. *J. Nanostruct.* **2015**, *7*, 145–151.
38. Qiao, H.; Wei, Z.; Yang, H.; Zhu, L.; Yan, X. Preparation and Characterization of NiO Nanoparticles by Anodic Arc Plasma Method. *J. Nanomater.* **2009**, *2009*, 1–5. [CrossRef]
39. Li, Y.; Zhang, W.; Niu, J.; Chen, Y. Mechanism of Photogenerated Reactive Oxygen Species and Correlation with the Antibacterial Properties of Engineered Metal-Oxide Nanoparticles. *ACS Nano* **2012**, *6*, 5164–5173. [CrossRef]
40. Iqbal, J.; Mahmood, T.; Abbasi, B.; Khalil, A.; Ali, B.; Kanwal, S.; Shah, A.; Ahmad, R. Role of dietary phytochemicals in modulation of miRNA expression: Natural swords combating breast cancer. *Asian Pac. J. Trop. Med.* **2018**, *11*, 501. [CrossRef]
41. Iqbal, J.; Abbasi, B.A.; Ahmad, R.; Batool, R.; Mahmood, T.; Ali, B.; Khalil, A.T.; Kanwal, S.; Shah, A.; Alam, M.M.; et al. Potential phytochemicals in the fight against skin cancer: Current landscape and future perspectives. *Biomed. Pharmacother.* **2019**, *109*, 1381–1393. [CrossRef] [PubMed]
42. Lingaraju, K.; Naika, H.R.; Nagabhushana, H.; Jayanna, K.; Devaraja, S.; Nagaraju, G. Biosynthesis of Nickel oxide Nanoparticles from Euphorbia heterophylla (L.) and their biological application. *Arab. J. Chem.* **2020**, *13*, 4712–4719. [CrossRef]
43. Dobrovolskaia, M.A.; Clogston, J.D.; Neun, B.W.; Hall, J.B.; Patri, A.K.; McNeil, S.E. Method for Analysis of Nanoparticle Hemolytic Properties in Vitro. *Nano Lett.* **2008**, *8*, 2180–2187. [CrossRef] [PubMed]
44. Prach, M.; Stone, V.; Proudfoot, L. Zinc oxide nanoparticles and monocytes: Impact of size, charge and solubility on activation status. *Toxicol. Appl. Pharmacol.* **2013**, *266*, 19–26. [CrossRef] [PubMed]

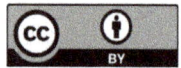

© 2020 by the authors. Licensee MDPI, Basel, Switzerland. This article is an open access article distributed under the terms and conditions of the Creative Commons Attribution (CC BY) license (http://creativecommons.org/licenses/by/4.0/).

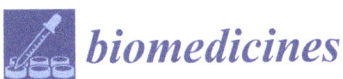

Review

Trametes versicolor (Synn. *Coriolus versicolor*) Polysaccharides in Cancer Therapy: Targets and Efficacy

Solomon Habtemariam

Pharmacognosy Research Laboratories & Herbal Analysis Services UK, University of Greenwich, Chatham-Maritime, Kent ME4 4TB, UK; s.habtemariam@herbalanalysis.co.uk; Tel.: +44-208-331-8302

Received: 5 May 2020; Accepted: 21 May 2020; Published: 25 May 2020

Abstract: *Coriolus versicolor* (L.) Quél. is a higher fungi or mushroom which is now known by its accepted scientific name as *Trametes versicolor* (L.) Lloyd (family Polyporaceae). The polysaccharides, primarily two commercial products from China and Japan as PSP and PSK, respectively, have been claimed to serve as adjuvant therapy for cancer. In this paper, research advances in this field, including direct cytotoxicity in cancer cells and immunostimulatory effects, are scrutinised at three levels: in vitro, in vivo and clinical outcomes. The level of activity in the various cancers, key targets (both in cancer and immune cells) and pharmacological efficacies are discussed.

Keywords: *Coriolus versicolor*; *Trametes*; cancer; polysaccharides; PSP; PSK; immunostimulation; adjuvant therapy

1. Introduction

According to the recent WHO figure [1], cancer is the second most leading cause of mortality in the world and accounts for an estimated 9.6 million deaths in 2018. Most of the cancer death (~70%) occur in developing or the so-called low- and middle-income countries where access to modern medicines are not widely available. The common cancer deaths are from the lung, colorectal, stomach, liver and breast cancers, respectively, while other common cancers include prostate and skin cancers [1]. The major control measure for cancer is chemotherapy by using a variety of small molecular weight compounds and biological agents. As always, nature has its fair share of abundance as a source of these agents and drugs like paclitaxel (Taxol®), podophyllotoxin derivatives and vinca alkaloids (vinblastine and vincristine) are our excellent examples for potential exploration of more novel anti-cancer agents from higher plants. On the other hand, doxorubicin, daunomycin, mitomycin C, and bleomycin are good representative examples of anti-cancer agents explored from fungal sources, particularly *Streptomyces*.

In addition to their nutritional value, medicinal mushrooms have emerged in recent years not only as a source of drugs but also as adjuvants to conventional chemo- or radiation-therapy to either enhance their potency or reduce their side effects (see [2] and references therein). In this regard, one of by far the best investigated medicinal mushroom in recent years is *Coriolus versicolor* (L.) Quél. (Syn. *Polyporus versicolor*) which is now known by its accepted scientific name as *Trametes versicolor* (L.) Lloyd (family Polyporaceae). Its most common name in the Western world is Turkey Tail, and its distinct morphological features include the concentric multicoloured zones on the upper side of the cap (no stalk) and spore-bearing polypores underside (Figure 1). The fungus is common in temperate Asia, North America and Europe, including the UK, where it has been recorded in all regions [3]. Its medicinal value as part of the Chinese traditional medicine dates back for at least 2000 years and includes general health-promoting effects [4], including endurance and longevity. Both in China and Japan, preparations such as dried powdered tea of the fungus are employed in traditional medicine practices. In this communication, the main components of the fungi, polysaccharides, that have given the fungi its medicinal value in cancer therapy are assessed by reviewing the chemistry, pharmacology and therapeutic potential at three levels: in vitro, in vivo and clinical studies. Readers should note that nearly all the published literature in this field is available under the name *Coriolus versicolor* (*Trametes versicolor*).

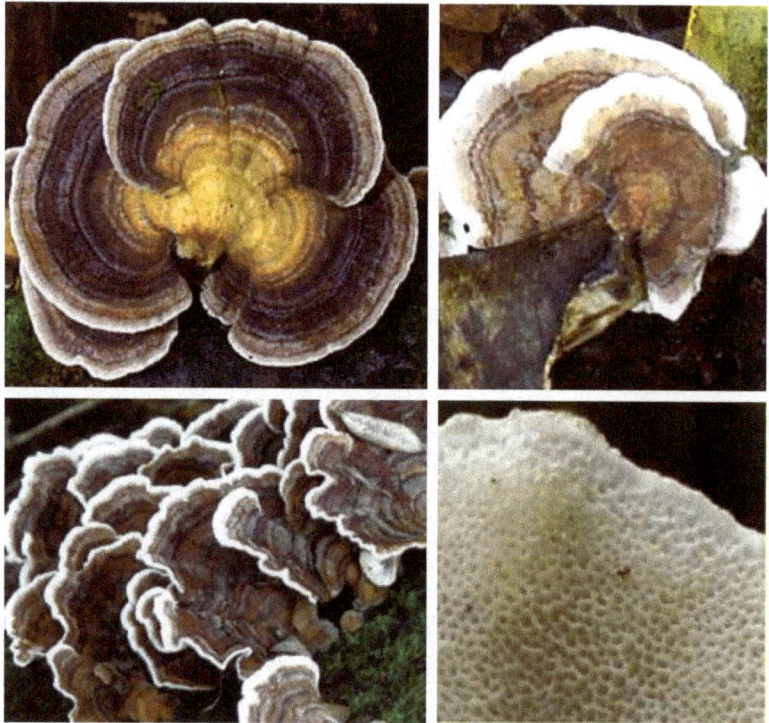

Figure 1. Morphological features of *Coriolus versicolor*. The various morphological features of the fungus grown in the UK are shown. While the upper surface shows concentric zones of colours (red, yellow, green, blue, brown, black, and white), the picture in the lower-right shows the polyporous nature of the underside portion of the fungus. Pictures are a kind gift of *first-nature.com* (https://www.first-nature.com/fungi/trametes-versicolor.php#distribution).

2. Overview of Chemistry

2.1. Small Molecular Weight Compounds

Like all other mushrooms, the fruiting body of *C. versicolor* is harvested for its nutritional and medicinal values. The bracket or shelf mushroom body in the wild or the mycelial biomass collected from the submerged fermentation could all be used for this purpose. In addition to the major macromolecules (proteins, carbohydrates, and lipids) and minerals, the fungus is known to contain potential pharmacologically active secondary metabolites belonging to small molecular weight compounds. The study by Wang et al. [5] reported the isolation of four new spiroaxane sesquiterpenes (Figure 2), tramspiroins A–D (1–4), one new rosenonolactone 15,16-acetonide (5), and the known drimane sesquiterpenes isodrimenediol (6) and funatrol D (7) from the cultures. Readers should bear in mind that these compounds isolated from the ethyl acetate fraction are non-polar and are not expected to be available in the polysaccharide fractions of the fungus (see below). Janjušević et al. [6] studied the phenolic composition of the fruiting body of *C. versicolor* of European origin. In their HPLC–MS/MS-based study, they identified 38 phenolic compounds belonging to the flavonoid (flavones, flavonols, flavanone, flavanols, biflavonoids, isoflavonoids) and hydroxy cinnamic acids. Although the ethanol and methanol extracts are generally the richest sources of these phenolic compounds, the water extracts were also shown to contain (μg/g dry weight) considerable amount of baicalein (21.60), baicalin (10.7), quercetin (31.20), isorhamnetin (14.60), catechin (17.20), amentoflavone (17.20), *p*-hydroxybenzoic acid (141.00) and cyclohexanecarboxylic acid (80.40). The biological activities of the water extracts of *C. versicolor*, especially in the antioxidant area, must, therefore, account for the cumulative effects of the phenolic compounds. These compounds are, however, not established as the main components of the fungus, and further research is required to establish their potential contribution to the known biological activities of *C. versicolor*.

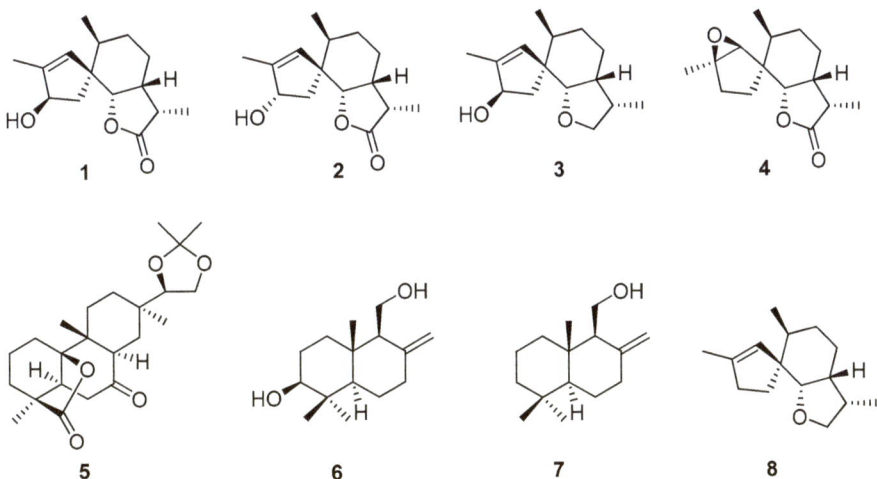

Figure 2. Terpenoids from *C. versicolor*.

2.2. Polysaccharides

Like other edible mushrooms, the fruiting body of *C. versicolor* is composed of carbohydrates, proteins, amino acids, and minerals. The main bioactive components of *C. versicolor* are the polysaccharopeptides (PSPs), which are isolated from the mycelium as well as fermentation broth. As a commercial product, the main sources of these PSPs are China and Japan that produce them from the strains of "COV-1" (PSP in China) and "CM-101" (polysaccharide K (PSP Krestin or PSK, in Japan), respectively. Both products have been approved as medicines primarily as adjuvants in cancer therapy. Given that over 100 strains of the fungi are known to occur, one must recognise the diversity of these products coming from different genetic and environmental sources, including the in vitro culture conditions of their mycelial production. They are made from polysaccharides covalently bonded to peptides through *O*- or *N*-glycosidic bonds. Numerous studies have established that D-glucose is the principal monosaccharide of PSP and PSK, although other sugars such as arabinose and rhamnose are also found in small amounts (e.g., [6–8]). One noticeable difference in these products could be the composition of polysaccharide:peptide ratio, and their relative molecular weight. The (PSK and PSP) are both proteoglucans of about 100 kDa with variations in the individual sugar compositions such as glucose, fucose, galactose, mannose, and xylose.

The distinction between the extracellular (EPS) and intracellular polysaccharides have also been made with respect to their backbone structure [7,8]. The EPS contains small amounts of galactose (Gal), mannose (Man), arabinose (Ara), xylose (Xyl) and predominantly glucose (Glc) and are composed of β-(1→3) and β-(1→6)-linked D-glucose molecules. On the other hand, PSP and PSK contain α-(1→4) and β-(1→3) glucosidic linkages in their polysaccharide moieties. D-glucose is the major monosaccharide present while fucose (Fru), Gal, Man, and Xyl are the other principal monosaccharides in PSK. Earlier studies [9] established the distinctive features of these two polysaccharides with the presence of fucose in the PSK and rhamnose and arabinose in PSP. Analysis of the polysaccharide moiety of PSP, showed the predominance of 1→4, 1→2 and 1→3 glucose linkages (molar ratio 3:1:2), together with small amounts of 1→3, 1→4 and 1→6 Gal, 1→3 and 1→6 Man, and 1→3 and 1→4 Ara linkages [9]. On the other hand, the peptide moiety of PSP contains 18 different amino acids, with aspartic and glutamic acid residues being most predominant [8]. More importantly, PSK and PSP polymers are soluble in water.

The complexity of *C. versicolor* can be seen from the detailed structural analysis, as shown for PSP-1b1 backbone by Wang et al. [10] as follows: "→4)-α-Gal$p$-(1→4)-α-Gal$p$-(1→2)-α-Man$p$-(1→4)-α-Gal$p$-(1→2)-α-Man$p$-(1→4)-α-Gal$p$-(1→4)-α-Gal$p$-(1→2)-α-Man$p$-(1→4)-α-Gal$p$-(1→2)-α-Man$p$-(1→4)→, with branches of α-1,6-Man$p$, β-1,6-Glc$p$, β-1,3,6-Glc$p$, α-1,3-Man$p$, α-1,6-Gal$p$, α-1,3-Fuc$p$, T-α-Glc$p$ and T-α-Gal$p$ on the O-6 position of α-Man$p$ of the main chain, and secondary branches linked to the O-6 position of β-Glc$p$ (β-glucose-pyranose(p)) of the major branch." Awadasseid et al. [11] also isolated a water-soluble glucan extracted from *C. versicolor* called CVG with the general backbone structure of [→6)−α−D−Glc$p$−(1→] n. In comparison to the PSK and PSP, CVG was small with a molecular weight of 8.8 Kda and carbohydrate composition of D-Fuc, D-Ara, D-Man, D-Gal and D-Glc, in a molar ratio of 1.0/1.1/3.0/3.9/350.7, respectively. The polysaccharide isolated by Zhang et al. [12] called β-1→3 was with the main chain consisting of β -D-1,4-Glc and β-D-1,3-Glc, and branch chains situated at β-D-1,3,6-Glc and β-D-1,4,6-Glc. More research is, however, required to identify the structures of all polysaccharides from this fungus.

3. Anticancer Effect through Direct Toxicity to Cancer Cells

Studies during the 1990s established that *C. versicolor* polysaccharides such as PSK could inhibit hepatic carcinogenesis in rats induced by 3'-methyl-4-dimethylaminoazobenzene [13]. The direct effect of PSK on gene expression profile in cancer cells was also established back in the 1980s [14]. Studies on combination therapy with radiation further showed the increased survival rate of mice bearing MM46 tumours [15]. Corriolan as a β-(1→3) polysaccharide with some (1→6) and no (1→4) branched glucan from *C. versicolor* was shown to be effective (100 mg/kg for 30 days) in suppressing sarcoma 180 tumours in mice [16]. Since then, the direct anticancer effect of *C. versicolor* polysaccharides has been demonstrated in the various experimental models in vitro, in vivo and clinical trials (see below).

3.1. Evidence of Efficacy through In Vitro Studies

The direct toxicity of *C. versicolor* polysaccharide preparations to cancer/tumour cells has been demonstrated in the various in vitro models [17–49] (Table 1). The number of cancer types that could be targeted by the polysaccharides is incredibly large and include breast (e.g., MCF-7, HBL-100, T-47D, ZR-75-30, MDA-MB-231 and Walker 256) [18,20,32,37,44,46], lung (e.g., A-549, and SWi573) [20,21], melanoma (e.g., SKMel-188 and B16) [17,31], colon (e.g., LoVo, HT-29, SW480, WiDr, LS174 and LS174-T) [19–26,48], leukaemia (e.g., Jukart, K562, THP-1, OCI-AML3, HL-60 and U937) [20,22,24–26,28, 30,35,36,38–40,48,49], cervix (e.g., HeLa [20,21], gastric cancer (e.g., AGS, KATOIII, SCG-7901 [24–26,48]), prostate (e.g., PC-3, JCA-1, LNCaP, DU-145 [29,43], glioma (e.g., C6) [42], hepatoma (e.g., HepG2) [45,48], and ovarian (e.g., H4-II-E) [47] cancers. The vast majority of studies are on the two known commercially available *C. versicolor* polysaccharides, PSP and PSK (Table 1), while others include small polypeptide of about 10 Kd [48], refined polysaccharide peptide fractions [23,45], and aqueous or alcoholic extract [19–21,31,35,37,41,43]. Given the high molecular weight nature of the polysaccharides and even most are crude products, their observed anticancer activity mostly demonstrated in less than 1 mg/mL concentrations should be considered good but many experiments even showed activity at concentrations less or equal to 100 µg/mL [17,19,24–26,28,32,36,38,41,46,48]. The inhibition of cell proliferation by *C. versicolor* is associated with cell cycle arrest which could vary depending on the concentration and cell type. For example, disruption of cell cycle progression and arrest at G0 phase [22],

G0/G1 phase [31,33] or G1/S and G2/M phases [36] have been reported. As a mode of cell death, induction of apoptosis has been shown for many cell types which was associated with caspase-3 activation via the mitochondrial pathway [24–26,28,36,39].

Table 1. Direct cytotoxic effects in vitro.

Preparation	Experimental Model	Key Findings	References
Protein-bound polysaccharides	Human SKMel-188 melanoma cells—100 and 200 µg/mL	Induces caspase-independent cytotoxicity; increases the intracellular level of ROS—effect inhibited by SP600125 (JNK inhibitor); cytotoxic effect abolished by receptor-interacting serine/threonine-protein kinase 1 inhibitor.	Pawlikowska et al. 2020 [17]
Immobilised fungal laccase on pH-responsive (and charge-switchable) Pluronic-stabilised silver nanoparticles (AgNPs^{Trp})	MCF-7 breast cancer cells	Inhibits cell proliferation through β-estradiol degradation and cell apoptosis; decreases in the mRNA levels of anti-apoptotic genes (BCL-2 and NF-kβ); increases the mRNA level of proapoptotic genes (p53).	Chauhan et al. 2019 [18]
Polysaccharide-rich extracts	Human colon carcinoma LoVo and HT-29 cells—proliferation; wound healing and invasion assays—10 or 100 µg/mL	Inhibits human colon cell proliferation and induces cytotoxicity; inhibits oncogenic potential, cell migration and invasion in colon cancer cells; suppresses MMP-2 enzyme activity; increases the expression of the E-cadherin.	Roca-Lema et al. 2019 [19]
Water extracts from mycelial biomass (strain It-1)—Russian origin—water and methanol extracts	Leukemia cell lines (Jukart, K562, and THP-1); solid tumors (A-549 and SWi573 (lung), HBL-100 and T-47D (breast), HeLa (cervix), and WiDr (colon)) cells—50 µg/mL	IC$_{50}$ between 0.7–3.6 µg/mL—antiproliferative effect against lung and cervix tumors.	Shnyreva et al. 2018 [20]
Dried mycelia of Serbian origin—96% ethanol extract	Human cervix adenocarcinoma (HeLa), human colon carcinoma (LS174) and human lung adenocarcinoma (A549) cell lines	Cytotoxic activity with IC$_{50}$ value between 60–90 µg/mL.	Knezevic et al. 2018 [21]
Polysaccharidic fraction, Tramesan (Patent number RM2012A000573)—extracted exopolysaccharide from fungal culture filtrate	Leukemic cell lines (human myeloid (OCI-AML3) and lymphoid (Jurkat) cell lines) and primary cells from AML patients—0.5–2 mg/mL	No cytotoxic effect on mononuclear cells from healthy donors; dose-dependent increase in G0 phase of cancer cells; decreases in both G1 and S phases; time- and dose-dependent induction of apoptosis in cancer cells	Ricciardi et al. 2017 [22]
Aqueous extract	Mouse mammary carcinoma 4T1 cells—0.125–2 mg/mL	No direct toxicity but inhibits cell migration and invasion; suppresses enzyme activities and protein levels of MMP-9	Luo et al. 2014 [23]

Table 1. Cont.

Preparation	Experimental Model	Key Findings	References
PSK	Human malignant cell lines (WiDr, HT29, SW480, KATOIII, AGS, HL-60 and U937)—30–100 µg/mL	Antiproliferative—most potent against HL-60 cells; activates caspase-3 and induces p38 MAPK phosphorylation; co-treatment with SB203580 (A p38 MAPK inhibitor) blocked apoptosis induction, caspase-3 activation and growth inhibition; apoptosis induction via mitochondrial pathway (effect on mitochondrial depolarization reversed by SB203580).	Hirahara et al. 2011, 2012, 2013 [24–26]
Ethanolic extracts	Human promyelocytic HL-60 cells	Suppresses cell growth; induces apoptosis; downregulates the phosphorylation of Rb; increases PARP cleavage; better effect in combination with *Ganoderma lucidum*.	Hsieh et al. 2013 [27]
PSK	HL-60 cells—100 µg/mL	Induces apoptosis without inducing cell differentiation; induces p38 MAPK phosphorylation; effect on induction of apoptosis, caspase-3 activation and growth inhibition abolished by SB203580 (p38 MAPK inhibitor).	Wang et al. 2012 [28]
PSP—Commercial source	Prostate cancer cell line PC-3—250 or 500 µg/mL	Suppresses PC-3 cell growth and in spheroid formation assay; see Table 2 for in vivo effect.	Luk et al. 2011 [29]
Polysaccharopeptide (PSP)—Commercial source—Winsor Health Products Ltd, Hong Kong	HL-60–25 µg/mL	Reduces cell proliferation; inhibits cell progression through both S and G2 phase; reduces ^{3}H-thymidine uptake and prolonged DNA synthesis time; enhances the cytotoxicity of camptothecin; no effect on normal human peripheral blood mononuclear cells.	Wan et al. 2010 [30]
Methanol extract of fruiting body of Serbian origin	B16 mouse melanoma cells—200 µg/mL	Induces cell cycle arrest in the G0/G1 phase, followed by both apoptotic and secondary necrotic cell death; see Table 2 for in vivo effect.	Harhaji et al. 2008 [31]
PSP	Human breast cancer (ZR-75-30) cells—50 µg/mL or with 5 µM of doxorubicin, etoposide or cytarabine	Enhances the cytotoxicity of doxorubicin and etoposide but not cytarabine; effect associated with S-phase trap; reduces the ratio of protein expression of Bcl-xL/Bax.	Wan et al. 2008 [32]
PSK	B16, A549, Hela, AGS, Jurkat, B9 and Ando-2 tumour cell lines—50 or 100 µg/mL	Inhibits cell growth; induces cell cycle arrest, with cell accumulation in G0/G1 phase; induces apoptosis and increases caspase-3 expression.	Jimenez-Medina et al. 2008 [33]

Table 1. Cont.

Preparation	Experimental Model	Key Findings	References
PSP	HepG2 cells	Non-toxic dose of PSP enhanced the cytotoxicity of cyclophosphamide; decreased cell viability by 22% at 10 µg/mL	Chan and Yeung 2006 [34]
Standardised aqueous ethanol extract	HL-60 cells	Suppresses cell proliferation in a dose-dependent manner (IC_{50} = 150.6 µg/mL); increases nucleosome production from apoptotic cells; increases Bax and downregulates Bcl-2 or increases Bax/Bcl-2 proteins ratio; increases the release of cytochrome-c from mitochondria to cytosol; other effects, see Table 2	Ho et al. 2006 [35]
PSP	Human leukemia HL-60 and U-937 cells—0.1–1 mg/mL	Inhibits cell proliferation and induces apoptosis; cell type-dependent disruption of the G1/S and G2/M phases of cell cycle progression; more cytotoxic to HL-60 cells; suppresses the expression of bcl-2 and survivin while increasing Bax and cytochrome-c; enhances cleavage of PARP from its native 112-kDa form to the 89-kDa truncated product; decreases in p65 and to a lesser degree p50 forms of NF-κB; reduces the expression of COX-2.	Hsieh et al. 2006 [36]
Standardised aqueous ethanol extract—commercial source, Hong Kong	MDA-MB-231, MCF-7 and T-47D cells—400 or 600 µg/mL	Suppresses cell proliferation—IC_{50} values in ascending order of T-47D, MCF-7, MDA-MB-231, and BT-20 least affected; increases nucleosome productions in apoptotic cells; downregulates Bcl-2 protein expression (MCF-7 and T-47D cells, but not in MDA-MB-231 cells); upregulates p53 protein only in T-47D cells	Ho et al. 2005 [37]
Polysaccharide peptide (PSP)	Human promyelocytic leukemia HL-60 cells—25–100 µg/mL	Dose-dependently enhances cell apoptosis induced by doxorubicin and etoposide, but not cytarabine (Ara-C); enhances the apoptotic machinery of Doxo and VP-16 in a cell cycle-dependent manner; modulates the regulatory checkpoint cyclin E and caspase 3.	Hui et al. 2005 [38]
Polysaccharide peptide (PSP)	HL-60 cells	Induces apoptosis HL-60 cells but not of normal human T-lymphocytes; decrease in Bcl-2/Bax ratio, drop in mitochondrial transmembrane potential, cytochrome c release, and activation of caspase −3, −8 and −9	Yang et al. 2005 [39]

Table 1. Cont.

Preparation	Experimental Model	Key Findings	References
Proteins and peptide bound polysaccharides (PSP)	HL-60 cells—400 µg/mL	Induces apoptosis; phosphorylated regulation of early transcription factors (AP-1, EGR1, IER2 and IER5) and downregulates NF-κB pathways; increases apoptotic or anti-proliferation genes (GADD45A/B and TUSC2) and the decrease of a batch of phosphatase and kinase genes; alters carcinogenesis-related gene transcripts (SAT, DCT, Melan-A, uPA and cyclin E1).	Zeng et al. 2005 [40]
Ethanol–water extract—commercial source (Hong Konk)	Raji, NB-4, and HL-60 cells—50 to 800 µg/mL	Suppresses cell proliferation; no cytotoxic effect on normal liver cell line WRL (IC_{50} > 800 µg/mL); increases nucleosome productions in cancer but not in normal cells.	Lau et al. 2004 [41]
Polysaccharopeptide (PSP)	C6 rat glioma cells exposed to radiation (4 Gy)—1 mg/mL	Inhibits ^{3}H-thymidine uptake; augments radiation-induced cancer cell damage though radiation efficacy did not increase.	Mao et al. 2001 [42]
Yunzhi (Windsor Wunxi)—a proprietary dietary supplement—ethanolic extracts (70%)	Hormone-responsive LNCaP and androgen-refractory JCA-1, PC-3, and DU-145 prostate cancer cells—0.5 mg/mL	Increases the levels STAT1 and STAT3 in JCA-1 but not LNCaP cells; reduces LNCaP cell growth, downregulates the levels of secreted but not intracellular prostate-specific antigen; no effect on level of the androgen receptor; less antiproliferative effect on PC-3 and DU-145 cells than LNCaP, and no effect on JCA-1 cells.	Hsieh and Wo 2001 [43]
PSK	MCF-7 cells—200 µg/mL	Inhibited DNA synthesis with IC_{50} value of 200 µg/mL.	Aoyagi et al. 1997 [44]
RPSP, a refined polysaccharide peptide fraction isolated by fast performance liquid chromatography (FPLC) from the crude powder of total peptide-bound polysaccharides of cultivated *Coriolus versicolor* Cov-1	Human hepatoma cell line (HepG2)	IC_{50} of 243 µg/mL for 3-day assay; no effect on normal human foetal hepatocytes.	Dong et al. 1996 [45]
PSK	NRK-49F (normal rat kidney) and H4-II-E ovarian cancer cells—100 µg/mL	Prevented cytotoxicity due to cisplatin toward NRK-49F, but enhanced the cytotoxicity on H4-II-E and human ovarian cancer cells; modulates cell-dependent effect on cisplatin-induced alteration in lipid peroxide and SOD activity.	Kobayashi et al. 1994 [46]

Table 1. *Cont.*

Preparation	Experimental Model	Key Findings	References
PSK	Walker 256 (fibrosarcoma) NRK-49F (rat normal kidney fibroblast), H4-II-E (rat hepatoma) and H4-II-E-C3 (rat hepatoma) cell lines—500 µg/mL	More pronounced antiproliferative effect in Walker 256 cells, which have more SOD activity; increased SOD activity in Walker 256 by 3.6 times and H_2O_2 by 2.56 times; no effect on CAT and GPx activity.	Kobayashi et al. 1994 [47]
Small polypeptide of about 10 Kd	HL-60 (leukaemia), LS174-T (colon), SMMU-7721 (hepatoma), and SCG-7901 (stomach)	Cytotoxicity against HL-60 (most sensitive cell line) with IC_{50} value of 30 µg/mL; more cytotoxic to leukemia and SCG-7901 cells than PSP or PSK.	Yang et al. 1992 [48]
PSK and four PSK subfractions	TNF-induced cytotoxicity in mouse L-929 fibroblast; interferon-γ-induced differentiation of human myelogenous leukemic U-937 and THP-1 cells.	Enhances the TNF-induced cytotoxicity against L-929 cells; induces cell differentiation; induces the expression of NBT-reducing and α-naphthyl acetate esterase activity; polysaccharides of over 200 kDa had the most potent stimulating activity.	Kim et al. 1990 [49]

Abbreviations: CAT, catalase; COX-2, cyclooxygenase 2; GPx, glutathione peroxidase; JNK, c-Jun N-terminal kinase; MAPK, mitogen-activated kinase; MMP, matrix metalloproteinase; NBT, nitroblue tetrazolium; NF-κB, nuclear factor κB; PARP, poly(ADP-ribose) polymerase; ROS, reactive oxygen species; SOD, superoxide dismutase; STAT, signal transducer and activator family of transcription.

As expected for apoptosis-inducing agents, genes and proteins that are associated with cancer cell survival (anti-apoptotic BCL-2, Bcl-xL, survivin) are shown to be suppressed while those markers of apoptosis (proapoptotic Bax) induction are upregulated by the *C. versicolor* polysaccharide preparations [18,32,35,36]. Induction of the intracellular level of reactive oxygen species (ROS) in cancer cells is a well-established mechanism of cell death by chemotherapeutic agents and this appears to be the case for *C. versicolor* in several cell lines [17,46]. The critical cell growth and death regulator mitogen-activated protein kinase (MAPK) is involved in the induction of cell death by *C. versicolor* polysaccharides, as shown by the enhancement of p38 MAPK phosphorylation [24–26,28]. Accordingly, the cytotoxicity of these polysaccharides in melanoma cells could be abolished in the presence of c-Jun N-terminal kinase (JNK) inhibitors [17] or the p38 MAPK inhibitor [24–26]. Key transcription factors that are involved in cancer development and metastasis could be inhibited by *C. versicolor* polysaccharides. This includes the well-defined cancer modulator, NF-κB, or its induced protein product, cyclooxygenase-2 (COX-2) [36,40]. The potential combination of *C. versicolor* polysaccharides with conventional chemotherapeutic agents has been demonstrated in vitro, as shown for camptothecin [30], doxorubicin and etoposide [32,38], and cisplatin [46]. Even at concentrations where direct toxicity was not observed, inhibition of cell migration and invasion was evident along with inhibition of key angiogenic enzymes such as matrix metalloprotease (MMP)-9 [23] or MMP-2 [19].

3.2. Evidence of Efficacy through Animal Models

Many in vitro experiments that showed promising effects in direct cytotoxicity study were also extended to animal models of tumour-bearing mice. This was based on the injection of the cancer cells into mice and assess the size and spread (metastasis) of the tumour in the presence or absence of *C. versicolor* polysaccharides. Table 2 has a good summary of these data with the description of the polysaccharides, their route of administration and main outcomes [14,23,29,31,37,42,45,50–55]. It appears that *C. versicolor* polysaccharides in the form of PSP, PSK, refined fractions, water or aqueous extracts exhibit anticancer effects in vivo when administered by either oral (p.o.), intraperitoneal (i.p.) or intravenous (i.v.) routes. In a combination approach, favourable responses were obtained with metronomic zoledronic acid [50] and docetaxel–taxane [51]. In addition to a reduction in the size and volume of the implanted tumours, the incidence of tumours [29,45] and angiogenesis via vascular endothelial cell growth factor (VEGF) expression have been shown to be inhibited.

Table 2. Direct antitumour effect in vivo.

Preparation	Experimental Model	Key Findings	References
Water extract of commercial source	Nude mice inoculated with human breast cancer cells - aqueous extract, metronomic zoledronic acid, or the combination of both for 4 week—1g/kg extract, p.o. daily), metronomic zoledronic acid group (0.0125 mg/kg, i.p. injected twice a week), or in combination.	Combination with metronomic zoledronic acid diminished tumor growth without increasing the incidence of lung and liver metastasis; combination therapy reserved the integrity of bones.	Ko et al. 2017 [50]
Aqueous extract	Mouse mammary carcinoma 4T1 tumour-bearing mice—1 g/kg, p.o. for 4 weeks	Decreased tumor weight by 36%, lung metastasis by 70.8%; protects bones from cancer-induced bone loss	Luo et al. 2014 [23]
PSK	Combination with taxanes for prostate transgenic adenocarcinoma of the mouse prostate (TRAMP)—C2-bearing mice—PSK with docetaxel—Mouse prostate tumor (TRAMP-C2) cells injected orthotopically—docetaxel (5 mg/kg, i.p. twice weekly); PSK (300 mg/kg daily p.o.) or in combination for 11–13 days	The combination increased more tumour suppression than either treatment alone—reduced tumor proliferation and enhanced apoptosis; other effects on immunomodulation (see Table 4).	Wenner et al. 2012 [51]
BreastDefend (BD)—extract that also contains several other mushrooms and herbal products	MDA-MB-231 cells implanted in female nude mice—100 mg/kg, ig., for 33 days.	Reduces tumour volume and anti-metastatic activity to the lungs; downregulates the expression of *PLAU* (uPA protein) and *CXCR4 genes* in breast tumors; no effect on genes associated with breast-to-lung cancer metastasis: ezrin (*EZR*), *HRAS*, *S100A4*, *CDKN1A* (protein p21) and *HTATIP2* (protein TIP30).	Jiang et al. 2012 [52]
PSP	Transgenic mice (TgMAP) mice that spontaneously develop prostate tumors—200 or 300 mg/kg p.o. 5 days per week for 20 weeks	Suppress tumourogenicity–chemopreventive property; see Table 1 for in vitro effect.	Luk et al. 2011 [29]
Methanol extract of fruiting body of Serbian origin	C57BL/6 mice inoculated with syngeneic B16 tumor cells—50 mg/kg, i.p. for 14 days	Inhibits tumor growth; peritoneal macrophages collected 21 days after tumor implantation; see Table 1 and Table 4 for other effects.	Harhaji et al. 2008 [31]
Standardised aqueous ethanol extract	Athymic nude mouse with HL-60 leukaemic xenograft model—100 mg/kg, p.o. for 28 days	Inhibits tumour growth; see Table 1 for in vitro effect.	Ho et al. 2006 [35]

Table 2. Cont.

Preparation	Experimental Model	Key Findings	References
VPS, a hot water extract	Swiss mice—as a 2% dose in the powdered diet for life and 1,2-dimethylhydrazine dihydrochloride (1,2-DMH) injection	No inhibitory effect on the development of large intestinal cancers; intestinal tumours and the total number of these tumors in the intestine not significantly different.	Coles et al. 2005 [53]
PSP	S180 tumor-bearing mouse model—murine sarcoma S180 cells implanted in subcutaneously in the back of each mouse—PSP solution in drinking water (35 µg/day/mouse) for 20 days	Suppress the expression of VEGF and angiogenesis and tumour markers.	Ho et al. 2004 [54]
PSP	Tumour bearing mice—radiation (8 Gy/mouse) or with PSP, i.p. 5 days before implantation and for 10 days after	Increase natural killer cell, lymphocyte and granulocyte counts in blood and spleen; no direct tumor reducing effect; see Table 1 for direct cytotoxic effect.	Mao et al. 2001 [42]
RPSP, a refined polysaccharide peptide fraction isolated by fast performance liquid chromatography from the crude powder of total peptide-bound polysaccharides of cultivated Coriolus versicolor Cov-1	Sarcoma 180 inoculated nude mice—1 mg, i.p. for 15 days	Reduces incidences of tumor growth; suppresses tumor mass; no pathological lesions in vital organs of animals such as heart, liver, spleen, lung and kidney.	Dong et al. 1996 [45]
PSK	N-methyl-N-nitrosourea-induced mammary gland tumors in rats—250 mg/kg twice a week for 3 weeks after tumour development	Inhibits tumour size and carcinogenesis	Fujii et al. 1995 [55]
PSK	Rat ascites hepatoma cell line (AH66) inoculated i.p. in rats—250 mg/kg, i.p. for 5 days before inoculation and 7 days after.	Direct effect on the transcription and translation of genens (pPIC1, pPIC2 and pPDC1).	Hirose et al. 1985 [14]

Abbreviations: VEGF, vascular endothelial cell growth factor.

3.3. Evidence of Efficacy through Clinical Trials

Chay et al. [56] employed a human study on *C. versicolor* extract by recruiting fifteen eligible cases of hepatocellular carcinoma patients in Singapore who failed or were unfit for standard therapy. The randomised placebo-controlled trial using 2.4 g as a daily treatment for ~5.9 weeks) showed a better quality of life without a significant difference in primary endpoint measure of the median time to progression. On the other hand, a pilot study of randomised, double-blind, and multidose study on dogs (not humans) revealed that treatment with PSP (e.g., 100 mg/kg capsules daily) could delay the progression of metastases of canine hemangiosarcoma [57]. The systematic review and meta-analysis studies by Eliza et al. [58] assessed the survival outcome in cancer patients from 13 clinical trials on *C. versicolor*. They reported an impressive result showing a significant survival advantage when compared with standard conventional anti-cancer agents alone. For example, a 9% absolute reduction in 5-year mortality was recorded with one additional patient alive for every 11 patients treated. They also reported a better 5-year survival rate in patients receiving combination treatment in cases of breast cancer, gastric cancer, or colorectal cancer. Database on ClinicalTrial.gov shows one terminated clinical trial on the potential benefit of *C. versicolor* for hepatocellular carcinoma and one currently recruiting for a vaginal gel based on *C. versicolor* medical device (PAPILOCARE) as a phase III trial. A further entry in this database is the USA (University of Minnesota), trial on *C. versicolor* extract in Stage I, Stage II, or Stage III breast cancer who have finished radiation therapy.

4. Anti-Cancer Effect Via Immunostimulation

Studies on the immunotherapeutic potential of the *C. versicolor* polysaccharides in cancer started in the late 1970s and accelerated in the 1980s and 1990s. In 1977, Kataoka et al. [59] reported that immuno-resistance in mice could be induced when protein-bound polysaccharides are administered together with L1210 murine leukemic cells. The suppression of TNF-α production in mice by cytotoxic antitumour agents (5-fluorouracil, cyclophosphamide and bleomycin) was shown to be ameliorated by PSK with an implication of immunotherapy potential [60]. The immunosuppressive effect of cyclophosphamide in rats could also be abolished by PSP [61]. Myelosuppressed mice due to chemotherapy could also be reversed by PSK, particularly when used in combination with granulocyte colony-stimulating factor (G-CSF), granulocyte/macrophage colony-stimulating factor (GM-CSF) or IL-3 [62]. These general immunostimulations or ameliorations of immunosuppression under cancer and depressed immune systems, either by cancer, splenectomy or other experimental agents, have been observed for *C. versicolor* polysaccharides [63–69].

Further studies in vitro showed the direct lymphocyte proliferative effect of PSP, while in mice, it reversed the inhibition of IL-2 production induced by cyclophosphamide along with restoration of the T-cell-mediated response [70]. The study by Kanoh et al. [71] also demonstrated that PSK could enhance the anti-tumour effects of IgG2a monoclonal antibody in the human colon cancer cell line, colo 205, both in vitro and in vivo via antibody-dependent macrophage-mediated cytotoxicity. Studies on PSK using mice bearing syngeneic plasmacytoma X5563 also showed that it enhances anti-tumour immunity by ameliorating the immunosuppressive activity of serum from tumour-bearing mice [72,73]. The tumour-induced immunosuppression could also be abolished by PSK in various cancer models in vivo [74]. Earlier in vitro studies further confirmed the direct effect of the polysaccharides on peritoneal macrophages [75], namely, interleukin-1 production by human peripheral blood mononuclear cells [76]. Further insight into the immunotherapeutic potential of *C. versicolor* polysaccharides is outlined below under the headings of in vitro, in vivo and human studies.

4.1. Evidence of Immunotherapy Potential through In Vitro Studies

Perhaps the best characterised pharmacological activity of *C. versicolor* relates to its immunostimulatory effects. Some of the key outcomes from in vitro studies with implications to cancer are shown in Table 3 [8,49,77–94]. The proliferative effect of the polysaccharides on mononuclear cells, such as lymphocytes [78,79,86,92], monocytes [85] or macrophages [77] and others, including splenocytes [81], has been shown for the polysaccharides. The immunostimulatory effect also includes activation of immune cells, as shown in the LPS-induced cytokine (interleukin (IL)-1β and IL-6) expression by peripheral blood mononuclear cells (PBMCs) [77] or by blood lymphocytes) [78]. Enhancement of antibody production such as IgM and IgG1 by splenocytes was reported [82], while activation of dendritic cells was evident from the expression level of surface markers in mature cells [84]. Increased level of IgM production in B cells by PSK has also been reported. Similarly, cytokines expression, including upregulation of TNF-α expression, leads to enhanced breast cancer cell killing) [79]. The production of IL-10 in mouse B cells could be enhanced by up to 60-fold for some preparations [86], while the antibody-mediated cytotoxicity of natural killer (NK) cells against cancer cells could be enhanced through IL-12-dependent and independent mechanisms [87]. Selective induction of cytokines expression that promotes Th1 and Th2 lymphocytes have been shown [92]. Also, increased nitric oxide (NO) production in polymorphonuclear cells (PMNs) or mononuclear cells such as U937 and THP-1 have been reported for PSK and its fractions [49,94].

Considerable levels of research have been devoted to understanding how *C. versicolor* polysaccharides interact with the immune cells. One of the established recognition sites for the polysaccharides is the toll-like receptors (TLRs), of which effects via TLR4 are well-documented. In mouse peritoneal macrophages, the expression of cytokines and NF-κB activation by PSP was shown to be coupled with TLR4 activation [81]. Furthermore, the induction of TNF-α and IL-6 secretion in J774A.1 cells and primary splenocytes by PSP via TLR4 has also been well established and correlated with its effect on NF-κB p65 transcription and phosphorylation of c-Jun [88]. The expression of both TLR4 and TLR5 by PSP was shown in PBMCs of human origin, while TLR9 and TLR10 appear to be downregulated [89]. Fractionation of PSK further led to the identification of two motifs: a β-glucan recognised by the Dectin-1 receptor and lipid fraction with agonistic activity towards TLR2.

Table 3. Immunomodulatory effects related to cancer: in vitro studies.

Preparation	Experimental Model	Key Findings	References
PSP	Normal and LPS-stimulated rat peripheral blood mononuclear cells (PBMCs—5–300 µg/mL	Enhances mitogenic activity and attenuates the induced cytokines (interleukin (IL)-1β and IL-6) production in stimulated macrophages; increases cell proliferation and pro-inflammatory cytokines release in unstimulated (LPS-free) macrophages.	Jedrzejewski et al. 2016 [77]
Protein-bound polysaccharides (PBP)	Blood lymphocytes and breast cancer cells (MCF-7)—100 and 300 µg/mL	Induces proliferative response on blood lymphocytes, as well as IL-1β and IL-6 mRNA expression; temperature of 39.5 °C blocks the PBP-induced cytotoxicity against MCF-7 cells, which correlates with reduction in TNFα level; see Table 4 for in vivo effect.	Pawlikowska et al. 2016 [78]
PSP	Breast cancer (MCF-7) cells and blood lymphocytes—100 µg/mL	Reduces cell growth; upregulates TNF-α-expression but not IL-1β and IL-6; enhances the proliferative response of blood lymphocytes associated with IL-6 and IL-1β mRNA upregulation.	Kowalczewska et al. 2016 [79]
PSK—isolation of TLR2 agonist activity from soluble β-glucan fraction—labeled the soluble β-glucan with fluorescein	Uptake of the labeled β-glucan in J774A macrophages and JAWSII dendritic cells—10–1000 µg/mL	Uptake inhibited by anti-Dectin-1 antibody but not by anti-TLR2 antibody; Dectin-1 is the receptor for β-glucan; lipid fraction enhances the uptake of the soluble β-glucan.	Quayle et al. 2015 [80]
PSP	Peritoneal macrophages from mice—25 µg/mL	Stimulates the expressions of cytokines, as well as TLR4, TRAF6, phosphorylation of NF-κB p65 and phosphorylation of c-Jun (a component of the transcription factor AP-1) in peritoneal macrophages from C57BL/10J (TLR4$^{+/+}$) mice but not from C57BL/10ScCr (TLR4$^{-/-}$) mice; see Table 4 for in vivo effect.	Wang et al. 2015 [81]
Polysaccharides—hot water extraction in house	Mouse splenocytes—high dose of 30 mg/mL	Stimulates splenocytes proliferation; fluorescence-labeled polysaccharides selectively stained mouse B cells but not T-cells; induces the production of IgM and IgG1 with or without exogenously added IL-4; membrane Ig (B cell antigen-receptor) acts as the polysaccharide binding protein; induces B-cell proliferation (inhibited by anti-mouse immunoglobulin (Ig) blocking antibody or in cells from TLR4-mutant mice; increases the phosphorylation of ERK-1/2 and p38 MAPK; enhances the nuclear translocation of the cytosolic NF-κB p65 subunit.	Yang et al. 2015 [82]

Table 3. Cont.

Preparation	Experimental Model	Key Findings	References
PSK as TLR2 agonist	PBMCs from healthy human donors—monocyte-derived DCs and tumor fusion cells	Upregulates MHC (class II and CD86) expression on DC/tumor; increases fusion efficiency; increases production of fusions derived IL-12p70; activates CD4$^+$ and CD8$^+$ T-cells to induce IFN-γ production; enhances induction of CTL activity specific for Mucin 1.	Koido et al. 2013 [83]
PSK	Mouse bone marrow-derived dendritic cells (DC)—5, 10, 20, 40, and 80 µg/mL	Induces DC maturation—dose-dependent increase in the expression of CD80, CD86, MHCII, and CD40; induces the production (mRNA and protein levels) of IL-12, TNF-α, and IL-6.	Engel et al. 2013 [84]
PSP	PBMCs—10 and 100 µg/mL	Increases monocytes counts (CD14$^+$/CD16$^-$) compared to controls—confirmed by CD14 and MHCII antibodies; no significant effect on proliferation of T-cells, NK, and B-cells.	Sekhon et al. 2013 [85]
Purified new protein—YZP is a 12-kDa non-glycosylated protein comprising 139 amino acids, including an 18-amino acids signal peptide	Mice lymphocyte proliferation—20 µg/mL	Induced a greater than 60-fold increase in IL-10 secretion in mice B lymphocytes; specifically triggers the differentiation of CD1d$^+$ B cells into IL-10-producing regulatory B cells (Bregs); enhances the expression of CD1d; activates Breg function via interaction with TLR2 and TLR4 and upregulation of the TLR-mediated signaling pathway.	Kuan et al. 2013 [86]
PSK	Human peripheral blood mononuclear cells—12–100 µg/mL	Activates NK cells to produce IFN-γ and to lyse K562 target cells; enhances trastuzumab-mediated antibody-dependent cell-mediated cytotoxicity ADCC against SKBR3 and MDA-MB-231 breast cancer cells; effect related to both direct and IL-12-dependent (indirect) mechanism.	Lu et al. 2011 [87]
PSK	J774A.1 cells and primary splenocytes—125 µg/mL	Induces TNF-α and IL-6 secretion by wild-type but not by TLR4-deficient peritoneal macrophages; TNFα secretion by J774A.1 cells and primary splenocytes effect inhibited by TLR4 blocking antibody.	Price et al. 2010 [88]
PSP	Human PBMCs—25 µg/mL	Upregulates the expression of (e.g., IFN-γ, CXCL10, TLR4, TLR5) while downregulating (e.g., TLR9, TLR10, SARM1, TOLLIP) other genes related with TLR signaling pathway; upregulated some cytokines (GCSF, GM-CSF, IL-1α, IL-6, IFN-γ) by more than 1.3 times; increases the mRNA levels of TRAM, TRIF, and TRAF6; increases the protein level of TRAF6.	Li et al. 2010 [89]
PSK	B-cells—human B-cell line BALL-1—1–100 µg/mL	Enhances IgM production in B-cells.	Maruyama et al. 2009 [90]
Polysaccharides from New Zealand isolate (Wr-74) and a patented strain (ATCC-20545) of *C. versicolor*—culture medium isolates	Murine splenocytes—extracellular polysaccharide (1150 µg/mL), and intracellular polysaccharide (IPS) (100 µg/mL)	Induces cytokine production (interleukin 12 and gamma interferon) in murine splenocytes.	Cui et al. 2007 [8]

Table 3. Cont.

Preparation	Experimental Model	Key Findings	References
PSP	Human T lymphocyte proliferation—100 or 500 μg/mL	Exhibits similar and additive inhibitory effects to ciclosporin to suppress activated T-cell proliferation, Th1 cytokines; reduces CD3$^+$/CD25$^+$ cell expression but not Th2 cytokine expression.	Lee et al. 2008 [91]
Ethanol–water extract—commercial source	Proliferation of murine (BALB/c mice) splenic lymphocytes—12.5–400 μg/mL	Enhances cell proliferation by up to 2.4-fold in a time- and dose-dependent manner; upregulates Th1-related cytokines (IL-2 and IL-12); enhanced the level of Th1-related cytokines (IFN-γ and IL-18) transiently (24 h, but not at 48 and 72 h) while Th2-(IL-4 and IL-6).	Ho et al. 2004 [92]
PSK	Dendritic cells derived from CD14-positive cells obtained from human peripheral blood monocytes	Increases the expression of HLA (class II antigen) and CD40; increases the number and expression of CD80-, CD86- and CD83-positive cells; decreases FITC-dextran uptake; augments IL-12 production and allogeneic mixed lymphocyte reaction; induces antigen-specific cytotoxicity.	Kanazawa et al. 2004 [93]
PSK	Mouse peritoneal PMNs—500 μg/ml	In combination with IFN-γ, increases NO production.	Asai et al. 2000 [94]
PSK and fractions (F1 <50 kDa; F2 50–100 kDa; F3 100–200 kDa; F4 >200 kDa)	U937 and THP-1 cells differentiation; TNF-induced cytotoxicity in L929 cells—5–500 μg/mL	In combination with IFN-γ, increases NO production and cell differentiation; enhances cytotoxicity in L929 cells; fraction F4 is the most active.	Kim et al. 1990 [49]

Abbreviations: ADCC, antibody-dependent cellular cytotoxicity; CTL, cytotoxic T lymphocytes; DC, dendritic cells; FITC, fluorescein isothiocyanate; HLA, human leukocyte antigen; IFN-γ, interferon-γ; LPS, lipopolysaccharides; MHC, major histocompatibility complex; PMBCs, peripheral blood mononuclear cells; PMN, polymorphonuclear cells; SARM, sterile-alpha and Armadillo motif-containing protein; TOLLIP, Toll interacting protein; TRIF, TIR domain-containing adaptor protein-inducing interferon β; TRAM, (TRIF)–related adaptor molecule; TRAF, tumor necrosis factor receptor (TNF-R)-associated factor.

4.2. Evidence of Immunotherapy Potential through In Vivo Studies

The animal studies on *C. versicolor* polysaccharides also support the general immunostimulatory effect (Table 4) [23,31,48,78,81,84,87,95–104]. Increased cytokine and ROS production and NF-κB activation have been reported in rats [95]. Through IL-10-dependent mechanism, an enhancement of cytokine production that was associated with T helper (Th2 and Th17 cells) (e.g., IL-2, -4, -6, -10, -17A and IFN-α and -γ) were observed for a glucan product of *C. versicolor* in cancer-bearing mice [96]. By increasing the level of IL-6, PSP could also increase the duration of endotoxin fever in rats [98]. The proinflammatory effect of *C. versicolor* is also evident from in vivo effect of PSP in inducing a writhing response in animals, which was associated with induction of the release of prostaglandin-E2 (PGE2), TNF-α, IL-1β, and histamine from macrophages and mast cells [101]. In agreement with the in vitro experiments, combination with acacia gum resulted in a selective increase in IgG level in mice treated by PSP while the IgA or IgE levels were not affected [97]. Small peptide fractions of the polysaccharides have also shown to increase IgG level in vivo as well as white blood cell (WBC) count in tumour-bearing nude mice [48]. The animal studies in rats also suggest that high temperature exposure (hyperthermia) could suppress the cytokine production by *C. versicolor* polysaccharides [78]. Furthermore, PSP has been shown to rapidly lower temperature in rats by elevating the level of TNFα [99].

The correlation between TLR4 activation by PSP and anti-tumour potential was studied in mice. This was substantiated from the fact that its anti-tumour effect and increased thymus index and spleen index were evident in tumour-bearing C57BL/10J (TLR4$^{+/+}$) mice but not in C57BL/10ScCr (TLR4$^-$) mice [81]. PSK could also enlarge lymph nodes, activate dendritic cells, and stimulate T-cells to produce cytokines, including IFN-γ, IL-2, and TNF-α [84]. The methanol extract of *C. versicolor* also induced a higher level of tumouricidal potential of peritoneal macrophage, as revealed by the study in mice subjected to melanoma cancer [31].

The beneficial effect of PSK in combination treatment with docetaxel in prostate-carrying mice was shown to be associated with immunostimulatory effects. In this case, the number of WBCs count under the combination treatment was much more favourable than docetaxel alone [51]. The potentiation effect of PSK in anti-HER2/neu mAb therapy of Neu transgenic mice with cancer was reported [87]. The potential application of PSP in potentiating radiation therapy has also been investigated where increased lymphocyte and granulocyte counts in the blood and spleen tissues were observed [102].

Table 4. Immunomodulatory effects related to cancer: in vivo studies.

Preparation	Experimental Model	Key Findings	References
Extract from *Coriolus versicolor* (Cov 1 strain)	Pre-injection in LPS-treated rats and PBMCs isolated—100 mg/kg, i.p.	Partially prevents endotoxin tolerance through maintaining febrile response; increases IL-6 and greater NF-κB activation in response to LPS stimulation ex vivo; enhances mitogenic effect of LPS and increases ROS generation.	Jedrzejewski et al. 2019 [95]
Glucan—home-made purification—[→6)-α-D-Glcp-(1→]$_n$.	Sarcoma 180-bearing mice—100 or 200 mg/kg for nine days, subcutaneously	Promotes the secretion of IL-2, -4, -6, -10, -17A and IFN-α and -γ; enhances cytokine production associated with T-helper Th2 and Th17 cells; effect dependent on IL-10.	Awadasseid et al. 2017 [96]
PSP	C57BL/6 male mice—50 mg/kg, p.o.	When combined with acacia gum, increased total IgG titre levels (day 4) while decreasing IgM titre had no effect on IgA or IgE titre levels.	Sekhon et al. 2016 [97]
Protein-bound polysaccharides (PBP)	Fever-range hyperthermia (FRH) combined with PBP in rats—100 mg/kg i.p.	Combination treatment of (FRH + PBP) decrease IL-1β, IL-6 and TNF-α mRNA expression in peripheral blood mononuclear cells; see Table 3 for in vitro effect.	Pawlikowska et al. 2016 [78]
PSP	Male Wistar rats—100 mg/kg, i.p. 2 h before LPS	Increases the duration of endotoxin fever; increases the blood level of IL-6 (3 or 14 h post-injection); effect inhibited by anti-IL-6 antibody (30 μg/rat).	Jedrzejewski et al. 2015 [98]
PSP	500 mg/kg/d by p.o. in mice for 25 days	Decreases the mean weights of tumors; increases thymus index and spleen index relative in tumour-bearing C57BL/10J (TLR4$^{+/+}$) mice but not in C57BL/10ScCr (TLR4$^-$) mice; see Table 3 for in vitro effect.	Wang et al. 2015 [81]
PSP	Male Wistar rats—50, 100 and 200 mg/kg, i.p.	Induces a rapid reduction in temperature; elevates TNF-α level; anti-TNF-α antibody abolish effect on temperature.	Jedrzejewski et al. 2014 [99]
Aqueous extract	Mouse mammary carcinoma 4T1 tumor bearing mice—1 g/kg, p.o. for 4 weeks	Increases IL-2, 6, 12, TNF-α and IFN-γ productions from the spleen lymphocytes; see Tables 1 and 2 for other effects	Luo et al. 2014 [23]
PSK	As an adjuvant to OVAp323-339 vaccine in vivo—DC activation 1000 μg—one injection by intradermal route	Enlarges draining lymph nodes with higher number of activated DC; stimulates the proliferation of OVA-specific T-cells, and induces T-cells that produce multiple cytokines (IFN-γ, IL-2, and TNF-α; see Table 3 for in vitro effect.	Engel et al. 2013 [84]

Table 4. Cont.

Preparation	Experimental Model	Key Findings	References
PSK	PSK with docetaxel- mouse prostate tumor (TRAMP-C2) cells injected orthotopically—docetaxel (5 mg/kg) injected i.p. twice weekly; PSK (300 mg/kg) daily by oral gavage or combination for 11–13 days	Lower level of decrease in number of white blood cells than docetaxel alone; increases numbers of tumor-infiltrating CD4+ and CD8+ T-cells; PSK with or without docetaxel enhance mRNA expression of IFN-γ—no effect on T-regulatory FoxP3 mRNA expression in tumors; augments the docetaxel-induced splenic natural killer cell cytolytic activity against YAC-1 target cells.	Wenner et al. 2012 [51]
PSK	Neu transgenic mice received subcutaneous implant of 1 million MMC cells—100 mg/kg, p.o. 3 times per week for up to 4 weeks	Potentiates the anti-tumour effect of anti-HER2/neu mAb therapy in neu-T mice; see Table 3 for in vitro effect.	Lu et al. 2011 [87]
Methanol extract of fruiting body of Serbian origin	C57BL/6 mice inoculated with syngeneic B16 tumor cells—50 mg/kg, i.p. for 14 days	Peritoneal macrophages collected 21 days after tumor implantation possess stronger tumouristatic activity ex vivo than those from untreated animals; see Tables 1 and 2 for other effects.	Harhaji et al. 2008 [31]
PSP—composed of 90% polysaccharides (74.6% glucose, 2.7% galactose, 1.5% mannose, 2.4% fucose and 4.8% xylose) and 10% peptides (18 different amino acids, mostly aspartic acid and glutamic acid)	Acetic acid-induced writhing model—0.2–2 µmol/kg, i.p. in hot-plate test; 2–4 µmol/kg, i.p. in acetic acid-induced writhing response; 0.05–4 µmol/kg, i.p. induction of writhing response by itself.	Decreased the number of acetic acid-induced writhing by 92.9%; PSP itself induces a dose-dependent writhing response; increased the release of PGE2, TNF-α, IL-1β, and histamine in mouse peritoneal macrophages and mast cells both in vivo and in vitro (1–100 µM).	Chan et al. 2006 [100]
Purified polysaccharide (CV-S2-Fr.I) of C. versicolor obtained by Sepharose CL-6B gel chromatography	Mouse peritoneal macrophage—100 µg/mL	Enhanced macrophage lysosomal enzyme activity by 250%; enhances the induction of NO production by interferon-γ (no effect by its own).	Jeong et al. 2006 [101]
PSP	Tumour bearing mice—radiation (8 Gy/mouse) or with PSP, i.p. 5 days before implantation and for 10 days after	Increases natural killer cell, lymphocyte and granulocyte counts in blood and spleen; no direct tumor reducing effect; see Table 1 for direct cytotoxic effect.	Mao et al. 2001 [102]
PSP	C57BL/6NIA mice—diets containing 0.1, 0.5 or 1.0% PSP for 1 month	No effect on mitogenic response to Con A, PHA or LPS, or on production of IL-1, IL-2, IL-4 and PGE2; induced higher delayed-type hypersensitivity response (1.0% PSP) in old but not in young mice.	Wu et al. 1998 [103]
Small polypeptide of about 10 Kd	Human tumour cells (SMMU-7721 or LS174-T) inculated into nude mice—2 mg, i.p. for 2 weeks.	Increases WBC and IgG levels; decreases the incidence of tumor mass.	Yang et al. 1992 [48]

Abbreviations: Con A, concanavalin A; IFN-γ, interferon-γ; LPS, lipopolysaccharide; NO, nitric oxide; PGE2, prostaglandin E2; PHA, phytohemagglutinin; WBC, white blood cell.

4.3. Evidence of Immunotherapy Potential through Human Studies

Perhaps the most promising immunostimulatory effect of C. versicolor polysaccharides resides on the reported promise in human cancer patients. In breast cancer patients, for example, PSP has been shown to upregulate cytokine genes for L-12, IL-6 and TNF-α in PBMCs [104]. A comprehensive study with 349 gastric cancer patients receiving PSK (3 g/day) as adjuvant immunotherapy also revealed a greatly improved 3-year recurrence-free survival (RFS) rates when patients were MHC class I-negative [105]. A freeze-dried mycelial powder preparation of the fungus was also reported to show the trend of increased lymphocyte counts when applied at 6 and 9 g/day doses [106]. Although only 9 women were involved in this experiment, dose-related increases in $CD8^+$ T-cells and $CD19^+$ B-cells (not $CD4^+$ T-cells or $CD16^+56^+$ NK cells) were reported. The application of PSK in gastric cancer —(Stage II/III) studied using large group (138 patients)—further revealed a relapse-free survival rate after post-operation or when compared to oral fluorinated pyrimidine anti-metabolites alone or in combination [107]. The double-blind placebo-controlled randomised trial study by Tsang et al. [108] employed 34 patients who had completed conventional treatment for advanced non-small cell lung cancer. They showed that PSP capsules of 340 mg each, 3× daily for 4 weeks, could lead to an improvement in blood leukocyte and neutrophil counts, serum IgG and IgM. Finally, Zhong et al. [109] undertook a meta-analysis study on randomised controlled trials of *C. versicolor* along with others. They reported that the treatment had a favorable effect on elevated levels of CD3 and CD4. Earlier studies in human cancer patients also substantiate this argument [110–113].

5. Other Benefits of *C. versicolor* Polysaccharides

Given oxidative stress is a prominent feature in cancer patients and experimental animals transplanted with tumours, the benefits of *C. versicolor* polysaccharides have also been tested as antioxidants. In both rats bearing with Walker 256 fibrosarcoma and human cancer patients, oral administration of PSK (daily dose of 3.0 g in humans and 50 mg/kg in rats) could normalise the disease-associated oxidative stress [114]. The immunostimulatory effect of *C. versicolor* polysaccharides has also been shown to be associated with increased superoxide dismutase (SOD) activities of lymphocytes and the thymus [115]. It is also worth noting that *C. versicolor* polysaccharides have been shown to ameliorate obesity [116] or experimental diabetes in rodents [117]. As anti-inflammatory agents, they further showed their benefit in experimental animal models of osteoarthritis [118], inflammatory bowel disease [119] or induction of analgesia [120]. Their organ protective effect was also proven through experimental models of alcoholic liver injury [10] and diabetic cardiomyopathy [121]. Their immunomodulatory effect in cancer is also extended in defenses against bacteria, including against intracellular parasites such as *Neisseria gonorrhoeae* [122].

While *C. versicolor* is regarded as an edible and medicinal mushroom, there is no report on sever toxicity induced by the fungus in humans. Experiments in rats using the standardised water extract has shown no mortality and signs of toxicity in acute and sub-chronic toxicity (up to 28 days) studies for doses up to 5000 mg/kg (p.o.) [123]. Monoclonal antibody against PSK has been developed [124], and, in principle, such antibodies could reduce the long-term use of the peptide-bound polysaccharides. For the doses indicated in the various animal experiments and human studies indicated herein, the toxicity of *C. versicolor* polysaccharides is not suggested as a concern.

6. General Summary and Conclusions

A great deal of attention has been given to medicinal mushrooms in recent years, with emphasis to their polysaccharide-active components. Most of these fungi are highly exploited as commercial products in far eastern countries such as Japan and China. In this regard, the edible mushroom *Dictyophora indusiata* (Vent. Ex. Pers.) Fischer (Syn. *Phallus indusiatus*) as a source of polysaccharides with main components as β-(→3)-D-glucan with side branches of β-(1→6)-glucosyl units have been established. Their chemistry, along with potential applications in cancer and immunotherapy, inflammatory and CNS diseases, among others, have been reviewed [2]. Another excellent example of the potential application of fungal polysaccharides in cancer therapy was demonstrated for *Ganoderma species*, which is reviewed by Cao et al. [125]. Similarly, PSP, PSK as well as other polysaccharides from *C. versicolor* have now been established to induce direct cytotoxicity to cancer/tumour cells. They also increase the release of cytokines such as TNF-α with direct implication to tumour cell killing. The overall, anti-cancer pharmacology of these polysaccharides through a direct effect on cancer cells and an indirect effect via immunostimulation is depicted in Figure 3.

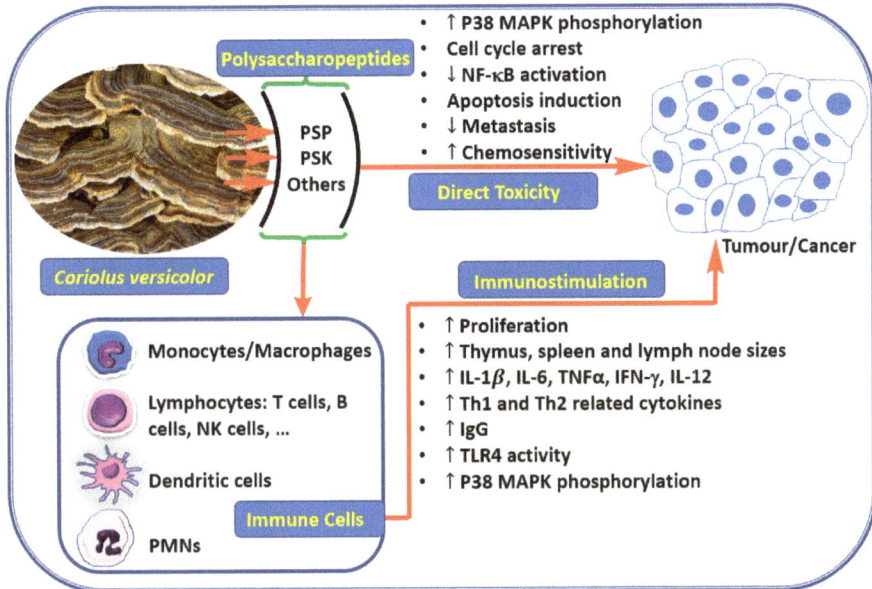

Figure 3. Anti-cancer potential of *C. versivolor* polysaccharides.

Overall, the polysaccharides of *C. versicolor* have been shown to induce direct cell growth inhibitory effect and apoptosis in cancer cells. Cell cycle arrest, even in some cases at concentrations lower than 100 μg/mL in vitro, has been observed. This moderate level of activity should be considered significant since the active components are large molecular weight compounds or mixtures. Given that carbohydrates taken through the oral route are subjected to hydrolysis by intestinal enzymes, there is always a question of whether they could maintain their therapeutic value *in vivo*. Interestingly, *C. versicolor* polysaccharides, including PSP and PSK, have been shown to demonstrate anti-cancer effect in vivo following oral administration. The other well-established mechanism of the anti-cancer effect by *C. versicolor* is via immunostimulant action, as evidenced by their ability to increase the production of cytokines such as IL-12, which is Th1 related. Th-lymphocyte subsets, including Th1, Th2, Th17 or Treg, mainly through the production of key cytokines and lymphocyte subsets (B-cells, CD4$^+$ and CD8$^+$ T-cells, NK cells, and different stages of differentiated T-cells), have been extensively studied for their response to *C. versicolor* polysaccharides. The further induction of cytokines such as IFN-γ in T cells was evident, which, together with TNF-α, induce cancer/tumour killing. Other cytokines, including IL-1 and IL-6, have been shown to be augmented by the polysaccharides. All these events appear to enhance antibody production in T-cells while enhancing the activity of other mononuclear cells, including monocytes/macrophages.

By interacting via the membrane Ig (B-cell antigen receptor) and TLR4, *C. versicolor* polysaccharides have been shown to activate B-cells via the phosphorylation of ERK 1/2 and p38 MAPK [82]. In human PBMCs, for example, PSP activates cells through TLRs family (e.g., TLR4, TLR5, TLR6 and TLR7) and their adaptor proteins (e.g., TICAM2, HRAS, HSPA4, HSPA6, and PELI2) leading to genes activation for key cytokines (including IFN-γ, G-CSF, GM-CSF, IL-1α, IL-6) and NF-κB and TRAF6 [89]. In the latter case, it appears that PSP appears to involve the TRAM-TRIF-TRAF6 pathway of immunomodulation. With TRAM acting as a bridge between TLRs (e.g., TLR4) and TRIF6, activation of mononuclear cells to orchestrate an inflammatory response has been well-established [126]. Other important cell surface receptors for the polysaccharides include the TLR2, and Dectin-1, which are shown to be linked to the immunogenic activity of PSK [80]. Dendritic cells being an important component of the immune system, they appear to be the target for *C. versicolor* polysaccharides. For example, PSK as an adjuvant to vaccines has been demonstrated to induce the production of cytokines (e.g., IL-12, TNF-α, and IL6) in these cells both in vitro and in vivo [84]. Hence, the immunostimulatory effect coupled with direct toxicity to cancer cells by *C. versicolor* polysaccharides implies application even more than an adjuvant therapy. The evidence for signal transduction pathways, including that for TLR4 as well as other cell surface recognition markers of the polysaccharides (e.g., Dectin-1 as a β-glucan receptor), are evolving current research. The structural moieties of the polysaccharides that attribute to the various pharmacological effects also need further research.

Funding: This research received no internal or external funding.

Conflicts of Interest: The author declares no conflict of interest.

References

1. WHO. Cancer. Available online: https://www.who.int/news-room/fact-sheets/detail/cancer (accessed on 1 May 2020).
2. Habtemariam, S. The chemistry, pharmacology and therapeutic potential of the edible mushroom *Dictyophora indusiata (Vent ex. Pers.) Fischer (Synn. Phallus indusiatus)*. *Biomedicines* **2019**, *7*, 98. [CrossRef] [PubMed]
3. NBNatlas. Trametes Versicolor (L.) Lloyd: Turkeytail. 2020. Available online: https://species.nbnatlas.org/species/nhmsys0001499939 (accessed on 1 May 2020).
4. Shen-Nong. Herbal Glossary—Chinese Herb List—Coriolus Versicolor. 2020. Available online: http://www.shen-nong.com/eng/herbal/yunzhi.html (accessed on 1 May 2020).
5. Wang, S.R.; Zhang, L.; Chen, H.P.; Li, Z.H.; Dong, Z.J.; Wei, K.; Liu, J.K. Four new spiroaxane sesquiterpenes and one new rosenonolactone derivative from cultures of Basidiomycete *Trametes versicolor*. *Fitoterapia* **2015**, *105*, 127–131. [CrossRef] [PubMed]
6. Janjušević, L.; Karaman, M.; Šibul, F.; Tommonaro, G.; Iodice, C.; Jakovljevic, D.M.; Pejin, B. The lignicolous fungus *Trametes versicolor* (L.) Lloyd (1920): A promising natural source of antiradical and AChE inhibitory agents. *J. Enzyme Inhib. Med. Chem.* **2017**, *32*, 355–362. [CrossRef]
7. Rau, U.; Kuenz, A.; Wray, V.; Nimtz, M.; Wrenger, J.; Cicek, H. Production and structural analysis of the polysaccharide secreted by *Trametes (Coriolus) versicolor* ATCC 200801. *Appl. Microbiol. Biotechnol.* **2009**, *81*, 827–837. [CrossRef]
8. Cui, J.; Goh, K.K.; Archer, R.; Singh, H. Characterisation and bioactivity of protein-bound polysaccharides from submerged-culture fermentation of *Coriolus versicolor* Wr-74 and ATCC-20545 strains. *J. Ind. Microbiol. Biotechnol.* **2007**, *34*, 393–402. [CrossRef]
9. Ng, T.B. A review of research on the protein-bound polysaccharide (polysaccharopeptide, PSP) from the mushroom *Coriolus versicolor* (Basidiomycetes: Polyporaceae). *Gen. Pharmacol.* **1998**, *30*, 1–4. [CrossRef]
10. Wang, K.L.; Lu, Z.M.; Mao, X.; Chen, L.; Gong, J.S.; Ren, Y.; Geng, Y.; Li, H.; Xu, H.Y.; Xu, G.H.; et al. Structural characterization and anti-alcoholic liver injury activity of a polysaccharide from *Coriolus versicolor* mycelia. *Int. J. Biol. Macromol.* **2019**, *137*, 1102–1111. [CrossRef]
11. Awadasseid, A.; Hou, J.; Gamallat, Y.; Xueqi, S.; Eugene, K.D.; Musa Hago, A.; Bamba, D.; Meyiah, A.; Gift, C.; Xin, Y. Purification, characterization, and antitumor activity of a novel glucan from the fruiting bodies of *Coriolus versicolor*. *PLoS ONE* **2017**, *12*, e0171270. [CrossRef]
12. Zhang, J.S.; Han, W.W.; Pan, Y.J. Studies on chemical structure of polysaccharide from fruit body of Coriolus versicolor. *Yao Xue Xue Bao* **2001**, *36*, 664–667.
13. Nakajima, T.; Ichikawa, S.; Uchida, S.; Komada, T. Effects of a protein-bound polysaccharide from a basidiomycetes against hepatocarcinogenesis induced by 3′-methyl-4-dimethylaminoazobenzene in rats. *Clin. Ther.* **1990**, *12*, 385–392.
14. Hirose, K.; Hakozaki, M.; Matsunaga, K.; Yoshikumi, C.; Hotta, T.; Yanagisawa, M.; Yamamoto, M.; Endo, H. Cloning of sequences induced and suppressed by administration of PSK, antitumor protein-bound polysaccharide. *Biochem. Biophys. Res. Commun.* **1985**, *126*, 884–892. [CrossRef]

15. Miyaji, C.; Ogawa, Y.; Imajo, Y.; Imanaka, K.; Kimura, S. Combination therapy of radiation and immunomodulators in the treatment of MM46 tumor transplanted in C3H/He mice. *Oncology* **1983**, *40*, 115–119. [CrossRef] [PubMed]
16. Ito, H.; Hidaka, H.; Sugiura, M. Effects of coriolan, an antitumor polysaccharide, produced by *Coriolus versicolor* Iwade. *Jpn. J. Pharmacol.* **1979**, *29*, 953–957. [CrossRef] [PubMed]
17. Pawlikowska, M.; Piotrowski, J.; Jedrzejewski, T.; Kozak, W.; Slominski, A.T.; Brozyna, A.A. *Coriolus versicolor*-derived protein-bound polysaccharides trigger the caspase-independent cell death pathway in amelanotic but not melanotic melanoma cells. *Phytother. Res.* **2020**, *34*, 173–183. [CrossRef] [PubMed]
18. Chauhan, P.S.; Kumarasamy, M.; Sosnik, A.; Danino, D. Enhanced thermostability and anticancer Activity in breast cancer cells of laccase immobilized on pluronic-stabilized nanoparticles. *ACS Appl. Mater. Interfaces* **2019**, *11*, 39436–39448. [CrossRef] [PubMed]
19. Roca-Lema, D.; Martinez-Iglesias, O.; Fernandez de Ana Portela, C.; Rodriguez-Blanco, A.; Valladares-Ayerbes, M.; Diaz-Diaz, A.; Casas-Pais, A.; Prego, C.; Figueroa, A. In vitro anti-proliferative and anti-invasive effect of polysaccharide-rich extracts from *Trametes versicolor* and *Grifola frondosa* in colon cancer cells. *Int. J. Med. Sci.* **2019**, *16*, 231–240. [CrossRef]
20. Shnyreva, A.V.; Shnyreva, A.A.; Espinoza, C.; Padron, J.M.; Trigos, A. Antiproliferative Activity and Cytotoxicity of some medicinal wood-destroying mushrooms from Russia. *Int. J. Med. Mushrooms* **2018**, *20*, 1–11. [CrossRef]
21. Knezevic, A.; Stajic, M.; Sofrenic, I.; Stanojkovic, T.; Milovanovic, I.; Tesevic, V.; Vukojevic, J. Antioxidative, antifungal, cytotoxic and antineurodegenerative activity of selected *Trametes species* from Serbia. *PLoS ONE* **2018**, *13*, e0203064. [CrossRef]
22. Ricciardi, M.R.; Licchetta, R.; Mirabilii, S.; Scarpari, M.; Parroni, A.; Fabbri, A.A.; Cescutti, P.; Reverberi, M.; Fanelli, C.; Tafuri, A. Preclinical Antileukemia Activity of Tramesan: A Newly Identified Bioactive Fungal Metabolite. *Oxid. Med. Cell Longev.* **2017**, *2017*, 5061639. [CrossRef]
23. Luo, K.W.; Yue, G.G.; Ko, C.H.; Lee, J.K.; Gao, S.; Li, L.F.; Li, G.; Fung, K.P.; Leung, P.C.; Lau, C.B. In vivo and in vitro anti-tumor and anti-metastasis effects of *Coriolus versicolor* aqueous extract on mouse mammary 4T1 carcinoma. *Phytomedicine* **2014**, *21*, 1078–1087. [CrossRef]
24. Hirahara, N.; Edamatsu, T.; Fujieda, A.; Fujioka, M.; Wada, T.; Tajima, Y. Protein-bound polysaccharide-K induces apoptosis via mitochondria and p38 mitogen-activated protein kinase-dependent pathways in HL-60 promyelomonocytic leukemia cells. *Oncol. Rep.* **2013**, *30*, 99–104. [CrossRef] [PubMed]
25. Hirahara, N.; Edamatsu, T.; Fujieda, A.; Fujioka, M.; Wada, T.; Tajima, Y. Protein-bound polysaccharide-K (PSK) induces apoptosis via p38 mitogen-activated protein kinase pathway in promyelomonocytic leukemia HL-60 cells. *Anticancer Res.* **2012**, *32*, 2631–2637. [PubMed]
26. Hirahara, N.; Fujioka, M.; Edamatsu, T.; Fujieda, A.; Sekine, F.; Wada, T.; Tanaka, T. Protein-bound polysaccharide-K (PSK) induces apoptosis and inhibits proliferation of promyelomonocytic leukemia HL-60 cells. *Anticancer Res.* **2011**, *31*, 2733–2738. [PubMed]
27. Hsieh, T.C.; Wu, J.M. Regulation of cell cycle transition and induction of apoptosis in HL-60 leukemia cells by the combination of *Coriolus versicolor* and *Ganoderma lucidum*. *Int. J. Mol. Med.* **2013**, *32*, 251–257. [CrossRef] [PubMed]
28. Wang, D.F.; Lou, N.; Li, X.D. Effect of *Coriolus versicolor* polysaccharide-B on the biological characteristics of human esophageal carcinoma cell line eca109. *Cancer Biol. Med.* **2012**, *9*, 164–167.
29. Luk, S.U.; Lee, T.K.; Liu, J.; Lee, D.T.; Chiu, Y.T.; Ma, S.; Ng, I.O.; Wong, Y.C.; Chan, F.L.; Ling, M.T. Chemopreventive effect of PSP through targeting of prostate cancer stem cell-like population. *PLoS ONE* **2011**, *6*, e19804. [CrossRef]
30. Wan, J.M.; Sit, W.H.; Yang, X.; Jiang, P.; Wong, L.L. Polysaccharopeptides derived from *Coriolus versicolor* potentiate the S-phase specific cytotoxicity of Camptothecin (CPT) on human leukemia HL-60 cells. *Chin. Med.* **2010**, *5*, 16. [CrossRef]
31. Harhaji, L.; Mijatovic, S.; Maksimovic-Ivanic, D.; Stojanovic, I.; Momcilovic, M.; Maksimovic, V.; Tufegdzic, S.; Marjanovic, Z.; Mostarica-Stojkovic, M.; Vucinic, Z.; et al. Anti-tumor effect of *Coriolus versicolor* methanol extract against mouse B16 melanoma cells: In vitro and in vivo study. *Food Chem. Toxicol.* **2008**, *46*, 1825–1833. [CrossRef]
32. Wan, J.M.; Sit, W.H.; Louie, J.C. Polysaccharopeptide enhances the anticancer activity of doxorubicin and etoposide on human breast cancer cells ZR-75-30. *Int. J. Oncol.* **2008**, *32*, 689–699. [CrossRef]

33. Jimenez-Medina, E.; Berruguilla, E.; Romero, I.; Algarra, I.; Collado, A.; Garrido, F.; Garcia-Lora, A. The immunomodulator PSK induces in vitro cytotoxic activity in tumour cell lines via arrest of cell cycle and induction of apoptosis. *BMC Cancer* **2008**, *8*, 78. [CrossRef]
34. Chan, S.L.; Yeung, J.H. Effects of polysaccharide peptide (PSP) from *Coriolus versicolor* on the pharmacokinetics of cyclophosphamide in the rat and cytotoxicity in HepG2 cells. *Food Chem. Toxicol.* **2006**, *44*, 689–694. [CrossRef] [PubMed]
35. Ho, C.Y.; Kim, C.F.; Leung, K.N.; Fung, K.P.; Tse, T.F.; Chan, H.; Lau, C.B. *Coriolus versicolor* (Yunzhi) extract attenuates growth of human leukemia xenografts and induces apoptosis through the mitochondrial pathway. *Oncol. Rep.* **2006**, *16*, 609–616. [CrossRef] [PubMed]
36. Hsieh, T.C.; Wu, P.; Park, S.; Wu, J.M. Induction of cell cycle changes and modulation of apoptogenic/anti-apoptotic and extracellular signaling regulatory protein expression by water extracts of I'm-Yunity (PSP). *BMC Complement. Altern. Med.* **2006**, *6*, 30. [CrossRef] [PubMed]
37. Ho, C.Y.; Kim, C.F.; Leung, K.N.; Fung, K.P.; Tse, T.F.; Chan, H.; Lau, C.B. Differential anti-tumor activity of *Coriolus versicolor* (Yunzhi) extract through p53- and/or Bcl-2-dependent apoptotic pathway in human breast cancer cells. *Cancer Biol. Ther.* **2005**, *4*, 638–644. [CrossRef] [PubMed]
38. Hui, K.P.; Sit, W.H.; Wan, J.M. Induction of S phase cell arrest and caspase activation by polysaccharide peptide isolated from *Coriolus versicolor* enhanced the cell cycle dependent activity and apoptotic cell death of doxorubicin and etoposide, but not cytarabine in HL-60 cells. *Oncol. Rep.* **2005**, *14*, 145–155.
39. Yang, X.; Sit, W.H.; Chan, D.K.; Wan, J.M. The cell death process of the anticancer agent polysaccharide-peptide (PSP) in human promyelocytic leukemic HL-60 cells. *Oncol. Rep.* **2005**, *13*, 1201–1210. [CrossRef]
40. Zeng, F.; Hon, C.C.; Sit, W.H.; Chow, K.Y.; Hui, R.K.; Law, I.K.; Ng, V.W.; Yang, X.T.; Leung, F.C.; Wan, J.M. Molecular characterization of *Coriolus versicolor* PSP-induced apoptosis in human promyelotic leukemic HL-60 cells using cDNA microarray. *Int. J. Oncol.* **2005**, *27*, 513–523. [CrossRef]
41. Lau, C.B.; Ho, C.Y.; Kim, C.F.; Leung, K.N.; Fung, K.P.; Tse, T.F.; Chan, H.H.; Chow, M.S. Cytotoxic activities of *Coriolus versicolor* (Yunzhi) extract on human leukemia and lymphoma cells by induction of apoptosis. *Life Sci.* **2004**, *75*, 797–808. [CrossRef]
42. Mao, X.W.; Green, L.M.; Gridley, D.S. Evaluation of polysaccharopeptide effects against C6 glioma in combination with radiation. *Oncology* **2001**, *61*, 243–253. [CrossRef]
43. Hsieh, T.C.; Wu, J.M. Cell growth and gene modulatory activities of Yunzhi (Windsor Wunxi) from mushroom Trametes versicolor in androgen-dependent and androgen-insensitive human prostate cancer cells. *Int. J. Oncol.* **2001**, *18*, 81–88. [CrossRef]
44. Aoyagi, H.; Iino, Y.; Takeo, T.; Horii, Y.; Morishita, Y.; Horiuchi, R. Effects of OK-432 (picibanil) on the estrogen receptors of MCF-7 cells and potentiation of antiproliferative effects of tamoxifen in combination with OK-432. *Oncology* **1997**, *54*, 414–423. [CrossRef]
45. Dong, Y.; Kwan, C.Y.; Chen, Z.N.; Yang, M.M. Antitumor effects of a refined polysaccharide peptide fraction isolated from *Coriolus versicolor*: In vitro and in vivo studies. *Res. Commun. Mol. Pathol Pharmacol.* **1996**, *92*, 140–148. [PubMed]
46. Kobayashi, Y.; Kariya, K.; Saigenji, K.; Nakamura, K. Enhancement of anti-cancer activity of cisdiaminedichloroplatinum by the protein-bound polysaccharide of *Coriolus versicolor* QUEL (PS-K) in vitro. *Cancer Biother.* **1994**, *9*, 351–358. [CrossRef] [PubMed]
47. Kobayashi, Y.; Kariya, K.; Saigenji, K.; Nakamura, K. Suppression of cancer cell growth in vitro by the protein-bound polysaccharide of *Coriolus versicolor* QUEL (PS-K) with SOD mimicking activity. *Cancer Biother.* **1994**, *9*, 63–69. [CrossRef] [PubMed]
48. Yang, M.M.; Chen, Z.; Kwok, J.S. The anti-tumor effect of a small polypeptide from *Coriolus versicolor* (SPCV). *Am. J. Chin. Med.* **1992**, *20*, 221–232. [CrossRef] [PubMed]
49. Kim, F.; Sakagami, H.; Tanuma, S.; Konno, K. Stimulation of interferon-gamma-induced human myelogenous leukemic cell differentiation by high molecular weight PSK subfraction. *Anticancer Res.* **1990**, *10*, 55–58.
50. Ko, C.H.; Yue, G.G.; Gao, S.; Luo, K.W.; Siu, W.S.; Shum, W.T.; Shiu, H.T.; Lee, J.K.; Li, G.; Leung, P.C.; et al. Evaluation of the combined use of metronomic zoledronic acid and Coriolus versicolor in intratibial breast cancer mouse model. *J. Ethnopharmacol.* **2017**, *204*, 77–85. [CrossRef]
51. Wenner, C.A.; Martzen, M.R.; Lu, H.; Verneris, M.R.; Wang, H.; Slaton, J.W. Polysaccharide-K augments docetaxel-induced tumor suppression and antitumor immune response in an immunocompetent murine model of human prostate cancer. *Int. J. Oncol.* **2012**, *40*, 905–913. [CrossRef]

52. Jiang, J.; Thyagarajan-Sahu, A.; Loganathan, J.; Eliaz, I.; Terry, C.; Sandusky, G.E.; Sliva, D. BreastDefend prevents breast-to-lung cancer metastases in an orthotopic animal model of triple-negative human breast cancer. *Oncol. Rep.* **2012**, *28*, 1139–1145. [CrossRef]
53. Coles, M.; Toth, B. Lack of prevention of large intestinal cancer by VPS, an extract of *Coriolus versicolor* mushroom. *In Vivo* **2005**, *19*, 867–871.
54. Ho, J.C.; Konerding, M.A.; Gaumann, A.; Groth, M.; Liu, W.K. Fungal polysaccharopeptide inhibits tumor angiogenesis and tumor growth in mice. *Life Sci.* **2004**, *75*, 1343–1356. [CrossRef]
55. Fujii, T.; Saito, K.; Matsunaga, K.; Oguchi, Y.; Ikuzawa, M.; Furusho, T.; Taguchi, T. Prolongation of the survival period with the biological response modifier PSK in rats bearing N-methyl-N-nitrosourea-induced mammary gland tumors. *In Vivo* **1995**, *9*, 55–57.
56. Chay, W.Y.; Tham, C.K.; Toh, H.C.; Lim, H.Y.; Tan, C.K.; Lim, C.; Wang, W.W.; Choo, S.P. *Coriolus versicolor* (Yunzhi) Use as Therapy in Advanced Hepatocellular Carcinoma Patients with Poor Liver Function or Who Are Unfit for Standard Therapy. *J. Altern. Complement. Med.* **2017**, *23*, 648–652. [CrossRef]
57. Brown, D.C.; Reetz, J. Single agent polysaccharopeptide delays metastases and improves survival in naturally occurring hemangiosarcoma. *Evid. Based Complement Alternat. Med.* **2012**, *2012*, 384301. [CrossRef]
58. Eliza, W.L.; Fai, C.K.; Chung, L.P. Efficacy of Yun Zhi (Coriolus versicolor) on survival in cancer patients: Systematic review and meta-analysis. *Recent Pat. Inflamm. Allergy Drug Discov.* **2012**, *6*, 78–87. [CrossRef]
59. Kataoka, T.; Oh-hashi, F.; Tsukagoshi, S.; Sakurai, Y. Enhanced induction of immune resistance by concanavalin A-bound L1210 vaccine and an immunopotentiator prepared from Coriolus versicolor. *Cancer Res.* **1977**, *37*, 4416–4419.
60. Mori, H.; Mihara, M.; Teshima, K.; Uesugi, U.; Xu, Q.; Sakamoto, O.; Koda, A. Effect of immunostimulants and antitumor agents on tumor necrosis factor (TNF) production. *Int. J. Immunopharmacol.* **1987**, *9*, 881–892. [CrossRef]
61. Qian, Z.M.; Xu, M.F.; Tang, P.L. Polysaccharide peptide (PSP) restores immunosuppression induced by cyclophosphamide in rats. *Am. J. Chin. Med.* **1997**, *25*, 27–35. [CrossRef]
62. Kohgo, Y.; Hirayama, Y.; Sakamaki, S.; Matsunaga, T.; Ohi, S.; Kuga, T.; Kato, J.; Niitsu, Y. Improved recovery of myelosuppression following chemotherapy in mice by combined administration of PSK and various cytokines. *Acta Haematol.* **1994**, *92*, 130–135. [CrossRef]
63. Fujii, T.; Kano, T.; Saito, K.; Kobayashi, Y.; Iijima, H.; Matsumoto, T.; Yoshikumi, C.; Taguchi, T. Effect of PSK on prohibited immunity of splenectomized mice. *Anticancer Res.* **1987**, *7*, 845–848.
64. Matsunaga, K.; Morita, I.; Oguchi, Y.; Fujii, T.; Yoshikumi, C.; Nomoto, K. Restoration of immune responsiveness by a biological response modifier, PSK, in aged mice bearing syngeneic transplantable tumor. *J. Clin. Lab. Immunol.* **1987**, *24*, 143–149.
65. Matsunaga, K.; Morita, I.; Oguchi, Y.; Fujii, T.; Yoshikumi, C.; Nomoto, K. Competitive effect of PSK against the immunosuppressive effect induced in the sera of mice bearing syngeneic tumors. *Gan To Kagaku Ryoho* **1986**, *13*, 3461–3467. [PubMed]
66. Matsunaga, K.; Morita, I.; Oguchi, Y.; Fujii, T.; Yoshikumi, C.; Nomoto, K. Restoration of immunologic responsiveness by PSK in tumor-bearing animals. *Gan To Kagaku Ryoho* **1986**, *13*, 3468–3475.
67. Matsunaga, K.; Morita, I.; Oguchi, Y.; Fujii, T.; Yoshikumi, C.; Nomoto, K. Restoration of depressed immune responses by PSK in C3H/He mice bearing the syngeneic X5563 tumor. *Gan To Kagaku Ryoho* **1986**, *13*, 3453–3460.
68. Hattori, T.; Hamai, Y.; Ikeda, T.; Takiyama, W.; Hirai, T.; Miyoshi, Y. Survival time of tumor-bearing rats as related to operative stress and immunopotentiators. *Jpn. J. Surg.* **1982**, *12*, 143–147. [CrossRef]
69. Mayer, P.; Drews, J. The effect of a protein-bound polysaccharide from *Coriolus versicolor* on immunological parameters and experimental infections in mice. *Infection* **1980**, *8*, 13–21. [CrossRef]
70. Li, X.Y.; Wang, J.F.; Zhu, P.P.; Liu, L.; Ge, J.B.; Yang, S.X. Immune enhancement of a polysaccharides peptides isolated from *Coriolus versicolor*. *Zhongguo Yao Li Xue Bao* **1990**, *11*, 542–545.
71. Kanoh, T.; Saito, K.; Matsunaga, K.; Oguchi, Y.; Taniguchi, N.; Endoh, H.; Yoshimura, M.; Fujii, T.; Yoshikumi, C. Enhancement of the antitumor effect by the concurrent use of a monoclonal antibody and the protein-bound polysaccharide PSK in mice bearing a human cancer cell line. *In Vivo* **1994**, *8*, 241–245. [PubMed]
72. Matsunaga, K.; Iijima, H.; Aota, M.; Oguchi, Y.; Fujii, T.; Yoshikumi, C.; Nomoto, K. Enhancement of effector cell activities in mice bearing syngeneic plasmacytoma X5563 by a biological response modifier, PSK. *J. Clin. Lab. Immunol.* **1992**, *37*, 21–37.

73. Matsunaga, K.; Morita, I.; Iijima, H.; Endoh, H.; Oguchi, Y.; Yoshimura, M.; Fujii, T.; Yoshikumi, C.; Nomoto, K. Effects of biological response modifiers with different modes of action used separately and together on immune responses in mice with syngeneic tumours. *J. Int. Med. Res.* **1992**, *20*, 406–421. [CrossRef] [PubMed]
74. Matsunaga, K.; Morita, I.; Iijima, H.; Endo, H.; Oguchi, Y.; Yoshimura, M.; Fujii, T.; Yoshikumi, C.; Nomoto, K. Competitive action of a biological response modifier, PSK, on a humoral immunosuppressive factor produced in tumor-bearing hosts. *J. Clin. Lab. Immunol.* **1990**, *31*, 127–136.
75. Liu, W.K.; Ng, T.B.; Sze, S.F.; Tsui, K.W. Activation of peritoneal macrophages by polysaccharopeptide from the mushroom, Coriolus versicolor. *Immunopharmacology* **1993**, *26*, 139–146. [CrossRef]
76. Sakagami, H.; Sugaya, K.; Utsumi, A.; Fujinaga, S.; Sato, T.; Takeda, M. Stimulation by PSK of interleukin-1 production by human peripheral blood mononuclear cells. *Anticancer Res.* **1993**, *13*, 671–675.
77. Jedrzejewski, T.; Pawlikowska, M.; Piotrowski, J.; Kozak, W. Protein-bound polysaccharides from Coriolus versicolor attenuate LPS-induced synthesis of pro-inflammatory cytokines and stimulate PBMCs proliferation. *Immunol. Lett.* **2016**, *178*, 140–147. [CrossRef]
78. Pawlikowska, M.; Jędrzejewski, T.; Piotrowski, J.; Kozak, W. Fever-range hyperthermia inhibits cells immune response to protein-bound polysaccharides derived from *Coriolus versicolor* extract. *Mol. Immunol.* **2016**, *80*, 50–57. [CrossRef]
79. Kowalczewska, M.; Piotrowski, J.; Jedrzejewski, T.; Kozak, W. Polysaccharide peptides from Coriolus versicolor exert differential immunomodulatory effects on blood lymphocytes and breast cancer cell line MCF-7 in vitro. *Immunol. Lett.* **2016**, *174*, 37–44. [CrossRef]
80. Quayle, K.; Coy, C.; Ztandish, L.; Lu, H. The TLR2 agonist in polysaccharide-K is a structurally distinct lipid which acts synergistically with the protein-bound beta-glucan. *J. Nat. Med.* **2015**, *69*, 198–208. [CrossRef]
81. Wang, Z.; Dong, B.; Feng, Z.; Yu, S.; Bao, Y. A study on immunomodulatory mechanism of Polysaccharopeptide mediated by TLR4 signaling pathway. *BMC Immunol.* **2015**, *16*, 34. [CrossRef]
82. Yang, S.F.; Zhuang, T.F.; Si, Y.M.; Qi, K.Y.; Zhao, J. *Coriolus versicolor* mushroom polysaccharides exert immunoregulatory effects on mouse B cells via membrane Ig and TLR-4 to activate the MAPK and NF-κB signaling pathways. *Mol. Immunol.* **2015**, *64*, 144–151. [CrossRef]
83. Koido, S.; Homma, S.; Okamoto, M.; Namiki, Y.; Takakura, K.; Takahara, A.; Odahara, S.; Tsukinaga, S.; Yukawa, T.; Mitobe, J.; et al. Combined TLR2/4-activated dendritic/tumor cell fusions induce augmented cytotoxic T lymphocytes. *PLoS ONE* **2013**, *8*, e59280. [CrossRef]
84. Engel, A.L.; Sun, G.C.; Gad, E.; Rastetter, L.R.; Strobe, K.; Yang, Y.; Dang, Y.; Disis, M.L.; Lu, H. Protein-bound polysaccharide activates dendritic cells and enhances OVA-specific T cell response as vaccine adjuvant. *Immunobiology* **2013**, *218*, 1468–1476. [CrossRef]
85. Sekhon, B.K.; Sze, D.M.; Chan, W.K.; Fan, K.; Li, G.Q.; Moore, D.E.; Roubin, R.H. PSP activates monocytes in resting human peripheral blood mononuclear cells: Immunomodulatory implications for cancer treatment. *Food Chem.* **2013**, *138*, 2201–2209. [CrossRef]
86. Kuan, Y.C.; Wu, Y.J.; Hung, C.L.; Sheu, F. *Trametes versicolor* protein YZP activates regulatory B lymphocytes—Gene identification through de novo assembly and function analysis in a murine acute colitis model. *PLoS ONE* **2013**, *8*, e72422. [CrossRef]
87. Lu, H.; Yang, Y.; Gad, E.; Inatsuka, C.; Wenner, C.A.; Disis, M.L.; Standish, L.J. TLR2 agonist PSK activates human NK cells and enhances the antitumor effect of HER2-targeted monoclonal antibody therapy. *Clin. Cancer Res.* **2011**, *17*, 6742–6753. [CrossRef]
88. Price, L.A.; Wenner, C.A.; Sloper, D.T.; Slaton, J.W.; Novack, J.P. Role for toll-like receptor 4 in TNF-alpha secretion by murine macrophages in response to polysaccharide Krestin, a *Trametes versicolor* mushroom extract. *Fitoterapia* **2010**, *81*, 914–919. [CrossRef]
89. Li, W.; Liu, M.; Lai, S.; Xu, C.; Lu, F.; Xiao, X.; Bao, Y. Immunomodulatory effects of polysaccharopeptide (PSP) in human PBMC through regulation of TRAF6/TLR immunosignal-transduction pathways. *Immunopharmacol. Immunotoxicol.* **2010**, *32*, 576–584. [CrossRef]
90. Maruyama, S.; Akasaka, T.; Yamada, K.; Tachibana, H. Protein-bound polysaccharide-K (PSK) directly enhanced IgM production in the human B cell line BALL-1. *Biomed. Pharmacother.* **2009**, *63*, 409–412. [CrossRef]
91. Lee, C.L.; Sit, W.H.; Jiang, P.P.; So, I.W.; Wan, J.M. Polysaccharopeptide mimics ciclosporin-mediated Th1/Th2 cytokine balance for suppression of activated human T cell proliferation by MAPKp38 and STAT5 pathways. *J. Pharm. Pharmacol.* **2008**, *60*, 1491–1499. [CrossRef]

92. Ho, C.Y.; Lau, C.B.; Kim, C.F.; Leung, K.N.; Fung, K.P.; Tse, T.F.; Chan, H.H.; Chow, M.S. Differential effect of *Coriolus versicolor* (Yunzhi) extract on cytokine production by murine lymphocytes in vitro. *Int. Immunopharmacol.* **2004**, *4*, 1549–1557. [CrossRef]
93. Kanazawa, M.; Mori, Y.; Yoshihara, K.; Iwadate, M.; Suzuki, S.; Endoh, Y.; Ohki, S.; Takita, K.; Sekikawa, K.; Takenoshita, S. Effect of PSK on the maturation of dendritic cells derived from human peripheral blood monocytes. *Immunol. Lett.* **2004**, *91*, 229–238. [CrossRef]
94. Asai, K.; Kato, H.; Hirose, K.; Akaogi, K.; Kimura, S.; Mukai, S.; Inoue, M.; Yamamura, Y.; Sano, H.; Sugino, S.; et al. PSK and OK-432-induced immunomodulation of inducible nitric oxide (NO) synthase gene expression in mouse peritoneal polymorphonuclear leukocytes and NO-mediated cytotoxicity. *Immunopharmacol. Immunotoxicol.* **2000**, *22*, 221–235. [CrossRef]
95. Jedrzejewski, T.; Piotrowski, J.; Pawlikowska, M.; Wrotek, S.; Kozak, W. Extract from Coriolus versicolor fungus partially prevents endotoxin tolerance development by maintaining febrile response and increasing IL-6 generation. *J. Therm. Biol.* **2019**, *83*, 69–79. [CrossRef]
96. Awadasseid, A.; Eugene, K.; Jamal, M.; Hou, J.; Musa Hago, A.; Gamallat, Y.; Meyiah, A.; Bamba, D.; Gift, C.; Abdalla, M.; et al. Effect of *Coriolus versicolor* glucan on the stimulation of cytokine production in sarcoma-180-bearing mice. *Biomed. Rep.* **2017**, *7*, 567–572. [CrossRef]
97. Sekhon, B.K.; Roubin, R.H.; Li, Y.; Devi, P.B.; Nammi, S.; Fan, K.; Sze, D.M. Evaluation of selected immunomodulatory glycoproteins as an adjunct to cancer immunotherapy. *PLoS ONE* **2016**, *11*, e0146881. [CrossRef]
98. Jedrzejewski, T.; Piotrowski, J.; Kowalczewska, M.; Wrotek, S.; Kozak, W. Polysaccharide peptide from Coriolus versicolor induces interleukin 6-related extension of endotoxin fever in rats. *Int. J. Hyperth.* **2015**, *31*, 626–634. [CrossRef]
99. Jedrzejewski, T.; Piotrowski, J.; Wrotek, S.; Kozak, W. Polysaccharide peptide induces a tumor necrosis factor-alpha-dependent drop of body temperature in rats. *J. Therm. Biol.* **2014**, *44*, 1–4. [CrossRef]
100. Chan, S.L.; Yeung, J.H. Polysaccharide peptides from COV-1 strain of *Coriolus versicolor* induce hyperalgesia via inflammatory mediator release in the mouse. *Life Sci.* **2006**, *78*, 2463–2470. [CrossRef]
101. Jeong, S.C.; Yang, B.K.; Kim, G.N.; Jeong, H.; Wilson, M.A.; Cho, Y.; Rao, K.S.; Song, C.H. Macrophage-stimulating activity of polysaccharides extracted from fruiting bodies of Coriolus versicolor (Turkey Tail Mushroom). *J. Med. Food* **2006**, *9*, 175–181. [CrossRef]
102. Mao, X.W.; Archambeau, J.O.; Gridley, D.S. Immunotherapy with low-dose interleukin-2 and a polysaccharopeptide derived from *Coriolus versicolor*. *Cancer Biother. Radiopharm.* **1996**, *11*, 393–403. [CrossRef]
103. Wu, D.; Han, S.N.; Bronson, R.T.; Smith, D.E.; Meydani, S.N. Dietary supplementation with mushroom-derived protein-bound glucan does not enhance immune function in young and old mice. *J. Nutr.* **1998**, *128*, 193–197. [CrossRef]
104. Wang, J.; Dong, B.; Tan, Y.; Yu, S.; Bao, Y.X. A study on the immunomodulation of polysaccharopeptide through the TLR4-TIRAP/MAL-MyD88 signaling pathway in PBMCs from breast cancer patients. *Immunopharmacol. Immunotoxicol.* **2013**, *35*, 497–504. [CrossRef] [PubMed]
105. Ito, G.; Tanaka, H.; Ohira, M.; Yoshii, M.; Muguruma, K.; Kubo, N.; Yashiro, M.; Yamada, N.; Maeda, K.; Sawada, T.; et al. Correlation between efficacy of PSK postoperative adjuvant immunochemotherapy for gastric cancer and expression of MHC class I. *Exp. Ther. Med.* **2012**, *3*, 925–930. [CrossRef] [PubMed]
106. Torkelson, C.J.; Sweet, E.; Martzen, M.R.; Sasagawa, M.; Wenner, C.A.; Gay, J.; Putiri, A.; Standish, L.J. Phase 1 Clinical trial of *Trametes versicolor* in women with breast cancer. *ISRN Oncol.* **2012**, *2012*, 251632. [CrossRef] [PubMed]
107. Tanaka, H.; Muguruma, K.; Kubo, N.; Amano, R.; Noda, E.; Yamada, N.; Yashiro, M.; Maeda, K.; Sawada, T.; Ohira, M.; et al. Effect of PSK on recurrence of stage II/III gastric cancer. *Gan To Kagaku Ryoho* **2010**, *37*, 2258–2260. [PubMed]
108. Tsang, K.W.; Lam, C.L.; Yan, C.; Mak, J.C.; Ooi, G.C.; Ho, J.C.; Lam, B.; Man, R.; Sham, J.S.; Lam, W.K. *Coriolus versicolor* polysaccharide peptide slows progression of advanced non-small cell lung cancer. *Respir. Med.* **2003**, *97*, 618–624. [CrossRef] [PubMed]
109. Zhong, L.; Yan, P.; Lam, W.C.; Yao, L.; Bian, Z. *Coriolus versicolor and Ganoderma* lucidum related natural products as an adjunct therapy for cancers: A systematic review and meta-analysis of randomized controlled trials. *Front. Pharmacol.* **2019**, *10*, 703. [CrossRef]

110. Wong, C.K.; Bao, Y.X.; Wong, E.L.; Leung, P.C.; Fung, K.P.; Lam, C.W. Immunomodulatory activities of Yunzhi and Danshen in post-treatment breast cancer patients. *Am. J. Chin. Med.* **2005**, *33*, 381–395. [CrossRef]
111. Wong, C.K.; Tse, P.S.; Wong, E.L.; Leung, P.C.; Fung, K.P.; Lam, C.W. Immunomodulatory effects of yun zhi and danshen capsules in health subjects–a randomized, double-blind, placebo-controlled, crossover study. *Int. Immunopharmacol.* **2004**, *4*, 201–211. [CrossRef]
112. Kariya, K.; Nakamura, K.; Nomoto, K.; Matama, S.; Saigenji, K. Mimicking of superoxide dismutase activity by protein-bound polysaccharide of *Coriolus versicolor* QUEL, and oxidative stress relief for cancer patients. *Mol. Biother.* **1992**, *4*, 40–46. [PubMed]
113. Maehara, Y.; Inutsuka, S.; Takeuchi, H.; Baba, H.; Kusumoto, H.; Sugimachi, K. Postoperative PSK and OK-432 immunochemotherapy for patients with gastric cancer. *Cancer Chemother. Pharmacol.* **1993**, *33*, 171–175. [CrossRef]
114. Kobayashi, Y.; Kariya, K.; Saigenji, K.; Nakamura, K. Oxidative stress relief for cancer-bearing hosts by the protein-bound polysaccharide of *Coriolus versicolor* QUEL with SOD mimicking activity. *Cancer Biother.* **1994**, *9*, 55–62. [CrossRef] [PubMed]
115. Wei, W.S.; Tan, J.Q.; Guo, F.; Ghen, H.S.; Zhou, Z.Y.; Zhang, Z.H.; Gui, L. Effects of *Coriolus versicolor* polysaccharides on superoxide dismutase activities in mice. *Zhongguo Yao Li Xue Bao* **1996**, *17*, 174–178. [PubMed]
116. Li, X.; Chen, P.; Zhang, P.; Chang, Y.; Cui, M.; Duan, J. Protein-Bound beta-glucan from *Coriolus versicolor* has potential for use against obesity. *Mol. Nutr. Food Res.* **2019**, *63*, e1801231. [CrossRef] [PubMed]
117. Xian, H.M.; Che, H.; Qin, Y.; Yang, F.; Meng, S.Y.; Li, X.G.; Bai, Y.L.; Wang, L.H. *Coriolus versicolor* aqueous extract ameliorates insulin resistance with PI3K/Akt and p38 MAPK signaling pathways involved in diabetic skeletal muscle. *Phytother. Res.* **2018**, *32*, 551–560. [CrossRef]
118. Wang, K.; Wang, Z.; Cui, R.; Chu, H. Polysaccharopeptide from *Trametes versicolor* blocks inflammatory osteoarthritis pain-morphine tolerance effects via activating cannabinoid type 2 receptor. *Int. J. Biol. Macromol.* **2019**, *126*, 805–810. [CrossRef]
119. Lim, B.O. *Coriolus versicolor* suppresses inflammatory bowel disease by Inhibiting the expression of STAT1 and STAT6 associated with IFN-gamma and IL-4 expression. *Phytother. Res.* **2011**, *25*, 1257–1261. [CrossRef]
120. Gong, S.; Zhang, H.Q.; Yin, W.P.; Yin, Q.Z.; Zhang, Y.; Gu, Z.L.; Qian, Z.M.; Tang, P.L. Involvement of interleukin-2 in analgesia produced by *Coriolus versicolor* polysaccharide peptides. *Zhongguo Yao Li Xue Bao* **1998**, *19*, 67–70.
121. Wang, Y.; Li, H.; Li, Y.; Zhao, Y.; Xiong, F.; Liu, Y.; Xue, H.; Yang, Z.; Ni, S.; Sahil, A.; et al. *Coriolus versicolor* alleviates diabetic cardiomyopathy by inhibiting cardiac fibrosis and NLRP3 inflammasome activation. *Phytother. Res.* **2019**, *33*, 2737–2748. [CrossRef]
122. Pramudya, M.; Wahyuningsih, S.P.A. Immunomodulatory potential of polysaccharides from *Coriolus versicolor* against intracellular bacteria *Neisseria gonorrhoeae*. *Vet. World* **2019**, *12*, 735–739. [CrossRef]
123. Hor, S.Y.; Ahmad, M.; Farsi, E.; Lim, C.P.; Asmawi, M.Z.; Yam, M.F. Acute and subchronic oral toxicity of *Coriolus versicolor* standardized water extract in Sprague-Dawley rats. *J. Ethnopharmacol.* **2011**, *137*, 1067–1076. [CrossRef]
124. Hoshi, H.; Saito, H.; Iijima, H.; Uchida, M.; Wada, T.; Ito, G.; Tanaka, H.; Sawada, T.; Hirakawa, K. Anti-protein-bound polysaccharide-K monoclonal antibody binds the active structure and neutralizes direct antitumor action of the compound. *Oncol. Rep.* **2011**, *25*, 905–913. [CrossRef] [PubMed]
125. Cao, Y.; Xu, X.; Liu, S.; Huang, L.; Gu, J. *Ganoderma*: A Cancer Immunotherapy Review. *Front Pharmacol.* **2018**, *9*, 1217. [CrossRef] [PubMed]
126. Verstak, B.; Stack, J.; Ve, T.; Mangan, M.; Hjerrild, K.; Jeon, J.; Stahl, R.; Latz, E.; Gay, N.; Kobe, B.; et al. The TLR signaling adaptor TRAM interacts with TRAF6 to mediate activation of the inflammatory response by TLR4. *J. Leukoc. Biol.* **2014**, *96*, 427–436. [CrossRef] [PubMed]

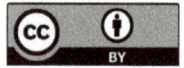

© 2020 by the author. Licensee MDPI, Basel, Switzerland. This article is an open access article distributed under the terms and conditions of the Creative Commons Attribution (CC BY) license (http://creativecommons.org/licenses/by/4.0/).

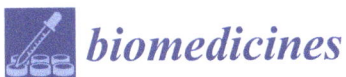

Article

Anti-Anaphylactic Activity of Isoquercitrin (Quercetin-3-O-β-D-Glucose) in the Cardiovascular System of Animals

Jinbong Park

Department of Pharmacology, College of Korean Medicine, Kyung Hee University, Seoul 02447, Korea; thejinbong@khu.ac.kr; Tel.: +82-2-961-2297

Received: 9 May 2020; Accepted: 27 May 2020; Published: 29 May 2020

Abstract: Effects of isoquercitrin (IQ) on anaphylactic responses were examined in cardiovascular systems of experimental animals. In pithed rats, IQ at 30 and 100 mg/kg (intravenous) significantly blunted both the initial hypertensive and the ensuing hypotensive responses during anaphylaxis. Death rate and tachycardia were also significantly inhibited after the same IQ doses in these rats. In isolated guinea pig hearts, IQ infusion at 30–100 μg/mL markedly reduced anaphylaxis-related coronary flow decrease, contractile force change, and heart rate responses (both tachycardia and arrhythmia). Cardiac histamine and creatine kinase releases were similarly diminished by IQ during anaphylaxis in the isolated guinea pig hearts. In two different isolated guinea pig vasculatures, the pulmonary artery and mesenteric arterial bed, anaphylactic vasoconstriction was reduced by IQ 30 and 100 μg/mL. It was observed that IQ had a marked inhibitory effect on histamine release from rat mast cells, and this mechanism was suggested as the major anti-anaphylactic mechanism. Direct inhibition of histamine-induced muscle contraction did not seem to be relevant, but IQ treatment successfully repressed intracellular calcium influx/depletion in mast cells. Overall, this study provided evidence for the beneficial effect of IQ on cardiac anaphylaxis, thus suggesting its potential applications in the treatment and prevention of related diseases.

Keywords: isoquercitrin; cardiovascular anaphylaxis; rats; guinea pigs; histamine

1. Introduction

Systemic anaphylaxis is a rare but a dramatic and fatal allergic disease with a prevalence of 0.05–2.0% in humans [1]. In anaphylaxis, cardiovascular systems play a critical role, both as a source and a target of various anaphylactoid mediators released during this highly life-threatening episode [2]. Heart functions fail as a result of arrhythmia and coronary vessel constriction, and the systemic blood vessels dilate, leading to worsened blood perfusion [3]. Appropriate pharmacological interventions can lead to an improved prevention and better recovery from anaphylactic symptoms, and natural substances can be good candidates to alleviate the damage arising from anaphylactic symptoms.

Flavonoids are plant-derived polyphenolic substances that are ubiquitously found in numerous herbal medicines, and quercetin is one of the most extensively studied substance of all flavonoids for its beneficial pharmacological activities [4]. However, quercetin (Q) occurs mostly as glycosides rather than in its aglycone form in nature. Typically found examples are quercitrin (Q-3-O-rhamnoside), rutin (Q-3-O-rutinoside), isoquercitrin (Q-3-O-glucoside), and hyperin (Q-3-O-galactoside).

Isoquercitrin (IQ) is frequently found in many plants including onions and numerous medicinal plants [5,6]. IQ was reported to have a variety of pharmacological actions, including anti-oxidant [7], anti-hypertensive [8], anti-cancer [9], and diuretic effects [10]. A few available studies hint the possibility that IQ could exert anti-anaphylactic activity because this glycoside inhibited certain biological processes known to be linked to allergic events [5,11].

In contrast to a wide range of reported beneficial activities of quercetin flavonoids, only limited information circumstantially suggests that IQ might be effective against allergic anaphylaxis. Furthermore, there are almost no studies on the preventive effect of flavonoids against cardiovascular anaphylaxis symptoms. In this study, the beneficial effect of IQ on ovalbumin (OVA)-induced cardiac anaphylaxis was evaluated to provide evidence for its use on allergic anaphylaxis.

2. Materials and Methods

2.1. Test Substance and Reagents

The test substance IQ was purchased from Sigma-Aldrich Inc. (St. Louis, MO, USA) (Product No. 00140585) and dissolved in the physiological buffers used in the in vitro experiments. For intravenous administration of IQ in pithed rats, IQ was dissolved in dimethylsulfoxide (DMSO) (Product No. 472301) and then injected slowly for about 1 min. DMSO ($\geq$ 99.9%) was used for vehicle treatment. All other reagents were also purchased from Sigma-Aldrich Inc.

2.2. Experimental Animals

Rats (specific pathogen-free) and guinea pigs were purchased from Damul Science (Daejon City, Korea) and maintained in rodent chambers at 21 $\pm$ 1 °C and 55 $\pm$ 2% relative humidity. Feeds and drinking water were supplied ad libitum. All experimental protocols involving the use of animals conformed to the NIH guidelines (Guide for the Care and Use of Laboratory Animals, 8th edition). The Animal Care and Use Committee of the Institutional Review Board of Kyung Hee University approved all animal experiments (confirmation number: KHUASP(SE)-12-036, date: 1 May 2016).

2.3. Cardiovascular Anaphylaxis in Pithed Rats

Male Wistar rats (220–250 g) were actively sensitized with 10 mg/head of OVA (turkey OVA, Grade IV) (Product No. SAB4200702) injected intraperitoneally on day 1 and 2, once daily. On day 20, the rats were lightly anesthetized with ethyl ether and a tracheal cannula was placed for artificial respiration (Harvard Apparatus, Holliston, MA, USA), which ran at 60 strokes/min and 1 mL/100 g body weight rates. A pithing rod (round copper 12 cm long, 1.5 mm diameter) was inserted through the right orbit, the brain, and down to the sacral region in the spinal cord. During this process, the brain tissues were maximally destroyed [12]. The right common carotid artery and jugular vein were respectively cannulated with PE-50 cannulae for cardiovascular monitoring and intravenous drug administration. Test substance IQ (dissolved in DMSO) was bolus administered 10 min before intravenous OVA injection (1 mg/rat). Cardiovascular parameters were recorded with a physiography (Letica Polygraph 4006, Barcelona, Spain).

2.4. Anaphylaxis in Isolated Guinea Pig Hearts

Passively sensitized anaphylactic animal models were produced with male Hartley guinea pigs weighing 300–350 g [13]. Anti-OVA serum was administered to naïve guinea pigs, 24 hr before the experiments. The guinea pigs were lightly anesthetized with ethyl ether and the hearts were rapidly removed. An aortic cannula was placed and the heart was setup into a Langendorff heart apparatus for coronary artery perfusion [14]. The hearts were perfused with Krebs-Henseleit solution (in mM, NaCl 118, KCl 4.7, $CaCl_2$ 2.5, $MgSO_4$ 1.6, $NaHCO_3$ 24.9. KH_2PO_4 1.2, glucose 2.5, pH 7.4) under a constant pressure of 60 cm H_2O at 37 °C. The perfusion solution was continuously saturated with 95% O_2–5% CO_2 gas. Cardiac contractility was continuously monitored with a TRI201 isometric transducer (Hugo-Sachs Electronik GmbH, March, Germany). Cardiac anaphylactic response was induced by delivering 1 mg of OVA into the perfusion buffer. When testing the effect of IQ, the IQ-containing buffer was infused to the heart for 10 min before anaphylaxis induction. Cardiac parameters were recorded with a physiography (Letica Polygraph 4006). Coronary effluent was collected at 1-min intervals for flow change monitoring and chemical analyses.

2.5. Anaphylaxis in Isolated Guinea Pig Mesenteric Arterial Beds

Male Hartley guinea pigs were passively sensitized in the same manner as in the isolated heart experiment. Under ether anesthesia, the animal was sacrificed by cervical exanguination and the mesenteric vascular bed was exposed through a midline incision on the abdomen. A stainless cannula was inserted into the superior mesenteric artery via the abdominal aorta. Blood remaining in the mesenteric arterial bed was disposed by perfusing with 20 mL Krebs–Henseleit buffer containing 2000 IU of heparin. The whole arterial bed was carefully isolated, keeping the surrounding arteriole-venule junctions intact [15]. The preparation was maintained in a 50-mL glass container at 37 °C, and continuously perfused with the Krebs-Henseleit buffer (saturated with 95% O_2–5% CO_2, pH 7.4) at 5 mL/min rate. Perfusion pressure was monitored with a pressure transducer (Letica). IQ was infused into the preparation 10 min prior to the OVA (1 mg) challenge.

2.6. Anaphylaxis in Isolated Guinea Pig Pulmonary Artery

From the same guinea pigs that were used for the mesenteric arterial beds, the pulmonary arteries were isolated. Excised artery was cut into ring segments of 2–3 mm. The segments were suspended using two stainless stirrups in a water jacked 10-mL organ bath maintained at 37 °C. Rings were submerged in Krebs–Henseleit buffer (pH 7.4) saturated with 95% O_2–5% CO_2. Constant tension of 1.0 g was applied to the rings and a TRI201 isometric transducer was connected for tension measurements. OVA (1 mg) was applied to the bath to elicit anaphylactic contraction. IQ was exposed to the artery, 10 min prior to anaphylaxis.

2.7. Histamine Release in Rat Peritoneal Mast Cells

Naïve male Wistar rats (250–300 g) were injected with 20 mL of phosphate-buffered saline (mM, NaCl 137, KCl 2.7, $CaCl_2$ 1.8, $MgCl_2$ 1.1, NaH_2PO_4 0.4, $NaHCO_3$ 11.9, glucose 5.5, HEPES 1.0, pH 7.4). The abdomen was gently massaged for a few minutes and the abdominal fluid was obtained. Mast cells were isolated by centrifugation of the fluid (200× g, 5 min) and suspended at 1×10^5 cells/mL, following Percoll density gradient method (Erenbeck and Svensson, 1980). The purity of the mast cells was ≥97%, when determined by a toluidine blue staining. After stabilization at 37 °C, histamine release was evoked by adding either 0.5 µM of compound 48/80 (Product No. C2313) or 1 µM of calcium ionophore A23187 (Product No. C7522). Releases were terminated by freezing the cells following 15-min incubation, in the presence or absence of IQ.

2.8. Antagonism of IQ Against Histamine in Isolated Guinea Pig Guinea Trachea and Ileum

Naïve male Hartley guinea pigs (350–380 g) were used to examine direct effects of IQ on histamine-induced muscle contractions. The tracheal strip was composed of two rings excised with 3 mm width, opened, and sutured together with a silk thread. The preparation was suspended in a 15-mL organ bath maintained at 37 °C [15]. Ring strips were submerged in Krebs–Henseleit buffer (saturated with 95% O_2–% CO_2, pH 7.4) and a resting tension of 500 mg was applied. Distal portion of the ileum was cut at 1.5 cm long and mounted in a 20-mL organ bath kept in the Tyrode's solution at 37 °C [16]. The solution was saturated with 95% O_2–5% CO_2 and 1 g resting tension was applied. Both muscles were exposed to IQ for 10 min, prior to histamine (1 µM) addition. Tension changes were measured with a TRI201 isometric transducer and strip chart recorder.

2.9. Analysis of Histamine Concentration and Creatine Kinase Activity

Histamine concentrations in the buffers of heart perfusion and mast cell incubation were performed [17]. The guinea pig heart perfusate was used directly for the histamine measurements. However, the mast cell culture was centrifuged (2000× g, 5 min, 3 °C) to obtain the medium for the released histamine. Mast cell pellets were boiled for 5 min and then used for intracellular histamine measurements. Released histamine was conjugated with o-phthalaldehyde (Product No. P1378) to produce a fluorescent product, and the fluorescence signals were measured with a fluorometer, at 360 nm excitation wavelengths and 450 nm emission wavelengths. The ratios were calculated from the two values. Creatine kinase activity in the guinea pig heart effluent was assessed using creatine phosphokinase from the rabbit muscle (Product No. C3755), as previously described [15].

2.10. Intracellular Calcium Level Measurement

The intracellular calcium was measured with the use of the fluorescence indicator Fura 2-AM (Product No. F0888). HMC-1 cells (1×10^5 cells) were pre-incubated with Fura 2-AM for 45 min at 37 °C. After being washed to remove the remaining Fura 2-AM, HMC-1 cells were treated with IQ (100 μg/mL) or cromolyn sodium (100 μM) (Product No. 1150502) for 20 min. Intracellular calcium depletion was measured by stimulation with 20 nM of phorbol 12-myristate 13-acetate (PMA) (Product No. P1585) and 1 μM of calcium ionophore A23187 treatment. The intracellular calcium influx was measured by applying calcium in the cell media. The signals were measured with excitation wavelengths of 340 and 380 nm, by a spectrofluorometer FluoroMax®-3 (Horiba Ltd., Kyoto, Japan).

2.11. Statistical Analysis

Data were expressed as mean ± standard error. Statistical significance between groups was analyzed with one-way analysis of variance, followed by Newman-Keul's *t*-test. *p*-values of 0.05 were used for the significance criteria.

3. Results

3.1. IQ Alleviates Cardiovascular Anaphylaxis in Pithed Rats

By pre-treatment with IQ, a dose-related reduction in mortality was noted (Figure 1). A drastic 3.5-fold decrease was observed in 100 mg/kg of IQ when compared to the vehicle-treated control rats. Figure 2 illustrates the effects of IQ on OVA-induced cardiovascular anaphylaxis in sensitized and pithed rats. Administration of 30 and 100 mg/kg IQ, prior to the OVA challenge reduced all functional cardiovascular changes, including the pressor response (Figure 2A), depressor response (Figure 2B), and tachycardia (Figure 2C). However, 10 mg/kg dose did not influence the parameters.

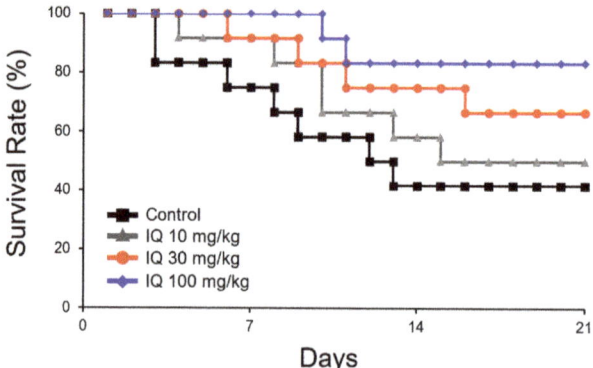

Figure 1. Effect of isoquercitrin (IQ) on mortality caused by cardiovascular anaphylaxis in pithed rats. Male Wistar rats (*n* = 12 per group) were intraperitoneally sensitized with 10 mg/head of ovalbumin (OVA) on day 1 and 2. Survival rate was observed for 20 days. DMSO was used as the control.

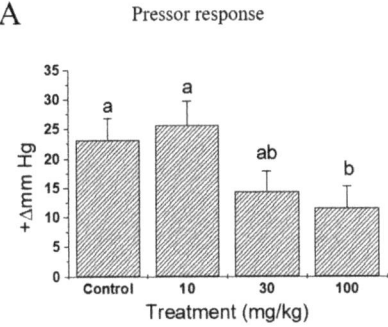
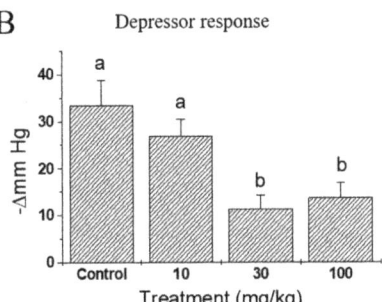
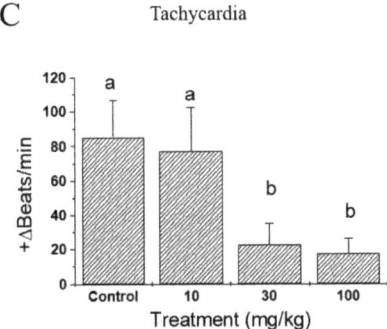

Figure 2. Effects of isoquercitrin (IQ) on cardiovascular anaphylaxis in the pithed rats. Male Wistar rats ($n = 12$ per group) were intraperitoneally sensitized with 10 mg/head of OVA on day 1 and 2. (**A**) Pressor response, (**B**) depressor response, and (**C**) the tachycardia rate were measured in the cardiovascular system of the pithed rats. DMSO was used as control. Different alphabets on the bars denote significantly different means at $p < 0.05$.

3.2. IQ Improves Cardiac Anaphylaxis in Isolated Guinea Pig Heart

As in vivo anti-anaphylactic effects were observed in rats, it was examined whether a similar protective activity was also present at the heart levels. OVA-treated guinea pig heart was selected as an ex vivo approach to evaluate the effect of IQ. In response to OVA, heart rate started to increase (tachycardia) markedly but lasted briefly (< 1 min), then it turned into an irregular rate (arrhythmia), which rarely disappeared during the 20-min observation period (data not shown). Infusion of the test substance IQ before the OVA challenge blunted these anaphylactic responses, i.e., coronary flow, contractility, and tachycardia in a concentration-dependent manner (Figure 3A–C). However, the lowest concentration (IQ 10 µg/mL) was ineffective in most parameters except on contractility changes. In the coronary flow, IQ 10 µg/mL was temporally effective on the recovery phase of flow (8–16 min post-OVA, Figure 3B). Arrhythmia onset time was not delayed by IQ (Figure 3D), however its duration was remarkably reduced by 30 and 100 µg/mL of IQ pre-treatment (Figure 3E).

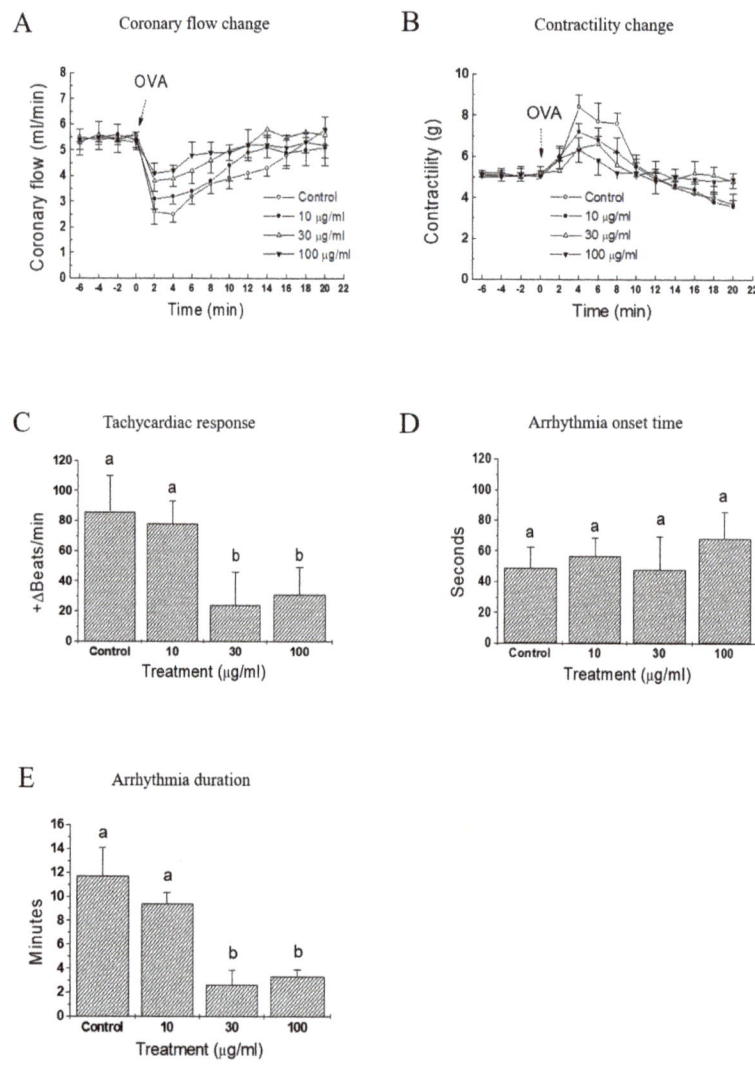

Figure 3. Effects of isoquercitrin (IQ) on cardiac anaphylaxis in isolated guinea pig hearts. (**A**) Coronary flow change, (**B**) contractility change, (**C**) tachycardiac response, (**D**) onset, and (**E**) duration time of arrhythmia were measured in OVA (1 mg)-treated isolated hearts from Hartley guinea pigs ($n = 10$ per group). DMSO was used as the control. Different alphabets on bars denote significantly different means at $p < 0.05$. Statistical significance was not shown for clarity purpose in the coronary flow change and contractility change.

3.3. IQ Ameliorates Anaphylaxis in Isolated Vasculatures of Guinea Pig Heart

Effects of IQ on anaphylactic responses were examined in sensitized isolated guinea pulmonary artery and mesenteric arterial beds (Figure 4). In both preparations, vasoconstrictive responses were monitored and the test substance IQ was effective in significantly blocking OVA-induced vasoconstriction—tension increase in pulmonary artery (Figure 4A) and perfusion pressure increase in mesenteric arterial beds (Figure 4B).

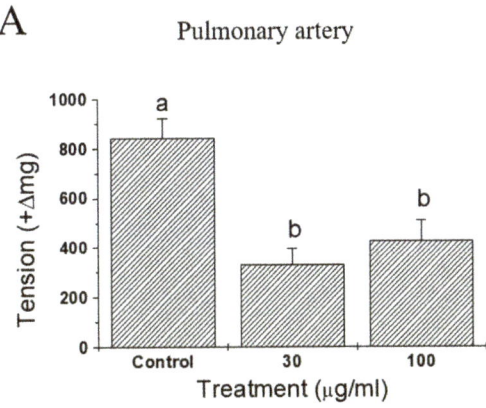

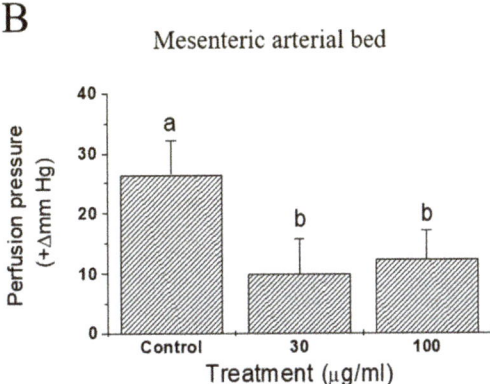

Figure 4. Effects of isoquercitrin (IQ) on anaphylactic responses in isolated guinea pig blood vessels. (**A**) Pulmonary artery tension and (**B**) pressure in mesenteric arterial bed were measured in isolated blood vessels from the Hartley guinea pigs ($n = 7$ per group). DMSO was used as the control. Different alphabets on the bars denote significantly different means at $p < 0.05$.

3.4. IQ Suppresses Histamine and Creatinine Release in Isolated Guinea Pig Heart and Rat Mast Cells

Concomitant with the functional changes that occurred during the anaphylactic event, histamine and creatine kinase levels markedly increased over their baselines. These elevations were also bunted by IQ in a concentration-dependent manner. Effects on creatine kinase activity by IQ was an indication that IQ possessed preventive activities against the myocardial damage occurring in anaphylaxis. As histamine concentration in the coronary effluent decreased by IQ in the isolated heart model, effects of IQ on histamine release was directly examined in the purified rat mast cells. Compound 48/80

(Figure 5C) or ionophore 23187 (Figure 5D) elicited histamine release and this release was significantly reduced by IQ at 30 and 100 µg/mL (>50% inhibition).

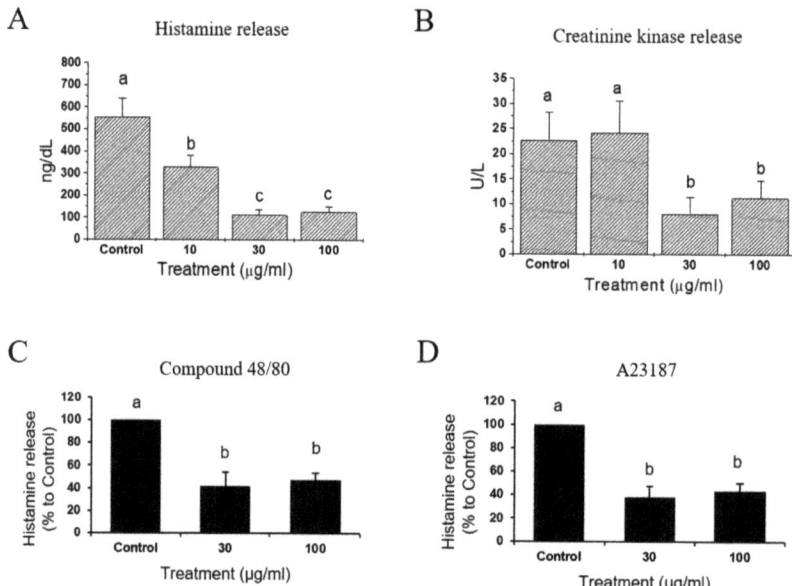

Figure 5. Effects of isoquercitrin (IQ) on histamine and creatinine kinase release. (**A**) Histamine and (**B**) creatinine kinase release were measured in OVA (1 mg)-treated isolated hearts from Hartley guinea pigs (n = 10 per group). Basal histamine and creatine kinase levels were 0–52 ng/dL and 0 IU/L during the resting and the pre-challenge periods, respectively. (**C**) Compound 48/80 (0.5 µM)-induced and (**D**) A23187 (1 µM)-induced histamine release in rat peritoneal mast cells were measured (n = 7 per group). DMSO was used as control. Different alphabets on the bars denoted significantly different means at $p < 0.05$.

3.5. IQ Did not Affect Direct Muscle Contraction by Histamine in Tissues Isolated from Guinea Pig

To examine if the test compound exerted direct inhibition on histamine, effects of IQ on histamine-induced contraction were assessed in the trachea and ileum of guinea pigs (Figure 6A and B). Surprisingly, IQ was not effective or were only marginally effective (significant inhibition with 100 µg/mL in trachea, $p = 0.04$) in influencing contractile responses in both of these muscle preparations.

3.6. IQ Stabilizes Mast Cells and Inhibits OVA-Stimulated Intracellular Calcium Release

Since IQ did not protect muscles from histamine stimulation but did inhibit histamine release, we next evaluated its effect on intracellular calcium levels. As shown in Figure 7, positive control cromolyn sodium inhibited calcium depletion caused by PMA + A23187 in HMC-1 cells. Similar results were observed by pre-treatment with IQ, and in addition, both cromolyn sodium and IQ suppressed calcium influx in mast cells as well.

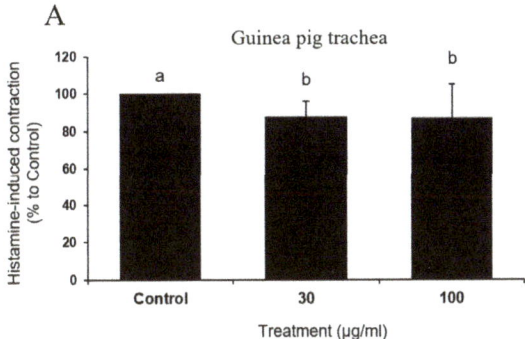
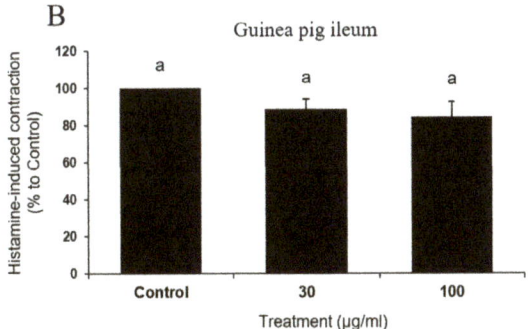

Figure 6. Effects of isoquercitrin (IQ) on histamine-induced muscle contractions. Histamine (1 µM)-induced muscle contraction in (**A**) trachea and (**B**) ileum tissues were measured ($n = 5$ per group). DMSO was used as the control. Different alphabets on the bars denote significantly different means at $p < 0.05$.

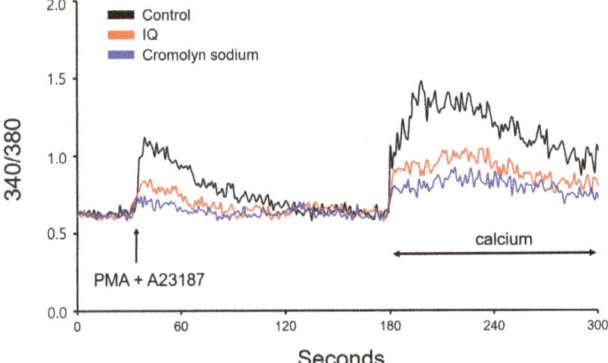

Figure 7. Effects of isoquercitrin (IQ) on PMA + A23187-induced intracellular calcium levels in HMC-1 cells. Intracellular calcium levels were measured for 300 s. PMA (20 nM) and A23187 (1 µM) was used to stimulate the HMC-1 cells. DMSO was used as a control.

4. Discussion

Pithed rats in the anaphylaxis study showed an advantage in the assessment of the overall cardiovascular changes under silent conditions, without the participation of compensatory reflex adjustments [12]. Anaphylactic responses in this in vivo animal model were characterized as a brief increase in blood pressure (pressor response), followed by a gradual decline (depressor response) that frequently led to death [12,15]. Heart rates increased (tachycardia) markedly and sustained at the elevated levels for several minutes. When IQ was treated at 10, 30, and 100 mg/kg, the treatment did not only decrease the overall mortality (Figure 1), but also alleviated pressure/depressor response and tachycardia in pithed rats (Figure 2), suggesting a dose-dependent improvement on cardiac anaphylaxis.

When the antigen OVA was injected into pre-sensitized, isolated guinea pig hearts, immediate and dramatic cardiac functional changes occurred [18]. Namely, the coronary flow diminished markedly and the contractile force increased initially (in about 2 min post-OVA challenge in this study), then both of these changes gradually returned to pre-challenge values. IQ pretreatment suppressed OVA-induced anaphylactic responses, including coronary flow, contractility, tachycardia, and duration of arrhythmia (Figure 3). These results clearly suggest the beneficial intervention of IQ during OVA-induced cardiac anaphylaxis. Moreover, when sensitized isolated guinea pulmonary artery and mesenteric arterial beds were used in the same manner as that of OVA treatment, IQ significantly reduced the tension or perfusion pressure in these two isolated vasculatures (Figure 4). These data had a meaning that it was possible to confirm the anti-anaphylactic activity of IQ at isolated blood vessel levels—the isolated pulmonary artery as a representative large vessel and the mesenteric arterial bed as a capillary blood vessel.

Dramatic functional changes in cardiac anaphylaxis were well-described [19] and such reactions reflected the biological actions of endogenous mediators released from cardiac tissues [20]. By IQ treatment of 10, 30, and 100 µg/mL in isolated guinea pig hearts and 30 and 100 µg/mL in primary cultured rat mast cells, histamine release by OVA (guinea pig heart) or Compound 48/80 and A23187 (rat mast cell) were significantly suppressed (Figure 5). While the release of histamine, an important anaphylactic mediator [19], was reduced by IQ at 10 µg/mL, this concentration failed to reduce creatine kinase output in the coronary effluent. Such discrepancy might be explained by the fact that histamine is not the only anaphylactic mediator in hearts [3]. However, in cardiovascular anaphylaxis, histamine is known to play the most important role, although other mast cell-derived mediators such as leukotrienes, platelet-activating factor, thromboxane A_2, and 5-hydroxytryptamine are also involved [21,22]. Thus, it is not unreasonable to assume that IQ could inhibit the release of other mediators in addition to histamine. Further study must evaluate the changes in such mediators in order to verify the specific action mechanism of IQ besides histamine. Notably, IQ did not affect the histamine-induced changes in guinea pig trachea/ileum (Figure 6), implying that most part of the anti-anaphylactic activities can be ascribed to inhibition of mediator release. IQ is known to directly antagonize leukotriene D_4- and carbachol-induced tracheal muscle contractions but not those induced by histamine [5].

Intracellular calcium is known to be the most important pathway of histamine release in mast cells [23]. Thus, mast cell stabilizers such as cromolyn sodium or nedocromil [24] work by blocking a calcium channel that is essential for the degranulation of mast cells. Since IQ treatment showed beneficial effects in cardiac anaphylaxis but could not repress muscle contraction through direct histamine treatment, another logical approach might be to check its effect on mast cell stabilization. The results in Figure 7 indicate that IQ exerts such effect at a similar level to cromolyn sodium, a widely used mast cell stabilizer [25]. Though a direct comparison on histamine-related anaphylaxis was not provided, the data suggests that IQ possesses the potential efficacy as a conventionally used medication for allergic responses. In addition, confirming the effect of IQ along with several anti-anaphylactic agents (adrenalines, H1 antihistamine, glucocorticosteroid, etc.) [26] would provide important information and might justify the application of IQ.

This study demonstrated that IQ is active against cardiovascular anaphylaxis not only in the whole animal, but also in isolated hearts or vessels. However, this study indeed had its own limitations. The action mechanism of IQ seemed to be the inhibition of histamine, the most important anaphylactic mediator, from mast cells although additional minor mechanism(s) are still unknown. There are some reports that suggest the possibility that quercetin or quercetin glycosides could be anti-allergic [27–29].

While most biological activities are attributable to the aglycone form quercetin, its glycoside IQ was more potent than quercetin in some pharmacological effects [6,30]. Yet, because there are several pathways in the upstream channel of histamine release, such as the Fc epsilon receptor pathway or IgE and interleukins [31: Respir Med. 2012 Jan; 106(1):9–14.], extensive investigation regarding the action mechanism of IQ must be carried out. Whether IQ regulated these signaling pathways was not fully elucidated in this study but rather proved the sole fact that IQ suppressed histamine release from mast cells and thus improved cardiac anaphylaxis. More importantly, effect on the mast cell-derived mediators that drive allergic reactions after degranulation, besides histamine, should be confirmed as well, before being accepted as an anti-anaphylaxis agent, at least provisionally.

In summary, as cardiovascular anaphylaxis is a highly detrimental allergic episode that could result in fatal consequences in humans, exploring phytochemical candidates against this disease would be meaningful. Being ubiquitously present in nature and widely consumed through diets, IQ deserves further investigation for invention of a preventive measure against cardiovascular anaphylaxis.

Author Contributions: Conceptualization, J.P.; methodology, J.P.; software, J.P.; validation, J.P.; formal analysis, J.P.; investigation, J.P.; resources, J.P.; data curation, J.P.; writing—original draft preparation, J.P.; writing—review and editing, J.P.; visualization, J.P.; project administration, J.P.; funding acquisition, J.P. All authors have read and agreed to the published version of the manuscript.

Funding: This research was funded by the National Research Foundation of Korea (NRF), grant number NRF-2020R1C1C1009721.

Conflicts of Interest: The author declares no conflict of interest.

References

1. Lieberman, P.; Camargo, C.A., Jr.; Bohlke, K.; Jick, H.; Miller, R.L.; Sheikh, A.; Simons, F.E.R. Epidemiology of anaphylaxis: Findings of the American College of Allergy, Asthma, and Immunology Epidemiology of Anaphylaxis Working Group. *Ann. Allergy Asthma Immunol.* **2006**, *97*, 596–602. [CrossRef] [PubMed]
2. Lucke, W.C.; Thomas, H. Anaphylaxis: Pathophysiology, clinical presentations, and treatment. *J. Emerg. Med.* **1983**, *1*, 83–95. [CrossRef]
3. Triggiani, M.; Patella, V.; Staiano, R.I.; Granata, F.; Marone, G. Allergy and the cardiovascular system. *Clin. Exp. Immunol.* **2008**, *153*, 7–11. [CrossRef] [PubMed]
4. Formica, J.; Regelson, W. Review of the biology of quercetin and related bioflavonoids. *Food Chem. Toxicol.* **1995**, *33*, 1061–1080. [CrossRef]
5. Fernández, J.; Reyes, R.; Ponce, H.; Oropeza, M.; van Calsteren, M.-R.; Jankowski, C.; Campos, M.G.; Reyes-Chilpa, R. Isoquercitrin from Argemone platyceras inhibits carbachol and leukotriene D4-induced contraction in guinea-pig airways. *Eur. J. Pharmacol.* **2005**, *522*, 108–115. [CrossRef]
6. Silva, C.; Raulino, R.; Cerqueira, D.; Mannarino, S.; Pereira, M.; Panek, A.; Silva, J.; Menezes, F.; Eleutherio, E.C.A. In vitro and in vivo determination of antioxidant activity and mode of action of isoquercitrin and Hyptis fasciculata. *Phytomedicine* **2009**, *16*, 761–767. [CrossRef]
7. Jung, S.H.; Kim, B.J.; Lee, E.H.; Osborne, N.N. Isoquercitrin is the most effective antioxidant in the plant Thuja orientalis and able to counteract oxidative-induced damage to a transformed cell line (RGC-5 cells). *Neurochem. Int.* **2010**, *57*, 713–721. [CrossRef]
8. Junior, A.G.; Junior, A.G.; Lourenço, E.L.B.; Crestani, S.; Stefanello, M.; Élida, A.; Salvador, M.; da Silva-Santos, J.E.; Marques, M.C.A.; Kassuya, C.A.L. Antihypertensive effects of isoquercitrin and extracts from Tropaeolum majus L.: Evidence for the inhibition of angiotensin converting enzyme. *J. Ethnopharmacol.* **2011**, *134*, 363–372. [CrossRef]
9. Amado, N.G.; Cerqueira, D.M.; Menezes, F.S.; da Silva, J.F.M.; Neto, V.M.; Abreu, J.G. Isoquercitrin isolated from Hyptis fasciculata reduces glioblastoma cell proliferation and changes β-catenin cellular localization. *Anti-Cancer Drugs* **2009**, *20*, 543–552. [CrossRef]
10. Junior, A.G.; Prando, T.B.L.; Leme, T.D.S.V.; Junior, A.G.; Lourenço, E.L.B.; Rattmann, Y.D.; Da Silva-Santos, J.E.; Kassuya, C.A.L.; Marques, M.C.A. Mechanisms underlying the diuretic effects of Tropaeolum majus L. extracts and its main component isoquercitrin. *J. Ethnopharmacol.* **2012**, *141*, 501–509. [CrossRef]

11. Itoh, T.; Ohguchi, K.; Nakajima, C.; Oyama, M.; Iinuma, M.; Nozawa, Y.; Akao, Y.; Ito, M. Inhibitory effects of flavonoid glycosides isolated from the peel of Japanese persimmon (Diospyros kaki Fuyu) on antigen-stimulated degranulation in rat basophilic leukaemia RBL-2H3 cells. *Food Chem.* **2011**, *126*, 289–294. [CrossRef]
12. Park, H.-H.; Lee, S.; Son, H.-Y.; Park, S.-B.; Kim, M.-S.; Choi, E.-J.; Singh, T.S.K.; Ha, J.-H.; Lee, M.-G.; Kim, J.-E.; et al. Flavonoids inhibit histamine release and expression of proinflammatory cytokines in mast cells. *Arch. Pharmacal Res.* **2008**, *31*, 1303–1311. [CrossRef] [PubMed]
13. Park, K.H.; Koh, D.; Kim, K.; Park, J.; Lim, Y. Antiallergic activity of a disaccharide isolated fromSanguisorba of? Cinalis. *Phytotherapy Res.* **2004**, *18*, 658–662. [CrossRef] [PubMed]
14. Park, K.H.; Rubin, L.E.; Gross, S.S.; Levi, R. Nitric oxide is a mediator of hypoxic coronary vasodilatation. Relation to adenosine and cyclooxygenase-derived metabolites. *Circ. Res.* **1992**, *71*, 992–1001. [CrossRef] [PubMed]
15. Lee, H.-S.; Park, K.-H.; Kwon, K.-B.; Mun, B.-S.; Song, C.-M.; Song, Y.-S.; Seo, E.-A.; Kim, Y.-S.; Kim, K.-J.; Ryu, -G. Anti-allergic Activity of the Sophorae Radix Water Extract in Experimental Animals. *Am. J. Chin. Med.* **2001**, *29*, 129–139. [CrossRef] [PubMed]
16. Park, K.H.; Long, J.P.; Cannon, J.G. Effects of serotonin1-like receptor agonists on autonomic neurotransmission. *Can. J. Physiol. Pharmacol.* **1991**, *69*, 1855–1860. [CrossRef] [PubMed]
17. Shore, P.; Burkhalter, A.; Cohn, V.H. A method for the fluorometric assay of histamine in tissues. *J. Pharmacol. Exp. Ther.* **1959**, *127*, 182–186.
18. Xu, F.; Zhuang, J.; Zhou, T.; Lee, L.-Y. Ovalbumin sensitization alters the ventilatory responses to chemical challenges in guinea pigs. *J. Appl. Physiol.* **2005**, *99*, 1782–1788. [CrossRef]
19. del Balzo, U.; Polley, M.J.; Levi, R. Cardiac anaphylaxis. Complement activation as an amplification system. *Circ. Res.* **1989**, *65*, 847–857. [CrossRef]
20. Feigen, G.; Prager, D.J. Experimental cardiac anaphylaxis. Physiologic, pharmacologic, and biochemical aspects of immune reactions in the isolated heart. *Am. J. Cardiol.* **1969**, *24*, 474–491. [CrossRef]
21. Levi, R.; Burke, J.; Corey, E.J. SRS-A, leukotrienes, and immediate hypersensitivity reactions of the heart. *Adv. Prostaglandin Thromboxane Leukot. Res.* **1982**, *9*, 215–222. [PubMed]
22. Vleeming, W.; van Rooij, H.H.; Werner, J.; Porsius, A.J. Characterization and Modulation of Antigen-Induced Effects in Isolated Rat Heart. *J. Cardiovasc. Pharmacol.* **1991**, *18*, 556–565. [CrossRef] [PubMed]
23. MacGlashan, D. Histamine. *J. Allergy Clin. Immunol.* **2003**, *112*, 53–59. [CrossRef]
24. Castillo, M.; Scott, N.; Mustafa, M.; Mustafa, M.S.; Azuara-Blanco, A. Topical antihistamines, and mast cell stabilisers for treating seasonal and perennial allergic conjunctivitis. *Cochrane Database Syst. Rev.* **2015**, *6*. [CrossRef]
25. Liao, C.-H.; Akazawa, H.; Tamagawa, M.; Ito, K.; Yasuda, N.; Kudo, Y.; Yamamoto, R.; Ozasa, Y.; Fujimoto, M.; Wang, P.; et al. Cardiac mast cells cause atrial fibrillation through PDGF-A–mediated fibrosis in pressure-overloaded mouse hearts. *J. Clin. Investig.* **2010**, *120*, 242–253. [CrossRef]
26. Ring, J.; Beyer, K.; Biedermann, T.; Bircher, A.; Duda, D.; Fischer, J.; Friedrichs, F.; Fuchs, T.; Gieler, U.; Jakob, T.; et al. Guideline for acute therapy and management of anaphylaxis. *Allergo J. Int.* **2014**, *23*, 96–112. [CrossRef]
27. Kahraman, A.; Erkasap, N.; Köken, T.; Serteser, M.; Aktepe, F.; Erkasap, S. The antioxidative and antihistaminic properties of quercetin in ethanol-induced gastric lesions. *Toxicology* **2003**, *183*, 133–142. [CrossRef]
28. Cruz, E.; Da-Silva, S.; Muzitano, M.; Silva, P.; Costa, S.S.; Rossi-Bergmann, B. Immunomodulatory pretreatment with Kalanchoe pinnata extract and its quercitrin flavonoid effectively protects mice against fatal anaphylactic shock. *Int. Immunopharmacol.* **2008**, *8*, 1616–1621. [CrossRef]
29. Matsumoto, T.; Horiuchi, M.; Kamata, K.; Seyama, Y. Effects of Bidens pilosa L. var. radiata SCHERFF treated with enzyme on histamine-induced contraction of guinea pig ileum and on histamine release from mast cells. *J. Smooth Muscle Res.* **2009**, *45*, 75–86. [CrossRef]
30. Kim, H.Y.; Yoon, J.H.; Yokozawa, T.; Sakata, K.; Lee, S. Protective activity of flavonoid and flavonoid glycosides against glucose-mediated protein damage. *Food Chem.* **2011**, *126*, 892–895. [CrossRef]

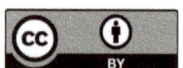 © 2020 by the author. Licensee MDPI, Basel, Switzerland. This article is an open access article distributed under the terms and conditions of the Creative Commons Attribution (CC BY) license (http://creativecommons.org/licenses/by/4.0/).

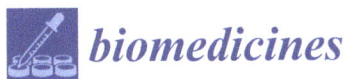

Article

β-Caryophyllene Reduces the Inflammatory Phenotype of Periodontal Cells by Targeting CB2 Receptors

Giacomo Picciolo [1,†], Giovanni Pallio [2,†], Domenica Altavilla [1], Mario Vaccaro [2], Giacomo Oteri [1], Natasha Irrera [2] and Francesco Squadrito [2,3,*]

1. Department of Biomedical, Dental, Morphological and Functional Imaging Sciences, University of Messina, Via C. Valeria, 98125 Messina, Italy; giacomopicciolo94@gmail.com (G.P.); daltavilla@unime.it (D.A.); oterig@unime.it (G.O.)
2. Department of Clinical and Experimental Medicine, University of Messina, Via C. Valeria, 98125 Messina, Italy; gpallio@unime.it (G.P.); vaccaro@unime.it (M.V.); nirrera@unime.it (N.I.)
3. SunNutraPharma, Academic Spin-Off Company of the University of Messina, Via C. Valeria, 98125 Messina, Italy
* Correspondence: fsquadrito@unime.it; Tel.: +39-0902213648
† These authors contributed equally to this work.

Received: 20 May 2020; Accepted: 15 June 2020; Published: 17 June 2020

Abstract: Human gingival fibroblasts (GF) and human oral mucosa epithelial cells (EC) with an inflammatory phenotype represent a valuable experimental paradigm to explore the curative activity of agents to be used in oral mucositis. The role of cannabinoid receptor 2 (CB2) has not yet been investigated in oral mucositis. The aim of this study was to evaluate the therapeutic potential of β-Caryophyllene (BCP), a CB2 agonist, in an in vitro model of oral mucositis. GF and EC were stimulated with LPS (2 µg/mL) alone or in combination with BCP; a group of LPS challenged GF and EC were treated with BCP and AM630, a CB2 antagonist. LPS increased the inflammatory cytokines TNF-α, IL-1β, IL-6 and IL-17A whereas it decreased the anti-inflammatory cytokine IL-13. The upstream signals were identified in an augmented expression of NF-κB and STAT-3 and in reduced mRNA levels of PPARγ and PGC-1α. BCP blunted the LPS-induced inflammatory phenotype and this effect was reverted by the CB2 antagonist AM630. These results suggest that CB2 receptors are an interesting target to develop innovative strategies for oral mucositis and point out that BCP exerts a marked curative effect in a preclinical model of oral mucositis which deserves to be confirmed in a clinical setting.

Keywords: β-Caryophyllene; CB2 receptors; inflammation; oral mucositis; periodontitis

1. Introduction

Oral mucositis (OM) is a clinical condition characterized by a marked inflammatory reaction that results in erythematous lesions, ulcers, dysphagia and inability to afford and ensure a physiological calories intake that ultimately leads to interrupting life-saving treatments in cancer patients [1–4]. Oral mucositis may also complicate and/or be a clinical manifestation of peri-implantitis a common complication of dental implants, showing a prevalence of at least 20% in patients that have undergone this surgical procedure [5–8]. As a direct consequence of this tremendous impact on public health, there is an urgent need to identify the exact physiopathology of this condition in order to facilitate the design of rational therapeutic strategies to cure this complication.

Indeed, the mechanism underlying oral mucositis has been, at least in part, clarified. Whatever the triggering event, either DNA damage as in the case of chemotherapy/radiation therapy or infectious stimuli and progressive bone loss as in peri-implantitis [9,10], a common pathway converges in an exaggerated production of reactive oxygen species (ROS) released by both epithelial cells and gingival fibroblasts [11]. In fact, ROS boosts the translocation to the nucleus of Nuclear Factor Kappa B (NF-κB) [12]. Once it reaches the nucleus, the transcription factor turns on genes that codify for inflammatory cytokines such as Tumor Necrosis Factor (TNF-α), Interleukin 1 beta (IL-1β) and IL-6; moreover at the same time, it silences genes priming anti-inflammatory signals, in particular IL-13 and the nuclear receptor called peroxisome proliferator-activated receptor gamma (PPAR-γ) [13,14]. Indeed, this NF-κB primed cytokine storm may be considered an important arm of the acute phase response, but it has also been reported to have a key role in driving the second wave of the acute response in mammals. This second step of the inflammatory cascade is a crucial phenomenon that, at least at the beginning, is positive and reinforces the host immune and inflammatory response. The master regulator of this second step of host response to inflammatory injury is the Signal Transducer and Activator of Transcription (STAT) 3 [12]. STAT3 belongs to the seven-member family of proteins that cause the transduction of hormonal information from the cell membrane to the nucleus. STAT3 primes the formation of T helper 2 (Th2) cells that release a large number of Th2 derived cytokines including IL-17A. Activation of STAT3 is induced by several hormones, being the best studied and analyzed the components of the IL-6 group of cytokines. More specifically IL-6 has been shown to cause a robust activation of STAT3, representing this molecular event either the triggering of the second phase and the pathophysiological link between the first wave and the second wave of the host immune-inflammatory reaction. However, if the second wave of the inflammatory response is not appropriately modulated, a transition may occur into a maladaptive response that transforms acute inflammation into a chronic inflammatory condition that is responsible for several disabling diseases.

Therefore, pharmacological modulation of either the first phase or the second phase of the host inflammatory response is a rational strategy for the treatment of oral mucositis.

Relevant bioassays are therefore needed to facilitate the preclinical screening of candidate molecules. In this context, human gingival fibroblasts (GF) and human oral mucosa epithelial cells (EC) with an inflammatory phenotype represent a valuable experimental paradigm to explore the potential curative activity of agents to be used in this clinical condition [15]. LPS boosts an inflammatory cascade that plays a pivotal role in the pathogenesis of this unpleasant disease. Indeed, LPS belongs to the pathogen associated molecular patterns (PAMPs) family, a group of molecules that orchestrate an exaggerated immune-inflammatory response. Therefore, LPS stimulation of epithelial cells and gingival fibroblasts is an appropriate model to study in vitro oral mucositis.

The endocannabinoid system has two classical receptors: the cannabinoid receptor of type 1 (CB1) and the cannabinoid receptor of type 2 (CB2). While the CB1 mediates the classical psychotropic effects, the CB2 is expressed in the immune system and exerts anti-inflammatory effects [16]. The endocannabinoid system, through the CB2 receptor, has a fundamental role in the modulation of the inflammatory signals during pathological conditions such as osteoarthritis and rheumatoid arthritis. CB2 receptor activation inhibits upstream and downstream molecules of the inflammatory process. In addition, stimulation of the CB2 receptors exerts analgesic activity that might be of clinical relevance in the management of patients suffering from oral mucositis. All these experimental evidences clearly suggest that the type 2 cannabinoid receptor is strategical for a rational innovative drug design. However, no study so far has investigated the hypothesis of targeting the CB2 receptor to modulate the inflammatory cascade that occurs in oral mucositis.

β-caryophyllene (BCP) is a Food Drug Administration (FDA) approved natural compound that engages cannabinoid CB2 receptors and causes anti-inflammatory and analgesic effects [17]. The aim of this study was to evaluate the therapeutic potential of BCP in an "in vitro" experimental paradigm of oral mucositis.

2. Materials and Methods

2.1. Cell Cultures

Human primary gingival fibroblasts (atcc-pcs-pcs201-018) and human oral mucosa epithelial cells (cticc1.8.3 sk0251) were obtained from LGC Standards S.r.l Milan, Italy and Clinisciences s.r.l. Rome, Italy, respectively. Cells were put in culture in a medium made by DMEM, 10% fetal calf serum, 1% antibiotic mixture and incubated at 37 °C with 5% of CO_2. AM630 was put in the cell culture 2 h before BCP. Cells and cell supernatants were collected following an incubation of 4 h with all the substances.

2.2. Treatments of Cells

GF and EC cells were cultured in six well culture plates at a density of 2.5×10^5 cells/well and were challenged with LPS (2 µg/mL; Escherichia coli serotype 055:B5; Sigma-Aldric, Milan, Italy) alone or with BCP (Sanherb Biotech Inc., China) at the dose of 10 µg/mL. A previous study showed that this dose represents the IC50 of the biomolecule at least in the experimental paradigm of LPS stimulated human chondrocytes and considering IL-1β as readout of this bioassay [18]. Furthermore, a set of LPS challenged GF and EC cells were treated with BCP (10 µg/mL) and AM630 (100 nM; Sigma-Aldric, Milan, Italy), an antagonist of the CB2 receptor. AM630 was added 2 h before BCP treatment. Cells were harvested after a 4 h of incubation with several treatments.

2.3. MTT Assay

Cell viability was evaluated by MTT assay. GF and EC cells were grown and then treated with LPS (2 µg/mL), LPS + BCP (10 µg/mL), LPS + BCP +AM630 (100 nM), when it reached confluence. In particular, LPS, LPS + BCP and LPS + BCP + AM360 were tested in a 96-well plate at a density of 8×10^4 cells/well for 24 h to evaluate the cytotoxic effect. The tetrazolium dye MTT 3-(4,5-dimethylthiazol-2-yl)-2,5-diphenyltetrazolium bromide (Sigma Aldrich, Milan, Italy) was dissolved in sterile filtered PBS, and 20 µL of the mixture were added into each well 5 h before the end of the 24 h of incubation. Medium was removed and the insoluble formazan crystals were dissolved with dimethyl sulfoxide (DMSO; 200 µL/well) following 5 h. The difference between the values obtained at 540 and 620 nm of absorbance was used to calculate the average of replicates and to evaluate cytotoxicity. Results were expressed as % of cell viability compared to untreated cells and reported as means and SD.

2.4. Measurements of Cytokines by Enzyme-Linked Immunosorbent Assay (ELISA)

TNF-α, IL-1β, IL-13, IL-6 and IL-17A were measured in the cell supernatants. The cytokines under investigation were evaluated using Enzyme-Linked Immunosorbent Assay (ELISA) kits (Abcam, Cambridge, UK) in agreement with the instructions reported by the manufacturer. All the samples were evaluated in duplicate and the obtained results were interpolated with the pertinent standard curves. To evaluate the sample, the means of the duplicated sample were used and expressed in pg/mL [19,20].

2.5. Real Time Quantitative PCR Amplification (RTqPCR)

Total RNA was extracted from GF and EC cells for RTqPCR using Trizol LS Reagent (Invitrogen, Carlsbad, CA, USA). Two micrograms of total RNA was reverse transcribed in a final volume of 20 µL using a Superscript VILO kit (Invitrogen). cDNA (1 µL) was added to the EvaGreen qPCR Master Mix (Biotium Inc., Fremont, CA, USA) (20 µL per well). The final primer concentration selected to perform the analysis was 10 µM. Samples were run in duplicate and β-actin was used as an endogenous control. Results were calculated using the $2^{-\Delta\Delta CT}$ method and expressed as n-fold increase in gene expression using the CTRL group as the calibrator [21]. Primers used for targets and reference genes are listed in Table 1.

Table 1. Primer list.

Gene	Sequence
β-actin	Fw:5′AGAGCTACGAGCTGCCTGAC3′
	Rw:5′AGCACTGTGTTGGCGTACAG3′
TNF-α	Fw:5′CAGAGGGCCTGTACCTCATC3′
	Rw:5′GGAAGACCCCTCCCAGATAG3′
IL-1β	Fw:5′TGAGCTCGCCAGTGAAATGA3′
	Rw:5′AGATTCGTAGCTGGATGCCG3′
IL-13	Fw:5′CATGGCGCTTTTGTTGACCA 3′
	Rw:5′AGCTGTCAGGTTGATGCTCC3′
NF-κB	Fw:5′CCTGGATGACTCTTGGGAAA3′
	Rw:5′TCAGCCAGCTGTTTCATGTC3′
PPAR-γ	Fw:5′TCGACCAGCTGAATCCAGAG3′
	Rw:5′GGGGGTGATGTGTTTGAACTTG3′
PGC-1α	Fw:5′CATGTGCAACCAGGACTCTGA3′
	Rw:5 GCGCATCAAATGAGGGCAAT3′
STAT3	Fw:5′GAGCTGCACCTGATCACCTT3′
	Rw:5′CCCAGAAGGAGAAGCCCTTG3′
IL-6	Fw:5′TTCGGTCCAGTTGCCTTCTC3′
	Rw:5′CAGCTCTGGCTTGTTCCTCA3′
IL-17A	Fw:5′CTGTCCCCATCCAGCAAGAG3′
	Rw:5′AGGCCACATGGTGGACAATC3′

2.6. Statistical Analysis

Results were statistically analyzed calculating standard deviation (SD). Data are expressed as the mean ± SD and the values reported are the results of at least five experiments performed in duplicate. All assays were repeated three times to ensure reproducibility. The different groups were compared and analyzed using one-way ANOVA with a Tukey post-test for comparison between the different groups. A p value < 0.05 was considered significant. Graphs were prepared using GraphPad Prism (version 5.0 for Windows, San Diego, CA, USA).

3. Results

3.1. BCP Reverts the Inflammatory Phenotype Induced by LPS in Gingival Fibroblasts and Oral Mucosa Epithelial Cells

LPS challenge resulted in a marked expression of TNF-α and IL-1β with a concomitant reduced mRNA of IL-13 in both gingival fibroblasts and oral mucosa epithelial cells (p < 0.0001 vs. CTRL; Figure 1). To confirm the full induction of the inflammatory phenotype, we measured the mature proteins in the cell supernatants. TNF-α and IL-1β were markedly increased, while IL-13 significantly diminished in the supernatants of GF and EC cells (p < 0.0001 vs. CTRL; Figure 2). BCP incubation in LPS stimulated GF and EC cells suppressed the increased mRNA for the inflammatory cytokines TNF-α and IL-1β and caused a marked enhancement in the expression of the message of the anti-inflammatory cytokine IL-13 (p < 0.0001 vs. LPS; Figure 1). Overlapping results were observed when mature proteins were used as readouts (p < 0.0001 vs. LPS; Figure 2). To dissect out the role of the CB2 receptors in the effect of BCP, we performed experiments in which a specific antagonist of this receptor subtype (AM630) was added in cell culture 2 h before BCP. Blockade of the CB2 receptor reverted the positive effect of the biomolecule on the inflammatory phenotype (Figures 1 and 2).

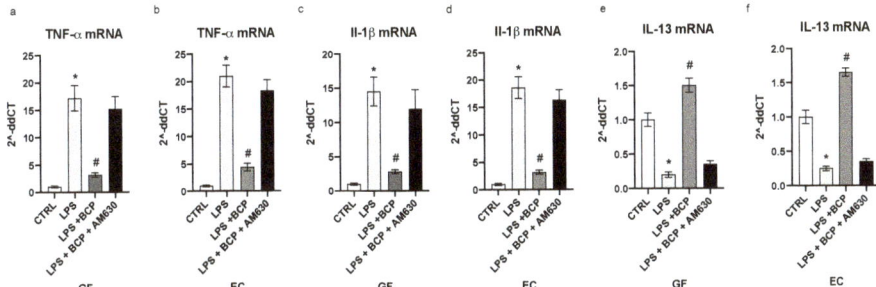

Figure 1. The graphs represent qPCR results of TNF-α (**a**), IL-1β (**c**), IL-13 (**e**) mRNA expression from GF cells and TNF-α (**b**), IL-1β (**d**), IL-13 (**f**) mRNA expression from EC cells. Values are expressed as the means and SD. * $p < 0.0001$ vs. CTRL; # $p < 0.0001$ vs. LPS.

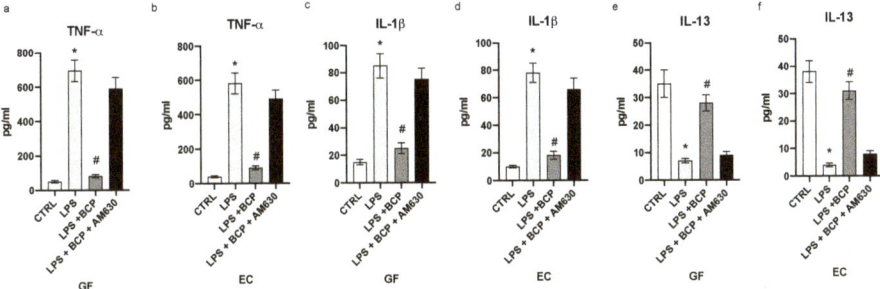

Figure 2. The graphs represent the levels of TNF-α (**a**), IL-1β (**c**) and IL-10 (**e**) in cell supernatants from GF cells and TNF-α (**b**), IL-1β (**d**), IL-13 (**f**) levels in cell supernatants from EC cells. Levels of cytokines were evaluated by immunosorbent assay (ELISA). Values are expressed as the means and SD. * $p < 0.0001$ vs. CTRL; # $p < 0.0001$ vs. LPS.

3.2. BCP Modulates Upstream Signals that Trigger the First Phase of the Inflammatory Response

The transcription factor NF-κB was markedly induced by the LPS challenge in both human gingival fibroblasts and oral mucosa epithelial cells ($p < 0.0001$ vs. CTRL; Figure 3a,b). BCP treatment in GF and EC cells suppressed the mRNA for the transcription factor and this effect was abrogated by AM630, a specific antagonist of CB2 receptors ($p < 0.0001$ vs. LPS; Figure 3a,b). LPS also produced a diminished PPARγ and PGC-1α expression in gingival fibroblasts ($p < 0.0001$ vs. CTRL; Figure 3c,e) and epithelial cells ($p < 0.0001$ vs CTRL; Figure 3d,f). BCP treatment prompted a marked enhancement in the expression of both the nuclear receptor and its co-activator when compared to cell cultures challenged with LPS alone ($p < 0.0001$ vs. LPS; Figure 3c–f). The antagonist of the CB2 receptor AM630 reverted the effects of BCP in GF and EC cells (Figure 3).

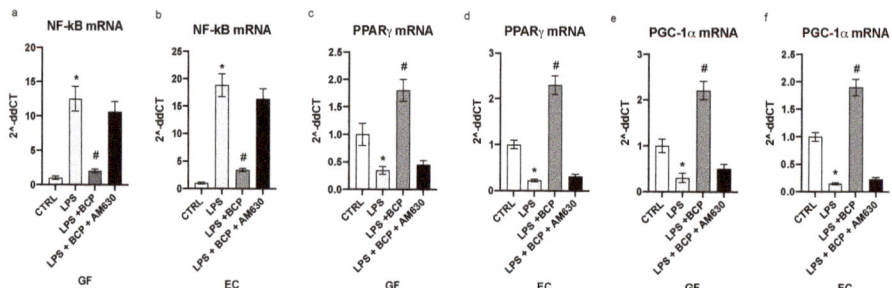

Figure 3. The graphs represent the qPCR results of NF-kB (**a**), PPARγ (**c**), PGC1α (**e**) mRNA expression from GF cells and NF-kB (**b**), PPARγ (**d**), PGC1α (**f**) mRNA expression from EC cells. Values are expressed as the means and SD. * $p < 0.0001$ vs. CTRL; # $p < 0.0001$ vs. LPS.

3.3. BCP Halts the Second Phase of the Inflammatory Response in Gingival Fibroblasts and Oral Mucosa Epithelial Cells

STAT-3 serves as a pathophysiological connection between the first and the second phase of the acute inflammatory response. LPS stimulation prompted a robust increase in the message for this upstream signal in both gingival fibroblasts and oral mucosa epithelial cells ($p < 0.0001$ Figure 4a,b). BCP incubation markedly dampened STAT-3 expression in both GF and EC cells and CB2 receptors blockade by AM630 cancelled the BCP effects ($p < 0.0001$ Figure 4a,b). IL-6 is released during the acute phase of the inflammatory reaction and it is the cytokine that promotes the transition from the first phase to the second wave of the acute inflammatory cascade. This step, if it is not adequately modulated, results in a chronic inflammatory condition. BCP was able to decrease the IL-6 message and mature protein, both markedly stimulated by LPS challenge in GF an EC cells ($p < 0.0001$ Figure 4c,d; Figure 5a,b). Again, the pharmacological blockade of the CB2 receptor brought about by AM630 reverted the BCP effects ($p < 0.0001$ Figure 4c,d; Figure 5a,b). Dysregulated activation of STAT-3 promotes an aberrant production of IL-17A, a cytokine that orchestrates the accumulation of inflammatory cells as neutrophils to the inflammatory scene. If the release is persistent, it may cause a negative remodeling of the inflamed tissue, thus sustaining and maintaining a chronic inflammation scenario. LPS challenge caused an elevation in both IL-17A mRNA and mature protein in both GF and EC cells ($p < 0.0001$ Figure 4c,f; Figure 5b,d). BCP incubation markedly reduced IL-17A expression and this effect was abolished by AM630, a cannabinoid CB2 receptor antagonist ($p < 0.001$ Figure 4e,f; Figure 5c,d). This experiment indicates that BCP efficiently interrupts the transition towards chronic inflammation.

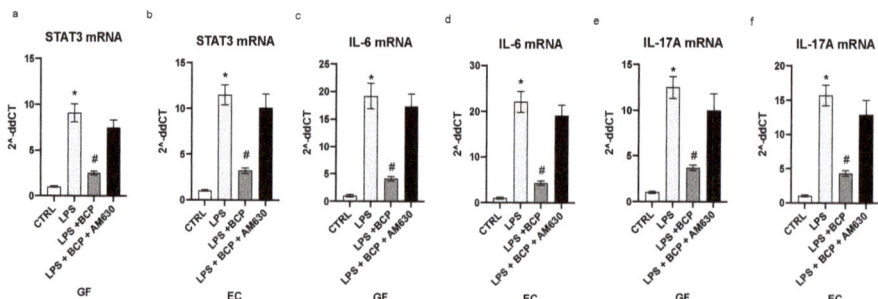

Figure 4. The graphs represent qPCR results of STAT3 (**a**), IL-6 (**c**), IL-17A (**e**) mRNA expression from GF cells and STAT3 (**b**), IL-6 (**d**), IL-17A (**f**) mRNA expression from EC cells. Values are expressed as the means and SD. * $p < 0.0001$ vs. CTRL; # $p < 0.0001$ vs. LPS.

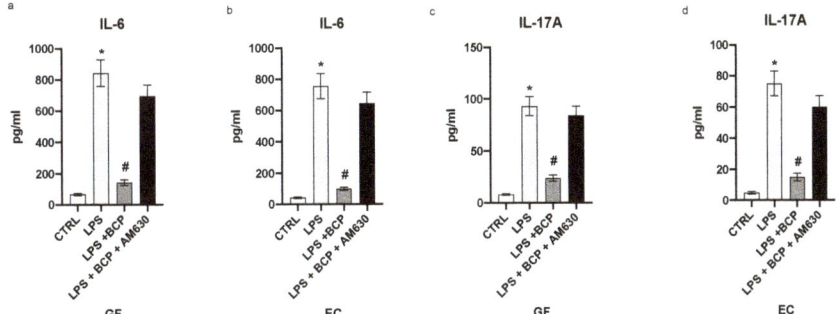

Figure 5. The graphs represent the levels of IL-6 (**a**), IL-17A (**c**) in cell supernatants from GF cells and IL-6 (**b**), IL-17A (**d**) levels in cell supernatants from EC cells. Levels of cytokines were evaluated by immunosorbent assay (ELISA). Values are expressed as the means and SD. * $p < 0.0001$ vs. CTRL; # $p < 0.0001$ vs. LPS.

3.4. BCP Does Not Affect Cell Viability

One hundred percent of viability was observed on control cells following 24 h. The incubation with β-caryophyllene did not affect GF and EC viability, thus demonstrating that this natural product does not have a cytotoxic effect and does not affect cell viability. Furthermore LPS incubation did not change cell viability (Figure 6a,b).

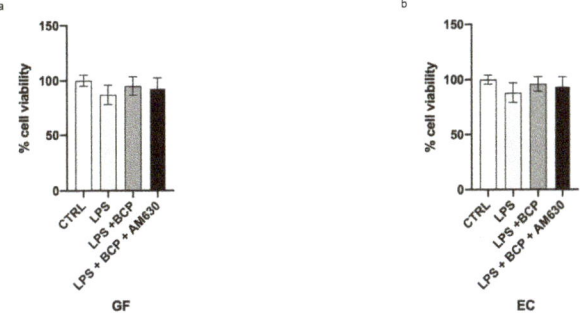

Figure 6. The graphs show the cytotoxicity assay at 24 h in GF cells (**a**) and EC cells (**b**). Values are expressed as the means and SD.

4. Discussion

In the present study we reproduced "in vitro" an experimental paradigm to mimic oral mucositis. To this aim we primed with LPS human gingival fibroblasts and oral mucosa epithelial cells, two main components of the periodontium. Both cell types acquired an inflammatory phenotype characterized by a sustained inflammatory cascade that was orchestrated by the transcription factors NF-κB and STAT3. Indeed, our experimental model is a slight modification of a previous published bioassay for oral mucositis [15]. However, we used LPS to trigger the inflammatory phenotype instead of recombinant cytokines, as in the previously published model [22].

LPS stimulation may have some theoretical advantages over cytokine stimulation: it may reproduce more closely the clinical scenario where infective stimuli and micro-organisms, at least in peri-implantitis, play an important role and may activate more efficiently the intracellular upstream signals that regulate and coordinate the inflammatory storm. In agreement with this reasoning it has been shown that in oral mucositis, pathogens are main participants in the triggering of the inflammatory cascade by engaging pathogen associated molecular patterns (PAMPs), such as the toll-like receptor that is targeted by LPS [23].

Oral mucositis management is theoretically easy to accomplish, but practically hard to implement in the clinical setting. Several therapeutics have been proposed for the treatment of oral mucositis: they include local antiseptic and cytoprotective agents, laser therapy and cryotherapy as well as pharmacological approaches such as anti-inflammatory drugs, recombinant cytokines and growth factors. Among these curative strategies, keratinocyte growth factor-1 is the only medicine that has received approval by the U.S. Food and Drug administration and by the European Medicine Agency for the management of oral mucositis, but its use is restricted to "at-high-risk" population [24,25]. Phyto-therapy has been suggested as a rationale strategy in the management of oral mucositis [26–28]. In this context BCP may represent an interesting molecule. It is a bicyclic sesquiterpene obtained by extraction from copaiba (Copaifera spp) and marijuana/hemp (Cannabis spp) that has gained the Food Drug Administration (FDA) authorization in light of its interesting curative profile. The compound has a long history of use in complementary therapy because of its ability to reduce inflammation and to cause analgesia [29]. β-caryophyllene engages with high affinity the cannabinoid CB2 receptors which are mainly localized in the immune system and immune-derived cells [30]. Since BCP does not bind the type 1 cannabinoid receptors, it is devoid of action at the Central Nervous System.

Several targets have been proposed to design a curative approach for oral mucositis, but so far, no attempt has been carried out to explore the feasibility of positively modulating the CB2 receptor. Our results suggest that BCP succeeded in turning off the inflammatory phenotype of GF and EC cells that is the main pathophysiological hallmark of oral mucositis [31]. BCP reduced relevant inflammatory cytokines such as TNF-α and IL-1β and augmented the expression of the anti-inflammatory IL-13. The positive effects brought about by BCP were abrogated by a specific antagonist of the CB2 receptor, thus clearly pointing out that this specific receptor subtype represents the mode of action of this natural compound. Furthermore, the results unmask for the first time that the CB2 receptor has potential for becoming a target candidate to allow an innovative drug design for medicines useful in the management of oral mucositis. We also explored the first steps of the intracellular biomolecular pathway that is modulated by the blockade of the CB2 receptor and we identified that the transcription factor NF-κB is the upstream molecular signal that is targeted by this therapeutic strategy. This result is of paramount importance: in fact, the transcription factor has been recognized as being one of the main actors in the initiation of oral mucositis and therefore the strategy of the CB2 blockade is able to intercept the very early event in the boosting of the inflammatory cascade. PPARγ is a nuclear receptor that may be considered as an "atypical transcription factor" able to activate anti-inflammatory signals. Indeed, pharmacological stimulation of PPARγ exerts beneficial activity in oral mucositis [13,14]. In agreement with these findings we also investigated PPARγ and its co-activator PGC-1α and we found that the expression of this intracellular signal was "downregulated" in our model of oral mucositis. Interestingly stimulation of the CB2 receptor by BCP also caused an upregulation of this protective intracellular signal, thus confirming previous studies suggesting the occurrence of a cross-talk between CB2 and PPAR-γ receptors [32].

Inflammation is a complex cascade of events that may lead to its resolution or, alternatively, to its stalling into a chronic condition that renders the management of the clinical condition hard to accomplish. The molecular events involved in this scenario are: an exaggerated production of IL-6 [33] and the consequent activation of the transcription factor STAT3 [34] that primes the production and release of several additional cytokines that sustain and maintain the inflammatory state. Among those cytokines, IL-17A is of paramount importance in the context of oral disease. Elevated levels of IL-17A have been measured in periodontal diseases characterized by high grade chronic inflammation [35,36]. In this clinical setting IL-17A orchestrates a coordinated recruitment of inflammatory cells that amplifies the maladaptive mechanisms underlying the maintenance of a persistent inflammation. Interestingly, BCP succeeded in counteracting this second wave of the host inflammatory response.

All these data, taken together highlight the great therapeutic potential of BCP for oral mucositis; in fact it possesses a dual mechanism of action; inhibition of NF-κB and activation of PPAR-γ that amplifies its efficacy in the first phase of inflammation and later it halts, by inhibiting STAT3, the second phase of the inflammatory response. Finally, it has been shown that BCP has an anti-cancer effect [37] that may enhance the appropriateness of this treatment, at least for oral mucositis due to chemotherapy or radiotherapy.

In conclusion, our data show for the first time that BCP has a marked efficacy in a preclinical in vitro model of oral mucositis: this effect, in light of its high translational potential, deserves to be confirmed in a clinical setting.

Author Contributions: Conceptualization: G.P. (Giacomo Picciolo) and G.P. (Giovanni Pallio); methodology: D.A. and N.I.; formal analysis and investigation: M.V. and G.O.; writing—original draft preparation: G.P. (Giacomo Picciolo) and G.P. (Giovanni Pallio); writing—review and editing: D.A.; funding acquisition: F.S.; resources; F.S.; supervision: F.S. All authors have read and agreed to the published version of the manuscript.

Funding: This work was supported by departmental funding assigned to Professor Francesco Squadrito.

Conflicts of Interest: The authors declare no conflicts of interest.

References

1. Elting, L.S.; Cooksley, C.D.; Chambers, M.S.; Garden, A.S. Risk, Outcomes, and Costs of Radiation-Induced Oral Mucositis Among Patients With Head-and-Neck Malignancies. *Int. J. Radiat. Oncol. Biol. Phys.* **2007**, *68*, 1110–1120. [CrossRef] [PubMed]
2. Elting, L.S.; Keefe, D.M.; Sonis, S.T.; Garden, A.S.; Spijkervet, F.K.; Barasch, A.; Tishler, R.B.; Canty, T.P.; Kudrimoti, M.K.; Vera-Llonch, M. Patient-reported measurements of oral mucositis in head and neck cancer patients treated with radiotherapy with or without chemotherapy. *Cancer* **2008**, *113*, 2704–2713. [CrossRef] [PubMed]
3. Murphy, B.A.; Beaumont, J.L.; Isitt, J.; Garden, A.S.; Gwede, C.K.; Trotti, A.M.; Meredith, R.F.; Epstein, J.B.; Le, Q.T.; Brizel, D.M. Mucositis-Related Morbidity and Resource Utilization in Head and Neck Cancer Patients Receiving Radiation Therapy With or Without Chemotherapy. *J. Pain Symptom Manag.* **2009**, *38*, 522–532. [CrossRef] [PubMed]
4. Lalla, R.V.; Sonis, S.T.; Peterson, D.E. Management of oral mucositis in patients who have cancer. *Dent. Clin. N. Am.* **2008**, *52*, 61–77. [CrossRef]
5. Pjetursson, B.E.; Asgeirsson, A.G.; Zwahlen, M.; Sailer, I. Improvements in implant dentistry over the last decade: Comparison of survival and complication rates in older and newer publications. *Int. J. Oral Maxillofac. Implants* **2014**, *29*, 308–324. [CrossRef] [PubMed]
6. Albrektsson, T.; Donos, N. Implant survival and complications. The third EAO consensus conference 2012. *Clin. Oral Implants Res.* **2012**, *6*, 63–65. [CrossRef]
7. Atieh, M.A.; Alsabeeha, N.H.M.; Faggion, C.M.; Druncan, W.J. The frequency of peri-implant diseases: A systematic review and metaanalysis. *J. Periodontol.* **2013**, *84*, 1586–1598.
8. Abrahamsson, I.; Berglundh, T. Effects of different implant surfaces and designs on marginal bone-level alterations: A review. *Clin. Oral Implants Res.* **2009**, *4*, 207–215. [CrossRef]
9. Sonis, S.T. New thoughts on the initiation of mucositis. *Oral Dis.* **2010**, *16*, 597–600. [CrossRef]
10. Mombelli, A.; Oosten, M.A.C.; Schürch, E., Jr.; Land, N.P. The microbiota associated with successful or failing osseointegrated titanium implants. *Oral Microbiol. Immunol.* **1987**, *2*, 145–151. [CrossRef]
11. Sardaro, N.; Della Vella, F.; Incalza, M.A.; Di Stasio, D.; Lucchese, A.; Contaldo, M.; Laudadio, C.; Petruzzi, M. Oxidative Stress and Oral Mucosal Diseases: An Overview. *In Vivo* **2019**, *33*, 289–296. [CrossRef] [PubMed]
12. Curra, M.; Pellicioli, A.C.; Filho, N.A.; Ochs, G.; Matte, U.; Filho, M.S.; Martins, M.A.; Martins, M.D. Photobiomodulation reduces oral mucositis by modulating NF-kB. *J. Biomed. Opt.* **2015**, *20*, 125008. [CrossRef] [PubMed]
13. Mangoni, M.; Sottili, M.; Gerini, C.; Desideri, I.; Bastida, C.; Pallotta, S.; Castiglione, F.; Bonomo, P.; Meattini, I.; Greto, D. A PPAR gamma agonist protects against oral mucositis induced by irradiation in a murine model. *Oral Oncol.* **2017**, *64*, 52–58. [CrossRef] [PubMed]

14. Sottili, M.; Mangoni, M.; Gerini, C.; Salvatore, G.; Castiglione, F.; Desideri, I.; Bonomo, P.; Meattini, I.; Greto, D.; Loi, M. Peroxisome proliferator activated receptor gamma stimulation for prevention of 5-fluorouracil-induced oral mucositis in mice. *Head Neck* **2018**, *40*, 577–583. [CrossRef] [PubMed]
15. Panahipour, L.; Nasserzare, S.; Amer, Z.; Brücke, F.; Stähli, A.; Kreissl, A.; Haiden, N.; Gruber, R. The anti-inflammatory effect of milk and dairy products on periodontal cells: An in vitro approach. *Clin. Oral Investig.* **2019**, *23*, 1959–1966. [CrossRef] [PubMed]
16. Russo, E.B. Beyond Cannabis: Plants and the Endocannabinoid System. *Trends Pharmacol. Sci.* **2016**, *37*, 594–605. [CrossRef]
17. Sharma, C.; Al Kaabi, J.M.; Nurulain, S.M.; Goyal, S.N.; Kamal, M.A.; Ojha, S. Polypharmacological Properties and Therapeutic Potential of β-Caryophyllene: A Dietary Phytocannabinoid of Pharmaceutical Promise. *Curr. Pharm. Des.* **2016**, *22*, 3237–3264. [CrossRef]
18. D'Ascola, A.; Irrera, N.; Ettari, R.; Bitto, A.; Pallio, G.; Mannino, F.; Atteritano, M.; Campo, G.M.; Minutoli, L.; Arcoraci, V. Exploiting curcumin synergy with natural products using quantitative analysis of doe-effect relationships in an in vitro model of osteoarthritis. *Front. Pharmacol.* **2019**, *10*, 1347. [CrossRef]
19. Marini, H.; Polito, F.; Altavilla, D.; Irrera, N.; Minutoli, L.; Calò, M.; Adamo, E.B.; Vaccaro, M.; Squadrito, F.; Bitto, A. Genistein aglycone improves skin repair in an incisional model of wound healing: A comparison with raloxifene and oestradiol in ovariectomized rats. *Br. J. Pharmacol.* **2010**, *160*, 1185–1194. [CrossRef]
20. Minutoli, L.; Marini, H.; Rinaldi, M.; Bitto, A.; Irrera, N.; Pizzino, G.; Pallio, G.; Calò, M.; Adamo, E.B.; Trichilo, V. A dual inhibitor of cyclooxygenase and 5-lipoxygenase protects against kainic acid-induced brain injury. *Neuromolecular Med.* **2015**, *17*, 192–201. [CrossRef]
21. Pizzino, G.; Irrera, N.; Bitto, A.; Pallio, G.; Mannino, F.; Arcoraci, V.; Aliquò, F.; Minutoli, L.; De Ponte, C.; D'Andrea, P. Cadmium-Induced Oxidative Stress Impairs Glycemic Control in Adolescents. *Oxid. Med. Cell Longev.* **2017**, *2017*, 6341671. [CrossRef] [PubMed]
22. Irrera, N.; D'Ascola, A.; Pallio, G.; Bitto, A.; Mazzon, E.; Mannino, F.; Squadrito, V.; Arcoraci, V.; Minutoli, L.; Campo, G.M. β-Caryophyllene Mitigates Collagen Antibody Induced Arthritis (CAIA) in Mice Through a Cross-Talk between CB2 and PPAR-γ Receptors. *Biomolecules* **2019**, *9*, 326. [CrossRef]
23. Tang, D.; Kang, R.; Coyne, C.B.; Zeh, H.J.; Lotze, M.T. PAMPs and DAMPs: Signal 0s that spur autophagy and immunity. *Immunol. Rev.* **2012**, *249*, 158–175. [CrossRef]
24. Hou, J.; Zheng, H.; Li, P.; Liu, H.; Zhou, H.; Yang, X. Distinct shifts in the oral microbiota are associated with the progression and aggravation of mucositis during radiotherapy. *Radiother. Oncol.* **2018**, *129*, 44–51. [CrossRef] [PubMed]
25. Lalla, R.V.; Bowen, J.; Barasch, A.; Elting, L.; Epstein, J.; Keefe, D.M.; McGuire, D.B.; Migliorati, C.; Nicolatou-Galitis, O.; Peterson, D.E. Mucositis Guidelines Leadership Group of the Multinational Association of Supportive Care in Cancer and International Society of Oral Oncology (MASCC/ISOO). MASCC/ISOO clinical practice guidelines for the management of mucositis secondary to cancer therapy. *Cancer* **2014**, *120*, 1453–1461. [CrossRef]
26. Li, C.L.; Huang, H.L.; Wang, W.C.; Hua, H. Efficacy and safety of topical herbal medicine treatment on recurrent aphthous stomatitis: A systemic review. *Drug Des. Devel. Ther.* **2016**, *10*, 107–115. [CrossRef] [PubMed]
27. Zhang, Y.; Ng, K.H.; Kuo, C.Y.; Wu, D.J. Chinese herbal medicine for recurrent aphthous stomatitis: A protocol for systematic review and meta-analysis. *Medicine* **2018**, *97*, e13681. [CrossRef] [PubMed]
28. Baharvand, M.; Jafari, S.; Mortazavi, H. Herbs in Oral Mucositis. *J. Clin. Diagn. Res.* **2017**, *11*, ZE05–ZE11. [CrossRef]
29. La Porta, C.; Bura, S.A.; Llorente-Onaindia, J.; Pastor, A.; Navarrete, F.; García-Gutiérrez, M.S.; De la Torre, R.; Manzanares, J.; Monfort, J.; Maldonado, R. Role of the endocannabinoid system in the emotional manifestations of osteoarthritis pain. *Pain* **2015**, *156*, 2001–2012. [CrossRef]
30. Machado, K.D.C.; Islam, M.T.; Ali, E.S.; Rouf, R.; Uddin, S.J.; Dev, S.; Shilpi, J.A.; Shill, M.C.; Reza, H.M.; Das, A.K. A systematic review on the neuroprotective perspectives of beta-caryophyllene. *Phytother. Res.* **2018**, *32*, 2376–2388. [CrossRef]
31. Sonis, S.T. Pathobiology of oral mucositis: Novel insights and opportunities. *J. Support. Oncol.* **2007**, *5* (Suppl. S4), 3–11.

32. Youssef, D.A.; El-Fayoumi, H.M.; Mahmoud, M.F. Beta-caryophyllene protects against diet-induced dyslipidemia and vascular inflammation in rats: Involvement of CB2 and PPAR-γ receptors. *Chem. Biol. Interact.* **2019**, *297*, 16–24. [CrossRef] [PubMed]
33. Hernández-Caldera, A.; Vernal, R.; Paredes, R.; Veloso-Matta, P.; Astorga, J.; Hernández, M. Human periodontal ligament fibroblasts synthesize C-reactive protein and Th-related cytokines in response to interleukin (IL)-6 trans-signalling. *Int. Endod. J.* **2018**, *51*, 632–640. [CrossRef]
34. Bharadwaj, U.; Kasembeli, M.M.; Robinson, P.; Tweardy, D.J. Targeting Janus Kinases and Signal Transducer and Activator of Transcription 3 to Treat Inflammation, Fibrosis, and Cancer: Rationale, Progress, and Caution. *Pharmacol. Rev.* **2020**, *72*, 486–526. [CrossRef] [PubMed]
35. Vernal, R.; Dutzan, N.; Chaparro, A.; Puente, J.; Antonieta Valenzuela, M.; Gamonal, J. Levels of interleukin-17 in gingival crevicular fluid and in supernatants of cellular cultures of gingival tissue from patients with chronic periodontitis. *J. Clin. Periodontol.* **2005**, *32*, 383–389. [CrossRef] [PubMed]
36. Mitani, A.; Niedbala, W.; Fujimura, T.; Mogi, M.; Miyamae, S.; Higuchi, N.; Abe, A.; Hishikawa, T.; Mizutani, M.; Ishihara, Y. Increased expression of interleukin (IL)-35 and IL-17, but not IL-27, in gingival tissues with chronic periodontitis. *J. Periodontol.* **2015**, *86*, 301–309. [CrossRef]
37. Irrera, N.; D'Ascola, A.; Pallio, G.; Bitto, A.; Mannino, F.; Arcoraci, V.; Rottura, M.; Ieni, A.; Minutoli, L.; Metro, D. β-Caryophyllene Inhibits Cell Proliferation through a Direct Modulation of CB2 Receptors in Glioblastoma Cells. *Cancers* **2020**, *23*, 12.

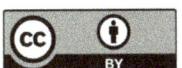

© 2020 by the authors. Licensee MDPI, Basel, Switzerland. This article is an open access article distributed under the terms and conditions of the Creative Commons Attribution (CC BY) license (http://creativecommons.org/licenses/by/4.0/).

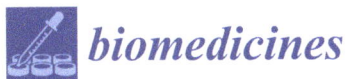

Article

A Mechanism by which Ergosterol Inhibits the Promotion of Bladder Carcinogenesis in Rats

Nobutomo Ikarashi [1,*,†], Motohiro Hoshino [2,†], Tetsuya Ono [2], Takahiro Toda [3], Yasuharu Yazawa [4] and Kiyoshi Sugiyama [5,*]

1. Department of Biomolecular Pharmacology, Hoshi University, 2-4-41 Ebara, Shinagawa-ku, Tokyo 142-8501, Japan
2. Department of Clinical Pharmacokinetics, Hoshi University, 2-4-41 Ebara, Shinagawa-ku, Tokyo 142-8501, Japan; hsnmt777-star@yahoo.co.jp (M.H.); onote20218@gmail.com (T.O.)
3. Division of Pharmacology, Faculty of Pharmaceutical Sciences, Teikyo Heisei University, 4-21-2 Nakano, Nakano-ku, Tokyo 164-8530, Japan; t.toda@thu.ac.jp
4. Department of Clinical Pharmaceutics, School of Pharmaceutical Sciences, University of Shizuoka, 52-1 Yada, Suruga-ku, Shizuoka 422-8526, Japan; yazawa@u-shizuoka-ken.ac.jp
5. Department of Functional Molecular Kinetics, Hoshi University, 2-4-41 Ebara, Shinagawa-ku, Tokyo 142-8501, Japan
* Correspondence: ikarashi@hoshi.ac.jp (N.I.); sugiyama@hoshi.ac.jp (K.S.); Tel.: +81-3-5498-5918 (N.I.)
† These authors contributed equally to this paper.

Received: 11 June 2020; Accepted: 25 June 2020; Published: 27 June 2020

Abstract: We previously showed that ergosterol has an inhibitory effect on bladder carcinogenesis. In this study, we aimed to elucidate the molecular mechanism by which ergosterol inhibits bladder carcinogenesis using a rat model of N-butyl-N-(4-hydroxybutyl)nitrosamine-induced bladder cancer. The messenger ribonucleic acid (mRNA) expression level of the cell cycle-related gene cyclin D1 and inflammation-related gene cyclooxygenase-2 in bladder epithelial cells was significantly increased in the carcinogenesis group compared with the control group. In contrast, in ergosterol-treated rats, these increases were significantly suppressed. Ergosterol did not affect the plasma testosterone concentration or the binding of dihydrotestosterone to androgen receptor (AR). The mRNA expression levels of 5α-reductase type 2 and AR were higher in the carcinogenesis group than in the control group but were significantly decreased by ergosterol administration. These results suggest that ergosterol inhibits bladder carcinogenesis by modulating various aspects of the cell cycle, inflammation-related signaling, and androgen signaling. Future clinical application of the preventive effect of ergosterol on bladder carcinogenesis is expected.

Keywords: ergosterol; cyclin D1; androgen receptor; 5α-reductase; bladder cancer

1. Introduction

Bladder cancer is one of the most common urological tumors. It mainly affects men, with an incidence approximately 10 times higher in men than in women [1]. Approximately 70% of bladder cancers are non-muscle-invasive, and transurethral resection (TUR) is a common treatment. Although the prognosis after TUR is good and the 5-year survival rate is at least 95%, the high recurrence rate is a clinical problem [2]. Treatment with anticancer agents [3,4] and bacillus Calmette-Guérin (BCG) infusion [5,6] into the bladder are performed after TUR. However, these treatments impose both a heavy burden on the patient and a large economic burden [7]. Therefore, a new preventive method that can solve these problems is strongly desired.

We previously screened traditional Kampo medicines via a short-term carcinogenicity test to identify preventive agents for superficial bladder cancer. Our results clarified that Choreito strongly inhibits the promotion of bladder carcinogenesis [8]. Choreito is composed of five crude drugs: *Polyporus sclerotium, Alisma rhizome, Poria sclerotium, Donkey glue,* and aluminum silicate hydrate with silicon dioxide. We clarified that among these components, *Polyporus sclerotium* has the strongest inhibitory effect on bladder carcinogenesis [9] and that the ergosterol contained in *Polyporus sclerotium* is the main active ingredient [10]. Furthermore, a long-term carcinogenicity test showed that when ergosterol was orally administered to rats in a model of bladder cancer for 25 weeks, the incidence of bladder tumors was decreased. In addition, experiments using castrated rats revealed that the action of ergosterol may be due to the suppression of androgen signaling by the active metabolite brassicasterol [11]. In this study, we aimed to elucidate the detailed molecular mechanism by which ergosterol inhibits bladder carcinogenesis. In brief, we focused on genes whose expression fluctuates from the early stage of bladder carcinogenesis and investigated the effect of ergosterol on the expression of these genes. In addition, we evaluated the effect of ergosterol on androgen, a hormone that promotes bladder carcinogenesis.

2. Experimental Section

2.1. Materials

Ergosterol and sodium saccharin (SS) were purchased from Wako Pure Chemicals (Osaka, Japan). *N*-butyl-*N*-(4-hydroxybutyl)nitrosamine (BHBN) was purchased from Tokyo Chemical Industry Co., Ltd. (Tokyo, Japan). Concanavalin A (Con A), α-methylmannoside (α-MM), and dextran-coated charcoal (DCC) were purchased from Sigma-Aldrich Corp. (St. Louis, MO, USA). An RNeasy Mini Kit was purchased from Qiagen (Valencia, CA, USA). A high-capacity complementary deoxyribonucleic acid (cDNA) synthesis kit was purchased from Applied Biosystems (Foster City, CA, USA). A testosterone enzyme immunoassay (EIA) kit was purchased from Cayman Chemical (Ann Arbor, MI, USA). The [1,2,4,5,6,7-^{3}H] 5α-dihydrotestosterone ([^{3}H]-DHT; 121 Ci/mmol) was purchased from GE Healthcare Bio-Sciences Corp. (Pittsburgh, PA, USA).

2.2. Animals

Male 5-week-old Wistar rats were obtained from Japan SLC, Inc. (Shizuoka, Japan). The care and handling of the animals were in accordance with the Hoshi University (approval no. 08-111).

2.3. Short-Term Carcinogenicity Study

A short-term carcinogenicity study was performed according to a previous method (Figure 1) [10,12]. In brief, rats were given an aqueous solution of 0.01% BHBN ad libitum for one week as the initiator. For the next three weeks, the rats in the control group were fed a normal diet alone, and those in the carcinogenesis and ergosterol-treated groups were fed a diet containing 5% SS as the promoter. Ergosterol (15 µg/kg/day) was administered orally once daily for three weeks to the rats in the ergosterol-treated group. The rats in the control and carcinogenesis groups received purified water containing 0.18% Tween 80. After the treatment, the rats were anesthetized, after which a blood sample was collected and the bladder was removed.

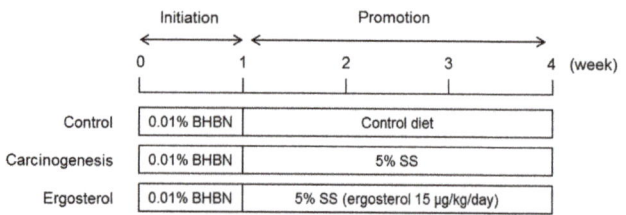

Figure 1. Experimental design.

2.4. Measurement of Plasma Testosterone Concentration

Blood samples were centrifuged (1000× g for 15 min at 4 °C), and the plasma was stored at −80 °C until the assays were performed. Free testosterone was obtained by centrifugation (12,000 × g for 90 s at 37 °C) using an ultrafiltration device (Ultracel YM-30, Millipore Corporation, Bedford, MA, USA). The plasma concentrations of total and free testosterone were enzymatically quantified using the Testosterone EIA kit.

2.5. Con A Agglutination Assay

A Con A agglutination assay was performed as described previously with slight modifications [13,14]. In brief, isolated cells from the removed bladders were collected by centrifugation. The cell suspension was mixed with Con A, with or without α-MM. Cell aggregates were counted with a hemocytometer.

2.6. Real-Time PCR

The expression levels of target genes were quantified using real-time RT-PCR analysis. Epithelial cells were isolated from rat bladders by scraping, and RNA was extracted with the RNeasy Mini Kit. The total RNA was reverse transcribed with high-capacity cDNA synthesis kit. The forward and reverse primers for target genes are listed in Table 1. The conditions for PCR were denaturation at 95 °C for 15 s, annealing at 56 °C for 30 s, and elongation at 72 °C for 30 s. The messenger ribonucleic acid (mRNA) expression levels were normalized to 18S ribosomal Ribonucleic acid (rRNA) expression levels.

Table 1. Primer sequences used for real-time PCR.

Gene	Forward	Reverse
Cyclin D1	CCAGCCGCAATGCTGTAG	TTGGGACGCCTCAGCTAAG
COX-1	AAGGAGATGGCCGCTGAGTT	AGGAGCCCCCATCTCTATCA
COX-2	GCTGATGACTGCCCAACTC	GATCCGGGATGAACTCTCTC
5α-R1	GCTGTACGAGTACATTCGTC	CCCTGATCAGAACCGGGAA
5α-R2	GGGAGCTCTAACCCAATTTC	CCTCTTCAGATCATACCGTG
AR	CCCTCCCATGGCACATTTTG	TTGGTTGGCACACAGCACAG
18S rRNA	GTCTGTGATGCCCTTAGATG	AGCTTATGACCCGCACTTAC

2.7. Androgen Receptor (AR) Binding Assay

Maltose binding protein-fused human AR ligand-binding domain (MBP-hAR-LBD; Toyobo Co., Ltd., Tokyo, Japan), [^{3}H]-DHT, and ergosterol or DHT were incubated at room temperature for 1 h. After the addition of DCC solution and reaction on ice for 10 min, DCC was removed by centrifugation. The supernatant was added to a liquid scintillation cocktail (Ultima Gold MV, PerkinElmer, Waltham, MA, USA), and the radioactivity of [^{3}H]-DHT was then measured in a liquid scintillation counter (TRI-CARB 3100TR, PerkinElmer).

2.8. Statistical Analysis

All quantitative results are presented as the means ± standard deviations (SDs). Means were compared using analysis of variance (ANOVA) with correction for multiple comparisons using Tukey's test for multiple comparisons. A p value of <0.05 was considered the level of significance.

3. Results

3.1. Inhibitory Effect of Ergosterol on Bladder Carcinogenesis

The inhibitory effect of ergosterol on bladder carcinogenesis was examined in a short-term carcinogenicity study using SS as the promoter [10,12] and evaluated in a Con A agglutination assay.

The number of Con A-dependent aggregates was significantly higher in the carcinogenic group than that in the control group. In contrast, the number of cell aggregates was significantly lower in rats treated with ergosterol compared to the carcinogenesis group (Table 2).

From the above results, it was confirmed that ergosterol exhibits inhibitory effect against bladder carcinogenesis, as in the previous reports [10,11].

Table 2. Inhibitory effect of ergosterol on bladder carcinogenesis.

Group	Number of Con A-Dependent Aggregates	Inhibition Rate (%)
Control	1 ± 1	-
Carcinogenesis	11 ± 3 *	-
Ergosterol	2 ± 1 #	90

The bladders were removed from rats in the control, carcinogenesis, and ergosterol-treated groups. Agglutination of urinary bladder cells in each group was induced by Concanavalin A (Con A), with or without α-methylmannoside (α-MM). Three assays, each on a pooled cell suspension from 2 rats, were carried out in each group of six rats. The data are presented as the means ± SDs. Tukey's test, * $p < 0.05$ vs. the control group, # $p < 0.05$ vs. the carcinogenesis group.

3.2. The mRNA Expression Level of Cyclin D1 in Bladder Epithelial Cells

During bladder carcinogenesis, the proliferation of epithelial cells is accelerated due to cell cycle dysregulation. Cyclin D1 is an important gene involved in cell cycle progression from G1 to S phase, and overexpression of cyclin D1 has been observed in various cancers, including bladder cancer [15,16]. Therefore, we investigated whether the inhibitory effect of ergosterol on bladder carcinogenesis is caused by a change in cyclin D1 expression.

The mRNA expression level of cyclin D1 in bladder epithelial cells in the carcinogenesis group was significantly increased by approximately two-fold compared with that in the control group. In contrast, cyclin D1 expression in the ergosterol-treated group was significantly lower than that in the carcinogenesis group and was almost the same as that in the control group (Figure 2).

The above results suggest that the inhibition of bladder carcinogenesis by ergosterol may be due to decreased expression of cyclin D1.

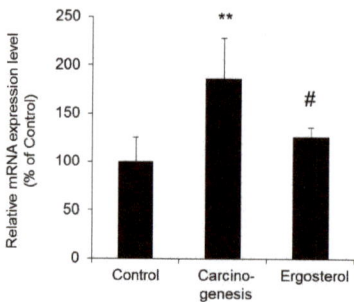

Figure 2. The mRNA expression level of cyclin D1 in bladder epithelial cells. The bladders were removed from rats in the control, carcinogenesis, and ergosterol-treated groups, and the mRNA expression level of cyclin D1 was measured using real-time RT-PCR and normalized to those of 18S rRNA. The data are presented as percentages of the mean value in the control group, which was set at 100%. The data show the mean ± SD from five rats per group. Tukey's test, ** $p < 0.01$ vs. the control group, # $p < 0.05$ vs. the carcinogenesis group.

3.3. The mRNA Expression Levels of Cyclooxygenase-1 (COX-1) and Cyclooxygenase-2 (COX-2) in Bladder Epithelial Cells

Inflammation in the bladder is considered to be one of the factors responsible for bladder cancer [17]. In general, when inflammation is induced, the expression of COX-2, the rate-limiting enzyme in prostaglandin E_2 (PGE$_2$) production, increases. Although COX-1 expression was not observed in bladder epithelial cells of rats in bladder cancer models, COX-2 expression was increased, which is considered a factor in bladder carcinogenesis [18,19]. Therefore, we investigated whether the change in COX-2 expression is involved in the inhibitory effect of ergosterol on bladder carcinogenesis.

The mRNA expression level of COX-1 in bladder epithelial cells in the carcinogenesis group was almost the same as that in the control group. In addition, no changes in COX-1 expression due to ergosterol administration were observed. On the other hand, the expression level of COX-2 in the carcinogenesis group was significantly increased by approximately two-fold compared with that in the control group. In contrast, the expression level of COX-2 in the ergosterol-treated group was significantly lower than that in the carcinogenesis group (Figure 3).

The above results suggest that ergosterol decreases the expression of COX-2 and suppresses the induction of inflammation.

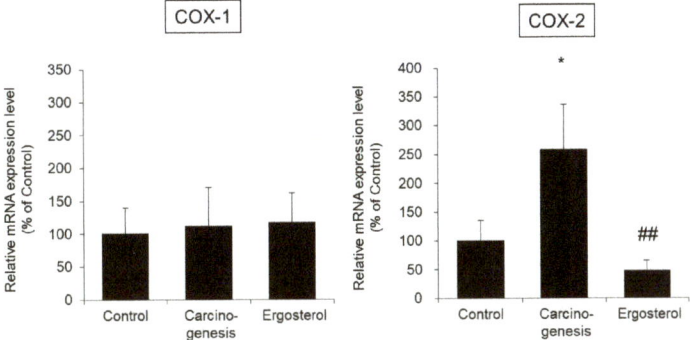

Figure 3. The mRNA expression levels of cyclooxygenase-1 (COX-1) and cyclooxygenase-2 (COX-2) in bladder epithelial cells. The bladders were removed from rats in the control, carcinogenesis, and ergosterol-treated groups, and the mRNA expression levels of COX-1 and COX-2 were measured using real-time RT-PCR and normalized to those of 18S rRNA. The data are presented as percentages of the mean value in the control group, which was set at 100%. The data show the mean ± SD from five rats per group. Tukey's test, * $p < 0.05$ vs. the control group, ## $p < 0.01$ vs. the carcinogenesis group.

3.4. Effect of Ergosterol on the Plasma Testosterone Concentration

Androgens have been reported to be involved in promoting bladder carcinogenesis [20]. Therefore, we investigated whether the plasma concentration of testosterone was changed by the administration of ergosterol.

In ergosterol-treated rats with BHBN-induced bladder cancer, the plasma concentrations of total and free testosterone were almost the same as those in the carcinogenesis group (Figure 4A,B). In addition, the ratio of the free testosterone concentration to the total testosterone concentration was not changed by ergosterol administration (Figure 4C).

The above results indicate that ergosterol is unlikely to suppress androgen signaling by affecting the blood testosterone concentration.

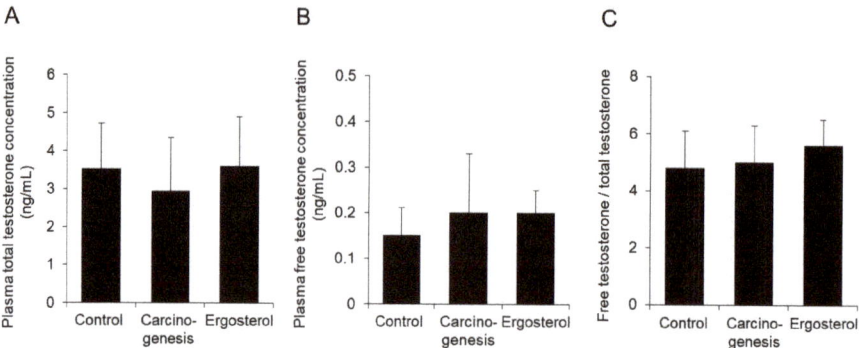

Figure 4. Effect of ergosterol on the plasma testosterone concentration. Plasma was obtained from rats in the control, carcinogenesis, and ergosterol-treated groups. The concentrations of total testosterone (**A**) and free testosterone (**B**) were measured. The ratio of the free testosterone concentration to the total plasma testosterone concentration was calculated (**C**). The data show the mean ± SD from five rats per group.

3.5. The mRNA Expression Levels of 5α-Reductase and AR in Bladder Epithelial Cells

After uptake by target tissues, testosterone is metabolized to DHT by 5α-reductase. DHT exerts an androgenic effect by binding to AR [20,21]. Therefore, we investigated whether ergosterol alters the expression levels of 5α-reductase and AR in bladder epithelial cells.

The mRNA expression level of 5α-reductase type 1 (5α-R1) in bladder epithelial cells was significantly higher in the carcinogenesis group than in the control group. The expression level of 5α-R1 in the ergosterol-treated group showed a trend of being lower than that in the carcinogenesis group. The expression levels of both 5α-reductase type 2 (5α-R2) and AR were significantly higher in the carcinogenesis group than in the control group. Treatment with ergosterol significantly suppressed these increases in expression (Figure 5).

The above results suggest that ergosterol may inhibit bladder carcinogenesis by decreasing the expression of 5α-reductase and AR and suppressing androgen signaling.

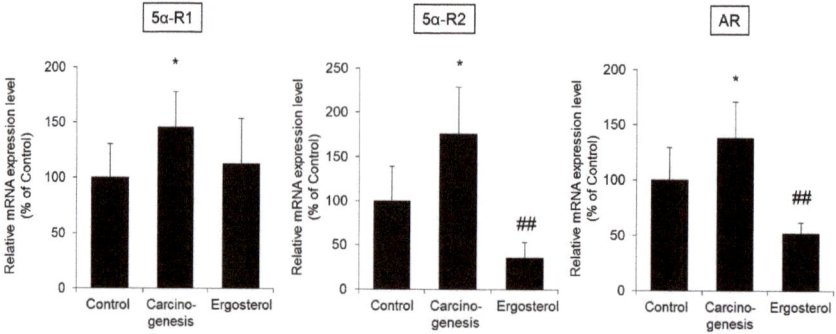

Figure 5. The mRNA expression levels of 5α-reductase and androgen receptor (AR) in bladder epithelial cells. The bladders were removed from rats in the control, carcinogenesis, and ergosterol-treated groups, and the mRNA expression levels of 5α-reductase type 1 (5α-R1), 5α-reductase type 2 (5α-R2), and AR were measured using real-time RT-PCR and normalized to those of 18S rRNA. The data are presented as percentages of the mean value in the control group, which was set at 100%. The data show the mean ± SD from five rats per group. Tukey's test, * $p < 0.05$ vs. the control group, ## $p < 0.01$ vs. the carcinogenesis group.

3.6. Effect of Ergosterol on the Binding Properties of AR and DHT

We investigated whether ergosterol competitively inhibits the binding of AR and DHT. Specifically, ergosterol was added in the presence of AR and [^{3}H]-DHT, and the extent of [^{3}H]-DHT exclusion from AR was evaluated.

DHT, used as the positive control, showed a concentration-dependent exclusion effect of [^{3}H]-DHT from AR. On the other hand, this exclusion effect was not observed with ergosterol (Figure 6).

The above results indicate that ergosterol is unlikely to inhibit the binding of AR and DHT to suppress androgen signaling.

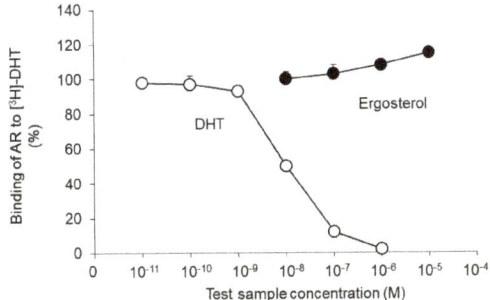

Figure 6. Effect of ergosterol on the binding properties of AR and dihydrotestosterone (DHT). Maltose binding protein-fused human AR ligand-binding domain (MBP-hAR-LBD) and [1,2,4,5,6,7-3H] 5α-dihydrotestosterone ([3H]-DHT) were incubated with ergosterol or DHT. The radioactivity of [^{3}H]-DHT bound to AR was measured using a liquid scintillation counter. The data show the mean ± SD from five experiments.

4. Discussion

We previously demonstrated that ergosterol, a component of the traditional Kampo medicine Choreito, strongly inhibits the promotion of bladder carcinogenesis [10] and that long-term administration of ergosterol reduces the incidence of carcinogenesis [11]. In this study, we aimed to elucidate the mechanism by which ergosterol inhibits bladder carcinogenesis.

Oral administration of ergosterol to rats in the BHBN-induced bladder carcinogenesis model reduced the Con A-induced cell aggregation rate by 90% (Table 2). This result is similar to that described in a previous report [10,11] and confirms that ergosterol exhibits inhibitory activity against bladder carcinogenesis. Therefore, we conducted a mechanistic analysis in this rat model.

During carcinogenesis, the cell cycle is dysregulated and cell proliferation is accelerated. Cyclin D1 is an important cell cycle mediator, and its expression has been reported to be increased in various cancers, including bladder cancer [15,16]. The expression level of cyclin D1 in bladder epithelial cells was significantly increased in the carcinogenesis group compared with the control group (Figure 2). In the rat model used in this study, carcinogenesis is at an earlier stage than in other rat models of bladder cancer in which increased expression of cyclin D1 has been reported [22,23]. Therefore, cyclin D1 may be one of the important genes whose expression is altered very early in bladder carcinogenesis. Ergosterol was found to suppress the increase in cyclin D1 expression observed in the carcinogenesis group, reducing cyclin D1 expression to a level similar to that in the control group (Figure 2). The above results suggest that suppression of cyclin D1 expression might be one of the mechanisms by which ergosterol inhibits bladder carcinogenesis.

Inflammation is one of the factors that induces the promotion of cell proliferation [17]. The enzyme COX-2 exhibits increased expression during inflammation and carcinogenesis and produces PGE$_2$, which has a promotive effect on cell proliferation [24,25]. COX-2 expression has been reported to be increased in bladder epithelial cells during bladder carcinogenesis in rats [18,19] and humans [26,27] and that PGE$_2$ has been reported to be involved in the development of bladder cancer [28]. The expression level of COX-2 in the carcinogenesis group was significantly increased compared to that in the control group, and ergosterol suppressed this increase (Figure 3). The above findings suggest that suppression of COX-2 expression might be one of the mechanisms by which ergosterol inhibits bladder carcinogenesis.

Why does ergosterol suppress cyclin D1 and COX-2 expression? Activation of nuclear factor-kappa B (NF-κB) is involved in mediating the increases in cyclin D1 and COX-2 expression during carcinogenesis [29,30], and ergosterol has been reported to suppress NF-κB activation [31,32]. Therefore, ergosterol may reduce the increase in cyclin D1 and COX-2 expression by suppressing the activation of NF-κB. In the future, it will be necessary to investigate the protein expression levels of these genes by Western blotting and immunohistochemistry and to clarify the inhibitory action of ergosterol on NF-κB activity and its mechanism.

Testosterone is metabolized to the active metabolite DHT by 5α-reductase and then binds to AR and exerts an androgenic effect. Flutamide, which has antiandrogenic activity, dose-dependently decreases the incidence of carcinogenesis in the rat model of BHBN-induced bladder carcinogenesis [33]. In addition, the progression of bladder carcinogenesis is suppressed in AR knockout mice [34]. We, therefore, investigated the effect of ergosterol on androgen signaling, which is important for bladder carcinogenesis. Our findings indicated that ergosterol does not affect the blood concentration of testosterone (Figure 4) or the binding of DHT to AR (Figure 6). On the other hand, ergosterol was found to decrease the expression level of 5α-R2 in rat bladder epithelial cells (Figure 5). The 5α-R1 is distributed in androgen-independent tissues such as liver and skin, and 5α-R2 is distributed in androgen-dependent tissues [35,36]. Therefore, we hypothesized that ergosterol reduces the expression level of 5α-R2, which might contribute to the suppression of androgen signaling. In addition, ergosterol was found to decrease AR expression in bladder epithelial cells (Figure 5). Therefore, ergosterol reduces the metabolic conversion of testosterone to DHT by decreasing the expression level of 5α-R2 in the bladder and decreases the expression of AR in bladder epithelial cells, thereby weakening androgen signaling. This finding suggests that the carcinogenesis is suppressed. It has been reported that the expression level of AR is upregulated by DHT [37]. Therefore, it is thought that the key to the suppression of bladder carcinogenesis due to ergosterol is the decrease in the expression of 5α-reductase, but there are many unclear points regarding its regulation mechanism. By investigating the DHT concentration in the bladder cells, we believe that the involvement of 5α-reductase in the suppressive action of bladder carcinogenesis by ergosterol will be clarified.

The results of this study clarified that ergosterol inhibits bladder carcinogenesis by modulating various aspects of the cell cycle, inflammation-related signaling, and androgen signaling. Reports have indicated that (1) high expression of cyclin D1 after TUR treatment shortens the time to recurrence in humans [38], (2) COX inhibitors may have a suppressive effect on bladder cancer [39], and (3) patients treated with antiandrogen therapy have a low rate of bladder cancer recurrence [40,41]. Although the prognosis of bladder cancer is relatively better than that of other carcinomas, the recurrence rate is very high. That is, bladder cancer repeatedly recurs, and when the disease progresses from superficial cancer to invasive cancer, the prognosis is poor. Therefore, preventing recurrence is an important issue. The action of ergosterol demonstrated in this study plays a very important role in preventing bladder cancer recurrence. Future clinical application of this preventive effect is expected.

Author Contributions: Conceptualization, K.S. methodology, N.I., M.H., and K.S.; formal analysis, N.I., M.H., T.O., T.T., and Y.Y.; writing—original draft preparation, N.I. and M.H.; writing—review and editing, K.S.; supervision, K.S. All authors have read and agreed to the published version of the manuscript.

Funding: This research received no external funding.

Conflicts of Interest: The authors declare no conflict of interest.

References

1. Torre, L.A.; Bray, F.; Siegel, R.L.; Ferlay, J.; Lortet-Tieulent, J.; Jemal, A. Global cancer statistics, 2012. *CA Cancer J. Clin.* **2015**, *65*, 87–108. [CrossRef]
2. DeGeorge, K.C.; Holt, H.R.; Hodges, S.C. Bladder cancer: Diagnosis and treatment. *Am. Fam. Physician* **2017**, *96*, 507–514.
3. Schlack, K.; Boegemann, M.; Steinestel, J.; Schrader, A.J.; Krabbe, L.M. The safety and efficacy of gemcitabine for the treatment of bladder cancer. *Expert Rev. Anticancer Ther.* **2016**, *16*, 255–271. [CrossRef]
4. Unda-Urzaiz, M.; Fernandez-Gomez, J.M.; Cozar-Olmo, J.M.; Juarez, A.; Palou, J.; Martinez-Pineiro, L. Update on the role of endovesical chemotherapy in nonmuscle-invasive bladder cancer. *Actas Urol. Esp.* **2018**, *42*, 73–76. [CrossRef] [PubMed]
5. Guallar-Garrido, S.; Julian, E. Bacillus calmette-guerin (bcg) therapy for bladder cancer: An update. *Immunotargets Ther.* **2020**, *9*, 1–11. [CrossRef]
6. Morales, A.; Eidinger, D.; Bruce, A.W. Intracavitary bacillus calmette-guerin in the treatment of superficial bladder tumors. *J. Urol.* **1976**, *116*, 180–183. [CrossRef]
7. Leal, J.; Luengo-Fernandez, R.; Sullivan, R.; Witjes, J.A. Economic burden of bladder cancer across the european union. *Eur. Urol.* **2016**, *69*, 438–447. [CrossRef] [PubMed]
8. Sugiyama, K.; Azuhata, Y.; Matsuura, D.; Kameda, Y.; Yokota, M. Antitumor-promoting effect of kampo formulations on rat urinary bladder carcinogenesis in a short-term test with concanavalin a. *J. Trad Med.* **1994**, *11*, 148–155.
9. Sugiyama, K.; Azuhata, Y.; Matsuura, D. Antitumor promoting effect of components of chorei-to on rat urinary bladder carcinogenesis in a short-term test with concanavalin a. *J. Trad Med.* **1994**, *11*, 214–219.
10. Yazawa, Y.; Yokota, M.; Sugiyama, K. Antitumor promoting effect of an active component of polyporus, ergosterol and related compounds on rat urinary bladder carcinogenesis in a short-term test with concanavalin a. *Biol. Pharm. Bull.* **2000**, *23*, 1298–1302. [CrossRef]
11. Yazawa, Y.; Ikarashi, N.; Hoshino, M.; Kikkawa, H.; Sakuma, F.; Sugiyama, K. Inhibitory effect of ergosterol on bladder carcinogenesis is due to androgen signaling inhibition by brassicasterol, a metabolite of ergosterol. *J. Nat. Med.* **2020**. [CrossRef] [PubMed]
12. Kakizoe, T.; Kawachi, T.; Okada, M. Concanavalin a agglutination of bladder cells of rats treated with bladder carcinogens; a rapid new test to detect bladder carcinogens. *Cancer Lett.* **1978**, *5*, 285–290. [CrossRef]
13. Kakizoe, T.; Hasegawa, F.; Kawachi, T.; Sugimura, T. Isolation of transitional epithelial cells from the rat urinary bladder. *Investig. Urol.* **1977**, *15*, 242–244.
14. Kakizoe, T.; Komatsu, H.; Niijima, T.; Kawachi, T.; Sugimura, T. Increased agglutinability of bladder cells by concanavalin a after administration of carcinogens. *Cancer Res.* **1980**, *40*, 2006–2009.
15. Lee, C.C.; Yamamoto, S.; Morimura, K.; Wanibuchi, H.; Nishisaka, N.; Ikemoto, S.; Nakatani, T.; Wada, S.; Kishimoto, T.; Fukushima, S. Significance of cyclin d1 overexpression in transitional cell carcinomas of the urinary bladder and its correlation with histopathologic features. *Cancer* **1997**, *79*, 780–789. [CrossRef]
16. Bringuier, P.P.; Tamimi, Y.; Schuuring, E.; Schalken, J. Expression of cyclin d1 and ems1 in bladder tumours; relationship with chromosome 11q13 amplification. *Oncogene* **1996**, *12*, 1747–1753.
17. Kantor, A.F.; Hartge, P.; Hoover, R.N.; Narayana, A.S.; Sullivan, J.W.; Fraumeni, J.F., Jr. Urinary tract infection and risk of bladder cancer. *Am. J. Epidemiol.* **1984**, *119*, 510–515. [CrossRef]
18. Shi, Y.; Cui, L.; Dai, G.; Chen, J.; Pan, H.; Song, L.; Cheng, S.; Wang, X. Elevated prostaglandin e2 level via cpla2–cox-2–mpges-1 pathway involved in bladder carcinogenesis induced by terephthalic acid-calculi in wistar rats. *Prostaglandins Leukot. Essent. Fat. Acids* **2006**, *74*, 309–315. [CrossRef]
19. Kitayama, W.; Denda, A.; Okajima, E.; Tsujiuchi, T.; Konishi, Y. Increased expression of cyclooxygenase-2 protein in rat urinary bladder tumors induced by n-butyl-n-(4-hydroxybutyl) nitrosamine. *Carcinogenesis* **1999**, *20*, 2305–2310. [CrossRef]
20. Li, Y.; Izumi, K.; Miyamoto, H. The role of the androgen receptor in the development and progression of bladder cancer. *Jpn. J. Clin. Oncol.* **2012**, *42*, 569–577. [CrossRef]

21. Chang, C.S.; Kokontis, J.; Liao, S.T. Molecular cloning of human and rat complementary DNA encoding androgen receptors. *Science* **1988**, *240*, 324–326. [CrossRef] [PubMed]
22. Cui, L.; Shi, Y.; Qian, J.; Dai, G.; Wang, Y.; Xia, Y.; Chen, J.; Song, L.; Wang, S.; Wang, X. Deregulation of the p16-cyclin d1/cyclin-dependent kinase 4-retinoblastoma pathway involved in the rat bladder carcinogenesis induced by terephthalic acid-calculi. *Urol. Res.* **2006**, *34*, 321–328. [CrossRef] [PubMed]
23. Lee, C.C.; Yamamoto, S.; Wanibuchi, H.; Wada, S.; Sugimura, K.; Kishimoto, T.; Fukushima, S. Cyclin d1 overexpression in rat two-stage bladder carcinogenesis and its relationship with oncogenes, tumor suppressor genes, and cell proliferation. *Cancer Res.* **1997**, *57*, 4765–4776. [PubMed]
24. Wang, D.; Buchanan, F.G.; Wang, H.; Dey, S.K.; DuBois, R.N. Prostaglandin e2 enhances intestinal adenoma growth via activation of the ras-mitogen-activated protein kinase cascade. *Cancer Res.* **2005**, *65*, 1822–1829. [CrossRef] [PubMed]
25. Pai, R.; Szabo, I.L.; Soreghan, B.A.; Atay, S.; Kawanaka, H.; Tarnawski, A.S. Pge(2) stimulates vegf expression in endothelial cells via erk2/jnk1 signaling pathways. *Biochem. Biophys. Res. Commun.* **2001**, *286*, 923–928. [CrossRef] [PubMed]
26. Shirahama, T. Cyclooxygenase-2 expression is up-regulated in transitional cell carcinoma and its preneoplastic lesions in the human urinary bladder. *Clin. Cancer Res.* **2000**, *6*, 2424–2430. [PubMed]
27. Mohammed, S.I.; Knapp, D.W.; Bostwick, D.G.; Foster, R.S.; Khan, K.N.; Masferrer, J.L.; Woerner, B.M.; Snyder, P.W.; Koki, A.T. Expression of cyclooxygenase-2 (cox-2) in human invasive transitional cell carcinoma (tcc) of the urinary bladder. *Cancer Res.* **1999**, *59*, 5647–5650.
28. Khan, M.A.; Thompson, C.S.; Mumtaz, F.H.; Jeremy, J.Y.; Morgan, R.J.; Mikhailidis, D.P. Role of prostaglandins in the urinary bladder: An update. *Prostaglandins Leukot. Essent. Fat. Acids* **1998**, *59*, 415–422. [CrossRef]
29. Shishodia, S.; Aggarwal, B.B. Nuclear factor-kappab activation: A question of life or death. *J. Biochem. Mol. Biol.* **2002**, *35*, 28–40.
30. Garg, A.; Aggarwal, B.B. Nuclear transcription factor-kappab as a target for cancer drug development. *Leukemia* **2002**, *16*, 1053–1068. [CrossRef]
31. Kim, J.A.; Tay, D.; de Blanco, E.C. Nf-kappab inhibitory activity of compounds isolated from cantharellus cibarius. *Phytother. Res.* **2008**, *22*, 1104–1106. [CrossRef] [PubMed]
32. Kobori, M.; Yoshida, M.; Ohnishi-Kameyama, M.; Shinmoto, H. Ergosterol peroxide from an edible mushroom suppresses inflammatory responses in raw264.7 macrophages and growth of ht29 colon adenocarcinoma cells. *Br. J. Pharmacol.* **2007**, *150*, 209–219. [CrossRef] [PubMed]
33. Imada, S.; Akaza, H.; Ami, Y.; Koiso, K.; Ideyama, Y.; Takenaka, T. Promoting effects and mechanisms of action of androgen in bladder carcinogenesis in male rats. *Eur. Urol.* **1997**, *31*, 360–364. [CrossRef] [PubMed]
34. Miyamoto, H.; Yang, Z.; Chen, Y.T.; Ishiguro, H.; Uemura, H.; Kubota, Y.; Nagashima, Y.; Chang, Y.J.; Hu, Y.C.; Tsai, M.Y.; et al. Promotion of bladder cancer development and progression by androgen receptor signals. *J. Natl. Cancer Inst.* **2007**, *99*, 558–568. [CrossRef] [PubMed]
35. Thigpen, A.E.; Silver, R.I.; Guileyardo, J.M.; Casey, M.L.; McConnell, J.D.; Russell, D.W. Tissue distribution and ontogeny of steroid 5 alpha-reductase isozyme expression. *J. Clin. Investig.* **1993**, *92*, 903–910. [CrossRef] [PubMed]
36. Normington, K.; Russell, D.W. Tissue distribution and kinetic characteristics of rat steroid 5 alpha-reductase isozymes. Evidence for distinct physiological functions. *J. Biol. Chem.* **1992**, *267*, 19548–19554.
37. Hata, S.; Ise, K.; Azmahani, A.; Konosu-Fukaya, S.; McNamara, K.M.; Fujishima, F.; Shimada, K.; Mitsuzuka, K.; Arai, Y.; Sasano, H.; et al. Expression of ar, 5alpha1 and 5alpha2 in bladder urothelial carcinoma and relationship to clinicopathological factors. *Life Sci.* **2017**, *190*, 15–20. [CrossRef]
38. Shin, K.Y.; Kong, G.; Kim, W.S.; Lee, T.Y.; Woo, Y.N.; Lee, J.D. Overexpression of cyclin d1 correlates with early recurrence in superficial bladder cancers. *Br. J. Cancer* **1997**, *75*, 1788–1792. [CrossRef]
39. Gakis, G. The role of inflammation in bladder cancer. *Adv. Exp. Med. Biol.* **2014**, *816*, 183–196.

40. Izumi, K.; Ito, Y.; Miyamoto, H.; Miyoshi, Y.; Ota, J.; Moriyama, M.; Murai, T.; Hayashi, H.; Inayama, Y.; Ohashi, K.; et al. Expression of androgen receptor in non-muscle-invasive bladder cancer predicts the preventive effect of androgen deprivation therapy on tumor recurrence. *Oncotarget* **2016**, *7*, 14153–14160. [CrossRef]
41. Izumi, K.; Taguri, M.; Miyamoto, H.; Hara, Y.; Kishida, T.; Chiba, K.; Murai, T.; Hirai, K.; Suzuki, K.; Fujinami, K.; et al. Androgen deprivation therapy prevents bladder cancer recurrence. *Oncotarget* **2014**, *5*, 12665–12674. [CrossRef] [PubMed]

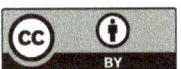 © 2020 by the authors. Licensee MDPI, Basel, Switzerland. This article is an open access article distributed under the terms and conditions of the Creative Commons Attribution (CC BY) license (http://creativecommons.org/licenses/by/4.0/).

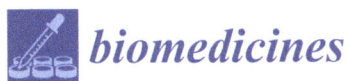

Article

Hemocyanins from *Helix* and *Rapana* Snails Exhibit in Vitro Antitumor Effects in Human Colorectal Adenocarcinoma

Ani Georgieva [1,*], Katerina Todorova [1], Ivan Iliev [1], Valeriya Dilcheva [1], Ivelin Vladov [1], Svetlozara Petkova [1], Reneta Toshkova [1], Lyudmila Velkova [2], Aleksandar Dolashki [2] and Pavlina Dolashka [2,*]

1. Institute of Experimental Morphology, Pathology and Anthropology with Museum, Bulgarian Academy of Sciences, Sofia 1113, Bulgaria; pda54@abv.bg (K.T.); taparsky@abv.bg (I.I.); val_dilcheva@yahoo.com (V.D.); iepparazit@yahoo.com (I.V.); svetlozarapetkova@abv.bg (S.P.); reneta.toshkova@gmail.com (R.T.)
2. Institute of Organic Chemistry with Centre of Phytochemistry, Bulgarian Academy of Sciences, Sofia 1113, Bulgaria; lyudmila_velkova@abv.bg (L.V.); adolashki@yahoo.com (A.D.)
* Correspondence: georgieva_any@abv.bg (A.G.); dolashka@orgchm.bas.bg (P.D.); Tel.: +359-029-792-384 (A.G.); +359 887-193-423 (P.D.)

Received: 10 June 2020; Accepted: 2 July 2020; Published: 5 July 2020

Abstract: Hemocyanins are oxygen-transporting glycoproteins in the hemolymph of arthropods and mollusks that attract scientific interest with their diverse biological activities and potential applications in pharmacy and medicine. The aim of the present study was to assess the in vitro antitumor activity of hemocyanins isolated from marine snail *Rapana venosa* (RvH) and garden snails *Helix lucorum* (HlH) and *Helix aspersa* (HaH), as well the mucus of *H. aspersa* snails, in the HT-29 human colorectal carcinoma cell line. The effects of the hemocyanins on the cell viability and proliferation were analyzed by 3-(4,5-dimethylthiazol-2-yl)-2,5-diphenyltetrazolium bromide (MTT) assay and the alterations in the tumor cell morphology were examined by fluorescent and transmission electron microscopy. The results of the MTT assay showed that the mucus and α-subunit of hemocyanin from the snail *H. aspersa* had the most significant antiproliferative activity of the tested samples. Cytomorphological analysis revealed that the observed antitumor effects were associated with induction of apoptosis in the tumor cells. The presented data indicate that hemocyanins and mucus from *H. aspersa* have an antineoplastic activity and potential for development of novel therapeutics for treatment of colorectal carcinoma.

Keywords: hemocyanin; snail *Rapana venosa*; snail *Helix lucorum*; snail *Helix aspersa*; antitumor activity; colorectal adenocarcinoma; apoptosis

1. Introduction

Neoplastic diseases are characterized as having high incidence and mortality and have significant health and social impacts. Conventional anticancer treatment includes a combination of surgery, radiation therapy, and chemotherapy [1]. However, traditional therapy has several drawbacks such as multidrug resistance, low selectivity, and toxicity to healthy tissues associated with severe side effects. Finding of selective and more efficient new drugs is one of the greatest challenges for pharmacology and medicine. Today, an extensive research effort has been focused on screening of compounds of natural origin with higher specificity and less adverse side effects [2]. In this context, bioactive compounds isolated from mollusk species attract a significant interest as good drug candidates for cancer therapeutic applications [3].

Numerous studies have indicated that hemocyanins, oxygen-carrying hemolymph metalloproteins, have a significant immunostimulatory and anticancer activity [4–7]. Molluscan hemocyanins are glycoproteins with high molecular masses and complex quaternary and oligosaccharide structures. They are usually composed of several structural subunits with approximate masses of 350–450 kDa, each consisting of seven or eight globular functional units connected by linker peptide strands, forming hollow cylinders [8]. The primary amino acid sequences of molluscan hemocyanins are highly divergent from mammalian sequences, which results in strong activation of the immune system. In addition, the carbohydrate moieties present in molluscan hemocyanins are considered responsible for their high immunogenicity. The carbohydrate structures of hemocyanins have been extensively studied in order to understand their organization, antigenicity, and biomedical properties [9,10]. The carbohydrate component of hemocyanins have been reported to be up to 9% (w/w) and contain diverse sugar moieties, including mannose, D-galactose, fucose, N-acetyl-D-galactosamine, and N-acetyl-glucosamine residues, as well as xylose, which is not usually present in animal proteins [11]. Hemocyanins are characterized with the presence of numerous N-glycosylation sites and limited number of O-glycosylation sites [12]. Due to these structural properties, hemocyanins stimulate the mammalian immune system nonspecifically by interacting with macrophages, polymorphonuclears, CD4+, and CD8+ cells and induce potent humoral and cellular immune response [11,13]. Moreover, significant direct antitumor effects of hemocyanins have been established in various in vitro and in vivo tumor models [4,14–16].

The present study aimed to assess the in vitro antitumor activity of hemocyanins isolated from *Helix aspersa*, *Helix lucorum*, and *Rapana venosa* against colorectal carcinoma cell line HT-29 and to investigate morphological and ultrastructural alterations in the tumor cells.

2. Materials and Methods

2.1. Materials

Membranes were purchased from Millipore Ultrafiltration Membrane Filters, regenerated cellulose. 3-(4,5-Dimethylthiazol-2-yl)-2,5-diphenyltetrazolium bromide (MTT), ethidium bromide (EB), and acridine orange (AO) were purchased from Sigma-Aldrich, Schnelldorf, Germany. All culture reagents, Dulbecco's modified Eagle's medium (DMEM; Sigma-Aldrich, Schnelldorf, Germany), fetal bovine serum (FBS; Gibso/BRL, Grand Island, NY), L-glutamine, penicillin, and streptomycin (LONZA, Cologne, Germany) were used as received. The disposable consumables were supplied by Orange Scientific, Braine-l'Alleud, Belgium. HT-29 cell line—human colorectal adenocarcinoma was obtained from American Type Cultures Collection (ATCC, Rockville, MD, USA).

2.2. Isolation of the Hemocyanin and Isoforms from Snail Rapana Venosa

The hemolymph was collected from *R. venosa* marine snails living in the Black Sea after cutting the foot muscles, and it was filtrated and centrifuged at 10,000 rpm and 4 °C for 20 min to remove rough particles and haemocytesas [17]. The crude hemolymph extract was ultrafiltrated (using membrane 100 kDa Millipore Ultrafiltration Membrane Filters) and the fraction above 100 kDa containing predominantly native RvH was ultracentrifugatied at 22,000 rpm and 4 °C for 180 min with rotor Kontron-Hermle A8.24 (centrifuge CENTRIKON). The sediment containing the native RvH was solubilized at a concentration of about 10% in 50 mM Tris buffer (pH 7.5) and was purified by gel filtration on column Sephadex G-200. Dissociation of native RvH was achieved by dialyzing the protein against 0.13 M glycine/NaOH buffer, pH 9.6. The structural subunits RvH1 and RvH2 were separated on an ion-exchange chromatography by a 16/10 Q Sepharose High Performance column equilibrated with 50 mM Tris/HCl buffer and 10 mM EDTA (pH 8.5) with a linear gradient of 0.0–0.5 M NaCl by FPLC system.

2.3. Isolation of the Native Hemocyanin and Isoforms from Snail H. Lucorum

The hemolymph was collected from the foot of garden snail *H. lucorum* and rough particles and hemocytes were removed after filtration and centrifuged at 10,000 rpm and 4 °C for 20 min [18].

After ultrafiltration of supernatant by membrane of 100 kDa (Millipore Ultrafiltration Membrane Filters, Regenerated cellulose), we applied the fraction with molecular mass above 100 kDa, containing mostly hemocyanin, to ultracentrifugation at 22,000 rpm and 4 °C for 180 min with rotor Kontron-Hermle A8.24 (centrifuge CENTRIKON). The sediment with total hemocyanin was solubilized in concentration of about 5% in 0.1 M sodium acetate buffer, pH 5.7.

The isoform βc-HlH was isolated after precipitation of native HlH during 4–5 days dialysis against 10 mM sodium acetate buffer (pH 5.1) at 4 °C and the buffer was renewed every 12 h. The βc-HlH was sedimented by centrifugation at 15,000 × g, at 4 °C for 30 min. The precipitate was dissolved in 100 mM sodium phosphate buffer (pH 6.5) and further purified by anion exchange chromatography on a 16/10 Q Sepharose High Performance column using a linear NaCl gradient (0.0–0.5 M) in 50 mM Tris–HCl buffer, pH 7.8.

Both subunits, $α_D$-HlH and $α_N$-HlH, dissolved in the supernatant, were purified by gel filtration chromatography on a Sephacryl S 300 column, were equilibrated and eluted with 50 mM Tris buffer (pH 7.5), and further concentrated by ultrafiltration (100 kDa, Millipore Ultrafiltration Membrane Filters, regenerated cellulose).

2.4. Isolation of the Native Hemocyanin and Mucus from Snail H. Aspersa

The native HaH was isolated after concenrtation of the hemolymph collected from the foot of garden snail *H. aspersa* by ultrafiltration (using 100 kDa, Amicon PM membranes) [4]. After ultracentrifugation at 22,000 rpm (rotor Kontron-Hermle A8.24, centrifuge CENTRIKON) and 4 °C for 3 h, the native HaH was sedimented. After removal of the supernatant, the precipitated HaH was solubilized in 50 mM Tris buffer (pH 7.5) containing 20 mM $CaCl_2$ and 10 mM $MgCl_2$ and further purified by gel filtration chromatography on a Sepharose 6B column (90 × 2.4 cm).

2.5. Separation of H. Aspersa Hemocyanin Isoforms

Three isoforms ($α_D$-HaH, $α_N$-HaH, and βc-HaH) were separated after 4 days of dialysis against 10 mM sodium acetate buffer (pH 5.3) at 4 °C, renewed every 12 h. The isoform βc-HaH precipitated after centrifugation and solubilized in 0.1 M sodium phosphate buffer (pH 6.5), and was further purified by gel filtration chromatography on a Sepharose 6B column and eluted with buffer of 50 mM Tris-HCl, pH 7.5. Two α-isoforms ($α_{D+N}$) in supernatant were concentrated by ultrafiltration (Millipore Ultrafiltration Membrane Filters, regenerated cellulose) and purified of FPLC-system by a 16/10 Q Sepharose High Performance column using a linear NaCl gradient (0.0–1.0 M) in 50 mM Tris–HCl buffer, pH 8.2.

The mucus was collected from the foot of *H. aspersa* snails that were grown in Bulgarian eco-farms. After several steps of purification and homogenization, including filtration and centrifugation for removal of rough particles, the crude mucus extract was obtained [19].

Mucus extract from *H. aspersa* was analyzed by sodium dodecyl sulphate polyacrylamide gel electrophoresis (SDS-PAGE) with the molecular weight marker ranging from 250 kDa to 10 kDa using a 5% stacking gel and 12% resolving gel, according to Laemmli method with modifications [20]. All tested hemocyanins and their isoforms were analyzed by 8% polyacrylamide gel electrophoresis under native conditions, as described [21].

2.6. Cell culture and Cell Viability

HT-29 and Balb/c 3T3 cells were cultured in 75 cm^2 tissue culture flasks in Dulbecco's modified Eagle's medium supplemented with 10% fetal calf serum, 2 mM glutamine, and the antibiotics penicillin (100 U mL^{-1}) and streptomycin (100 μg mL^{-1}) at 37 °C and 5% CO_2 and 90% relative humidity.

Cell viability was assessed by MTT (methyl thiazol tetrazolium bromide) assay, as described previously [22]. Briefly, cells were plated in a 96-well microtiter plate at a density of 1×10^4 cells per well in a final volume of 100 μL DMEM medium. HT-29 cells were treated with six different concentrations of the hemocyanin samples (31.25–1000 μg/mL) for 72 h. Parallel experiments with the same treatment and incubation regimen were performed on Balb/c 3T3 cells to assess the cytotoxic activity of the tested samples in non-tumor cells. After treatment, the cells were incubated with MTT dye at a concentration of 50 µg/100 µL for 3 h at 37 °C. The cells were thereafter lysed with DMSO/96% ethanol (1:1 v/v) solution. Absorbance of the reduced intracellular formazon product was read at 570 nm in a microtiter plate reader (TECAN, Sunrise, Groedig/Salzburg, Austria).

2.7. Fluorescent Microscopy

The morphological alterations in HT-29 cells induced by the test samples that showed higher cytotoxic activity were analyzed by fluorescent microscopy. HT-29 cells were cultured on 13 mm diameter cover glasses in 24-well plates and were treated for 24 h with hemocyanins in concentrations approximating the IC_{50} value established by the MTT test and concentrations lower and higher than the IC_{50} value. Cells treated with the standard anticancer drug doxorubicin were used as a positive control for the experiments. Doxorubicine was applied at concentrations equal to the IC_{50} value (2.7 µg/mL) established in our previous studies. The control and treated cells were stained by two different methods.

2.7.1. Acridine Orange/Ethidium Bromide Double Staining

Acridine orange (AO) and ethidium bromide (EB) (live/dead) staining was performed as previously described [23]. Briefly, cell preparations of HT-29 cells were stained with the fluorescent dyes AO (5 µg/mL) and EB (5 µg/mL) in phosphate-buffered saline (PBS) and mounted on microscope slides.

2.7.2. DAPI Staining

The alterations in the nuclear morphology of the tumor cells induced by hemocyanins were studied after staining with DNA binding dye 4′,6-diamidine-2′-phenylindole dihydrochloride (DAPI). The cells were fixed with methanol, incubated for 15 min in 1 µg/mL DAPI in methanol in the dark, and mounted with glycerol on microscope slides.

Stained cells were visualized and examined under a fluorescence microscope (Leica DM 5000B, Wetzlar, Germany).

2.8. Transmission Electron Microscopy (TEM)

Ultrastructural studies of cells exposed to bioactive compounds isolated from *Helix aspersa* at cytotoxic doses (concentrations equal or close to their IC_{50} values) were processed according to routine techniques for this type of assay. They were fixed for 1 h with 2.5% glutaraldehyde in 0.1 M pH 7.3 phosphate buffer, postfixed for 2 h in 1% OsO_4, dehydrated, and included in Durcupan ACM Fluka. Ultra-thin sections were prepared on Reichert Ultramicrotome and stained with 2% uranyl acetate and 2% lead citrate. For the TEM study, we used an Opton transmission electron microscope.

2.9. Statistical Analysis

Statistical analysis was performed by one-way ANOVA followed by Bonferroni's post hoc test (GraphPad Prism software package). $p < 0.05$ was accepted as the lowest level of statistical significance. Nonlinear regression (curve fit) analysis (GraphPad Prism) was applied to determine the concentrations inducing 50% inhibition of the cell growth (IC_{50} values).

3. Results

3.1. Isolation of Bioactive Compounds from the Three Mollusk Species

Total hemocyanins from garden snails *Helix aspersa* and *Helix lucorum* (HaH-total; HlH-total), their isoforms (subunits βc-HaH, α-HaH, βc-HlH, and α-HlH), *Helix aspersa* mucus, and subunits of *Rapana venosa* hemocyanin (RvH I and RvH II) were isolated and purified as previously described [4,17,18]. Hemocyanins are freely dissolved in the hemolymph of species in *Mollusca* and Arthropoda as a major protein constituent (90–98%) of this fluid. Specific absorption coefficient A_{278} nm = 1.413 mL·mg^{-1}·cm^{-1} for HaH was used for determination of the protein concentration [24].

The hemolymph was collected from *R. venosa* marine snails living in the Black Sea and garden snails *H. aspersa* and *H. lucorum* after cutting the foot muscles [17–19]. The hemocyanins with molecular mass ≈ 8 MDa were isolated from the crude hemolymph extract after ultrafiltration using membrane 100 kDa. Native RvH was obtained after ultracentrifugation at 22,000 rpm and 4 °C for 180 min and purified by gel filtration on column Sephadex G-200. After dissociation of native RvH by dialyzing the protein against 0.13 M glycine/NaOH buffer (pH 9.6) two structural subunits RvH1 and RvH2 were separated on an ion-exchange chromatography by a 16/10 Q Sepharose High Performance column equilibrated with 50 mM Tris/HCl buffer and 10 mM EDTA (pH 8.5) with a linear gradient of 0.0–0.5 M NaCl by FPLC system [17].

The native *H. lucorum* [18] and *H. aspersa* [4] hemocyanins are organized by three structural subunits (βc-HaH, α$_D$-HaH, and α$_N$-HaH) with molecular weight (MW) ≈ 450 kDa. The βc-isoforms were precipitated from the hemolymph and further purified by gel filtration chromatography on a Sepharose 6B column, and eluted with buffer 50 mM Tris-HCl, pH 7.5. After removal of βc-isoform, both α-isoforms in supernatant were purified of FPLC-system by gel filtration chromatography on a Sephacryl S 300 column, equilibrated and eluted with 50 mM Tris buffer, pH 7.5

The mucus collected from the foot of *H. aspersa* snails was purified after filtration and centrifugation of the crude mucus extract [19].

The tested hemocyanins were analyzed by 8% native PAGE (Figure 1) [21] to confirm their molecular masses and purity. As shown in Figure 1a, purity of total hemocyanin hemocyanins (line 2 of *H. aspersa*, line 5 of *R. venosa*, and line 8 of *H. lucorum*) and their structural subunits (lines 3, 4, 6, 7, and 10) is about 90%. Line 9 shows two main bands that correspond to the two isoforms αN-HlH and αD-HlH.

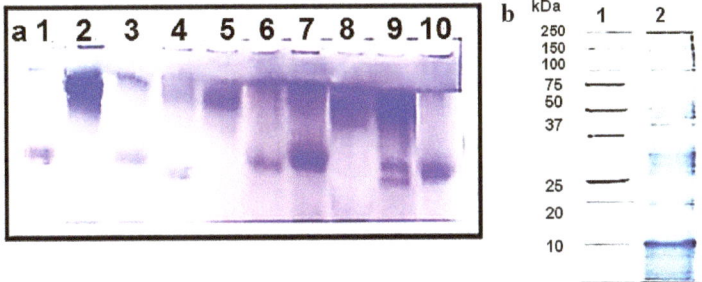

Figure 1. (a) The 8% native gel electrophoresis of the tested hemocyanins with Coomassie Blue G-250 dye: positions (1) standard ferritin (450 kDa); (2) total *Helix aspersa* hemocyanin; (3) two α-isoforms of *H. aspersa* hemocyanin; (4) structural subunit βc-HaH; (5) total *Rapana venosa* hemocyanin; (6) structural subunit RvH I; (7) structural subunit RvH II; (8) total *Helix lucorum* hemocyanin; (9) two α-isoforms of *H. lucorum* hemocyanin; (10) structural subunit βc-HlH. (b) The 12.0% SDS-PAGE analysis visualized by staining with Coomassie Blue G-250: (1) molecular weights of standard proteins from Bio-rad; (2) mucus extract from *H. aspersa*.

The 12% SDS-PAGE analysis of the mucus extract showed that the mucus is a complex mixture of various biological substances such as antimicrobial peptides and proteins (Figure 1b, line 2).

3.2. Effects of the Isolated Bioactive Compounds on the Viability and Proliferative Activity of HT-29 Tumor Cells

The effects of the hemocyanin samples on the viability and proliferative activity of the colorectal adenocarcinoma cells were assessed by MTT assay after 72 h of treatment (Figure 2).

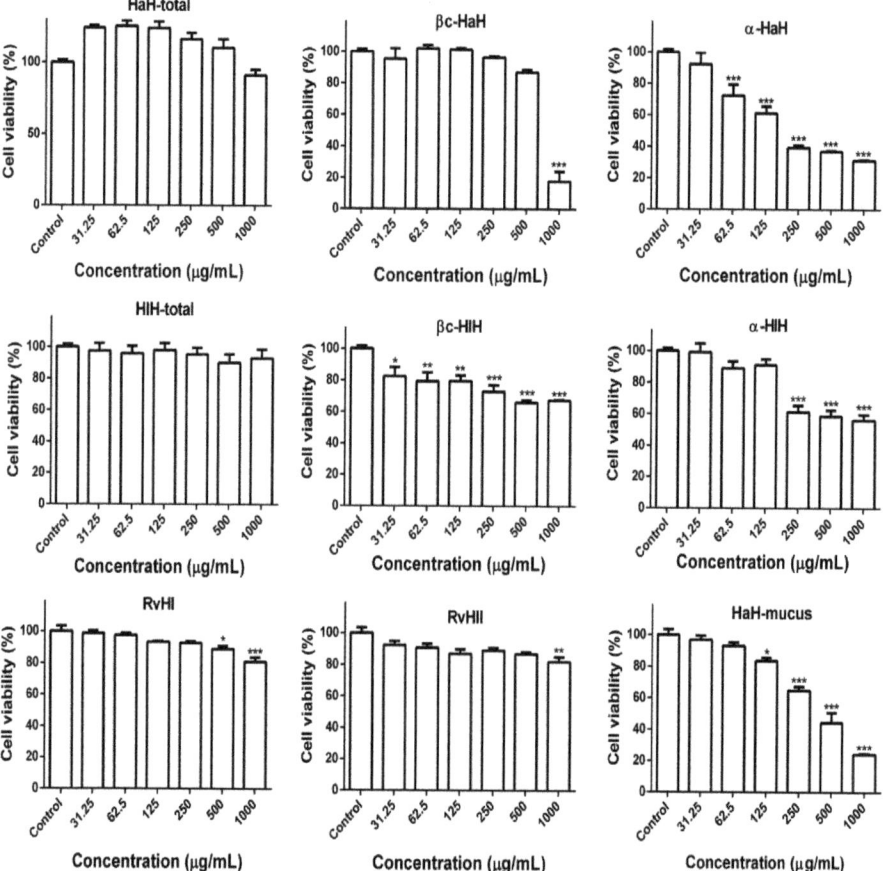

Figure 2. Antiproliferative effect of hemocyanins from *H. aspersa* (HaH-total) and its structural subunits βc-HaH and α-HaH; hemocyanin from *H. lucorum* (HlH-total) and its subunits βc-HlH and α-HlH; subunits RvH I and RvH II of hemocyanin from *R. venosa* (RvH); mucus extract of *Helix aspersa* on HT-29 colorectal carcinoma cell line. * $p < 0.05$; ** $p < 0.01$; *** $p < 0.001$

The results of the MTT assay showed that the total hemocyanins of *H. aspersa* and *H. lucorum* did not significantly affect the viability of the colon carcinoma cells. However, the isolated structural subunits α-HaH, βc-HlH, and α-HlH of hemocyanins as well the mucus from snail *H. aspersa* induced significant ($p < 0.001$ as compared to the untreated control) and dose-dependent reduction of the cell viability and proliferation.

The βc-HaH subunit induced the highest inhibition of cell viability at a concentration of 1000 μg/mL compared to the other tested subunits. Both subunits, RvH I and RvH II, of *R. venosa* hemocyanin significantly reduced ($p < 0.001$) the cell viability only at higher concentrations (500 and 1000 μg/mL, respectively). Of all tested samples, the subunits α-HaH and the mucus of snail *H. aspersa* showed the highest in vitro antitumor activity against HT-29 colon carcinoma cells. On the basis of the results of the MTT assay, we calculated the half-maximal inhibitory concentrations (IC_{50}) and compared them to the IC_{50} determined by MTT assay on Balb/c3T3 cells (Table 1).

Table 1. The half-maximal inhibitory concentrations (IC$_{50}$) of hemocyanins and their subunits isolated from *H. aspersa*, *H. lucorum*, and *R. venosa* determined by MTT assay on HT-29 and Balb/c3T3 cells.

IC$_{50}$ Values (µg/mL)	HT-29	Balb/c 3T3
HaH-total	>1000	934.1
Subunit βc-HaH	733.8	>1000
Subunits α-HaH	235.3	514.6
HlH-total	>1000	>1000
Subunit βc-HlH	>1000	>1000
Subunits α-HlH	>1000	>1000
Subunit RvH I	>1000	>1000
Subunit RvH II	>1000	>1000
Ha-mucus	415.7	825.1

The results showed that HT-29 cells were more sensitive to the aniproliferative and cytotoxic effects of the tested samples than Balb/c3T3 cells.

3.3. Apotogenic Effects of the Isolated Bioactive Compounds

3.3.1. Vital Double Staining of HT-29 Tumor Cells with Acridine Orange/Ethidium Bromide Acridin

For assessment of the apoptogenic potential of the selected samples, we examined the morphological alterations in HT-29 tumor cells. For this purpose, tumor cells were treated with three different concentrations of subunit α-HaH and *H. aspersa*. The changes in the cell morphology induced by the hemocyanins were examined under fluorescent microscope after staining with AO/EB (Figure 3).

Control cells were uniformly stained green and showed normal morphology and monolayer growth characteristics of the tumor cell line (Figure 3a). The positive control substance doxorubicin induced clearly pronounced apoptotic changes in the tumor cells (Figure 3b). Distinct dose-dependent morphological changes were found in HT-29 cells treated with α-HaH and the mucus of *H. aspersa*. The cell density of the monolayer was reduced and cells with intensive green fluorescence indicative of early apoptotic chromatin condensation changes were observed in treated cell cultures. In addition, late apoptotic cells with condensed chromatin, fragmented nuclei, and red-orange staining indicating the loss of membrane integrity and entry of ethidium bromide into the cell were also present.

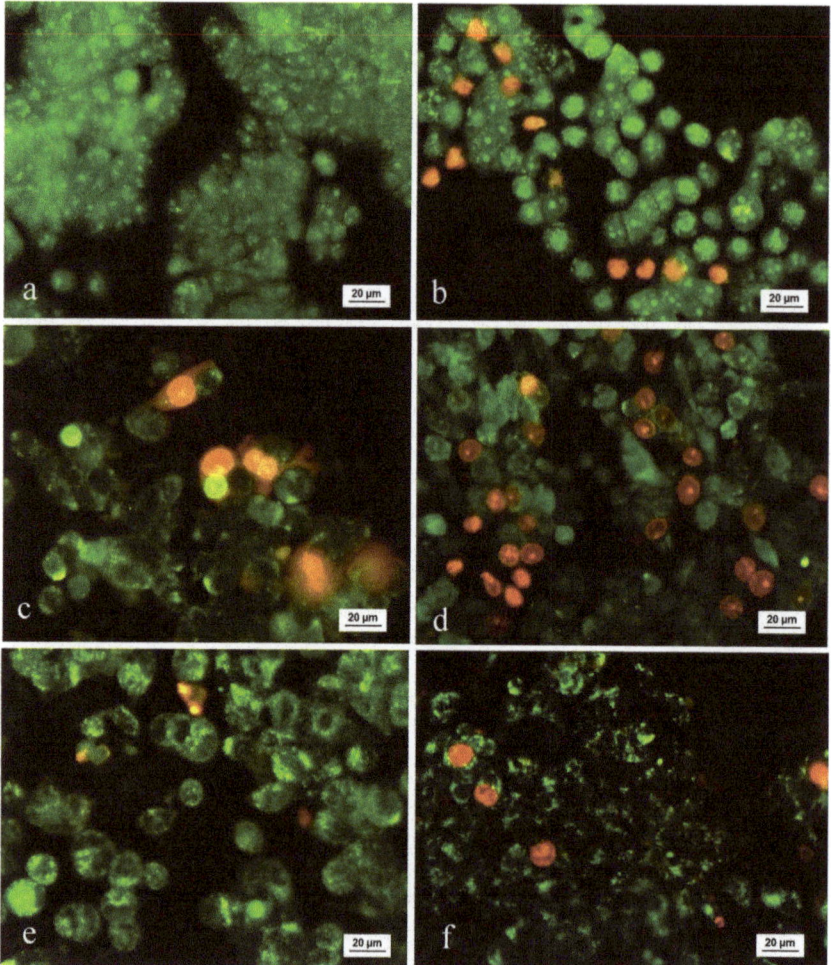

Figure 3. Fluorescence microscopic images of acridine orange (AO)/ethidium bromide (EB)-stained HT-29 colorectal carcinoma cells after treatment with bioactive compounds isolated from *H. aspersa*: (**a**) control; (**b**) doxorubicin 2.7 µg/mL; (**c**) subunit α-HaH 200 µg/mL; (**d**) subunit α-HaH 800 µg/mL; (**e**) *H. aspersa* mucus 400 µg/mL; (**f**) *H. aspersa* mucus 800 µg/mL.

3.3.2. DAPI Staining of HT-29 Tumor Cells

Further, the alterations in the nuclear morphology of the HT-29 cells induced by subunits α-HaH and the mucus were studied by fluorescent microscopy after staining with DNA-binding dye DAPI (Figure 4).

The control HT-29 tumor cells showed typical morphology of the nucleus with homogenous blue staining, and cells in mitosis phase were observed. The nuclei of the cells treated with the α-HaH subunits and the mucus were irregular in shape, more brightly colored, and had intense condensation of chromatin. Some treated cells showed nuclear fragmentation and formation of apoptotic bodies. Mitotic figures were not found in cells exposed to hemocyanin and mucus.

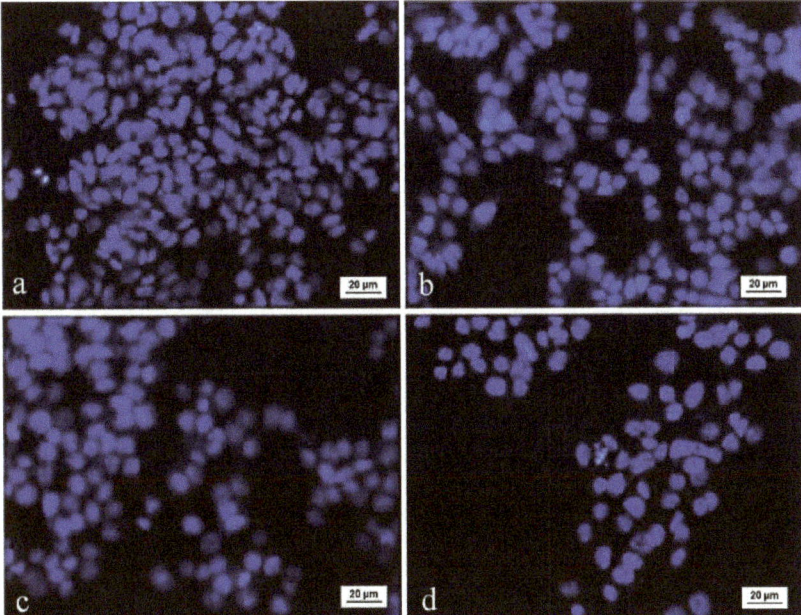

Figure 4. Fluorescence microscopic images of 4′,6-diamidine-2′-phenylindole dihydrochloride (DAPI)-stained HT-29 colorectal carcinoma cells after treatement with bioactive compounds isolated from garden snail *Helix aspersa*: (**a**) control; (**b**) *Helix aspersa* mucus 400 μg/mL; (**c**) subunit α-HaH 100 μg/mL; (**d**) subunit α-HaH 200 μg/mL.

3.4. Transmission Electron Microscopy

The ultrastructural alterations induced by the subunits α-HaH and the mucus from garden snail *H. aspersa* in HT-29 tumor cells were examined by transmission electron microscopy (Figure 5).

Our TEM observations of HT-29 cells in the control culture showed bipolar elongated cells with normal morphology (Figure 5a). The nucleus and the cytoplasm of the untreated cells had a normal structure, were relatively electronically dense, and were without cellular inclusions. The nucleus was more centrally located and several vesicles and the endoplasmic reticulum was peripherally observed. The cells' nuclei exhibited adenocarcinoma-specific appearance with prominent nucleoli. The notable superficial cellular membrane protrusions/microvilli evenly distributed on the surface of the plasmalemma are also typical for the carcinoma cells.

The ultrastructural aspects of the HT-29 cells treated with different test compounds showed mild to more pronounced changes (Figure 5b). The subunits α-HaH and the mucus extract seriously affected cell morphology. The lesions were mainly expressed in loss of polarity and rounded shapes. Numerous cytoplasmic vesicles were observed, being dispersed throughout the cytoplasm along with single electron-dense objects of a larger number and size (likely disorganization of the cytoskeleton and vacuolization of the organelles along the apoptosis pathway). No nuclear fragmentation was found after subunits' α-HaH exposure. The observed cells were also characterized by enlightened nuclei and cytoplasm, budding to form apoptotic bodies including parts of the cytoplasm.

The cells treated with the *Helix aspersa* mucus showed changes similar to the enlightened nuclei presented above, with separate small condensates of heterochromatin, focal perinuclear expansions of the membrane space of endoplasmic reticulum, and abundant organelle vacuolization (Figure 5c). The appearance of different electron-dense bodies and single autophagosomes or mitophagosome-like structures in cells were observed. Rare nuclear fragmentation, formation of apoptotic bodies with parts of the cytoplasm, and vacuoles within them were found as serious morphological alterations. In addition, extended nuclei were observed here, leading to changed nucleus–cytoplasm index.

4. Discussion

The search for novel, more effective, and safe antitumor medicines with natural origin is one of the main trends of contemporary oncology research. In this respect, hemocyanin oligomeric copper-containing glycoproteins that function as oxygen carriers in the hemolymph of mollusk and arthropod species represent significant interest because they combine strong immunostimulating activity and direct anticancer effects [5,6,25–27]. Among this class of compounds, the hemocyanin obtained from *Megathura crenulata*, known as keyhole limpet hemocyanin (KLH), has been most extensively studied and has found a number of biotechnological and medical applications. Clinical studies have shown that KLH treatment significantly reduces the tumor recurrence of patients with urinary bladder carcinoma [11]. It has also found an application as a bio-adjuvant and protein carrier in experimental antiviral and anticancer vaccines [16,28,29]. Moreover, KLH has been reported to induce significant reduction in the proliferation and viability of prostate cancer cells, estrogen-dependent breast and estrogen-independent breast cancer cells, and Barrett's esophageal adenocarcinoma cells [14,30].

The diverse biological activities and increasing biomedical applications of KLH have led to growing interest and a search of other hemocyanins with similar or more potent immunostimulatory and antitumor properties. In the present study, the antitumor activity of total hemocyanins isolated from *H. aspersa*, *H. lucorum*, and their subunits; subunits of *R. venosa* hemocyanin; and *H. aspersa* mucus was examined in the HT-29 human colorectal carcinoma cell line. The results showed that the total hemocyanins did not significantly affect the viability of the colorectal carcinoma cells, while the isolated hemocyanin subunits induced a statistically significant decrease of the tumor cell growth. Similarly, in a previous study, it was found that the subunits of *H. lucorum* hemocyanin induce stronger inhibition of the tumor growth of bladder carcinoma CAL-29 cells as compared to the effect of native HlH [26]. It could be supposed that the potent tumor inhibiting activity is due to the specific oligosaccharide structures, which are more easily accessible in the isolated structural subunits. In addition to hemocyanin subunits, the *H. aspersa* mucus also showed a significant anticancer effect against HT-29 carcinoma cells. The bioactive compounds, structural subunits α-HaH, βc-HaH, and mucus, isolated from garden snail *H. aspersa*, appeared to be the most active of all tested samples in inhibiting the colon cancer cell growth. This result is in agreement with the data reported by Matusiewicz et al., indicating that the application of extracts from lyophilized mucus and foot tissues of *H. aspersa* decrease the viability of the colon cancer cell line Caco-2 [31].

The reduction of the viability the HT-29 cells induced by treatment with HlH subunits was statistically significant with a clear dose dependency, but it was slightly weaker than those of HaH subunits. The subunits of *R. venosa* hemocyanin showed an antitumor effect only at the higher tested concentrations. Hemocyanins isolated from the land snail *H. pomatia* and marine snail *R. thomasiana* were previously found to express strong immunostimulatroy action and to inhibit tumor cell growth in a murine model of colon carcinoma [32]. These findings taken together with the results of the present study demonstrate that the hemocyanins isolated from different mollusk species have significant antitumor effects against colorectal carcinoma.

The tested bioactive substances, mucus and α-HaH from snail *H. aspersa*, which showed higher antiproliferative activity in the MTT assay, were further used in morphological studies that aimed to analyze the mechanisms that mediate their anticancer action and the nature of the cell death induced in HT-29 carcinoma cells. The fluorescent and transmission electron microscopy studies revealed typical apoptotic alterations in the cellular and nuclear morphology of the tumor cells treated with the tested samples. Apoptotic cell death is an important biological mechanism that contributes to the maintenance and integrity of multicellular organisms and an important factor in preventing cancer. Thus, the ability to induce apoptosis in tumor cells is a desired property of the anticancer therapeutics.

Our results are in line with the previously published data, indicating a significant proapoptotic activity of molluscan hemocyanins in various tumor cell lines [4,33–35] and suggesting their potential use in anticancer therapy.

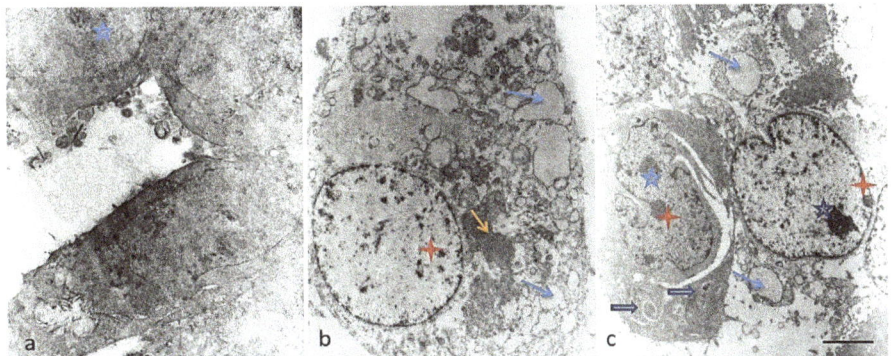

Figure 5. Transmission electron microscopy images of HT-29 cells after treatment with bioactive compounds isolated from *Helix aspersa*. (**a**) Control HT-29 cells with normal morphology: blue five-point star-nucleolus. (**b**) HT-29 cells treated with the subunits α-HaH with affected cell morphology: red four-point star—granules of highly condensed chromatin, thin blue arrow—numerous vacuoles, thin orange arrow—electron-dense cytoplasmic structures. (**c**) HT-29 cells treated with the mucus of *Helix aspersa* with impaired morphology: blue five-point star—nucleolus, red four-point star—granules of highly condensed chromatin, thin blue arrow—numerous vacuoles, blue filled arrow—presence of single autophagosomes or mitophagosome-like structures. TEM scale bar = 2 μm.

5. Conclusions

The tested hemocyanin samples isolated from garden snails *H. aspersa* and *H. lucorum*, marine snail *R. venosa*, as well as the mucus from garden snail *H. aspersa* significantly decreased the cell viability of HT-29 carcinoma cells. The mucus and α-HaH from snail *H. aspersa* were identified as bioactive substances with higher antiproliferative activity against HT-29 carcinoma cells. The mechanism of their antitumor activity includes the induction of apoptosis. In the combination with their already known immunogenic effect, these findings support further studies of molluscan hemocyanins as potential therapeutic agents against colorectal cancer.

Author Contributions: Conceptualization, P.D. and R.T.; methodology, A.D., L.V., A.G., and K.T.; validation, I.I. and I.V.; formal analysis, V.D.; investigation, A.G., K.T., I.I., R.T., and P.D.; resources, S.P., P.D., and R.T.; data curation, R.T.; writing—original draft preparation, A.G.; writing—review and editing, K.T., R.T., and P.D.; visualization, A.G. and K.T.; supervision, S.P., R.T., and P.D.; project administration, P.D. and S.P.; funding acquisition, P.D. and S.P. All authors have read and agreed to the published version of the manuscript.

Funding: Ministry of Education and Science of the Republic of Bulgaria supported by National Program "Innovative Low-Toxic and Biologically Active Means for Precision Medicine" – BioActiveMed, grant number Д01-217/30.11.2018, and Ministry of Education and Science of the Republic of Bulgaria and the Operational Program "Science and Education for Smart Growth" 2014-2020, co-financed by the European Union through the European Structural and Investment Funds, grant number BG05M2OP001-2.009-0019-C01/02.06.2017.

Acknowledgments: We thank Zdravka Stoichkova, Svetlana Vladova, and Boycho Nikolov (IEMPAM-BAS) for technical assistance.

Conflicts of Interest: The authors declare no conflict of interest. The funders had no role in the design of the study; in the collection, analyses, or interpretation of data; in the writing of the manuscript; or in the decision to publish the results.

Abbreviations

AO	Acridine orange
ATCC	4′,6-Diamidine-2′-phenylindole dihydrochloride
DMEM	Dulbecco's modified Eagle's medium
LD	Linear dichroism
DMSO	Dimethyl sulfoxide
EB	Ethidium bromide
HaH	Helix aspersa hemocyanin
HlH	Helix lucorum hemocyanin
KLH	Keyhole limpet hemocyanin
MTT	Methyl thiazol tetrazolium bromide
PBS	Phosphate-buffered saline
RvH	Rapana venosa hemocyanin
TEM	Transmission electron microscopy

References

1. Falzone, L.; Salomone, S.; Libra, M. Evolution of cancer pharmacological treatments at the turn of the third millennium. *Front. Pharmacol.* **2018**, *9*, 1300. [CrossRef] [PubMed]
2. Cragg, G.M.; Pezzuto, J.M. Natural products as a vital source for the discovery of cancer chemotherapeutic and chemopreventive agents. *Med. Princ. Pract.* **2016**, *25*, 41–59. [CrossRef] [PubMed]
3. Wang, L.; Dong, C.; Li, X.; Han, W.; Su, X. Anticancer potential of bioactive peptides from animal sources. *Oncol. Rep.* **2017**, *38*, 637–651. [CrossRef] [PubMed]
4. Antonova, O.; Toncheva, D.; Rammensee, H.G.; Floetenmeyer, M.; Stevanovic, S.; Dolashka, P. In vitro antiproliferative effect of *Helix aspersa* hemocyanin on multiple malignant cell lines. *Zeitschrift für Naturforschung C* **2014**, *69*, 325–334. [CrossRef]
5. Becker, M.I.; Arancibia, S.; Salazar, F.; Del Campo, M.; De Ioannes, A. Mollusk Hemocyanins as Natural Immunostimulants in Biomedical Applications, in Immune Response Activation. Duc, G.H.T., Ed.; InTech: Croatia, Rijeka, 2014; pp. 45–72.
6. Pizarro-Bauerle, J.; Maldonado, I.; Sosoniuk-Roche, E.; Vallejos, G.; López, M.N.; Salazar-Onfray, F.; Aguilar-Guzmán, L.; Valck, C.; Ferreira, A.; Becker, M.I. Molluskan hemocyanins activate the classical pathway of the human complement system through natural antibodies. *Front. Immunol.* **2017**, *8*, 188. [CrossRef]
7. Mora, J.J.; Del Campo, M.; Villar, J.; Paolini, F.; Curzio, G.; Venuti, A.; Jara, L.; Ferreira, J.; Murgas, P.; Lladser, A.; et al. Immunotherapeutic potential of mollusk hemocyanins in combination with human vaccine adjuvants in murine models of oral cancer. *J. Immunol. Res.* **2019**, *2019*, 7076942.
8. Kato, S.; Matsui, T.; Gatsogiannis, C.; Tanaka, Y. Molluscan hemocyanin: Structure, evolution, and physiology. *Biophysical Rev.* **2018**, *10*, 191–202. [CrossRef]
9. Paccagnella, M.; Bologna, L.; Beccaro, M.; Micetic, I.; Di Muro, P.; Salvato, B. Structural subunit organization of molluscan hemocyanins. *Micron* **2004**, *35*, 21–22. [CrossRef]
10. Sandra, K.; Dolashka-Angelova, P.; Devreese, B.; Van Beeumen, J. New insights in *Rapana venosa* hemocyani N-glycosylation resulting from on-line mass spectrometric analyses. *Glycobiology* **2007**, *17*, 141–156. [CrossRef]
11. Arancibia, S.; Salazar, F.; Becker, M.I. Hemocyanins in the immunotherapy of superficial bladder cancer. In *Bladder Cancer-From Basic Science to Robotic Surgery*; Canda, A.E., Ed.; InTech: Croatia, Rijeka, 2012; pp. 221–242.
12. Dolashka, P.; Velkova, L.; Shishkov, S.; Kostova, K.; Dolashki, A.; Dimitrov, I.; Atanasov, B.; Devreese, B.; Voelter, W.; Van Beeumen, J. Glycan structures and antiviral effect of the structural subunit RvH2 of *Rapana* hemocyanin. *Carbohydr. Res.* **2010**, *345*, 2361–2367. [CrossRef]
13. Zhong, T.-Y.; Arancibia, S.; Born, R.; Tampe, R.; Villar, J.; Del Campo, M.; Manubens, A.; Becker, M.I. Hemocyanins stimulate innate immunity by inducing different temporal patterns of proinflammatory cytokine expression in macrophages. *J. Immunol.* **2016**, *196*, 4650–4662. [CrossRef]

14. Riggs, D.R.; Jackson, B.J.; Vona-Davis, L.; Nigam, A.; McFadden, D.W. In vitro effects of keyhole limpet hemocyanin in breast and pancreatic cancer in regards to cell growth, cytokine production, and apoptosis. *Am. J. Surg.* **2005**, *189*, 680–684. [CrossRef] [PubMed]
15. Dolashka, P.; Velkova, L.; Iliev, I.; Beck, A.; Dolashki, A.; Yossifova, L.; Toshkova, R.; Voelter, W.; Zacharieva, S. Antitumor activity of glycosylated molluscan hemocyanins via Guerin ascites tumor. *Immunol. Invest.* **2011**, *40*, 130–149. [CrossRef]
16. Salazar, M.L.; Jiménez, J.M.; Villar, J.; Rivera, M.; Báez, M.; Manubens, A.; Becker, M. N-Glycosylation of mollusk hemocyanins contributes to their structural stability and immunomodulatory properties in mammals. *J. Biol. Chem.* **2019**, *294*, 19546–19564. [CrossRef] [PubMed]
17. Dolashka-Angelova, P.; Schwarz, H.; Dolashki, A.; Stevanovic, S.; Fecker, M.; Saeed, M.; Voelter, W. Oligomeric stability of Rapana venosa hemocyanin (RvH) and its structural subunits. *Biochim. Biophys. Acta.* **2003**, *1646*, 77–85. [CrossRef]
18. Velkova, L.; Dimitrov, I.; Schwarz, H.; Stevanovic, S.; Voelter, W.; Salvato, B.; Dolashka-Angelova, P. Structure of hemocyanin from garden snail Helix lucorum. *Comp. Biochem. Physiol.* **2010**, *157*, 16–25. [CrossRef] [PubMed]
19. Dolashki, A.; Nissimova, A.; Daskalova, E.; Velkova, L.; Topalova, Y.; Hristova, P.; Traldi, P.; Voelter, W.; Dolashka, P. Structure and antibacterial activity of isolated peptides from the mucus of garden snail *Cornu aspersum*. *Bulg. Chem. Commun.* **2018**, *50C*, 195–200.
20. Laemmli, U.K. Cleavage of Structural Proteins during the Assembly of the Head of Bacteriophage T4. *Nature* **1970**, *227*, 680–685. [CrossRef]
21. Schägger, H.; von Jagow, G. Blue Native Electrophoresis for Isolation of Membrane Protein Complexes in Enzymatically Active Form. *Anal. Biochem.* **1991**, *199*, 223–231. [CrossRef]
22. Mossmann, T. Rapid colorimetric assay of cellular growth and survival: Application to proliferation and cytotoxicity assays. *J. Immunol. Methods* **1983**, *65*, 55–63. [CrossRef]
23. Wahab, I.; Abdul, A.; Alzubairi, A.; Elhassan, M.; Mohan, S. In vitro ultramorphological assessment of apoptosis induced by zerumbone on (HeLa). *J. Biomed. Biotechnol.* **2009**, *2009*, 769568. [PubMed]
24. Gielens, C.; De Sadeleer, J.; Preaux, G.; Lontie, R. Identification, separation and cheracterization of the hemocyanin components of *Helix aspersa*. *Comp. Biochem. Phys. Part B* **1987**, *88*, 181–186. [CrossRef]
25. Luo, W.; Yang, G.; Luo, W.; Cao, Z.; Liu, Y.; Qiu, J.; Chen, G.; You, L.; Zhao, F.; Zheng, L.; et al. Novel therapeutic strategies and perspectives for metastatic pancreatic cancer: Vaccine therapy is more than just a theory. *Cancer Cell Int.* **2020**, *20*, 66. [CrossRef] [PubMed]
26. Dolashki, A.; Dolashka, P.; Stenzl, A.; Stevanovic, S.; Aicher, W.K.; Velkova, L.; Velikova, R.; Voelter, W. Antitumour activity of *Helix* hemocyanin against bladder carcinoma permanent cell lines. *Biotech. Biotech. Equip.* **2019**, *33*, 1–13. [CrossRef]
27. Dolashka-Angelova, P.; Stefanova, T.; Livaniou, E.; Velkova, L.; Klimentzou, P.; Stevanovic, S.; Salvato, B.; Neychev, H.; Voelter, W. Immunological potential of Helix vulgaris and Rapana venosa hemocyanins. *Immunol. Invest.* **2008**, *37*, 822–840. [CrossRef] [PubMed]
28. Miles, D.; Roché, H.; Martin, M.; Perren, T.J.; Cameron, D.A.; Glaspy, J.; Dodwell, D.; Parker, J.; Mayordomo, J.; Tres, A.; et al. Phase III multicenter clinical trial of the sialyl-TN (STn)-keyhole limpet hemocyanin (KLH) vaccine for metastatic breast cancer. *Oncologist* **2011**, *16*, 1092–1100. [CrossRef]
29. Gilewski, T.A.; Ragupathi, G.; Dickler, M.; Powell, S.; Bhuta, S.; Panageas, K.; Koganty, R.R.; Chin-Eng, J.; Hudis, C.; Norton, L.; et al. Immunization of high-risk breast cancer patients with clustered sTn-KLH conjugate plus the immunologic adjuvant QS-21. *Clin. Cancer Res.* **2007**, *13*, 2977–2985. [CrossRef]
30. McFadden, D.W.; Riggs, D.R.; Jackson, B.J.; Vona-Davis, L. Keyhole limpet hemocyanin, a novel immune stimulant with promising anticancer activity in Barrett's esophageal adenocarcinoma. *Am. J. Surg.* **2003**, *186*, 552–555. [CrossRef]
31. Matusiewicz, M.; Kosieradzka, I.; Niemiec, T.; Grodzik, M.; Antushevich, H.; Strojny, B.; Gołębiewska, M. In Vitro Influence of Extracts from Snail *Helix aspersa* Müller on the Colon Cancer Cell Line Caco-2. *Int. J. Mol. Sci.* **2018**, *19*, 1064. [CrossRef]
32. Gesheva, V.; Chausheva, S.; Mihaylova, N.; Manoylov, I.; Doumanova, L.; Idakieva, K.; Tchorbanov, A. Anti-cancer properties of gastropodan hemocyanins in murine model of colon carcinoma. *BMC Immunol.* **2014**, *15*, 34. [CrossRef]

33. Stenzl, A.; Dolashki, A.; Stevanovic, S.; Voelter, W.; Aicher, W.; Dolashka, P. Cytotoxic effects of *Rapana venosa* hemocyanin on bladder cancer permanent cell lines. *J. US China Med. Sci.* **2016**, *13*, 79–188.
34. Antonova, O.; Yossifova, L.; Staneva, R.; Stevanovic, S.; Dolashka, P.; Toncheva, D. Changes in the gene expression profile of the bladder cancer cell lines after treatment with Helix lucorum and Rapana venosa hemocyanin. *J. Buon.* **2015**, *20*, 180–187. [PubMed]
35. Somasundar, P.; Riggs, D.R.; Jackson, B.J.; McFadden, D.W. Inhibition of melanoma growth by hemocyanin occurs via early apoptotic pathways. *Am. J. Surg.* **2005**, *190*, 713–716. [CrossRef] [PubMed]

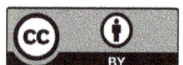

© 2020 by the authors. Licensee MDPI, Basel, Switzerland. This article is an open access article distributed under the terms and conditions of the Creative Commons Attribution (CC BY) license (http://creativecommons.org/licenses/by/4.0/).

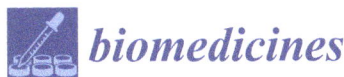

Review

Resveratrol Modulates Transforming Growth Factor-Beta (TGF-β) Signaling Pathway for Disease Therapy: A New Insight into Its Pharmacological Activities

Milad Ashrafizadeh [1], Masoud Najafi [2], Sima Orouei [3], Amirhossein Zabolian [4], Hossein Saleki [4], Negar Azami [4], Negin Sharifi [4], Kiavash Hushmandi [5], Ali Zarrabi [6,7,*] and Kwang Seok Ahn [8,*]

1. Department of Basic Science, Faculty of Veterinary Medicine, University of Tabriz, Tabriz 5166616471, Iran; dvm.milad73@yahoo.com
2. Radiology and Nuclear Medicine Department, School of Paramedical Sciences, Kermanshah University of Medical Sciences, Kermanshah 6715847141, Iran; najafi_ma@yahoo.com
3. Department of Genetics, Tehran Medical Sciences, Islamic Azad University, Tehran 1916893813, Iran; Sima.orouei@gmail.com
4. Young Researchers and Elite Club, Tehran Medical Sciences, Islamic Azad University, Tehran 1916893813, Iran; Fzr2000_0007@yahoo.com (A.Z.); hosseinsaleki2015@gmail.com (H.S.); negarazami77@gmail.com (N.A.); Negin.sharifi87@gmail.com (N.S.)
5. Department of Food Hygiene and Quality Control, Division of Epidemiology & Zoonoses, Faculty of Veterinary Medicine, University of Tehran, Tehran 1417414418, Iran; houshmandi.kia7@ut.ac.ir
6. Sabanci University Nanotechnology Research and Application Center (SUNUM), Tuzla, 34956 Istanbul, Turkey
7. Center of Excellence for Functional Surfaces and Interfaces (EFSUN), Faculty of Engineering and Natural Sciences, Sabanci University, Tuzla, 34956 Istanbul, Turkey
8. Department of Science in Korean Medicine, College of Korean Medicine, Kyung Hee University, 24 Kyungheedae-ro, Dongdaemun-gu, Seoul 02447, Korea
* Correspondence: alizarrabi@sabanciuniv.edu (A.Z.); ksahn@khu.ac.kr (K.S.A.)

Received: 23 June 2020; Accepted: 28 July 2020; Published: 31 July 2020

Abstract: Resveratrol (Res) is a well-known natural product that can exhibit important pharmacological activities such as antioxidant, anti-diabetes, anti-tumor, and anti-inflammatory. An evaluation of its therapeutic effects demonstrates that this naturally occurring bioactive compound can target different molecular pathways to exert its pharmacological actions. Transforming growth factor-beta (TGF-β) is an important molecular pathway that is capable of regulating different cellular mechanisms such as proliferation, migration, and angiogenesis. TGF-β has been reported to be involved in the development of disorders such as diabetes, cancer, inflammatory disorders, fibrosis, cardiovascular disorders, etc. In the present review, the relationship between Res and TGF-β has been investigated. It was noticed that Res can inhibit TGF-β to suppress the proliferation and migration of cancer cells. In addition, Res can improve fibrosis by reducing inflammation via promoting TGF-β down-regulation. Res has been reported to be also beneficial in the amelioration of diabetic complications via targeting the TGF-β signaling pathway. These topics are discussed in detail in this review to shed light on the protective effects of Res mediated via the modulation of TGF-β signaling.

Keywords: resveratrol; transforming growth factor-beta (TGF-β); chronic diseases; fibrosis; cancer; diabetes; therapy

1. Resveratrol

From immemorial times, plant-derived natural compounds have been under attention in the treatment of different disorders such as inflammatory diseases, cancers, pulmonary diseases, metabolic disorders, neurological disorders (NDs) including Alzheimer's disease (AD) and Parkinson's disease (PD), infertility, and so on [1–10]. Phytochemicals can exhibit beneficial actions against diseases due to their excellent pharmacological activities [11–14]. These benefits have resulted in extensive research into finding new natural compounds and revealing their potential mechanisms of actions [15–17]. Resveratrol (Res) is a dietary phytochemical that has been reported to be efficacious treatment for various ailments by targeting diverse molecular pathways [18–21]. The role of Res in the treatment of chronic diseases was established in early 1990s when it was found that this phytochemical possesses significant cardioprotective benefits [22]. This ascending trend toward Res research led to the revelation of its significant biological and therapeutic activities. The first report about anti-tumor activity of Res dates back to 1997, when Jang and his colleagues reported its inhibitory effect on leukemia [23].

Currently, Res can be derived from various plants including *Arachis hypogea*, *Cassia* sp., *Eucalyptus* sp., *Morus rubra*, and so on using a number of different isolation techniques [24]. High-performance liquid chromatography is the best strategy [25–28]. Over the past decades, Res has been applied in the treatment of various diseases such as osteoarthritis [29–31], NDs [32], cancer [33–35], diabetes [36], cardiovascular diseases [37], liver disorders [38], and so on. An increasing amount of evidence is in agreement with the fact that Res affects different molecular pathways to exhibit its protective effects [39–41]. Hence, the identification of these targets can promote further studies for investigating molecular pathways and the mechanisms of its therapeutic actions in depth. For instance, anti-inflammation is one of the most important biological effects of Res treatment. To function as an anti-inflammatory molecule, Res can effectively inhibit the activation of pro-inflammatory transcription factors such as nuclear factor-kappaB (NF-kB). It seems that the anti-inflammatory actions of Res are not only mediated via inhibitory actions on the NF-kB signaling pathway, but they also rely on its action as a PARP-γ agonist [42]. The anti-inflammatory activities of Res are also characterized by decreased levels of interleukin (IL)-6, IL-8, and tumor necrosis factor-α (TNF-α), etc. [43]. The production of pro-inflammatory lipid mediators from arachidonic acid can be mediated by the cyclooxygenase (COX) pathway. A number of anti-inflammatory drugs have been developed based on their inhibitory effect on COX-1 and COX-2 [44,45]. Res is capable of binding to the active site of COX-1 and thus causing anti-inflammatory effects. In addition to targeting inflammation, Res attaches to the active site of COX-2 to suppress cancer proliferation [46–49]. It is noteworthy that the inhibitory effect of Res on COX has been noted to follow a dose-dependent kinetics [50].

Obesity is one of the challenges faced in today's world. Res has demonstrated great potential in reducing weight and exerting anti-obesity activity. Res changes white adipose tissue (WAT) into brown adipose tissue (BAT), which in turn decreases weight and improves insulin resistance [51]. The inhibitory action of Res on lipid accumulation leads to its effect on cardiovascular disorders. Res stimulates PARP-α/γ to activate ATP binding cassette (ABC) transporter A1/G1-mediated cholesterol efflux, resulting in a decrease in lipid accumulation and cholesterol levels. These effects can lead to a significant amelioration of atherosclerosis [52]. Based on the effect of Res on amyloid-beta (Aβ), this plant-derived natural compound is of importance in treating NDs. For instance, Res is able to inhibit inflammation and the microglial activation caused by Aβ. This results in the alleviation of inflammation (down-regulation of TNF-α and IL-6) and a diminution in apoptosis (caspase-1 down-regulation) [53]. The antioxidant activity of Res provides its protective effect during kidney injury. In rats exposed to nicotine, an increase occurs in oxidative stress markers via the down-regulation of glutathione. The administration of Res has been also correlated with improving the antioxidant defense system that protects renal cells against oxidative injury [54]. A newly published study also demonstrates the effect of Res on stem cells. Res can stimulate stem cell function to ameliorate pancreatic injury such as fibrosis and apoptosis [55]. Overall, these reports exhibit that Res has diverse therapeutic effects that have resulted in its extensive application in the treatment of various disorders [56–58]. In the current review, we specifically focus on the therapeutic effects of Res mediated by its regulatory action on the transforming growth factor-β (TGF-β) signaling pathway.

1.1. Resveratrol: Limitations and Applied Strategies

In spite of the excellent pharmacological activities of plant-derived natural compounds, very soon it was found that a number of issues limit their efficacy in disease treatment. Increasing evidence shows that phytochemicals are able to exert their therapeutic effects predominantly under in vitro settings. However, when their efficiency is examined for in vivo experiments, a decrease occurs in their therapeutic efficacy due to their potential poor bioavailability. The difficulty is more prominent in clinical trials, leading to a limited application of phytochemicals in clinic. This holds also true for Res, and various formulations of this agent have been tested to enhance its therapeutic capabilities. Res has a lipophilic nature and can be dissolved in fruit or vegetable juices or given in capsule form. The administration frequency of Res is variable from one to three times a day, and its reported doses are at the range of 0.073 mg to 5 g [59,60]. The reports also demonstrated that the most efficient strategy in promoting the bioavailability and protective effects of Res is using nanoparticles [61]. The encapsulation of Res by nanoparticles protects against degradation and improves its intestinal absorption and blood circulation time [62–66]. These benefits lead to the promoted bioavailability of Res and an improvement in its therapeutic effects [67,68]. It has been reported that loading Res on lipid carriers can significantly increase its anti-tumor activity and cytotoxicity against breast cancer cells by providing targeted delivery and enhancing its intracellular internalization [69]. Lipid nanocarriers containing Res can be administered through the oral route. The oral administration of Res-loaded lipid nanostructures is more beneficial in reducing the levels of pro-inflammatory cytokines and induction of anti-inflammatory activity compared to Res alone [70]. The enhanced release of Res in the intestine by nanoparticles is of importance in elevating its cytotoxicity against cancer cells [71]. Overall, various studies reveal that nanostructures can be considered as potential delivery systems for Res and fortunately, a significant number of studies have been performed in this field. The findings are in line with the fact that these nano-based strategies can remarkably enhance both the bioavailability and therapeutic capability of Res [72–74]. However, more studies are needed to design different effective nanocarriers to facilitate an optimum delivery of Res.

1.2. Pharmacokinetics of Resveratrol: A Brief Explanation

Increasing evidence demonstrates that the dosage forms and conditions of patients can affect the absorption of Res. However, the gastrointestinal (GI) tract is involved in the absorption of Res after oral administration with a peak at plasma concentration after 30 min and 1.5–2 h [75–77]. The absorption of Res undergoes an increase via grape consumption and using other forms such as micronized form [78–82]. After absorption, Res can be distributed in different organs, such as the brain, liver, intestine, and fat [83]. For metabolism, enterocytes and hepatocytes play the most important role after oral administration. Notably, Res influx occurs through the passive diffusion and carrier-mediated process [84,85]. The metabolism of Res also confirms its distribution in liver, so that it has been reported that Res is a substrate of hepatic sulfotransferase and glucuronosyltransferase, and it extensively accumulates in liver [86]. The interesting point is that metabolism of Res relies on dose. Low doses (5–50 mg) of Res are bio-transformed into glucuronides, while high doses (more than 250 mg) are bio-transformed into monosulfates [87–91]. Facial areas and urine are responsible for the elimination of Res. It has been noted that the administration form of Res may affect its elimination, which can be delayed when micronized Res is used [92–96].

1.3. Toxicity of Resveratrol

Similar to other compounds, plant-derived natural compounds have a number of drawbacks. Although Res is safe and well-tolerated at normal doses, there are toxicities associated with the application of high doses of Res [97]. The willingness toward using high doses of Res is due to its poor bioavailability, which restricts its therapeutic usage. Therefore, providing information about the toxicity of Res is advantageous for directing further studies toward using normal and safe doses of Res. It is worth mentioning that the toxicity of Res has been evaluated in both in vivo and clinical trials. It appears that high doses of Res—as much as 3 g/kg/day in rats—may result in nephrotoxicity. Although there are few studies that have demonstrated that Res can negatively affect liver and enhance levels of liver enzymes such as aspartate aminotransferase, others have reported that it may not exhibit any significant toxicity on the liver [98,99]. The administration of 750 mg/kg/day of Res for 3 months is well-tolerated in rats [100]. Studies in humans show that Res is completely safe and only a few adverse effects including blood electrolyte changes, nasopharyngitis, and erythematous rash can be observed after the administration of 400 mg of Res. Headache, myalgia, epididymitis, and dizziness were other commonly reported adverse effects of Res [101–103].

2. TGF-β: Signaling Pathways and Pathological Role

2.1. Members and Receptors of TGF-β Family

There are three distinct members of TGF-β in mammals including TGF-β1, TGF-β2, and TGF-β3 that are homologous in terms of structure, but they demonstrate different biological activities, temporal, and spatial expression patterns [104–108]. The number of genes that can encode members of the TGF-β family are numerous, but a number of them can be mentioned as *activin, nodal, bone morphogenetic proteins (BMPs)*, and *growth and differentiation factors (GDFs)* [109]. The TGF-β signaling pathway possesses a regulatory effect on different cellular events such as growth, survival, differentiation, cell fate specification, angiogenesis, and so on [110–115]. TGF-β signaling is initiated by the attachment of a ligand onto cell surface receptors, which in turn triggers a cascade that mediates the translocation of TGF-β into the nucleus. In humans, there are 12 cell surface receptors that are affected by ligand, including type I receptors (ALK1-7) and type II receptors (TβRII, ActRII, ActRIIB, BMPRII, and AMHRII) [116,117]. After attachment of a certain type of TGF-β into type II receptors, these receptors are stimulated, which subsequently phosphorylates the glycine-serine-rich domain (GS domain) of type I receptors. In the canonical pathway of TGF-β, type I receptors mediate the formation of Smad complex via phosphorylation at carboxyl termini.

2.2. TGF-β Signaling Pathway

The *TGF-β* gene encodes a pro-precursor peptide consisting of 390 amino acids that undergoes proteolytic processing to produce mature TGF-β. This mature TGF-β has two distinct sections including amino-terminal and carboxy-terminal sections [118]. The amino-terminal fragment is known as latency associated peptide (LAP) with non-covalent attachment into TGF-β [119,120]. The cleavage of LAP by proteases or mechanical forces by cell surface integrins contributes to the release of mature and active TGF-β [121,122]. The activated TGF-β is a dimeric protein with disulfide bonds and molecular weight of 25 kDa that can bind into cell surface receptors. As described above, then, the binding of a ligand into a receptor leads to the phosphorylation of type I receptors by type II ones [123]. Then, TGF-βRI as a type I receptor can stimulate Smad2 and Smad3 via phosphorylation, resulting in the formation of a complex with Smad4. This complex translocates into the nucleus to affect target genes such as *plasminogen activator inhibitor 1* (*PAI1*). Among them, only Smad4 and Smad3 can bind to DNA. It is worth mentioning that the affinity of Smad3 and Smad4 for attachment to DNA is low and they need to collaborate with other DNA-binding transcription factors to promote gene expression [124,125]. This is the canonical pathway of TGF-β, and there is another pathway, which is known as the non-canonical pathway. In this pathway, activated receptors target different molecular pathways such as PI3K as well as JNK, P38, extracellular signal-regulated kinase (ERK), and mitogen-activated protein kinase (MAPK). For instance, PI3K can be activated by stimulated receptors to induce Akt/mTOR axis, resulting in the stimulation of S6K and regulate protein translation (Figure 1) [106].

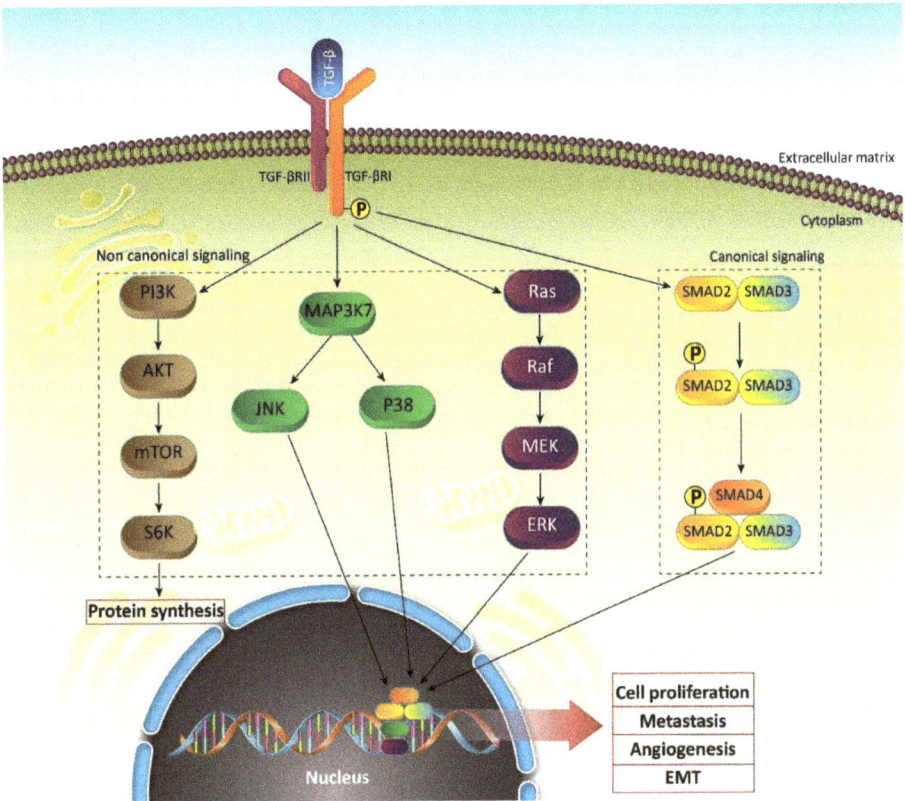

Figure 1. A schematic presentation of transforming growth factor-beta (TGF-β) signaling pathways. This pathway consists of two distinct modules: canonical signaling and non-canonical signaling. Canonical signaling, as shown in the figure, is a result of the formation of a complex containing Smad2, Smad3, and Smad4. Then, these molecules can translocate into the nucleus to trigger the expression of genes that are responsible for the proliferation and metastasis of cancer cells. Non-canonical signaling is Smad-independent and involves different signaling pathways such as PI3K/Akt, MAP3K7, Ras, and so on. However, final aim of these two signaling pathways is to promote aberrant growth and malignancy of cancer cells.

2.3. TGF-β in Cancer, Diabetes, and Other Pathological Events

A number of studies have highlighted that the abnormal expression of TGF-β may pave the road for generating pathological events. The role of the TGF-β signaling pathway in cancer cells has been extensively investigated. Increasing evidence demonstrates that TGF-β mediates the migration and invasion of cancer cells. For enhancing cancer cell metastasis, TGF-β induces epithelial-to-mesenchymal transition (EMT), which significantly promotes the migratory ability of cancer cells [126]. Interestingly, molecular pathways that negatively regulate the metastasis of cancer cells can reduce the expression of TGF-β. It has been revealed that sirtuin 7 (SIRT7) can suppress the migration of cancer cells through inhibiting TGF-β signaling via Smad4 degradation. Therefore, the Smad complex may be disrupted, and its nuclear translocation can be inhibited [127]. In addition to metastasis, TGF-β signaling induces angiogenesis, which is a mechanism that is vital for the proliferation and migration of cancer cells. The stimulatory effect of TGF-β on angiogenesis can be mediated via the phosphorylation of Smad3 [128]. TGF-β is able to stabilize the Nrf2 signaling pathway via p21 induction, thus leading to the chemoresistance of cancer cells [129]. Moreover, numerous studies are in agreement with the fact that TGF-β can act as a positive factor for the proliferation and migration of cancer cells, and a negative factor for cancer prognosis. In addition to cancer, TGF-β contributes to the development of other malignancies. Diabetes mellitus (DM) is a chronic metabolic disorder in which insulin resistance can be obtained and glucose metabolism undergoes dysregulation [130,131]. Myocardial injury and fibrosis may result from DM, and studies have demonstrated that TGF-β is involved in this process. In DM, TGF-β activates Smad2 to facilitate its nuclear translocation. Then, an increase occurs in fibrosis, thereby providing conditions for deteriorating DM. Mesenchymal stem cell-derived exosomes are able to improve DM fibrosis via the inhibition of the TGF-β/Smad2 axis [132]. The TGF-β/Smad3 axis may be also involved in DM fibrosis. Thus, the stimulation of TGF-β and the nuclear translocation of Smad3 provide conditions for the development of renal fibrosis during DM. It has been found that the administration of retinoic acid can alleviate DM-promoted fibrosis via the inhibition of TGF-β/Smad3 [133]. It is noteworthy that a number of phytochemicals have shown potential in the regulation of the TGF-β signaling pathway, which is of immense importance for disease therapy [134,135]. In the present review, we focus on modulation of the TGF-β signaling pathway by Res and its potential impact for disease therapy [136–138].

3. Resveratrol and TGF-β Signaling Pathway

In this section, we will highlight the modulatory effects of Res on TGF-β levels in different chronic diseases. For example, Res can suppress the TGF-β signaling pathway and its downstream targets such as Smads. It can also reduce TGF-β-mediated EMT in fibrosis. It has been reported that for the inhibition of EMT, Res can down-regulate matrix metalloproteinase-9 (MMP-9), leading to the alleviation of fibrosis. MicroRNAs (miRs) such as miR-31 can also be affected by Res in targeting TGF-β in disease therapy. The inhibitory effect of Res on the TGF-β signaling pathway can lead to the suppression of intra-abdominal adhesion formation, since TGF-β can enhance fibrin accumulation [139–149]. These modulatory effects of Res are discussed in the following sections.

3.1. Resveratrol and Fibrosis

Pulmonary fibrosis (PF) is a common disorder of the lung that is characterized with hypoxemia, restrictive functional ventilatory disturbance, and chronic fibrosis. Clinical manifestations of PF include wheezing, difficulties in breathing, and dry coughs [150]. The pathogenesis of PF is still not completely understood, but it appears that the TGF-β signaling pathway plays a significant role in PF development [151]. Thus, the administration of Res may be an ideal strategy in the amelioration of PF, and different molecular pathways may be involved. Normally, microRNA (miR)-21 can induce PF via the activation of TGF-β signaling and providing Smad7 nuclear translocation. TGF-β provides a positive feedback loop, so TGF-β enhances the expression of miR-21 and AP-1. The administration of Res down-regulates the expression of miR-21 via inhibition of the MAPK/AP-1 axis. This leads to a diminution in TGF-β expression and inhibition of Smad7, resulting in the alleviation of PF [152]. Accumulating data demonstrate that during the inhibition of fibrosis, Res affects the TGF-β signaling pathway via the modulation of miRs. Myocardial fibrosis (MF) is caused by the accumulation of collagen fibers, enhanced collagen content, and alteration in collagen composition. Systolic and diastolic functions of the heart can be negatively affected by MF [153]. TGF-β is one of the key players regulating MF [154]. The TGF-β/Smad7 axis can also contribute to the development of MF. The administration of Res can up-regulate the expression of miR-17, which in turn remarkably reduces levels of Smad7, leading to an improvement in MF [155].

In addition to PF and MF, renal fibrosis (RF) can arise as a result of the activation of the TGF-β signaling pathway. It has been reported that the inhibition of the TGF-β signaling pathway by natural products such as bardoxolone and nimbolide is of importance in RF therapy [156,157]. It is worth mentioning that Res can target the TGF-β signaling pathway, thereby causing an amelioration of RF. In RF treatment, fibroblast–myofibroblast differentiation (FMD), EMT, and the proliferation of tubular epithelial cells (TECs) should be targeted. The administration of Res can disrupt Smad2/3 activation by TGF-β and consequently suppress the proliferation of TECs, FMD, and EMT [158]. Increasing evidence demonstrates that EMT may be involved in renal fibrogenesis, and its activation can facilitate the development of RF [159–162]. Res is capable of suppressing EMT-mediated RF. It seems that TGF-β1 functions as an upstream mediator of EMT, and Res suppresses EMT and RF through inhibiting TGF-β1 [163]. In fact, in the stimulation of anti-fibrotic activity, Res affects the proliferation and survival of fibroblasts. It has been shown that Res can stimulate apoptosis in fibroblasts and suppress their growth as well. An investigation of the molecular pathways demonstrates that in targeting fibroblasts, Res can suppress TGF-β and the Smad2/3/4 complex, and it can also upregulate Smad7 [164].

It is worth mentioning that the anti-fibrotic activity of Res is dose-dependent, and using low doses is preferred as compared to higher doses. An experiment has evaluated the role of dose in the anti-fibrotic activity of Res. TGF-β induces fibrosis via formation of the Smad3/4 complex and subsequent stimulation of EMT. The administration of Res has been correlated with the deacetylation of Smad3 and Smad4 via sirtuin 1 (SIRT1). According to in vitro results, low doses of Res (5–20 mM) effectively exerted anti-fibrotic activity, while high doses (more than 40 mM) did not demonstrate any substantial anti-fibrotic activity. The in vivo findings are in line with in vitro results, so that low doses of Res (less than 25 mg/kg) improve fibrosis, while high doses of Res (more than 50 mg/kg) deteriorated the condition [165]. This study confirms the dose-related toxicity of Res. Overall, these studies demonstrate that TGF-β can function as a key player in the development of fibrosis and Res can suppress the TGF-β signaling pathway and its downstream targets such as Smads to alleviate fibrosis [166,167].

The TGF-β signaling pathway contributes to the development of fibrosis in different vital organs of body such as the lung and heart. The interesting point to highlight is the possible epigenetic regulation of TGF-β by miRs in the development of fibrosis. Res is capable of suppressing miR and TGF-β interaction in fibrosis therapy. MiR-17 and miR-21 are two important miRs that contribute to the emergence of myocardial and pulmonary fibrosis via TGF-β induction. The regulation of TGF-β by miRs is suppressed upon Res administration. RF also occurs by the function of TGF-β and subsequent induction of EMT. The TGF-β/EMT axis is inhibited by Res to alleviate RF. It is noteworthy that in the amelioration of fibrosis, components of TGF-β signaling such as Smad7 and Smad4 can also be down-regulated. Therefore, TGF-β is a versatile agent in the amelioration of fibrosis.

3.2. Resveratrol and Cancer Therapy

Accumulating data exhibit that the TGF-β signaling pathway can regulate both the proliferation and metastasis of cancer cells, and its inhibition is a promising strategy in cancer therapy [168–173]. Metastasis is an increasing challenge in the effective treatment of cancer. Cancer cells are able to migrate into neighboring and distant tissues, demanding novel strategies in the inhibition of their metastasis. EMT is one of the mechanisms that can promote invasion via the transformation of static epithelial cells into migratory mesenchymal ones [174]. A number of different molecular pathways have been recognized as regulators of EMT [175,176], and it has been found that TGF-β is capable of elevating migration via EMT induction. In breast cancer, TGF-β can stimulate EMT via Smad2 and Smad3 activation, leading to an increase in N-cadherin and vimentin levels, and a decrease in E-cadherin levels. The administration of Res suppresses the metastasis of breast cancer (under both in vitro and in vivo conditions) via the inhibition of TGF-β1 and down-regulation of Smad2 and Smad3 [177]. TGF-β also contributes to the migration and malignant behavior of lung cancer. In addition to breast cancer, Res targets TGF-β to inhibit EMT in lung cancer. By suppressing levels of TGF-β, Res down-regulates the levels of vimentin and fibronectin, while it enhances E-cadherin levels, leading to an inhibition of EMT and metastasis of lung cancer cells [178]. It is noteworthy that EMT induction enhances viability via the stimulation of cancer stem cell markers such as Bmi1 and Sox2. By inhibition of the TGF-β/Smad axis, Res not only inhibits EMT and migration, but also interferes with the proliferation and survival of cancer cells [179]. So, Res can function as a potential modulator of EMT in cancer cells to negatively affect their proliferation and metastasis.

Accumulating data also show that Res is able to diminish levels of TGF-β that in turn, suppresses the development of renal carcinoma [180]. These studies are in agreement with the fact that the inhibition of TGF-β by Res is of interest in suppressing tumor growth and metastasis [181]. Moreover, a dual relationship has been found between TGF-β and programmed cell death-1 (PD-1). For instance, PD-1 overexpression is associated with the induction of TGF-β, and TGF-β can regulate PD-1 expression [182,183]. This dual relationship is of importance in cancer therapy. Res can suppress the proliferation of oral cancer cells via the down-regulation of TGF-β and subsequent inhibition of PD-1. L-thyroxine as a thyroid hormone can also modulate the anti-tumor activity of Res via regulating the TGF-β/PD-1 axis [179].

Overall, the regulation of TGF-β by Res in cancer is of importance in terms of suppressing both migration and proliferation. The most well-known mechanism targeted by TGF-β is EMT, which can promote cancer metastasis. In addition, TGF-β can activate the signaling pathways such as PD-1 and Sox2 to ensure the growth and survival of cancer cells. Upon Res administration, TGF-β and its downstream targets are inhibited to pave the road for effective cancer therapy.

3.3. Resveratrol and Lung Injury

Injuries to vascular endothelium and alveolar epithelium by inflammatory factors can lead to the emergence of acute lung injury (ALI) [184]. Infections are able to generate ALI and among them, *Pseudomonas aerogenosa*, *Candidate albicans*, and *staphylococcal enterotoxin* B (SEB) are of importance [185–187]. In the amelioration of SEB-mediated lung injury, Res can target the TGF-β signaling pathway. Res can down-regulate the expression of miR-193a to inhibit TGF-β2 and TGFβR3, thus resulting in a decrease in levels of inflammatory cytokines and T cell infiltration [188]. The enhanced level of TGF-β has been associated with the development of asthma and lung injury [189]. In fact, the administration of Res may alleviate lung injury and asthma via decreasing levels of TGF-β [190]. Chronic obstructive pulmonary disease (COPD) is one of the most common disorders of lung tissue. Cigarette smoking is the most well-known reason for COPD [191]. Pulmonary inflammation, airflow obstruction, and remodeling are features of COPD [192]. Chronic inflammation can result in the development of COPD, and TGF-β has been found to play an important role in the pathogenesis of this disease [193,194]. Therefore, based on the modulatory impact of Res on TGF-β, the administration of this naturally occurring compound can be advantageous in the amelioration of COPD. It was also found that Res can decrease fibrotic response and inhibit mucus hypersecretion via the down-regulation of TGF-β [195].

It seems that via the regulation of TGF-β, Res is capable of reducing inflammation in lung and preventing the development of pathological events such as ALI, COPD, and asthma. Interestingly, Res inhibits inflammation via reducing the infiltration of cytokines and T cells. COPD is also emerged via pulmonary inflammation and fibrosis. Based on the effect of Res on TGF-β and subsequent decrease in fibrotic response and mucus hypersecretion, it can be beneficial in the treatment of COPD.

3.4. Resveratrol and Brain Injury

Cerebral hemorrhage is a leading cause of brain injury and vasospasm [196]. This malignancy results in ischemic/reperfusion and the induction of apoptosis in cancer cells [197,198]. The TGF-β signaling pathway has been correlated with brain injury [199]. Interestingly, the administration of Res was found to improve the blood–brain barrier (BBB) and inhibit apoptosis in neuronal cells. These protective effects of Res were found to be mediated via the inhibition of TGF-β-mediated ERK [200]. Moreover, it was found that exposing rats to alcohol is associated with an increase in levels of cytokines such as TGF-β. An administration of Res (10 and 20 mg/kg) can significantly improve cognitive deficits and reduces brain injury via decreasing TGF-β levels [201]. So, the alleviation of cognitive deficits and maintaining the integrity of BBB are functions of Res that can be mediated by TGF-β modulation.

3.5. Resveratrol and DM

During DM, microvascular complications can lead to hyperglycemia that accounts for the emergence of diabetic nephropathy (DN). Interestingly, an enhanced level of oxidative stress, renal polyol formation, protein kinase C induction, and activation of AMPK as well as the accumulation of advanced glycation end-products (AGEs) are responsible for DN [202,203]. TGF-β1 is considered as one of the potential pathways involved in the emergence of DN [204]. A combination of Res and rosuvastatin (RSU) was found to be beneficial in the alleviation of DN via the down-regulation of TGF-β1 [205]. The in vivo studies have also indicated that the administration of Res is a promising strategy in alleviating DN. It was observed that Res could diminish urinary albumin excretion, glomerular hypertrophy, and the deposition of fibronectin and collagen type IV to ameliorate DN. Moreover, an investigation of molecular pathways demonstrated that Res can alleviate TGF-β expression as well as the phosphorylation of Smad2 and Smad3 for DN alleviation (Table 1, Figure 2) [206]. The most important effect of Res during DN is reducing fibrosis, which can be mediated via TGF-β inhibition.

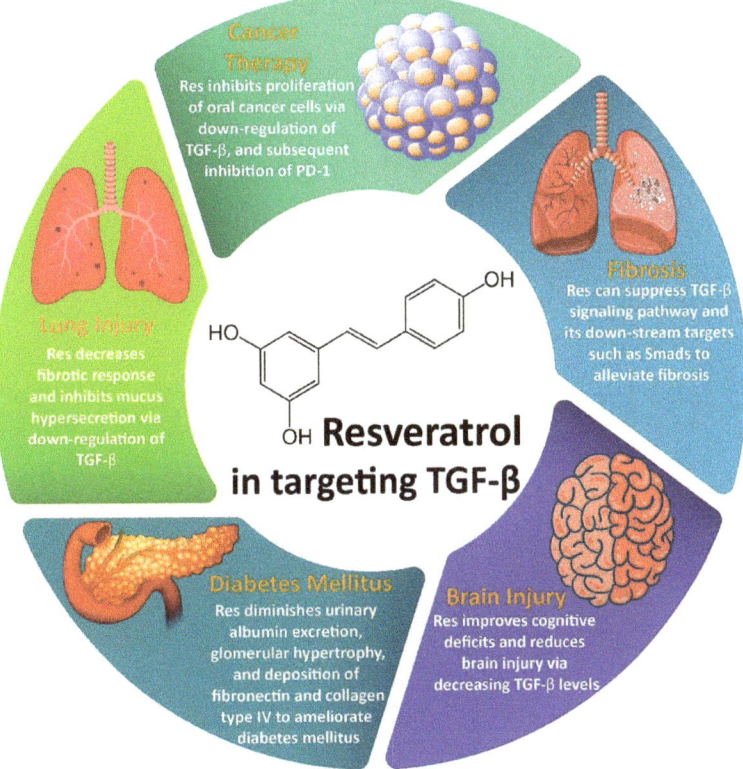

Figure 2. Regulation of TGF-β signaling by Res and its association with therapeutic effects.

Table 1. Res targets TGF-β signaling pathway in disease therapy.

Drug	In Vitro/In Vivo	Disease	Dose	Duration of Experiment	Administration Route	Effect on TGF-β	Results	References
Resveratrol Fenofibrate	In vivo (animal model of steatohepatitis)	Steatohepatitis	70 mg/kg	12 weeks	Diet	Inhibition	Alleviation of nonalcoholic steatohepatitis	[207]
Resveratrol	In vitro (rat mesangial cells) In vivo (rat model of diabetic nephropathy)	Diabetes	25 μM 20 mg/kg	24 h 4 weeks	Oral	Inhibition	Reducing mesangial cell viability, fibronectin secretion, and amelioration of diabetic nephropathy	[208]
Resveratrol	In vivo (diabetic mice)	Diabetes	5 and 25 mg/kg/day	2 months	Intragastric	Inhibition	Improving fibrosis via inhibition of ROS/ERK/TGF-β	[209]
Resveratrol	In vivo (diabetic rats)	Diabetes	10 mg/kg/day	30 days	Intraperitoneal	Inhibition	Alleviation of diabetic nephropathy and reducing epithelial desquamation, swelling, intracytoplasmic vacuolization, brush border loss, and peritubular infiltration	[210]
Resveratrol	In vivo (diabetic rats)	Diabetes	50 mg/kg	8 weeks	Gavage	Inhibition	Amelioration of renal damage and reducing collagen deposition	[211]
Resveratrol	In vivo (diabetic model)	Diabetes	10 mg/kg	8 weeks	Oral gavage	Inhibition	Reducing collagen deposition	[212]
Resveratrol	In vivo (diabetic rats)	Diabetes	10 mg/kg	4 weeks	Drinking water	Inhibition	Improving vascular dysfunction and reducing oxidative stress	[213]
Resveratrol	In vivo (rat model of chronic prostatitis)	Chronic prostatitis	10 mg/kg	10 days	Oral	Inhibition	Alleviation of prostate fibrosis via mast cell suppression	[214]
Resveratrol	In vivo (rat model of chronic prostatitis)	Chronic prostatitis	10 mg/kg	10 days	Oral	Inhibition	Reducing prostate fibrosis and urinary dysfunction via inhibition of TGF-β/Wnt/β-catenin	[215]
Resveratrol	In vitro (Human colorectal cancer cell line LoVo) In vivo (mice with orthotopic transplantation tumor)	Cancer	6 and 12 μM 50, 100, and 150 mg/kg	24 h 3 weeks	Intragastric	Inhibition	Suppressing metastasis of cancer cells by EMT inhibition via down-regulation of TGF-β/Smad signaling pathway	[216]
Resveratrol	In vitro (MCF-7 cells)	Cancer	5, 25, 50, 100, and 200 μM	48 h	-	Inhibition	Sensitizing cancer cells into chemotherapy via inhibition of TGF-β-mediated EMT	[217]
Resveratrol	In vitro (A431 human epidermoid carcinoma cells)	Cancer	50–100 μM	24 h	-	Inhibition	Suppressing ultraviolet-induced tumor proliferation	[218]
Resveratrol analogue (HS-1793)	In vivo (tumor bearing mice)	Cancer	0.5 and 1 mg/kg	3 weeks	Intraperitoneal	Inhibition	Enhancing efficacy of radiotherapy	[219]
Resveratrol	Murine model of LPS-induced pulmonary fibrosis	Pulmonary fibrosis	0.3 mg/kg	28 days	Intraperitoneal	Inhibition	Improving pulmonary fibrosis and inhibition of EMT via the down-regulation of TGF-β1/Smad	[216]

Table 1. *Cont.*

Drug	In Vitro/In Vivo	Disease	Dose	Duration of Experiment	Administration Route	Effect on TGF-β	Results	References
Resveratrol	In vivo (SIRT3-knock out mice)	Fibrosis	1.8 mg/kg	8 weeks	Diet	Inhibition	Improving cardiac fibrosis and suppressing fibroblast-to-myoblast transformation	[220]
Resveratrol	In vivo (chronic asthma model)	Asthma	10 and 50 mg/kg	3 months	Oral gavage	Inhibition	Inhibition of Smad2/3 phosphorylation, amelioration of airway inflammation and structural changes	[221]
Resveratrol	In vitro (human retinal pigment epithelial cells)	Eye disease	25, 50, 100, 200, 400, and 800 μM	24 h	-	Inhibition	Suppressing Smad2 and Smad3 phosphorylation leads to the inhibition of EMT and collagen deposition	[222]
Resveratrol	In vivo (mouse model of Duchene muscular dystrophy)	Muscular dystrophy	4 g/kg	32 weeks	Diet	Inhibition	Decreasing reactive oxygen species generation, fibronectin production, and enhancing expressions of α-SMA and SIRT1	[223]
Resveratrol	In vitro (rhabdomyosarcoma)	Rhabdomyosarcoma	5, 10, 20, 40, or 80 μmol/L	24, 48, and 72 h	-	Inhibition	Induction of G1 and S phases cell cycle arrest and down-regulation of Smad4	[224]
Resveratrol	In vivo (Male C57BL/6J mice)	-	5 mg/kg	2 days after surgery	Intraperitoneal	Inhibition	Reducing levels of collagen IV and fibronectin	[225]

TGF-β, transforming growth factor-beta; ROS, reactive oxygen species; ERK, extracellular signal-regulated kinase; EMT, epithelial-to-mesenchymal transition; α-SMA, α-smooth muscle actin; SIRT1, sirtuin 1.

4. Conclusions and Future Directions

Currently, extensive research is being performed for possible applications of natural products for the therapy of chronic diseases, as these agents can regulate multiple molecular targets and transcription factors [226–233]. In the present review, a comprehensive discussion of possible impact of Res on the TGF-β signaling pathway, which is one of the important cascades involved in the regulation of biological mechanisms and the generation of pathological events, is provided. TGF-β acts as an upstream inducer of EMT, and this not only enhances the metastasis of cancer cells, but also mediates fibrosis in cells. Res inhibits TGF-β/EMT in suppressing both cancer and fibrosis. Through inhibiting TGF-β, Res diminishes the accumulation of collagen and fibrin, and reduces organ adhesion. Interestingly, Res dually targets both upstream (such as miRs) and downstream (Smads, PD-1, and EMT) mediators of TGF-β signaling in disease therapy. In addition to anti-tumor and anti-fibrotic activities, Res can also exert neuroprotective, lung protective, and anti-diabetic effects via the down-regulation of TGF-β, which was also highlighted in this article. Moreover, to circumvent the issue of poor bioavailability, the application of nanoparticles can enhance the modulatory effects of Res on the TGF-β signaling pathway. Besides, genetic manipulations such as small interfering RNA (siRNA) can also be co-applied for Res to promote its potential modulatory actions on TGF-β for therapeutic uses.

More studies are needed to find the optimal dose of Res in disease therapy via targeting TGF-β. Chemical modification of the Res structure and using nanoparticles can promote its efficacy in TGF-β regulation as well as its potential against various malignancies. More importantly, these findings are more valuable when they are translated into clinic. So, clinical studies are vital to approve the results of in vitro and in vivo experiments.

Funding: This work was also supported by a National Research Foundation of Korea (NRF) grant funded by the Korean government (MSIP) (NRF-2018R1D1A1B07042969).

Conflicts of Interest: The authors declare no conflict of interest. The funders had no role in the design of the study; in the collection, analyses, or interpretation of data; in the writing of the manuscript; or in the decision to publish the results.

Abbreviations

NDs	neurological disorders
AD	Alzheimer's disease
PD	Parkinson's disease
TCM	Traditional Chinese Medicine
Res	resveratrol
NF-kB	nuclear factor-kappaB
IL	interleukin
TNF-α	tumor necrosis factor-α
WAT	white adipose tissue
BAT	brown adipose tissue
ABC	ATP binding cassette
Aβ	amyloid-beta
TGF-β	transforming growth factor-β
GI	gastrointestinal
CPC	centrifugal partition chromatography
BMPs	bone morphogenetic proteins
GDFs	growth and differentiation factors
LAP	latency associated peptide
PAI1	plasminogen activator inhibitor 1
EMT	epithelial-to-mesenchymal transition
SIRT7	sirtuin 7

DM	diabetes mellitus
MMP-9	matrix metalloproteinase-9
PF	pulmonary fibrosis
miR	microRNA
MF	myocardial fibrosis
RF	renal fibrosis
FMD	fibroblast-myofibroblast differentiation
TECs	tubular epithelial cells
SIRT1	sirtuin 1
PD-1	programmed cell death-1
ALI	acute lung injury
SEB	staphylococcal enterotoxin B
COPD	chronic obstructive pulmonary disease
BBB	blood-brain barrier
DN	diabetic nephropathy
ERK	extracellular signal-regulated kinase
MAPK	mitogen-activated protein kinase
AGEs	advanced glycation end-products
RSU	rosuvastatin

References

1. Mohan, C.D.; Rangappa, S.; Preetham, H.D.; Chandra Nayaka, S.; Gupta, V.K.; Basappa, S.; Sethi, G.; Rangappa, K.S. Targeting STAT3 signaling pathway in cancer by agents derived from Mother Nature. *Semin. Cancer Biol.* **2020**. [CrossRef] [PubMed]
2. Aggarwal, V.; Tuli, H.S.; Thakral, F.; Singhal, P.; Aggarwal, D.; Srivastava, S.; Pandey, A.; Sak, K.; Varol, M.; Khan, M.A.; et al. Molecular mechanisms of action of hesperidin in cancer: Recent trends and advancements. *Exp. Biol. Med.* **2020**, *245*, 486–497. [CrossRef] [PubMed]
3. Baek, S.H.; Ko, J.H.; Lee, H.; Jung, J.; Kong, M.; Lee, J.W.; Lee, J.; Chinnathambi, A.; Zayed, M.E.; Alharbi, S.A.; et al. Resveratrol inhibits STAT3 signaling pathway through the induction of SOCS-1: Role in apoptosis induction and radiosensitization in head and neck tumor cells. *Phytomedicine Int. J. Phytother. Phytopharm.* **2016**, *23*, 566–577. [CrossRef] [PubMed]
4. Dai, X.; Zhang, J.; Arfuso, F.; Chinnathambi, A.; Zayed, M.E.; Alharbi, S.A.; Kumar, A.P.; Ahn, K.S.; Sethi, G. Targeting TNF-related apoptosis-inducing ligand (TRAIL) receptor by natural products as a potential therapeutic approach for cancer therapy. *Exp. Biol. Med.* **2015**, *240*, 760–773. [CrossRef] [PubMed]
5. Prasannan, R.; Kalesh, K.A.; Shanmugam, M.K.; Nachiyappan, A.; Ramachandran, L.; Nguyen, A.H.; Kumar, A.P.; Lakshmanan, M.; Ahn, K.S.; Sethi, G. Key cell signaling pathways modulated by zerumbone: Role in the prevention and treatment of cancer. *Biochem. Pharmacol.* **2012**, *15*, 1268–1276. [CrossRef]
6. Tan, S.M.; Li, F.; Rajendran, P.; Kumar, A.P.; Hui, K.M.; Sethi, G. Identification of beta-escin as a novel inhibitor of signal transducer and activator of transcription 3/Janus-activated kinase 2 signaling pathway that suppresses proliferation and induces apoptosis in human hepatocellular carcinoma cells. *J. Pharmacol. Exp. Ther.* **2010**, *334*, 285–293. [CrossRef]
7. Lee, J.H.; Chinnathambi, A.; Alharbi, S.A.; Shair, O.H.M.; Sethi, G.; Ahn, K.S. Farnesol abrogates epithelial to mesenchymal transition process through regulating Akt/mTOR pathway. *Pharmacol. Res.* **2019**, *150*, 104504. [CrossRef]
8. Wong, A.L.A.; Hirpara, J.L.; Pervaiz, S.; Eu, J.Q.; Sethi, G.; Goh, B.C. Do STAT3 inhibitors have potential in the future for cancer therapy? *Expert Opin. Investig. Drugs* **2017**, *26*, 883–887. [CrossRef]
9. Ochiai, A.; Kuroda, K. Preconception resveratrol intake against infertility: Friend or foe? *Reprod. Med. Biol.* **2019**, *19*, 107–113. [CrossRef]
10. McSweeney, K.R.; Gadanec, L.K.; Qaradakhi, T.; Gammune, T.M.; Kubatka, P.; Caprnda, M.; Fedotova, J.; Radonak, J.; Kruzliak, P.; Zulli, A. Impridone enhances vascular relaxation via FOXO1 pathway. *Clin. Exp. Pharmacol. Physiol.* **2020**. [CrossRef]

11. Kashyap, D.; Tuli, H.S.; Yerer, M.B.; Sharma, A.; Sak, K.; Srivastava, S.; Pandey, A.; Garg, V.K.; Sethi, G.; Bishayee, A. Natural product-based nanoformulations for cancer therapy: Opportunities and challenges. *Semin. Cancer Biol.* **2019**. [CrossRef] [PubMed]
12. Shanmugam, M.K.; Manu, K.A.; Ong, T.H.; Ramachandran, L.; Surana, R.; Bist, P.; Lim, L.H.; Kumar, A.P.; Hui, K.M.; Sethi, G. Inhibition of CXCR4/CXCL12 signaling axis by ursolic acid leads to suppression of metastasis in transgenic adenocarcinoma of mouse prostate model. *Int. J. Cancer* **2011**, *129*, 1552–1563. [CrossRef] [PubMed]
13. Ramachandran, L.; Manu, K.A.; Shanmugam, M.K.; Li, F.; Siveen, K.S.; Vali, S.; Kapoor, S.; Abbasi, T.; Surana, R.; Smoot, D.T.; et al. Isorhamnetin inhibits proliferation and invasion and induces apoptosis through the modulation of peroxisome proliferator-activated receptor γ activation pathway in gastric cancer. *J. Biol. Chem.* **2012**, *287*, 38028–38040. [CrossRef]
14. Varughese, R.S.; Lam, W.S.-T.; Marican, A.A.b.H.; Viganeshwari, S.H.; Bhave, A.S.; Syn, N.L.; Wang, J.; Wong, A.L.-A.; Kumar, A.P.; Lobie, P.E.; et al. Biopharmacological considerations for accelerating drug development of deguelin, a rotenoid with potent chemotherapeutic and chemopreventive potential. *Cancer* **2019**, *125*, 1789–1798. [CrossRef]
15. Siveen, K.S.; Mustafa, N.; Li, F.; Kannaiyan, R.; Ahn, K.S.; Kumar, A.P.; Chng, W.J.; Sethi, G. Thymoquinone overcomes chemoresistance and enhances the anticancer effects of bortezomib through abrogation of NF-kappaB regulated gene products in multiple myeloma xenograft mouse model. *Oncotarget* **2014**, *5*, 634–648. [CrossRef] [PubMed]
16. Li, F.; Shanmugam, M.K.; Chen, L.; Chatterjee, S.; Basha, J.; Kumar, A.P.; Kundu, T.K.; Sethi, G. Garcinol, a polyisoprenylated benzophenone modulates multiple proinflammatory signaling cascades leading to the suppression of growth and survival of head and neck carcinoma. *Cancer Prev. Res.* **2013**, *6*, 843–854. [CrossRef] [PubMed]
17. Rajendran, P.; Li, F.; Shanmugam, M.K.; Vali, S.; Abbasi, T.; Kapoor, S.; Ahn, K.S.; Kumar, A.P.; Sethi, G. Honokiol inhibits signal transducer and activator of transcription-3 signaling, proliferation, and survival of hepatocellular carcinoma cells via the protein tyrosine phosphatase SHP-1. *J. Cell. Physiol.* **2012**, *227*, 2184–2195. [CrossRef] [PubMed]
18. Huang, X.-T.; Li, X.; Xie, M.-L.; Huang, Z.; Huang, Y.-X.; Wu, G.-X.; Peng, Z.-R.; Sun, Y.-N.; Ming, Q.-L.; Liu, Y.-X. Resveratrol: Review on its discovery, anti-leukemia effects and pharmacokinetics. *Chem. Biol. Interact.* **2019**, *306*, 29–38. [CrossRef]
19. Ko, J.-H.; Sethi, G.; Um, J.-Y.; Shanmugam, M.K.; Arfuso, F.; Kumar, A.P.; Bishayee, A.; Ahn, K.S. The Role of Resveratrol in Cancer Therapy. *Int. J. Mol. Sci.* **2017**, *18*, 2589. [CrossRef]
20. Shanmugam, M.K.; Warrier, S.; Kumar, A.P.; Sethi, G.; Arfuso, F. Potential Role of Natural Compounds as Anti-Angiogenic Agents in Cancer. *Curr. Vasc. Pharmacol.* **2017**, *15*, 503–519. [CrossRef]
21. Frazzi, R.; Guardi, M. Cellular and molecular targets of resveratrol on lymphoma and leukemia cells. *Molecules* **2017**, *22*, 885. [CrossRef] [PubMed]
22. Garg, A.K.; Buchholz, T.A.; Aggarwal, B.B. Chemosensitization and radiosensitization of tumors by plant polyphenols. *Antioxid. Redox Signal.* **2005**, *7*, 1630–1647. [CrossRef]
23. Jang, M.; Cai, L.; Udeani, G.O.; Slowing, K.V.; Thomas, C.F.; Beecher, C.W.; Fong, H.H.; Farnsworth, N.R.; Kinghorn, A.D.; Mehta, R.G. Cancer chemopreventive activity of resveratrol, a natural product derived from grapes. *Science* **1997**, *275*, 218–220. [CrossRef]
24. Aggarwal, B.B.; Bhardwaj, A.; Aggarwal, R.S.; Seeram, N.P.; Shishodia, S.; Takada, Y. Role of resveratrol in prevention and therapy of cancer: Preclinical and clinical studies. *Anticancer Res.* **2004**, *24*, 2783–2840. [PubMed]
25. Ragab, A.S.; Van Fleet, J.; Jankowski, B.; Park, J.-H.; Bobzin, S.C. Detection and quantitation of resveratrol in tomato fruit (*Lycopersicon esculentum* Mill.). *J. Agric. Food Chem.* **2006**, *54*, 7175–7179. [CrossRef] [PubMed]
26. Lo, C.; Le Blanc, J.Y.; Yu, C.K.; Sze, K.; Ng, D.C.; Chu, I.K. Detection, characterization, and quantification of resveratrol glycosides in transgenic arabidopsis over-expressing a sorghum stilbene synthase gene by liquid chromatography/tandem mass spectrometry. *Rapid Commun. Mass Spectrom. Int. J. Devoted Rapid Dissem. Minute Res. Mass Spectrom.* **2007**, *21*, 4101–4108. [CrossRef]
27. Loizzo, M.R.; Nigro, S.; De Luca, D.; Menichini, F. Detection of ochratoxin A and cis-and trans-resveratrol in red wines and their musts from Calabria (Italy). *Food Addit. Contam. Part A* **2011**, *28*, 1561–1568. [CrossRef] [PubMed]

28. Koga, C.C.; Becraft, A.R.; Lee, Y.; Lee, S.Y. Taste detection thresholds of resveratrol. *J. Food Sci.* **2015**, *80*, S2064–S2070. [CrossRef]
29. Xu, X.; Liu, X.; Yang, Y.; He, J.; Gu, H.; Jiang, M.; Huang, Y.; Liu, X.; Liu, L. Resveratrol inhibits the development of obesity-related osteoarthritis via the TLR4 and PI3K/Akt signaling pathways. *Connect. Tissue Res.* **2019**, *60*, 571–582. [CrossRef]
30. Ebrahim, H.A.; Alzamil, N.M.; Al-Ani, B.; Haidara, M.A.; Kamar, S.S.; Dawood, A.F. Suppression of knee joint osteoarthritis induced secondary to type 2 diabetes mellitus in rats by resveratrol: Role of glycated haemoglobin and hyperlipidaemia and biomarkers of inflammation and oxidative stress. *Arch. Physiol. Biochem.* **2020**, 1–8. [CrossRef]
31. Zhang, G.; Zhang, H.; You, W.; Tang, X.; Li, X.; Gong, Z. Therapeutic effect of Resveratrol in the treatment of osteoarthritis via the MALAT1/miR-9/NF-κB signaling pathway. *Exp. Ther. Med.* **2020**, *19*, 2343–2352. [CrossRef] [PubMed]
32. Cosín-Tomàs, M.; Senserrich, J.; Arumí-Planas, M.; Alquézar, C.; Pallàs, M.; Martín-Requero, Á.; Suñol, C.; Kaliman, P.; Sanfeliu, C. Role of Resveratrol and Selenium on Oxidative Stress and Expression of Antioxidant and Anti-Aging Genes in Immortalized Lymphocytes from Alzheimer's Disease Patients. *Nutrients* **2019**, *11*, 1764. [CrossRef]
33. Yuan, L.; Zhou, M.; Huang, D.; Wasan, H.S.; Zhang, K.; Sun, L.; Huang, H.; Ma, S.; Shen, M.; Ruan, S. Resveratrol inhibits the invasion and metastasis of colon cancer through reversal of epithelial- mesenchymal transition via the AKT/GSK-3β/Snail signaling pathway. *Mol. Med. Rep.* **2019**, *20*, 2783–2795. [CrossRef] [PubMed]
34. Jang, Y.G.; Go, R.E.; Hwang, K.A.; Choi, K.C. Resveratrol inhibits DHT-induced progression of prostate cancer cell line through interfering with the AR and CXCR4 pathway. *J. Steroid Biochem. Mol. Biol.* **2019**, *192*, 105406. [CrossRef] [PubMed]
35. Kiskova, T.; Kubatka, P.; Büsselberg, D.; Kassayova, M. The Plant-Derived Compound Resveratrol in Brain Cancer: A Review. *Biomolecules* **2020**, *10*, 161. [CrossRef] [PubMed]
36. Rašković, A.; Ćućuz, V.; Torović, L.; Tomas, A.; Gojković-Bukarica, L.; Ćebović, T.; Milijašević, B.; Stilinović, N.; Cvejić Hogervorst, J. Resveratrol supplementation improves metabolic control in rats with induced hyperlipidemia and type 2 diabetes. *Saudi Pharm. J. SPJ Off. Publ. Saudi Pharm. Soc.* **2019**, *27*, 1036–1043. [CrossRef]
37. Hong, M.; Li, J.; Li, S.; Almutairi, M.M. Resveratrol Derivative, Trans-3, 5, 4'-Trimethoxystilbene, Prevents the Developing of Atherosclerotic Lesions and Attenuates Cholesterol Accumulation in Macrophage Foam Cells. *Mol. Nutr. Food Res.* **2020**, *64*, e1901115. [CrossRef]
38. Yu, B.; Qin, S.Y.; Hu, B.L.; Qin, Q.Y.; Jiang, H.X.; Luo, W. Resveratrol improves CCL4-induced liver fibrosis in mouse by upregulating endogenous IL-10 to reprogramme macrophages phenotype from M(LPS) to M(IL-4). *Biomed. Pharmacother.* **2019**, *117*, 109110. [CrossRef]
39. Tewari, D.; Nabavi, S.F.; Nabavi, S.M.; Sureda, A.; Farooqi, A.A.; Atanasov, A.G.; Vacca, R.A.; Sethi, G.; Bishayee, A. Targeting activator protein 1 signaling pathway by bioactive natural agents: Possible therapeutic strategy for cancer prevention and intervention. *Pharm. Res.* **2018**, *128*, 366–375. [CrossRef]
40. Deng, S.; Shanmugam, M.K.; Kumar, A.P.; Yap, C.T.; Sethi, G.; Bishayee, A. Targeting autophagy using natural compounds for cancer prevention and therapy. *Cancer* **2019**, *125*, 1228–1246. [CrossRef]
41. Mishra, S.; Verma, S.S.; Rai, V.; Awasthee, N.; Chava, S.; Hui, K.M.; Kumar, A.P.; Challagundla, K.B.; Sethi, G.; Gupta, S.C. Long non-coding RNAs are emerging targets of phytochemicals for cancer and other chronic diseases. *Cell. Mol. Life Sci. CMLS* **2019**, *76*, 1947–1966. [CrossRef] [PubMed]
42. Ben Lagha, A.; Andrian, E.; Grenier, D. Resveratrol attenuates the pathogenic and inflammatory properties of Porphyromonas gingivalis. *Mol. Oral Microbiol.* **2019**, *34*, 118–130. [CrossRef] [PubMed]
43. Farzanegan, A.; Shokuhian, M.; Jafari, S.; Shirazi, F.S.; Shahidi, M. Anti-histaminic Effects of Resveratrol and Silymarin on Human Gingival Fibroblasts. *Inflammation* **2019**, *42*, 1622–1629. [CrossRef] [PubMed]
44. Calamini, B.; Ratia, K.; Malkowski, M.G.; Cuendet, M.; Pezzuto, J.M.; Santarsiero, B.D.; Mesecar, A.D. Pleiotropic mechanisms facilitated by resveratrol and its metabolites. *Biochem. J.* **2010**, *429*, 273–282. [CrossRef] [PubMed]
45. Hwang, S.H.; Wecksler, A.T.; Wagner, K.; Hammock, B.D. Rationally designed multitarget agents against inflammation and pain. *Curr. Med. Chem.* **2013**, *20*, 1783–1799. [CrossRef] [PubMed]

46. Lançon, A.; Frazzi, R.; Latruffe, N. Anti-oxidant, anti-inflammatory and anti-angiogenic properties of resveratrol in ocular diseases. *Molecules* **2016**, *21*, 304. [CrossRef]
47. Cheng, T.M.; Chin, Y.T.; Ho, Y.; Chen, Y.R.; Yang, Y.N.; Yang, Y.C.; Shih, Y.J.; Lin, T.I.; Lin, H.Y.; Davis, P.J. Resveratrol induces sumoylated COX-2-dependent anti-proliferation in human prostate cancer LNCaP cells. *Food Chem. Toxicol. Int. J. Publ. Br. Ind. Biol. Res. Assoc.* **2018**, *112*, 67–75. [CrossRef]
48. Gong, W.H.; Zhao, N.; Zhang, Z.M.; Zhang, Y.X.; Yan, L.; Li, J.B. The inhibitory effect of resveratrol on COX-2 expression in human colorectal cancer: A promising therapeutic strategy. *Eur. Rev. Med. Pharmacol. Sci.* **2017**, *21*, 1136–1143.
49. Zykova, T.A.; Zhu, F.; Zhai, X.; Ma, W.Y.; Ermakova, S.P.; Lee, K.W.; Bode, A.M.; Dong, Z. Resveratrol directly targets COX-2 to inhibit carcinogenesis. *Mol. Carcinog.* **2008**, *47*, 797–805. [CrossRef]
50. Latruffe, N.; Lançon, A.; Frazzi, R.; Aires, V.; Delmas, D.; Michaille, J.J.; Djouadi, F.; Bastin, J.; Cherkaoui-Malki, M. Exploring new ways of regulation by resveratrol involving miRNAs, with emphasis on inflammation. *Ann. N. Y. Acad. Sci.* **2015**, *1348*, 97–106. [CrossRef]
51. Kim, O.Y.; Chung, J.Y.; Song, J. Effect of resveratrol on adipokines and myokines involved in fat browning: Perspectives in healthy weight against obesity. *Pharm. Res.* **2019**, *148*, 104411. [CrossRef] [PubMed]
52. Ye, G.; Chen, G.; Gao, H.; Lin, Y.; Liao, X.; Zhang, H.; Liu, X.; Chi, Y.; Huang, Q.; Zhu, H.; et al. Resveratrol inhibits lipid accumulation in the intestine of atherosclerotic mice and macrophages. *J. Cell. Mol. Med.* **2019**, *23*, 4313–4325. [CrossRef] [PubMed]
53. Feng, L.; Zhang, L. Resveratrol Suppresses Aβ-Induced Microglial Activation Through the TXNIP/TRX/NLRP3 Signaling Pathway. *DNA Cell Biol.* **2019**, *38*, 874–879. [CrossRef] [PubMed]
54. Ramalingam, A.; Santhanathas, T.; Shaukat Ali, S.; Zainalabidin, S. Resveratrol Supplementation Protects Against Nicotine-Induced Kidney Injury. *Int. J. Environ. Res. Public Health* **2019**, *16*, 4445. [CrossRef]
55. Chen, T.S.; Kuo, C.H.; Day, C.H.; Pan, L.F.; Chen, R.J.; Chen, B.C.; Padma, V.V.; Lin, Y.M.; Huang, C.Y. Resveratrol increases stem cell function in the treatment of damaged pancreas. *J. Cell. Physiol.* **2019**, *234*, 20443–20452. [CrossRef]
56. Wang, Y.; Wang, B.; Qi, X.; Zhang, X.; Ren, K. Resveratrol Protects Against Post-Contrast Acute Kidney Injury in Rabbits With Diabetic Nephropathy. *Front. Pharmacol.* **2019**, *10*, 833. [CrossRef]
57. Lieben Louis, X.; Raj, P.; Meikle, Z.; Yu, L.; Susser, S.E.; MacInnis, S.; Duhamel, T.A.; Wigle, J.T.; Netticadan, T. Resveratrol prevents palmitic-acid-induced cardiomyocyte contractile impairment. *Can. J. Physiol. Pharmacol.* **2019**, *97*, 1132–1140. [CrossRef]
58. Gimeno-Mallench, L.; Mas-Bargues, C.; Inglés, M.; Olaso, G.; Borras, C.; Gambini, J.; Vina, J. Resveratrol shifts energy metabolism to increase lipid oxidation in healthy old mice. *Biomed. Pharmacother.* **2019**, *118*, 109130. [CrossRef]
59. Amri, A.; Chaumeil, J.; Sfar, S.; Charrueau, C. Administration of resveratrol: What formulation solutions to bioavailability limitations? *J. Control. Release* **2012**, *158*, 182–193. [CrossRef]
60. Chauhan, A.S. Dendrimer nanotechnology for enhanced formulation and controlled delivery of resveratrol. *Ann. N. Y. Acad. Sci.* **2015**, *1348*, 134–140. [CrossRef]
61. Santos, A.C.; Pereira, I.; Pereira-Silva, M.; Ferreira, L.; Caldas, M.; Collado-González, M.; Magalhães, M.; Figueiras, A.; Ribeiro, A.J.; Veiga, F. Nanotechnology-based formulations for resveratrol delivery: Effects on resveratrol in vivo bioavailability and bioactivity. *Colloids Surf. B Biointerfaces* **2019**, *180*, 127–140. [CrossRef] [PubMed]
62. Huang, M.; Liang, C.; Tan, C.; Huang, S.; Ying, R.; Wang, Y.; Wang, Z.; Zhang, Y. Liposome co-encapsulation as a strategy for the delivery of curcumin and resveratrol. *Food Funct.* **2019**, *10*, 6447–6458. [CrossRef] [PubMed]
63. Ravikumar, P.; Katariya, M.; Patil, S.; Tatke, P.; Pillai, R. Skin delivery of resveratrol encapsulated lipidic formulation for melanoma chemoprevention. *J. Microencapsul.* **2019**, *36*, 535–551. [CrossRef] [PubMed]
64. Intagliata, S.; Modica, M.N.; Santagati, L.M.; Montenegro, L. Strategies to Improve Resveratrol Systemic and Topical Bioavailability: An Update. *Antioxidants* **2019**, *8*, 244. [CrossRef]
65. Hu, Y.; Wang, Z.; Qiu, Y.; Liu, Y.; Ding, M.; Zhang, Y. Anti-miRNA21 and resveratrol-loaded polysaccharide-based mesoporous silica nanoparticle for synergistic activity in gastric carcinoma. *J. Drug Target.* **2019**, *27*, 1135–1143. [CrossRef]
66. Machado, N.D.; Fernández, M.A.; Díaz, D.D. Recent Strategies in Resveratrol Delivery Systems. *ChemPlusChem* **2019**, *84*, 951–973. [CrossRef]

67. Rugină, D.; Ghiman, R.; Focșan, M.; Tăbăran, F.; Copaciu, F.; Suciu, M.; Pintea, A.; Aștilean, S. Resveratrol-delivery vehicle with anti-VEGF activity carried to human retinal pigmented epithelial cells exposed to high-glucose induced conditions. *Colloids Surf. B Biointerfaces* **2019**, *181*, 66–75. [CrossRef]
68. Kang, J.H.; Ko, Y.T. Enhanced Subcellular Trafficking of Resveratrol Using Mitochondriotropic Liposomes in Cancer Cells. *Pharmaceutics* **2019**, *11*, 423. [CrossRef]
69. Poonia, N.; Kaur Narang, J.; Lather, V.; Beg, S.; Sharma, T.; Singh, B.; Pandita, D. Resveratrol loaded functionalized nanostructured lipid carriers for breast cancer targeting: Systematic development, characterization and pharmacokinetic evaluation. *Colloids Surf. B Biointerfaces* **2019**, *181*, 756–766. [CrossRef]
70. de Oliveira, M.T.P.; de Sá Coutinho, D.; Tenório de Souza, É.; Stanisçuaski Guterres, S.; Pohlmann, A.R.; Silva, P.M.R.; Martins, M.A.; Bernardi, A. Orally delivered resveratrol-loaded lipid-core nanocapsules ameliorate LPS-induced acute lung injury via the ERK and PI3K/Akt pathways. *Int. J. Nanomed.* **2019**, *14*, 5215–5228. [CrossRef]
71. Rostami, M.; Ghorbani, M.; Aman Mohammadi, M.; Delavar, M.; Tabibiazar, M.; Ramezani, S. Development of resveratrol loaded chitosan-gellan nanofiber as a novel gastrointestinal delivery system. *Int. J. Biol. Macromol.* **2019**, *135*, 698–705. [CrossRef] [PubMed]
72. Yang, C.; Wang, Y.; Xie, Y.; Liu, G.; Lu, Y.; Wu, W.; Chen, L. Oat protein-shellac nanoparticles as a delivery vehicle for resveratrol to improve bioavailability in vitro and in vivo. *Nanomedicine* **2019**, *14*, 2853–2871. [CrossRef] [PubMed]
73. Ha, E.S.; Sim, W.Y.; Lee, S.K.; Jeong, J.S.; Kim, J.S.; Baek, I.H.; Choi, D.H.; Park, H.; Hwang, S.J.; Kim, M.S. Preparation and Evaluation of Resveratrol-Loaded Composite Nanoparticles Using a Supercritical Fluid Technology for Enhanced Oral and Skin Delivery. *Antioxidants* **2019**, *8*, 554. [CrossRef] [PubMed]
74. Sharma, B.; Iqbal, B.; Kumar, S.; Ali, J.; Baboota, S. Resveratrol-loaded nanoemulsion gel system to ameliorate UV-induced oxidative skin damage: From in vitro to in vivo investigation of antioxidant activity enhancement. *Arch. Dermatol. Res.* **2019**, *311*, 773–793. [CrossRef] [PubMed]
75. Chukwumah, Y.; Walker, L.; Vogler, B.; Verghese, M. In vitro absorption of dietary trans-resveratrol from boiled and roasted peanuts in Caco-2 cells. *J. Agric. Food Chem.* **2011**, *59*, 12323–12329. [CrossRef]
76. Soleas, G.J.; Angelini, M.; Grass, L.; Diamandis, E.P.; Goldberg, D.M. Absorption of trans-resveratrol in rats. In *Methods in Enzymology*; Elsevier: Amsterdam, The Netherlands, 2001; Volume 335, pp. 145–154.
77. Willenberg, I.; Michael, M.; Wonik, J.; Bartel, L.C.; Empl, M.T.; Schebb, N.H. Investigation of the absorption of resveratrol oligomers in the Caco-2 cellular model of intestinal absorption. *Food Chem.* **2015**, *167*, 245–250. [CrossRef]
78. Walle, T.; Hsieh, F.; DeLegge, M.H.; Oatis, J.E.; Walle, U.K. High absorption but very low bioavailability of oral resveratrol in humans. *Drug Metab. Dispos.* **2004**, *32*, 1377–1382. [CrossRef]
79. Delmas, D.; Aires, V.; Colin, D.J.; Limagne, E.; Scagliarini, A.; Cotte, A.K.; Ghiringhelli, F. Importance of lipid microdomains, rafts, in absorption, delivery, and biological effects of resveratrol. *Ann. N. Y. Acad. Sci.* **2013**, *1290*, 90–97. [CrossRef]
80. Polonini, H.C.; de Almeida Bastos, C.; de Oliveira, M.A.L.; da Silva, C.G.A.; Collins, C.H.; Brandão, M.A.F.; Raposo, N.R.B. In vitro drug release and ex vivo percutaneous absorption of resveratrol cream using HPLC with zirconized silica stationary phase. *J. Chromatogr. B* **2014**, *947*, 23–31. [CrossRef]
81. Biasutto, L.; Marotta, E.; Mattarei, A.; Beltramello, S.; Caliceti, P.; Salmaso, S.; Bernkop-Schnürch, A.; Garbisa, S.; Zoratti, M.; Paradisi, C. Absorption and metabolism of resveratrol carboxyesters and methanesulfonate by explanted rat intestinal segments. *Cell. Physiol. Biochem.* **2009**, *24*, 557–566. [CrossRef]
82. Basavaraj, S.; Betageri, G.V. Improved oral delivery of resveratrol using proliposomal formulation: Investigation of various factors contributing to prolonged absorption of unmetabolized resveratrol. *Expert Opin. Drug Deliv.* **2014**, *11*, 493–503. [CrossRef] [PubMed]
83. Andres-Lacueva, C.; Macarulla, M.T.; Rotches-Ribalta, M.; Boto-Ordóñez, M.; Urpi-Sarda, M.; Rodríguez, V.M.; Portillo, M.P. Distribution of resveratrol metabolites in liver, adipose tissue, and skeletal muscle in rats fed different doses of this polyphenol. *J. Agric. Food Chem.* **2012**, *60*, 4833–4840. [CrossRef]
84. Bertelli, A.; Baccalini, R.; Battaglia, E.; Falchi, M.; Ferrero, M. Resveratrol inhibits TNF alpha-induced endothelial cell activation. *Therapie* **2001**, *56*, 613–616. [PubMed]
85. Lançon, A.; Hanet, N.; Jannin, B.; Delmas, D.; Heydel, J.-M.; Lizard, G.; Chagnon, M.-C.; Artur, Y.; Latruffe, N. Resveratrol in human hepatoma HepG2 cells: Metabolism and inducibility of detoxifying enzymes. *Drug Metab. Dispos.* **2007**, *35*, 699–703. [CrossRef] [PubMed]

86. De Santi, C.; Pietrabissa, A.; Spisni, R.; Mosca, F.; Pacifici, G. Sulphation of resveratrol, a natural product present in grapes and wine, in the human liver and duodenum. *Xenobiotica* **2000**, *30*, 609–617. [CrossRef] [PubMed]
87. Murias, M.; Miksits, M.; Aust, S.; Spatzenegger, M.; Thalhammer, T.; Szekeres, T.; Jaeger, W. Metabolism of resveratrol in breast cancer cell lines: Impact of sulfotransferase 1A1 expression on cell growth inhibition. *Cancer Lett.* **2008**, *261*, 172–182. [CrossRef]
88. Azorín-Ortuño, M.; Yáñez-Gascón, M.J.; Vallejo, F.; Pallarés, F.J.; Larrosa, M.; Lucas, R.; Morales, J.C.; Tomás-Barberán, F.A.; García-Conesa, M.T.; Espín, J.C. Metabolites and tissue distribution of resveratrol in the pig. *Mol. Nutr. Food Res.* **2011**, *55*, 1154–1168. [CrossRef]
89. Bode, L.M.; Bunzel, D.; Huch, M.; Cho, G.-S.; Ruhland, D.; Bunzel, M.; Bub, A.; Franz, C.M.; Kulling, S.E. In vivo and in vitro metabolism of trans-resveratrol by human gut microbiota. *Am. J. Clin. Nutr.* **2013**, *97*, 295–309. [CrossRef]
90. El-Sherbeni, A.A.; El-Kadi, A.O. Characterization of arachidonic acid metabolism by rat cytochrome P450 enzymes: The involvement of CYP1As. *Drug Metab. Dispos.* **2014**, *42*, 1498–1507. [CrossRef]
91. Xiao, X.; Wu, Z.-C.; Chou, K.-C. A multi-label classifier for predicting the subcellular localization of gram-negative bacterial proteins with both single and multiple sites. *PLoS ONE* **2011**, *6*, e20592. [CrossRef]
92. Ortuño, J.; Covas, M.-I.; Farre, M.; Pujadas, M.; Fito, M.; Khymenets, O.; Andres-Lacueva, C.; Roset, P.; Joglar, J.; Lamuela-Raventós, R.M. Matrix effects on the bioavailability of resveratrol in humans. *Food Chem.* **2010**, *120*, 1123–1130. [CrossRef]
93. Rotches-Ribalta, M.; Andres-Lacueva, C.; Estruch, R.; Escribano, E.; Urpi-Sarda, M. Pharmacokinetics of resveratrol metabolic profile in healthy humans after moderate consumption of red wine and grape extract tablets. *Pharmacol. Res.* **2012**, *66*, 375–382. [CrossRef] [PubMed]
94. Vickers, N.J. Animal Communication: When I'm Calling You, Will You Answer Too? *Curr. Biol.* **2017**, *27*, R713–R715. [CrossRef] [PubMed]
95. De Bock, M.; Thorstensen, E.B.; Derraik, J.G.; Henderson, H.V.; Hofman, P.L.; Cutfield, W.S. Human absorption and metabolism of oleuropein and hydroxytyrosol ingested as olive (Olea europaea L.) leaf extract. *Mol. Nutr. Food Res.* **2013**, *57*, 2079–2085. [CrossRef]
96. Menet, M.-C.; Marchal, J.; Dal-Pan, A.; Taghi, M.; Nivet-Antoine, V.; Dargère, D.; Laprévote, O.; Beaudeux, J.-L.; Aujard, F.; Epelbaum, J. Resveratrol Metabolism in a Non-Human Primate, the Grey Mouse Lemur (Microcebus murinus), Using Ultra-High-Performance Liquid Chromatography–Quadrupole Time of Flight. *PLoS ONE* **2014**, *9*, e91932. [CrossRef]
97. Cottart, C.H.; Nivet-Antoine, V.; Laguillier-Morizot, C.; Beaudeux, J.L. Resveratrol bioavailability and toxicity in humans. *Mol. Nutr. Food Res.* **2010**, *54*, 7–16. [CrossRef]
98. Crowell, J.A.; Korytko, P.J.; Morrissey, R.L.; Booth, T.D.; Levine, B.S. Resveratrol-associated renal toxicity. *Toxicol. Sci.* **2004**, *82*, 614–619. [CrossRef]
99. Juan, M.E.; Vinardell, M.P.; Planas, J.M. The daily oral administration of high doses of trans-resveratrol to rats for 28 days is not harmful. *J. Nutr.* **2002**, *132*, 257–260. [CrossRef]
100. Williams, L.D.; Burdock, G.A.; Edwards, J.A.; Beck, M.; Bausch, J. Safety studies conducted on high-purity trans-resveratrol in experimental animals. *Food Chem. Toxicol.* **2009**, *47*, 2170–2182. [CrossRef]
101. Boocock, D.J.; Faust, G.E.; Patel, K.R.; Schinas, A.M.; Brown, V.A.; Ducharme, M.P.; Booth, T.D.; Crowell, J.A.; Perloff, M.; Gescher, A.J. Phase I dose escalation pharmacokinetic study in healthy volunteers of resveratrol, a potential cancer chemopreventive agent. *Cancer Epidemiol. Prev. Biomark.* **2007**, *16*, 1246–1252. [CrossRef]
102. Vaz-da-Silva, M.; Loureiro, A.; Falcao, A.; Nunes, T.; Rocha, J.; Fernandes-Lopes, C.; Soares, E.; Wright, L.; Almeida, L.; Soares-da-Silva, P. Effect of food on the pharmacokinetic profile of trans-resveratrol. *Int. J. Clin. Pharm.* **2008**, *46*, 564–570. [CrossRef]
103. Almeida, L.; Vaz-da-Silva, M.; Falcão, A.; Soares, E.; Costa, R.; Loureiro, A.I.; Fernandes-Lopes, C.; Rocha, J.F.; Nunes, T.; Wright, L. Pharmacokinetic and safety profile of trans-resveratrol in a rising multiple-dose study in healthy volunteers. *Mol. Nutr. Food Res.* **2009**, *53*, S7–S15. [CrossRef] [PubMed]
104. Hao, Y.; Baker, D.; ten Dijke, P. TGF-β-mediated epithelial-mesenchymal transition and cancer metastasis. *Int. J. Mol. Sci.* **2019**, *20*, 2767. [CrossRef] [PubMed]
105. Boguslawska, J.; Kryst, P.; Poletajew, S.; Piekielko-Witkowska, A. TGF-β and microRNA Interplay in Genitourinary Cancers. *Cells* **2019**, *8*, 1619. [CrossRef] [PubMed]
106. Colak, S.; ten Dijke, P. Targeting TGF-β signaling in cancer. *Trends Cancer* **2017**, *3*, 56–71. [CrossRef]

107. Van Der Kraan, P.M. The changing role of TGFβ in healthy, ageing and osteoarthritic joints. *Nat. Rev. Rheumatol.* **2017**, *13*, 155. [CrossRef]
108. Chen, S.; Liu, S.; Ma, K.; Zhao, L.; Lin, H.; Shao, Z. TGF-β signaling in intervertebral disc health and disease. *Osteoarthr. Cartil.* **2019**, *27*, 1109–1117. [CrossRef]
109. Yu, Y.; Feng, X.-H. TGF-β signaling in cell fate control and cancer. *Curr. Opin. Cell Biol.* **2019**, *61*, 56–63. [CrossRef]
110. Chung, C.-L.; Tai, S.-B.; Hu, T.-H.; Chen, J.-J.; Chen, C.-L. Roles of Myosin-Mediated Membrane Trafficking in TGF-β Signaling. *Int. J. Mol. Sci.* **2019**, *20*, 3913. [CrossRef]
111. Muñoz, M.; Sánchez-Capelo, A. TGF-β/Smad3 Signalling Modulates GABA Neurotransmission: Implications in Parkinson's Disease. *Int. J. Mol. Sci.* **2020**, *21*, 590. [CrossRef]
112. Liarte, S.; Bernabé-García, Á.; Nicolás, F.J. Role of TGF-in Skin Chronic Wounds: A Keratinocyte Perspective. *Cells* **2020**, *9*, 306. [CrossRef] [PubMed]
113. Samarakoon, R.; Higgins, S.P.; Higgins, C.E.; Higgins, P.J. The TGF-β1/p53/PAI-1 Signaling Axis in Vascular Senescence: Role of Caveolin-1. *Biomolecules* **2019**, *9*, 341. [CrossRef] [PubMed]
114. Tzavlaki, K.; Moustakas, A. TGF-β Signaling. *Biomolecules* **2020**, *10*, 487. [CrossRef]
115. Suriyamurthy, S.; Baker, D.; ten Dijke, P.; Iyengar, P.V. Epigenetic reprogramming of TGF-β signaling in breast cancer. *Cancers* **2019**, *11*, 726. [CrossRef] [PubMed]
116. Massagué, J. TGFβ signalling in context. *Nat. Rev. Mol. Cell Biol.* **2012**, *13*, 616–630. [CrossRef]
117. Derynck, R.; Miyazono, K. *The Biology of the TGF-β Family*; Cold Spring Harbor Laboratory Press: New York, NY, USA, 2017.
118. Derynck, R.; Jarrett, J.A.; Chen, E.Y.; Eaton, D.H.; Bell, J.R.; Assoian, R.K.; Roberts, A.B.; Sporn, M.B.; Goeddel, D.V. Human transforming growth factor-β complementary DNA sequence and expression in normal and transformed cells. *Nature* **1985**, *316*, 701–705. [CrossRef]
119. Sha, X.; Yang, L.; Gentry, L.E. Identification and analysis of discrete functional domains in the pro region of pre-pro-transforming growth factor beta 1. *J. Cell Biol.* **1991**, *114*, 827–839. [CrossRef]
120. Shi, M.; Zhu, J.; Wang, R.; Chen, X.; Mi, L.; Walz, T.; Springer, T.A. Latent TGF-β structure and activation. *Nature* **2011**, *474*, 343–349. [CrossRef]
121. Cheifetz, S.; Hernandez, H.; Laiho, M.; Ten Dijke, P.; Iwata, K.K.; Massagué, J. Distinct transforming growth factor-beta (TGF-beta) receptor subsets as determinants of cellular responsiveness to three TGF-beta isoforms. *J. Biol. Chem.* **1990**, *265*, 20533–20538.
122. Dong, X.; Zhao, B.; Iacob, R.E.; Zhu, J.; Koksal, A.C.; Lu, C.; Engen, J.R.; Springer, T.A. Force interacts with macromolecular structure in activation of TGF-β. *Nature* **2017**, *542*, 55–59. [CrossRef]
123. Marafini, I.; Troncone, E.; Salvatori, S.; Monteleone, G. TGF-β activity restoration and phosphodiesterase 4 inhibition as therapeutic options for inflammatory bowel diseases. *Pharmacol. Res.* **2020**, 104757. [CrossRef] [PubMed]
124. Heldin, C.-H.; Moustakas, A. Role of Smads in TGFβ signaling. *Cell Tissue Res.* **2012**, *347*, 21–36. [CrossRef]
125. Schmierer, B.; Hill, C.S. TGFβ–SMAD signal transduction: Molecular specificity and functional flexibility. *Nat. Rev. Mol. Cell Biol.* **2007**, *8*, 970–982. [CrossRef]
126. Zhang, L.; Zhou, F.; García de Vinuesa, A.; de Kruijf, E.M.; Mesker, W.E.; Hui, L.; Drabsch, Y.; Li, Y.; Bauer, A.; Rousseau, A.; et al. TRAF4 promotes TGF-β receptor signaling and drives breast cancer metastasis. *Mol. Cell* **2013**, *51*, 559–572. [CrossRef]
127. Tang, X.; Shi, L.; Xie, N.; Liu, Z.; Qian, M.; Meng, F.; Xu, Q.; Zhou, M.; Cao, X.; Zhu, W.G.; et al. SIRT7 antagonizes TGF-β signaling and inhibits breast cancer metastasis. *Nat. Commun.* **2017**, *8*, 318. [CrossRef]
128. Muppala, S.; Xiao, R.; Krukovets, I.; Verbovetsky, D.; Yendamuri, R.; Habib, N.; Raman, P.; Plow, E.; Stenina-Adognravi, O. Thrombospondin-4 mediates TGF-β-induced angiogenesis. *Oncogene* **2017**, *36*, 5189–5198. [CrossRef]
129. Oshimori, N.; Oristian, D.; Fuchs, E. TGF-β promotes heterogeneity and drug resistance in squamous cell carcinoma. *Cell* **2015**, *160*, 963–976. [CrossRef]
130. Movahed, A.; Raj, P.; Nabipour, I.; Mahmoodi, M.; Ostovar, A.; Kalantarhormozi, M.; Netticadan, T. Efficacy and Safety of Resveratrol in Type 1 Diabetes Patients: A Two-Month Preliminary Exploratory Trial. *Nutrients* **2020**, *12*, 161. [CrossRef]

131. Bahmanzadeh, M.; Goodarzi, M.T.; Rezaei Farimani, A.; Fathi, N.; Alizadeh, Z. Resveratrol supplementation improves DNA integrity and sperm parameters in streptozotocin-nicotinamide-induced type 2 diabetic rats. *Andrologia* **2019**, *51*, e13313. [CrossRef]
132. Lin, Y.; Zhang, F.; Lian, X.F.; Peng, W.Q.; Yin, C.Y. Mesenchymal stem cell-derived exosomes improve diabetes mellitus-induced myocardial injury and fibrosis via inhibition of TGF-β1/Smad2 signaling pathway. *Cell. Mol. Biol.* **2019**, *65*, 123–126. [CrossRef]
133. Sierra-Mondragon, E.; Rodríguez-Muñoz, R.; Namorado-Tonix, C.; Molina-Jijon, E.; Romero-Trejo, D.; Pedraza-Chaverri, J.; Reyes, J.L. All-Trans Retinoic Acid Attenuates Fibrotic Processes by Downregulating TGF-β1/Smad3 in Early Diabetic Nephropathy. *Biomolecules* **2019**, *9*, 525. [CrossRef]
134. Hsu, W.H.; Liao, S.C.; Chyan, Y.J.; Huang, K.W.; Hsu, S.L.; Chen, Y.C.; Siu, M.L.; Chang, C.C.; Chung, Y.S.; Huang, C.F. Graptopetalum paraguayense Inhibits Liver Fibrosis by Blocking TGF-β Signaling In Vivo and In Vitro. *Int. J. Mol. Sci.* **2019**, *20*, 2592. [CrossRef]
135. Ma, J.Q.; Sun, Y.Z.; Ming, Q.L.; Tian, Z.K.; Yang, H.X.; Liu, C.M. Ampelopsin attenuates carbon tetrachloride-induced mouse liver fibrosis and hepatic stellate cell activation associated with the SIRT1/TGF-β1/Smad3 and autophagy pathway. *Int. Immunopharmacol.* **2019**, *77*, 105984. [CrossRef]
136. Razali, N.; Agarwal, R.; Agarwal, P.; Froemming, G.R.A.; Tripathy, M.; Ismail, N.M. IOP lowering effect of topical trans-resveratrol involves adenosine receptors and TGF-β2 signaling pathways. *Eur. J. Pharmacol.* **2018**, *838*, 1–10. [CrossRef]
137. Yang, R.C.; Zhu, X.L.; Zhang, H.Q.; Li, W.D. Study of resveratrol suppressing TGF-beta1 induced transdifferentiation of podocytes. *Zhongguo Zhong Xi Yi Jie He Za Zhi Zhongguo Zhongxiyi Jiehe Zazhi Chin. J. Integr. Tradit. West. Med.* **2013**, *33*, 1677–1682.
138. Suenaga, F.; Hatsushika, K.; Takano, S.; Ando, T.; Ohnuma, Y.; Ogawa, H.; Nakao, A. A possible link between resveratrol and TGF-beta: Resveratrol induction of TGF-beta expression and signaling. *FEBS Lett.* **2008**, *582*, 586–590. [CrossRef]
139. Garcia, P.; Schmiedlin-Ren, P.; Mathias, J.S.; Tang, H.; Christman, G.M.; Zimmermann, E.M. Resveratrol causes cell cycle arrest, decreased collagen synthesis, and apoptosis in rat intestinal smooth muscle cells. *Am. J. Physiol. Gastrointest. Liver Physiol.* **2012**, *302*, G326–G335. [CrossRef]
140. Trotta, V.; Lee, W.H.; Loo, C.Y.; Haghi, M.; Young, P.M.; Scalia, S.; Traini, D. In vitro biological activity of resveratrol using a novel inhalable resveratrol spray-dried formulation. *Int. J. Pharm.* **2015**, *491*, 190–197. [CrossRef]
141. Rahal, K.; Schmiedlin-Ren, P.; Adler, J.; Dhanani, M.; Sultani, V.; Rittershaus, A.C.; Reingold, L.; Zhu, J.; McKenna, B.J.; Christman, G.M.; et al. Resveratrol has antiinflammatory and antifibrotic effects in the peptidoglycan-polysaccharide rat model of Crohn's disease. *Inflamm. Bowel Dis.* **2012**, *18*, 613–623. [CrossRef]
142. Wei, G.; Chen, X.; Wang, G.; Fan, L.; Wang, K.; Li, X. Effect of Resveratrol on the Prevention of Intra-Abdominal Adhesion Formation in a Rat Model. *Cell. Physiol. Biochem. Int. J. Exp. Cell. Physiol. Biochem. Pharmacol.* **2016**, *39*, 33–46. [CrossRef]
143. He, Y.; Zeng, H.; Yu, Y.; Zhang, J.; Liu, Q.; Yang, B. Resveratrol improved detrusor fibrosis induced by mast cells during progression of chronic prostatitis in rats. *Eur. J. Pharmacol.* **2017**, *815*, 495–500. [CrossRef]
144. Alrafas, H.R.; Busbee, P.B.; Nagarkatti, M.; Nagarkatti, P.S. Resveratrol Downregulates miR-31 to Promote T Regulatory Cells during Prevention of TNBS-Induced Colitis. *Mol. Nutr. Food Res.* **2020**, *64*, e1900633. [CrossRef]
145. Xiao, Z.; Chen, C.; Meng, T.; Zhang, W.; Zhou, Q. Resveratrol attenuates renal injury and fibrosis by inhibiting transforming growth factor-β pathway on matrix metalloproteinase 7. *Exp. Biol. Med.* **2016**, *241*, 140–146. [CrossRef]
146. Ishikawa, K.; He, S.; Terasaki, H.; Nazari, H.; Zhang, H.; Spee, C.; Kannan, R.; Hinton, D.R. Resveratrol inhibits epithelial-mesenchymal transition of retinal pigment epithelium and development of proliferative vitreoretinopathy. *Sci. Rep.* **2015**, *5*, 16386. [CrossRef]
147. Rosa, P.M.; Martins, L.A.M.; Souza, D.O.; Quincozes-Santos, A. Glioprotective Effect of Resveratrol: An Emerging Therapeutic Role for Oligodendroglial Cells. *Mol. Neurobiol.* **2018**, *55*, 2967–2978. [CrossRef]
148. Losso, J.N.; Truax, R.E.; Richard, G. trans-resveratrol inhibits hyperglycemia-induced inflammation and connexin downregulation in retinal pigment epithelial cells. *J. Agric. Food Chem* **2010**, *58*, 8246–8252. [CrossRef]

149. Das, S.K.; Mukherjee, S.; Gupta, G.; Rao, D.N.; Vasudevan, D.M. Protective effect of resveratrol and vitamin E against ethanol-induced oxidative damage in mice: Biochemical and immunological basis. *Indian J. Biochem. Biophys.* **2010**, *47*, 32–37.
150. Leppäranta, O.; Sens, C.; Salmenkivi, K.; Kinnula, V.L.; Keski-Oja, J.; Myllärniemi, M.; Koli, K. Regulation of TGF-β storage and activation in the human idiopathic pulmonary fibrosis lung. *Cell Tissue Res.* **2012**, *348*, 491–503. [CrossRef]
151. Bellaye, P.S.; Yanagihara, T.; Granton, E.; Sato, S.; Shimbori, C.; Upagupta, C.; Imani, J.; Hambly, N.; Ask, K.; Gauldie, J.; et al. Macitentan reduces progression of TGF-β1-induced pulmonary fibrosis and pulmonary hypertension. *Eur. Respir. J.* **2018**, *52*. [CrossRef]
152. Wang, J.; He, F.; Chen, L.; Li, Q.; Jin, S.; Zheng, H.; Lin, J.; Zhang, H.; Ma, S.; Mei, J.; et al. Resveratrol inhibits pulmonary fibrosis by regulating miR-21 through MAPK/AP-1 pathways. *Biomed. Pharmacother.* **2018**, *105*, 37–44. [CrossRef]
153. Gao, C.; Howard-Quijano, K.; Rau, C.; Takamiya, T.; Song, Y.; Shivkumar, K.; Wang, Y.; Mahajan, A. Inflammatory and apoptotic remodeling in autonomic nervous system following myocardial infarction. *PLoS ONE* **2017**, *12*, e0177750. [CrossRef]
154. Gao, H.; Bo, Z.; Wang, Q.; Luo, L.; Zhu, H.; Ren, Y. Salvanic acid B inhibits myocardial fibrosis through regulating TGF-β1/Smad signaling pathway. *Biomed. Pharmacother.* **2019**, *110*, 685–691. [CrossRef]
155. Zhang, Y.; Lu, Y.; Ong'achwa, M.J.; Ge, L.; Qian, Y.; Chen, L.; Hu, X.; Li, F.; Wei, H.; Zhang, C.; et al. Resveratrol Inhibits the TGF-β1-Induced Proliferation of Cardiac Fibroblasts and Collagen Secretion by Downregulating miR-17 in Rat. *Biomed. Res. Int.* **2018**, *2018*, 8730593. [CrossRef]
156. Annaldas, S.; Saifi, M.A.; Khurana, A.; Godugu, C. Nimbolide ameliorates unilateral ureteral obstruction-induced renal fibrosis by inhibition of TGF-β and EMT/Slug signalling. *Mol. Immunol.* **2019**, *112*, 247–255. [CrossRef]
157. Song, M.K.; Lee, J.H.; Ryoo, I.G.; Lee, S.H.; Ku, S.K.; Kwak, M.K. Bardoxolone ameliorates TGF-β1-associated renal fibrosis through Nrf2/Smad7 elevation. *Free Radic. Biol. Med.* **2019**, *138*, 33–42. [CrossRef]
158. Zhang, X.; Lu, H.; Xie, S.; Wu, C.; Guo, Y.; Xiao, Y.; Zheng, S.; Zhu, H.; Zhang, Y.; Bai, Y. Resveratrol suppresses the myofibroblastic phenotype and fibrosis formation in kidneys via proliferation-related signalling pathways. *Br. J. Pharmacol.* **2019**, *176*, 4745–4759. [CrossRef]
159. Liu, Y. New insights into epithelial-mesenchymal transition in kidney fibrosis. *J. Am. Soc. Nephrol.* **2010**, *21*, 212–222. [CrossRef]
160. Alpers, C.E.; Hudkins, K.L.; Floege, J.; Johnson, R.J. Human renal cortical interstitial cells with some features of smooth muscle cells participate in tubulointerstitial and crescentic glomerular injury. *J. Am. Soc. Nephrol.* **1994**, *5*, 201–209.
161. Bi, W.; Xu, G.; Lv, L.; Yang, C. The ratio of transforming growth factor-β1/bone morphogenetic protein-7 in the progression of the epithelial-mesenchymal transition contributes to rat liver fibrosis. *Genet. Mol. Res.* **2014**, *13*, 1005–1014. [CrossRef]
162. Kalluri, R.; Weinberg, R.A. The basics of epithelial-mesenchymal transition. *J. Clin. Investig.* **2009**, *119*, 1420–1428. [CrossRef]
163. Bai, Y.; Lu, H.; Wu, C.; Liang, Y.; Wang, S.; Lin, C.; Chen, B.; Xia, P. Resveratrol inhibits epithelial-mesenchymal transition and renal fibrosis by antagonizing the hedgehog signaling pathway. *Biochem. Pharmacol.* **2014**, *92*, 484–493. [CrossRef]
164. Zhai, X.X.; Ding, J.C.; Tang, Z.M. Resveratrol Inhibits Proliferation and Induces Apoptosis of Pathological Scar Fibroblasts Through the Mechanism Involving TGF-β1/Smads Signaling Pathway. *Cell Biochem. Biophys.* **2015**, *71*, 1267–1272. [CrossRef]
165. Liu, S.; Zhao, M.; Zhou, Y.; Wang, C.; Yuan, Y.; Li, L.; Bresette, W.; Chen, Y.; Cheng, J.; Lu, Y.; et al. Resveratrol exerts dose-dependent anti-fibrotic or pro-fibrotic effects in kidneys: A potential risk to individuals with impaired kidney function. *Phytomedicine* **2019**, *57*, 223–235. [CrossRef]
166. Chávez, E.; Reyes-Gordillo, K.; Segovia, J.; Shibayama, M.; Tsutsumi, V.; Vergara, P.; Moreno, M.G.; Muriel, P. Resveratrol prevents fibrosis, NF-kappaB activation and TGF-beta increases induced by chronic CCl4 treatment in rats. *J. Appl. Toxicol. JAT* **2008**, *28*, 35–43. [CrossRef]
167. Ding, S.; Wang, H.; Wang, M.; Bai, L.; Yu, P.; Wu, W. Resveratrol alleviates chronic "real-world" ambient particulate matter-induced lung inflammation and fibrosis by inhibiting NLRP3 inflammasome activation in mice. *Ecotoxicol. Environ. Saf.* **2019**, *182*, 109425. [CrossRef]

168. Sun, D.Y.; Wu, J.Q.; He, Z.H.; He, M.F.; Sun, H.B. Cancer-associated fibroblast regulate proliferation and migration of prostate cancer cells through TGF-β signaling pathway. *Life Sci.* **2019**, *235*, 116791. [CrossRef]
169. Cruz-Bermúdez, A.; Laza-Briviesca, R.; Vicente-Blanco, R.J.; García-Grande, A.; Coronado, M.J.; Laine-Menéndez, S.; Alfaro, C.; Sanchez, J.C.; Franco, F.; Calvo, V.; et al. Cancer-associated fibroblasts modify lung cancer metabolism involving ROS and TGF-β signaling. *Free Radic. Biol. Med.* **2019**, *130*, 163–173. [CrossRef]
170. Bierie, B.; Moses, H.L. TGF-beta and cancer. *Cytokine Growth Factor Rev.* **2006**, *17*, 29–40. [CrossRef]
171. Zhao, M.; Mishra, L.; Deng, C.X. The role of TGF-β/SMAD4 signaling in cancer. *Int. J. Biol. Sci.* **2018**, *14*, 111–123. [CrossRef]
172. Camerlingo, R.; Miceli, R.; Marra, L.; Rea, G.; D'Agnano, I.; Nardella, M.; Montella, R.; Morabito, A.; Normanno, N.; Tirino, V.; et al. Conditioned medium of primary lung cancer cells induces EMT in A549 lung cancer cell line by TGF-ß1 and miRNA21 cooperation. *PLoS ONE* **2019**, *14*, e0219597. [CrossRef]
173. Liu, X.S.; Lin, X.K.; Mei, Y.; Ahmad, S.; Yan, C.X.; Jin, H.L.; Yu, H.; Chen, C.; Lin, C.Z.; Yu, J.R. Regulatory T Cells Promote Overexpression of Lgr5 on Gastric Cancer Cells via TGF-beta1 and Confer Poor Prognosis in Gastric Cancer. *Front. Immunol.* **2019**, *10*, 1741. [CrossRef] [PubMed]
174. Hyun Lee, J.; Dhananjaya Mohan, C.; Deivasigamani, A.; Yun Jung, Y.; Rangappa, S.; Basappa, S.; Chinnathambi, A.; Awad Alahmadi, T.; Ali Alharbi, S.; Garg, M.; et al. Brusatol suppresses STAT3-driven metastasis by downregulating epithelial-mesenchymal transition in hepatocellular carcinoma. *J. Adv. Res.* **2020**. [CrossRef]
175. Cheng, J.-T.; Wang, L.; Wang, H.; Tang, F.-R.; Cai, W.-Q.; Sethi, G.; Xin, H.-W.; Ma, Z. Insights into Biological Role of LncRNAs in Epithelial-Mesenchymal Transition. *Cells* **2019**, *8*, 1178. [CrossRef] [PubMed]
176. Loh, C.-Y.; Chai, J.Y.; Tang, T.F.; Wong, W.F.; Sethi, G.; Shanmugam, M.K.; Chong, P.P.; Looi, C.Y. The E-Cadherin and N-Cadherin Switch in Epithelial-to-Mesenchymal Transition: Signaling, Therapeutic Implications, and Challenges. *Cells* **2019**, *8*, 1118. [CrossRef] [PubMed]
177. Sun, Y.; Zhou, Q.M.; Lu, Y.Y.; Zhang, H.; Chen, Q.L.; Zhao, M.; Su, S.B. Resveratrol Inhibits the Migration and Metastasis of MDA-MB-231 Human Breast Cancer by Reversing TGF-β1-Induced Epithelial-Mesenchymal Transition. *Molecules* **2019**, *24*, 1131. [CrossRef]
178. Wang, H.; Zhang, H.; Tang, L.; Chen, H.; Wu, C.; Zhao, M.; Yang, Y.; Chen, X.; Liu, G. Resveratrol inhibits TGF-β1-induced epithelial-to-mesenchymal transition and suppresses lung cancer invasion and metastasis. *Toxicology* **2013**, *303*, 139–146. [CrossRef]
179. Song, Y.; Chen, Y.; Li, Y.; Lyu, X.; Cui, J.; Cheng, Y.; Zheng, T.; Zhao, L.; Zhao, G. Resveratrol Suppresses Epithelial-Mesenchymal Transition in GBM by Regulating Smad-Dependent Signaling. *Biomed. Res. Int.* **2019**, *2019*, 1321973. [CrossRef]
180. Kabel, A.M.; Atef, A.; Estfanous, R.S. Ameliorative potential of sitagliptin and/or resveratrol on experimentally-induced clear cell renal cell carcinoma. *Biomed. Pharmacother.* **2018**, *97*, 667–674. [CrossRef]
181. Zhang, Y.; Yang, S.; Yang, Y.; Liu, T. Resveratrol induces immunogenic cell death of human and murine ovarian carcinoma cells. *Infect. Agents Cancer* **2019**, *14*, 27. [CrossRef]
182. Rekik, R.; Belhadj Hmida, N.; Ben Hmid, A.; Zamali, I.; Kammoun, N.; Ben Ahmed, M. PD-1 induction through TCR activation is partially regulated by endogenous TGF-β. *Cell. Mol. Immunol.* **2015**, *12*, 648–649. [CrossRef]
183. Celada, L.J.; Kropski, J.A.; Herazo-Maya, J.D.; Luo, W.; Creecy, A.; Abad, A.T.; Chioma, O.S.; Lee, G.; Hassell, N.E.; Shaginurova, G.I.; et al. PD-1 up-regulation on CD4(+) T cells promotes pulmonary fibrosis through STAT3-mediated IL-17A and TGF-β1 production. *Sci. Transl. Med.* **2018**, *10*. [CrossRef] [PubMed]
184. Johnson, E.R.; Matthay, M.A. Acute lung injury: Epidemiology, pathogenesis, and treatment. *J. Aerosol Med. Pulm. Drug Deliv.* **2010**, *23*, 243–252. [CrossRef] [PubMed]
185. Sawa, T. The molecular mechanism of acute lung injury caused by Pseudomonas aeruginosa: From bacterial pathogenesis to host response. *J. Intensive Care* **2014**, *2*, 10. [CrossRef] [PubMed]
186. Kubota, Y.; Iwasaki, Y.; Harada, H.; Yokomura, I.; Ueda, M.; Hashimoto, S.; Nakagawa, M. Role of alveolar macrophages in Candida-induced acute lung injury. *Clin. Diagn. Lab. Immunol.* **2001**, *8*, 1258–1262. [CrossRef] [PubMed]
187. Savransky, V.; Rostapshov, V.; Pinelis, D.; Polotsky, Y.; Korolev, S.; Komisar, J.; Fegeding, K. Murine lethal toxic shock caused by intranasal administration of staphylococcal enterotoxin B. *Toxicol. Pathol.* **2003**, *31*, 373–378. [CrossRef] [PubMed]

188. Alghetaa, H.; Mohammed, A.; Sultan, M.; Busbee, P.; Murphy, A.; Chatterjee, S.; Nagarkatti, M.; Nagarkatti, P. Resveratrol protects mice against SEB-induced acute lung injury and mortality by miR-193a modulation that targets TGF-β signalling. *J. Cell. Mol. Med.* **2018**, *22*, 2644–2655. [CrossRef] [PubMed]
189. Karagiannidis, C.; Akdis, M.; Holopainen, P.; Woolley, N.J.; Hense, G.; Rückert, B.; Mantel, P.Y.; Menz, G.; Akdis, C.A.; Blaser, K.; et al. Glucocorticoids upregulate FOXP3 expression and regulatory T cells in asthma. *J. Allergy Clin. Immunol.* **2004**, *114*, 1425–1433. [CrossRef]
190. Alharris, E.; Alghetaa, H.; Seth, R.; Chatterjee, S.; Singh, N.P.; Nagarkatti, M.; Nagarkatti, P. Resveratrol Attenuates Allergic Asthma and Associated Inflammation in the Lungs Through Regulation of miRNA-34a That Targets FoxP3 in Mice. *Front. Immunol.* **2018**, *9*, 2992. [CrossRef]
191. Wollin, L.; Pieper, M. Tiotropium bromide exerts anti-inflammatory activity in a cigarette smoke mouse model of COPD. *Pulm. Pharmacol. Ther.* **2010**, *23*, 345–354. [CrossRef]
192. Tamimi, A.; Serdarevic, D.; Hanania, N.A. The effects of cigarette smoke on airway inflammation in asthma and COPD: Therapeutic implications. *Respir. Med.* **2012**, *106*, 319–328. [CrossRef]
193. Busse, P.J.; Zhang, T.F.; Srivastava, K.; Lin, B.P.; Schofield, B.; Sealfon, S.C.; Li, X.-M. Chronic exposure to TNF-α increases airway mucus gene expression in vivo. *J. Allergy Clin. Immunol.* **2005**, *116*, 1256–1263. [CrossRef] [PubMed]
194. Numasaki, M.; Tomioka, Y.; Takahashi, H.; Sasaki, H. IL-17 and IL-17F modulate GM-CSF production by lung microvascular endothelial cells stimulated with IL-1β and/or TNF-α. *Immunol. Lett.* **2004**, *95*, 175–184. [CrossRef] [PubMed]
195. Chen, J.; Yang, X.; Zhang, W.; Peng, D.; Xia, Y.; Lu, Y.; Han, X.; Song, G.; Zhu, J.; Liu, R. Therapeutic Effects of Resveratrol in a Mouse Model of LPS and Cigarette Smoke-Induced COPD. *Inflammation* **2016**, *39*, 1949–1959. [CrossRef] [PubMed]
196. Al-Mufti, F.; Amuluru, K.; Changa, A.; Lander, M.; Patel, N.; Wajswol, E.; Al-Marsoummi, S.; Alzubaidi, B.; Singh, I.P.; Nuoman, R.; et al. Traumatic brain injury and intracranial hemorrhage-induced cerebral vasospasm: A systematic review. *Neurosurg. Focus* **2017**, *43*, E14. [CrossRef]
197. Shoamanesh, A.; Kwok, C.S.; Lim, P.A.; Benavente, O.R. Postthrombolysis intracranial hemorrhage risk of cerebral microbleeds in acute stroke patients: A systematic review and meta-analysis. *Int. J. Stroke Off. J. Int. Stroke Soc.* **2013**, *8*, 348–356. [CrossRef]
198. Bugeme, M.; Mukuku, O. Neuropsychiatric manifestations revealing cerebral subarachnoid hemorrhage caused by electrification accident about a case and review of literature. *Pan Afr. Med. J.* **2014**, *18*, 201. [CrossRef]
199. Logan, T.T.; Villapol, S.; Symes, A.J. TGF-β superfamily gene expression and induction of the Runx1 transcription factor in adult neurogenic regions after brain injury. *PLoS ONE* **2013**, *8*, e59250. [CrossRef]
200. Zhao, R.; Zhao, K.; Su, H.; Zhang, P.; Zhao, N. Resveratrol ameliorates brain injury via the TGF-β-mediated ERK signaling pathway in a rat model of cerebral hemorrhage. *Exp. Ther. Med.* **2019**, *18*, 3397–3404. [CrossRef]
201. Tiwari, V.; Chopra, K. Resveratrol prevents alcohol-induced cognitive deficits and brain damage by blocking inflammatory signaling and cell death cascade in neonatal rat brain. *J. Neurochem.* **2011**, *117*, 678–690. [CrossRef]
202. Forbes, J.M.; Cooper, M.E.; Oldfield, M.D.; Thomas, M.C. Role of advanced glycation end products in diabetic nephropathy. *J. Am. Soc. Nephrol.* **2003**, *14*, S254–S258. [CrossRef]
203. Yamagishi, S.-i.; Matsui, T. Advanced glycation end products, oxidative stress and diabetic nephropathy. *Oxidative Med. Cell. Longev.* **2010**, *3*, 101–108. [CrossRef] [PubMed]
204. Mima, A. Inflammation and oxidative stress in diabetic nephropathy: New insights on its inhibition as new therapeutic targets. *J. Diabetes Res.* **2013**, *2013*, 8. [CrossRef] [PubMed]
205. Hussein, M.M.; Mahfouz, M.K. Effect of resveratrol and rosuvastatin on experimental diabetic nephropathy in rats. *Biomed. Pharmacother.* **2016**, *82*, 685–692. [CrossRef] [PubMed]
206. Chen, K.H.; Hung, C.C.; Hsu, H.H.; Jing, Y.H.; Yang, C.W.; Chen, J.K. Resveratrol ameliorates early diabetic nephropathy associated with suppression of augmented TGF-β/smad and ERK1/2 signaling in streptozotocin-induced diabetic rats. *Chem. Biol. Interact.* **2011**, *190*, 45–53. [CrossRef] [PubMed]
207. Abd El-Haleim, E.A.; Bahgat, A.K.; Saleh, S. Resveratrol and fenofibrate ameliorate fructose-induced nonalcoholic steatohepatitis by modulation of genes expression. *World J. Gastroenterol.* **2016**, *22*, 2931–2948. [CrossRef]

208. Qiao, Y.; Gao, K.; Wang, Y.; Wang, X.; Cui, B. Resveratrol ameliorates diabetic nephropathy in rats through negative regulation of the p38 MAPK/TGF-β1 pathway. *Exp. Ther. Med.* **2017**, *13*, 3223–3230. [CrossRef]
209. Wu, H.; Li, G.N.; Xie, J.; Li, R.; Chen, Q.H.; Chen, J.Z.; Wei, Z.H.; Kang, L.N.; Xu, B. Resveratrol ameliorates myocardial fibrosis by inhibiting ROS/ERK/TGF-β/periostin pathway in STZ-induced diabetic mice. *BMC Cardiovasc. Disord.* **2016**, *16*, 5. [CrossRef]
210. Elbe, H.; Vardi, N.; Esrefoglu, M.; Ates, B.; Yologlu, S.; Taskapan, C. Amelioration of streptozotocin-induced diabetic nephropathy by melatonin, quercetin, and resveratrol in rats. *Hum. Exp. Toxicol.* **2015**, *34*, 100–113. [CrossRef]
211. Wenbin, Z.; Guojun, G. Resveratrol Ameliorates Diabetes-induced Renal Damage through Regulating the Expression of TGF-β1, Collagen IV and Th17/Treg-related Cytokines in Rats. *West Indian Med. J.* **2014**, *63*, 20–25. [CrossRef]
212. Liu, J.; Zhuo, X.; Liu, W.; Wan, Z.; Liang, X.; Gao, S.; Yuan, Z.; Wu, Y. Resveratrol inhibits high glucose induced collagen upregulation in cardiac fibroblasts through regulating TGF-β1-Smad3 signaling pathway. *Chem. Biol. Interact.* **2015**, *227*, 45–52. [CrossRef]
213. Hammad, A.S.A.; Ahmed, A.F.; Heeba, G.H.; Taye, A. Heme oxygenase-1 contributes to the protective effect of resveratrol against endothelial dysfunction in STZ-induced diabetes in rats. *Life Sci.* **2019**, *239*, 117065. [CrossRef] [PubMed]
214. Zeng, H.; He, Y.; Yu, Y.; Zhang, J.; Zeng, X.; Gong, F.; Liu, Q.; Yang, B. Resveratrol improves prostate fibrosis during progression of urinary dysfunction in chronic prostatitis by mast cell suppression. *Mol. Med. Rep.* **2018**, *17*, 918–924. [CrossRef] [PubMed]
215. He, Y.; Zeng, H.Z.; Yu, Y.; Zhang, J.S.; Duan, X.; Zeng, X.N.; Gong, F.T.; Liu, Q.; Yang, B. Resveratrol improves prostate fibrosis during progression of urinary dysfunction in chronic prostatitis. *Environ. Toxicol. Pharmacol.* **2017**, *54*, 120–124. [CrossRef] [PubMed]
216. Zhang, Y.Q.; Liu, Y.J.; Mao, Y.F.; Dong, W.W.; Zhu, X.Y.; Jiang, L. Resveratrol ameliorates lipopolysaccharide-induced epithelial mesenchymal transition and pulmonary fibrosis through suppression of oxidative stress and transforming growth factor-β1 signaling. *Clin. Nutr.* **2015**, *34*, 752–760. [CrossRef] [PubMed]
217. Shi, X.P.; Miao, S.; Wu, Y.; Zhang, W.; Zhang, X.F.; Ma, H.Z.; Xin, H.L.; Feng, J.; Wen, A.D.; Li, Y. Resveratrol sensitizes tamoxifen in antiestrogen-resistant breast cancer cells with epithelial-mesenchymal transition features. *Int. J. Mol. Sci.* **2013**, *14*, 15655–15668. [CrossRef] [PubMed]
218. Kim, K.H.; Back, J.H.; Zhu, Y.; Arbesman, J.; Athar, M.; Kopelovich, L.; Kim, A.L.; Bickers, D.R. Resveratrol targets transforming growth factor-β2 signaling to block UV-induced tumor progression. *J. Investig. Dermatol.* **2011**, *131*, 195–202. [CrossRef]
219. Kim, J.S.; Jeong, S.K.; Oh, S.J.; Lee, C.G.; Kang, Y.R.; Jo, W.S.; Jeong, M.H. The resveratrol analogue, HS-1793, enhances the effects of radiation therapy through the induction of anti-tumor immunity in mammary tumor growth. *Int. J. Oncol.* **2020**, *56*, 1405–1416. [CrossRef]
220. Chen, T.; Li, J.; Liu, J.; Li, N.; Wang, S.; Liu, H.; Zeng, M.; Zhang, Y.; Bu, P. Activation of SIRT3 by resveratrol ameliorates cardiac fibrosis and improves cardiac function via the TGF-β/Smad3 pathway. *Am. J. Physiol. Heart Circ. Physiol.* **2015**, *308*, H424–H434. [CrossRef]
221. Lee, H.Y.; Kim, I.K.; Yoon, H.K.; Kwon, S.S.; Rhee, C.K.; Lee, S.Y. Inhibitory Effects of Resveratrol on Airway Remodeling by Transforming Growth Factor-β/Smad Signaling Pathway in Chronic Asthma Model. *Allergyasthma Immunol. Res.* **2017**, *9*, 25–34. [CrossRef]
222. Chen, C.L.; Chen, Y.H.; Tai, M.C.; Liang, C.M.; Lu, D.W.; Chen, J.T. Resveratrol inhibits transforming growth factor-β2-induced epithelial-to-mesenchymal transition in human retinal pigment epithelial cells by suppressing the Smad pathway. *Drug Des. Dev. Ther.* **2017**, *11*, 163–173. [CrossRef]
223. Hori, Y.S.; Kuno, A.; Hosoda, R.; Tanno, M.; Miura, T.; Shimamoto, K.; Horio, Y. Resveratrol ameliorates muscular pathology in the dystrophic mdx mouse, a model for Duchenne muscular dystrophy. *J. Pharmacol. Exp. Ther.* **2011**, *338*, 784–794. [CrossRef] [PubMed]
224. Yang, H.; Yuan, Y.; Luo, C.; He, H.; Zhou, Y. Inhibitory Effects of Resveratrol on the Human Alveolar Rhabdomyosarcoma Cell Line PLA-802 through Inhibition of the TGF-β1/Smad Signaling Pathway. *Pharmacology* **2016**, *98*, 35–41. [CrossRef] [PubMed]

225. Li, J.; Qu, X.; Ricardo, S.D.; Bertram, J.F.; Nikolic-Paterson, D.J. Resveratrol inhibits renal fibrosis in the obstructed kidney: Potential role in deacetylation of Smad3. *Am. J. Pathol.* **2010**, *177*, 1065–1071. [CrossRef] [PubMed]
226. Liskova, A.; Koklesova, L.; Samec, M.; Smejkal, K.; Samuel, S.M.; Varghese, E.; Abotaleb, M.; Biringer, K.; Kudela, E.; Danko, J.; et al. Flavonoids in Cancer Metastasis. *Cancers* **2020**, *12*, 1498. [CrossRef] [PubMed]
227. Manu, K.A.; Shanmugam, M.K.; Ramachandran, L.; Li, F.; Siveen, K.S.; Chinnathambi, A.; Zayed, M.E.; Alharbi, S.A.; Arfuso, F.; Kumar, A.P.; et al. Isorhamnetin augments the anti-tumor effect of capeciatbine through the negative regulation of NF-κB signaling cascade in gastric cancer. *Cancer Lett.* **2015**, *363*, 28–36. [CrossRef]
228. Varghese, E.; Liskova, A.; Kubatka, P.; Samuel, S.M.; Büsselberg, D. Anti-Angiogenic Effects of Phytochemicals on miRNA Regulating Breast Cancer Progression. *Biomolecules* **2020**, *10*, 191. [CrossRef]
229. Manu, K.A.; Shanmugam, M.K.; Li, F.; Chen, L.; Siveen, K.S.; Ahn, K.S.; Kumar, A.P.; Sethi, G. Simvastatin sensitizes human gastric cancer xenograft in nude mice to capecitabine by suppressing nuclear factor-kappa B-regulated gene products. *J. Mol. Med.* **2014**, *92*, 267–276. [CrossRef]
230. Siveen, K.S.; Ahn, K.S.; Ong, T.H.; Shanmugam, M.K.; Li, F.; Yap, W.N.; Kumar, A.P.; Fong, C.W.; Tergaonkar, V.; Hui, K.M.; et al. γ-tocotrienol inhibits angiogenesis-dependent growth of human hepatocellular carcinoma through abrogation of AKT/mTOR pathway in an orthotopic mouse model. *Oncotarget* **2014**, *5*, 1897–1911. [CrossRef]
231. Shanmugam, M.K.; Kannaiyan, R.; Sethi, G. Targeting cell signaling and apoptotic pathways by dietary agents: Role in the prevention and treatment of cancer. *Nutr. Cancer* **2011**, *63*, 161–173. [CrossRef]
232. Sawhney, M.; Rohatgi, N.; Kaur, J.; Shishodia, S.; Sethi, G.; Gupta, S.D.; Deo, S.V.; Shukla, N.K.; Aggarwal, B.B.; Ralhan, R. Expression of NF-kappaB parallels COX-2 expression in oral precancer and cancer: Association with smokeless tobacco. *Int. J. Cancer* **2007**, *120*, 2545–2556. [CrossRef]
233. Ahn, K.S.; Sethi, G.; Jain, A.K.; Jaiswal, A.K.; Aggarwal, B.B. Genetic deletion of NAD(P)H:quinone oxidoreductase 1 abrogates activation of nuclear factor-kappaB, IkappaBalpha kinase, c-Jun N-terminal kinase, Akt, p38, and p44/42 mitogen-activated protein kinases and potentiates apoptosis. *J. Biol. Chem.* **2006**, *281*, 19798–19808. [CrossRef] [PubMed]

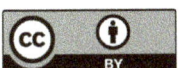

© 2020 by the authors. Licensee MDPI, Basel, Switzerland. This article is an open access article distributed under the terms and conditions of the Creative Commons Attribution (CC BY) license (http://creativecommons.org/licenses/by/4.0/).

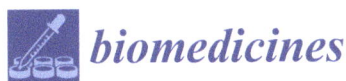

Review

Tackling Antibiotic Resistance with Compounds of Natural Origin: A Comprehensive Review

Francisco Javier Álvarez-Martínez [1], Enrique Barrajón-Catalán [1,*] and Vicente Micol [1,2]

[1] Institute of Research, Development and Innovation in Health Biotechnology of Elche (IDiBE), Universitas Miguel Hernández (UMH), 03202 Elche, Spain; f.alvarez@umh.es (F.J.Á.-M.); vmicol@umh.es (V.M.)
[2] CIBER, Fisiopatología de la Obesidad y la Nutrición, CIBERobn, Instituto de Salud Carlos III (CB12/03/30038), 28220 Madrid, Spain
* Correspondence: e.barrajon@umh.es; Tel.: +34-965222586

Received: 18 September 2020; Accepted: 9 October 2020; Published: 11 October 2020

Abstract: Drug-resistant bacteria pose a serious threat to human health worldwide. Current antibiotics are losing efficacy and new antimicrobial agents are urgently needed. Living organisms are an invaluable source of antimicrobial compounds. The antimicrobial activity of the most representative natural products of animal, bacterial, fungal and plant origin are reviewed in this paper. Their activity against drug-resistant bacteria, their mechanisms of action, the possible development of resistance against them, their role in current medicine and their future perspectives are discussed. Electronic databases such as PubMed, Scopus and ScienceDirect were used to search scientific contributions until September 2020, using relevant keywords. Natural compounds of heterogeneous origins have been shown to possess antimicrobial capabilities, including against antibiotic-resistant bacteria. The most commonly found mechanisms of antimicrobial action are related to protein biosynthesis and alteration of cell walls and membranes. Various natural compounds, especially phytochemicals, have shown synergistic capacity with antibiotics. There is little literature on the development of specific resistance mechanisms against natural antimicrobial compounds. New technologies such as -omics, network pharmacology and informatics have the potential to identify and characterize new natural antimicrobial compounds in the future. This knowledge may be useful for the development of future therapeutic strategies.

Keywords: natural antimicrobial; antimicrobial resistance; polyphenols; future medicine; natural origin; antibacterial compound; phytochemicals

1. Introduction

Antimicrobial resistance (AMR) and the inexorable advance of superbacteria poses a great threat to human health worldwide. If this problem is not tackled, the antibiotics we have used with great success so far could become substances unable to help us against infections caused by bacteria, going back to a worrying pre-antibiotic era. According to data from the United Kingdom government [1], 10 million deaths could happen annually due to antibiotic resistance by 2050, becoming one of the leading causes of death in the world (Figure 1).

This problem is known to scientists and institutions around the world, which are organizing to establish protocols to address the problem of antibiotic-resistant microbes. Proof of this was the 2012 Chennai Declaration of India, in which international experts and representatives of medical entities met to draw up action plans in the face of the inexorable advance of the superbugs [2]. Similar initiatives have been promoted from private and public institutions worldwide.

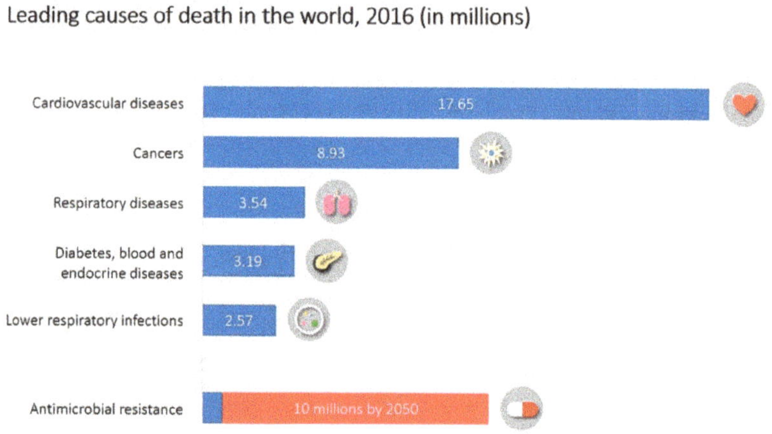

Leading causes of death in the world, 2016 (in millions)

- Cardiovascular diseases: 17.65
- Cancers: 8.93
- Respiratory diseases: 3.54
- Diabetes, blood and endocrine diseases: 3.19
- Lower respiratory infections: 2.57
- Antimicrobial resistance: 10 millions by 2050

Figure 1. Leading causes of death in the world in 2016 (blue bars) and prognosis for antimicrobial resistance (AMR) related deaths in 2050 (red bar).

Bacteria use their genetic plasticity to resist attack by antibiotics through mutations, acquisition of genetic material, and alteration of the expression of their genome [3]. In this way, bacteria that survive the attack of an antibiotic become the precursors of the next bacterial generations, further aggravating the problem of resistance. Once antibiotic resistance genes are acquired, they can be passed from one bacterium to another through division processes or by horizontal gene transfer [4]. Horizontal gene transfer processes can occur by transformation, transduction or conjugation with other bacteria. These mechanisms can transfer antibiotic resistance to bacteria that have not been subjected to antibiotic selection pressure, creating reservoirs of resistant bacteria in the environment [5]. In addition, the epistasis of the receptor bacteria plays a fundamental role in the process of acquisition of resistance genes, determining whether these bacteria are capable of maintaining, accumulating and propagating the genetic material [6].

Antibiotic resistance is an example of the enormous capacity for natural evolution and adaptation of bacteria to different environments [7,8]. Although this process seems inevitable, humans have accelerated it through various anthropogenic activities [9,10]. The causes behind the increase in the number of antimicrobial-resistant bacteria in recent years include the misuse of antibiotics in humans and animals, inadequate control of infections in hospitals and clinics or poor hygiene and sanitation [9–11]. In addition to the causes mentioned, the problem worsens as there is a drought in the discovery of new antibiotics. The increase in resistance rates in bacteria leads to a decrease in the effectiveness of existing antibiotics, making research in this field unattractive to companies that decide to invest in other types of fields with greater chances of success and benefits [12,13]. This concerning trend can be observed in Figure 2.

In view of this scenario, research on alternative or complementary therapies to traditional antibiotics has emerged strongly. Antimicrobial products of natural origin have been positioned as compounds of great scientific interest due to their enormous chemical variety and intrinsic properties that have promoted their study as a possible therapeutic tool in recent years.

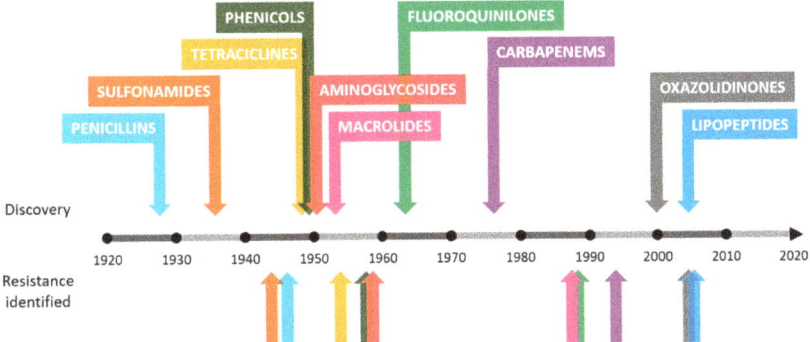

Figure 2. Approximate dates of discovery of new classes of antibiotics and identification of bacterial resistance.

2. Methodology

Electronic databases such as PubMed, Scopus and ScienceDirect were used to search scientific contributions until September 2020, using relevant keywords. Search terms included "natural antimicrobial", "antimicrobial resistance", "polyphenols", "future medicine", "natural origin", "antibacterial compound", "phytochemical" and their combinations. Literature focusing on the antimicrobial activity of natural origin compounds against bacteria focusing on antibiotic-resistant strains were identified and summarized.

The term "antimicrobial activity" is used throughout this work to refer to the process of killing or inhibiting the growth of microbes. Usually, this activity is expressed as MIC (minimum inhibitory concentration) values for a given agent. The methods to test microbial susceptibility compiled in this work are in accordance with the guidelines of the European Committee on Antimicrobial Susceptibility Testing (EUCAST) and The Clinical and Laboratory Standards Institute (CLSI). Following the EUCAST guidelines for the reproducibility and reliability of antimicrobial assays, broth dilution or microdilution methods should be used to test microbial susceptibility [14].

3. Results

3.1. Use of Natural Products as Antimicrobials

Natural products (NPs) make up a heterogeneous group of chemical entities that possess diverse biological activities with various uses in fields such as human and veterinary medicine, agriculture and industry. Molecules from the secondary metabolism of animals, vegetables, bacteria and fungi are classified as NPs, which are not crucial for the producer's survival under laboratory conditions, but which give him a clear advantage over his competitors in his native habitat [15]. Since the discovery of penicillin, more than 23,000 new NPs have been characterized, many of which have proven to be valuable tools in the field of pharmacology, herbicides, insecticides and more [16].

One of the main sources of antimicrobial NPs is plants. Plant organisms make up most of the biosphere on planet Earth, whose biomass accounts for a percentage greater than 80% of the total biomass [17]. Since their appearance, plants have survived, evolved and adapted to all types of ecosystems and adverse conditions. This adaptive process has led them to develop complex and effective defense systems against external aggressions: predators, abiotic stress and, of course, infections. Being sessile organisms that cannot escape their threats, plants have developed a splendid chemical arsenal in the form of secondary metabolites capable of coping with the most dangerous pathogens [18]. Humanity has made use of the medicinal properties of plants for thousands of years. There is evidence that in the year 5000 BC. the Sumerians already used thyme for its beneficial health properties [19]. The Egyptian Ebers Papyrus dating from around 1500 BC already attributed medicinal properties to plants and spices such as aloe vera, castor bean, garlic, hemp, anise or mustard [20,21]. Other texts such as the Atharva Veda, the Rig Veda and the Sushruta Samhita belonging to Indian Ayurveda, also spoke of the pharmacological properties of plant substances such as turmeric or cannabis [22,23]. Current technology allows us to study the bases of this ancestral knowledge and find therapeutic applications adapted to our time, making plants a source of invaluable therapeutic potential.

Bacteria are another of the main sources of antimicrobial NPs with radical importance during the 20th century. Most of the antibiotics used today in the clinic were discovered thanks to the Waksman platform in the 1940s. Waksman and his students dedicated themselves to growing soil microorganisms to detect and isolate antimicrobial substances. Through this method, they discovered very important antibiotics such as neomycin or streptomycin, for which Waksman received the Nobel Prize in 1952 for Physiology or Medicine [24]. Despite these successes, it should be noted that most existing bacteria are not cultivable in the laboratory using traditional methods. We could find an immense amount of opportunities for the isolation of new antibiotic compounds using a method like Waksman's combined with new technologies not present decades ago. From this idea, the Small World Initiative was born in 2012, a project in which students from all over the world collect soil samples and look for antibiotic-producing microorganisms in them [25].

Many of the NPs with antibiotic activity have been isolated from bacteria, especially from the genus actinomycetes. In the so-called "Golden Age" of the discovery of new antibiotics, which began in the 40s of the twentieth century, natural products were the star. The isolation of streptomycin from *Streptomyces griseus* in 1944 caused a worldwide surge in which numerous research groups struggled to identify new NPs, especially from samples of soil bacteria. The media were very limited, both in technology and in access to soil samples from remote places. However, another great milestone occurred in 1952, when a sample of soil sent from Borneo allowed *Streptomyces orientalis* to grow, from which vancomycin was extracted. Six years later, vancomycin was used in patients with great success. Unfortunately, this prolific period of discovery of valuable compounds ended the appearance and spread of bacteria resistant to these NPs, such as methicillin-resistant *Staphylococcus aureus* (MRSA) or glycopeptide-resistant enterococci (GREs), since the compounds that worked in the past stopped working with the desired efficiency [26], as observed in Figure 2.

In the 1990s, the pharmaceutical industry concentrated its efforts on other more sophisticated methods of identifying antimicrobial compounds, such as high-throughput screening of synthetic chemical libraries against specific therapeutic targets, many of them discovered from the Human Genome Project. Currently, there is a renewed interest in the discovery of new NPs of different sources since it has a much more advanced technology than that available during the "Golden Age". Advances in genomics, bioinformatics and mass spectrometry, among others, have elucidated that many of the sources of classical NPs were surprisingly under-exploited and have an enormous and unknown potential for the discovery of new NPs to be used for the discovery of present and tomorrow's antibiotics [15].

Given the existing problems in the field of antibiotics, in recent years alternative and complementary therapies have emerged that make use of different strategies to deal with new generations of resistant bacteria. The growing interest in this area is reflected in the ascending number of publications related to natural antimicrobials available in the PubMed search engine over the past recent years (Figure 3).

As abovementioned, the molecules with antimicrobial function present in nature have been molded by thousands of years of evolution to maintain their efficacy and selectivity, since they are a key piece for the development of the life of any organism exposed to bacteria. Thanks to these processes of continuous physicochemical adaptation driven by selective pressure, it has been demonstrated that antimicrobial compounds of natural origin generally have a greater capacity for cell penetration, being able to use active bacterial transporters and, in addition, passively pass through the cell membrane [27]. These and other properties that will be discussed below, make NPs a tool of great potential value for the development of novel and effective antibiotic therapies against AMR bacteria.

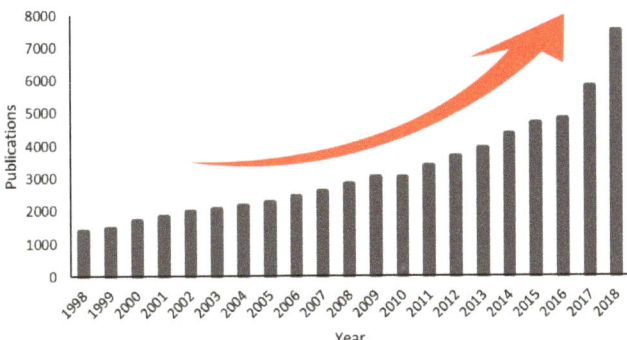

Figure 3. The number of research articles available in PubMed by searching "Natural Antimicrobial" from 1998 to 2018. The red arrow represents a growing trend.

3.2. Main Classes of Natural Antimicrobial Products

NPs are extremely diverse in terms of their chemical structures, properties and mechanisms of action. These agents can be classified according to their original source: animal, bacterial, fungal or vegetal.

3.2.1. Animal Origin

Animals have colonized virtually the entire planet Earth. For thousands of years, they have lived closely with different kinds of bacteria and have faced not a few pathogenic microorganisms. Evolution has shaped animal defense systems to deal with these microscopic threats. In recent years, attention has been focused on identifying which molecules confer resistance and allow certain animals to live in hostile environments with high pollution and pathogenic load, as is the case with certain insects such as cockroaches.

Currently, animals, and especially insects, are one of the main sources of antimicrobial proteins or peptides (AMPs). Since the discovery of AMPs in 1974, more than 150 new AMPs have been isolated or identified, the majority being cationic peptides between 20 and 50 residues in length. These molecules mainly have antimicrobial capacity mediated by disruption of the bacterial plasma membrane, most probably by forming pores or ion channels [28]. Some AMPs also have shown antifungal, antiparasitic or antiviral properties [29]. These AMPs can be divided into four subfamilies with different structures and sequences: the α-helical peptides, such as cecropin, which has a broad spectrum of antimicrobial activity against bacteria of both Gram-positive and Gram-negative bacteria; cysteine-rich peptides, such as insect defensins, which are mainly active against Gram-positive bacteria; proline-rich peptides, such as lebocins, which are active against both Gram-positive and Gram-negative bacteria and some fungi; and finally glycine-rich peptides or proteins, such as attacin, which are effective against Gram-negative bacteria and especially against *Escherichia coli*. These AMPs present a promising basis for the development of medical therapies, however, additional work must be developed to make them more powerful and stable [30]. Moreover, the intrinsic antimicrobial capacity of AMPs can be enhanced by a fusion of peptides to create more potent hybrid ones, such as in the case of attacin from *Spodoptera exigua* and a coleoptericin-like protein from *Protaetia brevitarsis seulensis*, which, when fused, exhibited a greater antimicrobial capacity than its two original peptides [31].

The study of antimicrobial molecules existent in cockroaches (*Periplaneta americana*) has revealed that extracts derived from its brain have a great antimicrobial capacity against MRSA and neuropathogenic *E. coli* K1. Although not all the components of the extract could be accurately identified, a great variety of molecules with known biological activity were found, such as isoquinolines, flavanones, sulfonamides and imidazone among others. A hypothesis about the production of this antimicrobial cocktail in the cockroach brain suggests that there could be a constitutive expression of these antimicrobials to protect the animal's neural system, since it is the central axis of its survival and a key piece to protect when it is lived in an environment of high pollution and exposure to pathogens and even superbugs [32]. Another example of insect producing antimicrobial molecules against resistant bacteria is *Lucilia cuprina* blowfly maggots. The extract obtained from excretions and secretions from maggots showed mild bacterial growth inhibition. However, using subinhibitory concentrations of this extract in combination with the antibiotic ciprofloxacin enhanced its activity, further delaying the appearance of bacteria resistant to it. The properties of this extract, including the presence of defensins and phenylacetaldehyde, make maggot debridement therapy a promising tool in the treatment of MRSA-infected wounds acquired in hospital [33].

One of the most popular insect-related products worldwide is honey. In addition to its nutritional properties and culinary values, it has antimicrobial capacity against Gram-negative bacteria, such as *E. coli* or *Pseudomonas aeruginosa*, and against Gram-positive bacteria, such as *Bacillus subtilis* or *S. aureus*, including MRSA. The key factors of honey's antimicrobial activity appear to be the presence of H_2O_2, bee defensin-1 and methylglyoxal. The diverse molecular composition of the different honey types that depends on the producing species and the raw material used, exerts also different antimicrobial activities and mechanisms [34]. Another substance produced by bees is propolis, a resinous substance produced by honeybees from plant matter, such as buds or sap. This substance has been used since ancient times, up to 3000 years BC in Egypt thanks to its various biological properties. The main components responsible for its activity are flavonoids, terpene derivatives and phenolic acids, although its composition is variable depending on the geographical area where it occurs. Ethanol extract of propolis produced by *Apis mellifera* in Brazil has demonstrated significant antibacterial capacity against *S. aureus*, *E. coli* and *Enterococcus sp.* [35]. Canadian propolis has also been shown to possess antibacterial capacity against *E. coli* and *S. aureus*, being more effective against the latter [36]. Another product with antimicrobial properties derived from honeybees is royal jelly. It is produced from the mandibular salivary and hypopharyngeal glands of bees aged between 5 and 14 days. Its composition is based on a complex mixture of carbohydrates, proteins, lipids, vitamins and minerals that varies with regional conditions, season, bee's genetics and postharvest storage conditions. Royal jelly shows antimicrobial activity against both Gram-positive and Gram-negative bacteria, including MDR bacteria such as MRSA. The compounds isolated from royal jelly with activity against Gram-positive bacteria are the peptide royalisin [37], the peptide family of jelleines and 10-hydroxy-2-decenoic acid (10-HDA), also known as queen bee acid [38]. Melittin, a major component from the venom of *A. mellifera*, has also shown interesting antimicrobial activity, including in in vivo experiments with mice infected with MRSA [39].

Other animals that can live in contaminated environments and exposed to infections are reptiles, such as snakes that are able to ingest rodents infected with germs and not develop a disease. Results suggest that animals exposed to huge amounts of pathogens can be a valuable source of antimicrobial molecules. However, to further study and identification of the key molecules responsible for the activity, it is necessary to know if they would be candidates for drugs with real applicability in therapies [40]. There are studies in Black cobra (*Naja naja karachiensis*) that show that plasma lysates and certain organs have a potent antimicrobial capacity against *E. coli* K1, MRSA, *P. aeruginosa*, *Streptococcus pneumoniae*, *Acanthamoeba castellanii*, and *Fusarium solani*. Against *E. coli* K1, solutions containing 25% and 50% of plasma from the blood of the Black cobra showed a bactericidal activity of 85% and 93% respectively with respect to the effect of the antibiotic gentamicin. Against MRSA, concentrations of 25% and 50% of plasma showed activity of 90% and 93%, respectively. Lung and gallbladder lysates also showed high antimicrobial capacity against MRSA. Antimicrobial molecules can also be extracted from the venom produced by certain species of snakes, such as cathelicidines or toxins. A cathelicidin-like antimicrobial peptide (cathelicidin-BF) isolated from the venom of *Bungarus fasciatus* has shown high antimicrobial activity, including drug-resistant bacteria [41]. *Crotalus adamanteus* toxin-II (CaTx-II) exerted a strong antimicrobial effect against *S. aureus*, *Burkholderia pseudomallei* and *Enterobacter aerogenes* by causing pores and damaging their membranes. Interestingly, this compound showed no cytotoxicity against lung (MRC-5), skin fibroblast (HEPK) cells or treated mice [42].

Molecules with great antimicrobial capacity have also been found in crustaceans, coming from their immune system. The anti-lipopolysacchride factor of red claw crayfish *Cherax quadricarinatus* has shown low minimum bactericidal concentrations (MBC) against Gram-negative *Shigella flexneri* (MBC < 6 µM) and Gram-positive *S. aureus* (MBC < 12 µM), meaning a high antimicrobial capacity. Studies showed that the mechanism of action of this compound does not appear to be related to the bacterial plasma membrane alteration, requiring more studies to find its specific mechanism [43].

The venom of *Vaejovis mexicanus*, a mexican scorpion, has an AMP called vejovine, which presents a high antimicrobial capacity against MDR Gram-negative bacteria with MIC values between 4.4 µM and 50 µM [44].

3.2.2. Bacterial Origin

Bacteria are the most prolific source of NPs with antimicrobial activity found so far, especially those of the actinomycetes class. Their great diversity, competitiveness and colonization capacity have led them to the development of secondary metabolites capable of giving them great advantages over other bacterial species. As described in previous sections, the detection and isolation of these bacterial antimicrobial NPs propelled medical science vertiginously in the middle of the last century. Some of the most relevant are described below.

Some of the most important antimicrobial molecules produced by bacteria of the actinomyces class are: vancomycin, baulamycin, fasamycin A and orthoformimycin. Vancomycin is a naturally occurring tricyclic glycopeptide extracted from *Streptococcus orientalis* that has reaped great success as an antibiotic against Gram-positive bacteria, especially against threats that are resistant to other treatments such as MRSA and penicillin-resistant pneumococci among others [45]. Vancomycin forms hydrogen bonds with the terminal dipeptide of the nascent peptidoglycan chain during biosynthesis of the bacterial cell wall. This union prevents the action of penicillin-binding proteins (PBPs), interrupting further wall formation and finally activating autolysin-triggered cell rupture and cell death [46]. Another important bacterial NP is produced by actinomyces is baulamycin, which is an isolated molecule of the marine bacterium *Streptomyces tempisquensis* that can inhibit the biosynthesis of iron-chelating siderophores in *S. aureus* (targeting staphylopherrin B) and *Bacillus anthracis* (targeting petrobactin), helping to treat MRSA and anthrax infections, respectively. In addition, it was also able to inhibit the growth of Gram-negative bacteria such as *S. flexneri* and *E. coli*, turning baulamycin and its derivatives into potential broad-spectrum antibiotics [47]. Fasamycin A is a polyketide isolated from *Streptomyces albus* that shows specific antimicrobial activity against Gram-positive bacteria such as vancomycin-resistant Enterococci (VRE) and MRSA with MIC values of 0.8 and 3.1 µg/mL, respectively. This molecule targets FabF in the initial condensation step of the elongation cycle from the lipidic biosynthetic bacterial metabolism [48]. Orthoformimycin is a molecule produced by *S. griseus* which can inhibit bacterial translation by more than 80% in the case of *E. coli*. Although the mechanism of action is not clear now, one hypothesis is the decoupling of mRNA and aminoacyl-tRNA in the bacterial ribosome [49].

The actinobacteria class is also prolific in the production of antimicrobial molecules. One example is kibdelomycin, which is a potent inhibitor of DNA synthesis that was isolated from *Kibdelosporangium* sp., MA7385. Its complex structure and its infrequent function as an inhibitor of bacterial DNA gyrase and IV topoisomerase make kibdelomycin the first bacterial type II topoisomerase inhibitor discovered from natural sources in more than 60 years [50]. This molecule has a broad-spectrum antimicrobial activity against aerobic bacteria, including antibiotic-resistant bacteria such as MRSA, with a MIC value of 0.25 µg/mL. In addition, this molecule has a very low resistance development rate due to its structure and way of binding with its target, at levels of other successful antibiotics such as ciprofloxacin [51]. Another example is pyridomycin, a molecule isolated from *Dactylosporangium fulvum* which has a great antimicrobial capacity against mycobacteria, a bacterium that causes tuberculosis. This disease is becoming relevant due to the appearance of bacteria resistant to the main antibiotics used for its treatment such as the InhA inhibitor isoniazid. Pyridomycin acts on the cell wall of *Mycobacterium tuberculosis* by inhibiting the production of mycolic acid by targeting NADH-dependent enoyl- (Acyl-Carrier-Protein) reductase InhA even in strains resistant to isoniazid. Pyridomycin showed minimum bactericidal concentration (MBC) values between 0.62 and 1.25 µg/mL against *M. tuberculosis* [52].

In addition to the two classes mentioned above, there are other classes of bacteria such as deltaproteobacteria, cyanophyceae or betaproteobacteria from which antimicrobial molecules have also been isolated. Myxovirecin is a macrocyclic secondary metabolite isolated from myxobacteria (deltaproteobacteria class) that possesses broad-spectrum antibacterial capacity. It seems to inhibit the production of type II signal peptidase by blocking Lpp lipoprotein processing. Myxovirecin showed very potent activity against *E. coli* DW37 with a MIC of 0.063 µg/mL [53]. Spirohexenolide A is a natural spirotetronate originally isolated from *Spirulina platensis* of the cyanophyceae class that shows antimicrobial activity against methicillin-resistant *S. aureus* by disrupting the cytoplasmic membrane, collapsing the proton motive force [54]. Teixobactin is a naturally occurring molecule produced by *Eleftheria terrae* of the betaproteobacteria class that possesses antibacterial capacity against antibiotic-resistant pathogens in infection animal models. It acts by binding to the precursors of the bacterial wall teicoic acid, causing the digestion of the cell wall by autolysins [55].

Lypoglycopeptides isolated from different bacteria show antimicrobial activity by inhibiting signal peptidase type IB (SpsB), which is a membrane-localized serine protease that cleaves the amino-terminal signal peptide from most secreted proteins. One example is actinocarbasin, a molecule isolated from *Actinoplanes ferrugineus* strain MA7383. Moreover, this molecule enhances the activity of β-lactam antibiotics against MRSA, sensitizing it to those drugs. Arylomycin is another lipoglycopeptide with bacterial type I signal peptidase inhibitory capacity which showed antibacterial activity witch MIC values in the range of 4–64 µM against Gram-positive and 8–64 µM against Gram-negative bacteria. Krisynomycin is also a lypoglycopeptide, isolated from *Streptomyces fradiae* strain MA7310, with the capacity of inhibition of SpsB [56].

In addition to the natural bacteria molecules with direct antimicrobial activity, there are also others capable of attacking the virulence factors caused by bacterial infections. Skyllamycins B and C are cyclic depsipeptides isolated from marine bacterial fractions with *P. aeruginosa* biofilm inhibition and dispersal activity. The ability to prevent the formation of biofilms or to disperse those already formed is of great importance since these biofilms are one of the major causes of drug resistance in nosocomial infections. These molecules do not possess a bactericidal capacity per se, but they are effective in combination with antibiotics that are not able to act in the presence of biofilms, causing them to recover their activity as in the case of azithromycin [57].

3.2.3. Fungal Origin

Fungi are eukaryotic-type living things, such as mushrooms, yeasts, and molds. Currently, the existence of some 120,000 species of fungi has been accepted, however, it is estimated that the number of different species of fungi present on earth could be between 2.2 and 3.8 million [58]. This relatively unexplored kingdom is a source of antimicrobial NPs and has great potential to be studied in the future as new species are discovered and identified.

Aspergillomarasmine A is a polyaminoacid naturally produced by *Aspergillus versicolor* capable of inhibiting antibiotic resistance enzymes in Gram-negative pathogenic bacteria, such as *Enterobacteriaceae*, *Acinetobacter spp.*, *Pseudomonas spp.* and *Klebsiella pneumoniae*. This compound has been used successfully to reverse resistance in mice infected with meropenem-resistant *K. pneumoniae* thanks to the NDM-I protein, making the bacterium sensitive to the antibiotic and ending the infection [59].

Mirandamycin is a quinol of fungal origin capable of inhibiting the growth of both Gram-negative and Gram-positive bacteria, being more effective against the latter group, including antibiotic-resistant strains such as MRSA or carbapenemase-producing *K. pneumoniae*. Its mechanism of action consists in the inhibition of the bacterial metabolism of sugars, interfering with their fermentation and transport [60].

There is evidence of the antibacterial capacity of various fungal species against Gram-positive bacteria. Extracts of *Ganoderma lucidum*, *Ganoderma applanatum*, *Meripilus giganteus*, *Laetiporus sulphureus*,

Flammulina velutipes, *Coriolus versicolor*, *Pleurotus ostreatus* and *Panus tigrinus* demonstrated antimicrobial activity in Kirby–Bauer assays against Gram-positive bacteria, such as *S. auerus* and *B. luteus* [61].

In recent times, molecules produced by various species of marine fungi have been studied, especially those that cohabit with sponges or corals. Fungal compounds with activity against antibiotic resistant bacteria have been isolated, such as lindgomycin and ascosetin, with MIC values of 5.1 µM and 3.2 µM against MRSA, respectively. These molecules were isolated from the mycelium and the *Lindgomycetae spp* culture broth from sponges found in the Baltic and Antarctic Sea [62]. Another marine fungus capable of producing antimicrobial molecules is *Pestalotiopsis* sp., isolated from the coral *Sarcophyton* sp. This fungus produces (±)-pestalachloride D, a chlorinated benzophenone derivative, which has shown antibacterial capacity against *E. coli*, *Vibrio anguillarum* and *Vibrio parahaemolyticus* with MIC values of 5, 10 and 20 µM, respectively [63]. *Trichoderma sp.* is a sponge-derived fungus from which different aminolipopeptide classes, called trichoderins, have been isolated. These molecules have a potent antimycobacterial capacity showing MIC values between 0.02 and 2.0 µg/mL against *Mycobacterium smegmatis*, *Mycobacterium bovis* BCG, and *M. tuberculosis* H37Rv in different aerobic and hypoxic conditions [64].

3.2.4. Plant Origin

Plants are a great source of biomolecules with various interesting properties for humans thanks to their enormous diversity and proven safety for human health [65]. Being sessile organisms, evolution has shaped its metabolism to produce certain molecules to cope with external aggressions and infections, since they cannot flee or defend themselves [66]. The Dictionary of Natural Products lists approximately 200,000 secondary plant metabolites, of which 170,000 have unique chemical structures [67]. Some of the families of molecules with antimicrobial capacity produced by plants are alkaloids, terpenoids, and polyphenols [68].

Plants that have been used in traditional medicine in various countries of the world for thousands of years. They are currently being studied at the molecular and functional level, rediscovering their properties and explaining their mechanisms of action.

Alkaloids have been shown to possess antimicrobial capacity against various bacterial species. Although studies of the antimicrobial capacity of pure alkaloids are limited, there are several studies on the antimicrobial activity of plant extracts that contain alkaloids as their main components. Different extracts rich in alkaloids obtained from *Papaver rhoeas* have shown activity against *S. aureus*, *Staphylococcus epidermidis* and *K. pneumoniae*, the main active component being roemerine [69]. Raw alkaloid-rich extracts of *Annona squamosa* seeds and *Annona muricata* root have also shown moderate antimicrobial capacity against *E. coli* and *S. aureus* [70].

Terpenoids, along with other families of compounds, are part of plant essential oils, many of which possess antimicrobial activity. Various in vitro studies affirm that terpenoids do not possess significant antimicrobial activity per se [71]. However, they can contribute to the antimicrobial activity of complete essential oils thanks to their hydrophobic nature and a low molecular weight that allow them to disrupt the cell wall and facilitate the action of the rest of the active components [72].

Polyphenols are molecules present in plants with a function of defense against stress and have one or more phenolic groups in their chemical structure as a common feature. There is abundant literature on the antimicrobial capacity of polyphenols and extracts of plants rich in them that have bactericidal and bacteriostatic capacity against many pathogens, both Gram-positive and Gram-negative. The potential use of polyphenols as antimicrobials is widely studied to be applied in different areas such as agriculture [73], food preservation [74] and medicine [75].

There are several subfamilies within the group of polyphenols according to their differentiated chemical structures: flavonoids, hydrolyzable tannins, lignans, phenolic acids and stilbenes. In turn, the flavonoid group can be subdivided into other subfamilies: anthocyanidins, flavanones, flavones, flavonols and isoflavones [76]. Examples of flavonoids with antimicrobial activity are quercetin [77], kaempferol [78], morin [79], myricetin [80] epigallocatechin gallate [81] or galangin [82] among many others [76,83]. Other known polyphenols with good antimicrobial activity are punicalagin, which exerts both antibacterial and antibiofilm effect against *S. aureus* [80,84], and resveratrol, which has antimicrobial activity against a wide range of bacteria [75].

The growing relevance of the study of polyphenols in the clinical setting is due to their antimicrobial synergy between polyphenols and antibiotics for clinical use. Polyphenols in subinhibitory concentrations enhance the action of an antibiotic against a bacterium that was originally resistant to its effect. For example, kaempferol and quercetin, two flavonols with antimicrobial activity on their own, have also shown to increase the efficacy of the rifampicin antibiotic against rifampicin-resistant MRSA strains by 57.8% and 75.8%, respectively. The study authors blame this increase in the activity to which these polyphenols are able to inhibit the catalytic activity of topoisomerases, inhibiting DNA synthesis, with a mechanism similar to that of the ciprofloxacin antibiotic, with which they have also shown to have a synergistic activity [85]. Epicatechin gallate (ECg), a flavanol, is capable of sensitizing strains of MRSA against β-lactam antibiotics such as penicillin or oxacillin. This polyphenol can bind to the MRSA cytoplasmic membrane and cause large changes in its structure and reducing its fluidity, decoupling the functioning mechanism of the enzyme PBP2a, which is the protein responsible for resistance to β-lactam antibiotics. In addition, ECg can reduce biofilm formation and protein secretion associated with virulence factors [86]. (-)-Epigallocatechin gallate (EGCg) is another flavanol with a great capacity to enhance the effect of antibiotics that acts mainly on the cell wall directly or indirectly and on some virulence factors, such as the production of penicillinases [87].

Another example of synergy between polyphenols and antibiotics is the case of the combination of catechin and epicatechin gallate extracted from *Fructus crataegi* and ampicillin, ampicillin/sulbactam, cefazolin, cefepime, and imipenem/cilastatin antibiotics, which are usually ineffective against MRSA. These combinations were effective against MRSA in both in vitro and in vivo assays using mice with an established infection model. The authors stressed that the possible mechanism of action of the combination of these two polyphenols to enhance the effect of antibiotics was the accumulation of antibiotics inside the cell thanks to the inhibition of the efflux pump gene [88].

In addition to synergy with antibiotics, there are also studies that point to the synergy between the polyphenols themselves, such as that between EGCg and quercetin against MRSA, attributed to a co-permeabilization process that would facilitate the activity of the compounds inside of the cell [89]. Synergic activity has also been found between the polyphenols quercetin-3-glucoside, punicalagin, ellagic acid and myricetin in different proportions and combinations against *S. aureus* CECT 59 [80].

Apart from the antimicrobial use of concrete molecules of plant origin, the use of complex extracts made from different parts of plants is common and effective. Plant extracts have a great diversity in their composition, since even from the same plant multiple completely different extracts can be obtained varying the extraction conditions. Time, temperature, solvents, pressure and other parameters such as the use of ultrasound or microwave have a huge impact on the final extract composition [90]. There is numerous evidence of the antimicrobial activity of plant extracts [76,91] and the synergistic effect that exists between different phytochemicals [80] when acting against different bacteria. An example of a plant extract with potent activity against AMR bacteria are extracts from *Lantana camara* leaves against clinical isolates of MRSA, *Streptococcus pyogenes*, VRE, *Acinetobacter baumannii*, *Citrobacter freundii*, *Proteus mirabilis*, *Proteus vulgaris* and *P. aeruginosa* [92]. The ethanolic extracts of *Anthocephalus cadamba*, *Pterocarpus santalinus* and *Butea monosperma* Lam. they have also demonstrated antimicrobial activity against MDR clinical isolates of 10 different microbial species: *S. aureus*, *Acinetobacter sp.*, *C. freundii*, *Chromobacterium violeceum*, *E. coli*, *Klebsiella sp.*, *Proteus sp.*, *P. aeruginosa*, *Salmonella typhi* and *Vibrio cholerae* [93,94]. In the case of *B. monosperma* Lam., antimicrobial activity was also found in the extract made with hot water from leaf.

3.2.5. Summary

As a summary, Table 1 contains all the NPs mentioned above together with their producing organism, type, target bacteria, mechanism of action, main use and references. Figure 4 shows the main molecular targets of the most relevant antimicrobial NPs.

Table 1. Alphabetically ordered natural products (NPs) with their properties and capabilities. Grey shaded cells mean effectiveness against AMR bacteria. Asterisk (*) means no antimicrobial activity alone.

Natural Product	Productor Organism	Type of Organism	Activity Against	Mechanism of Action	Main Use	Reference
Actinorhodin	*Streptomyces coelicolor*	Actinomycete	Gram-positive, including multidrug-resistant *S. aureus*	ROS production inside bacterial cells	Research	[95]
Albomycin	*Streptomyces sp.* ATCC 700974	Actinomycete	Gram-negative and Gram-positive, including MRSA	Seryl t-RNA synthetase inhibition	Medicine	[96,97]
Amphomycin	*Streptomyces canus*	Actinomycete	Gram-positive, including MRSA, VRE and MDR *S. pneumoniae*	Inhibition of peptidoglycan and wall teichoic acid biosyntheses	Medicine	[98]
Apramycin	*Streptoalloteicus hindustanus*	Actinomycete	Gram-negative, including MDR *A. baumannii* and *P. aeruginosa*	Inhibition of protein synthesis	Veterinary	[99]
Arlomycins	*Streptomyces sp.* Tü 6075	Actinomycete	Gram-positive and Gram-negative	Inhibition of type I bacterial signal peptidase	In research for medical use	[100]
Aspergillomarasmine A *	*A. versicolor*	Fungus	Sensitivizes carbapenem-resistant bacteria	Inhibition of bacterial metallo-β-lactamases	In research for medical use	[59]
Carbomycin	*Streptomyces halstedii*	Actinomycete	Gram-positive and *Mycoplasma*	Inhibition of protein synthesis	Medicine	[101]
Cathelicidin-BF	*Bungarus fasciatus*	Reptile	Mainly Gram-negative, including MDR strains	Damage in microbial cytoplasmic membrane	Research	[44]
CaTx-II	*C. adamanteus*	Reptile	Gram-positive and Gram-negative	Membrane pore formation and cell wall disintegration	Research	[12]
Cecropin A	*Aedes aegypti*	Insect	Gram-negative	Disruption of the cytoplasmic membrane	In research for medical use	[102]
Cephalosporin	*Cephalosporium acremonium*	Fungus	Gram-positive and Gram-negative	Inhibition of cell wall synthesis	Medicine	[103]
Cephamycin C	*Streptomyces clavuligerus*	Actinomycete	Gram-positive and Gram-negative	Inhibition of cell wall synthesis	Medicine and veterinary	[104]
Chloramphenicol	*Streptomyces venezuelae*	Actinomycete	Gram-positive and Gram-negative	Inhibition of protein synthesis	Medicine and veterinary	[105]
Chloroeremomycin	*Amycolatopsis orientalis*	Actinomycete	Gram-positive, including VRE	Inhibition of bacterial cell wall formation	Medicine	[106]
Clavulanic acid *	*S. clavuligerus*	Actinomycete	Sensitivizes β-lactam-resistant bacteria	β-lactamase inhibitor	Medicine and veterinary	[107]
Clorobiocin	*Streptomyces roseochromogenes*	Actinomycete	Gram-positive	Inhibitors of DNA gyrase	Medicine	[108]
Coumermycin	*Streptomyces rishiriensis*	Actinomycete	Mainly Gram-positive	Inhibition of DNA gyrase	Research	[109,110]
Dalbavancin	*Nonomuraea sp.*	Actinomycete	Gram-positive, including MRSA	Inhibition of cell wall synthesis	Medicine	[111]
Daptomycin	*Streptomyces roseosporus*	Actinomycete	Gram-positive	Inhibition of protein, DNA and RNA synthesis	Medicine	[112]
Epigallocatechin gallate	Abundant in *Camellia sinensis*	Plant	Gram-positive and Gram-negative	Damage in microbial cytoplasmic membrane	In research for medical use	[81,113]

Table 1. *Cont.*

Natural Product	Producer Organism	Type of Organism	Activity Against	Mechanism of Action	Main Use	Reference
Erythromycin	*Saccharopolyspora erythraea*	Actinomycete	Gram-positive	Inhibition of protein synthesis	Medicine	[114]
Fosfomycin	*Streptomyces wedmorensis*	Actinomycete	Gram-positive and Gram-negative	Inhibition of cell wall synthesis	Medicine	[115]
Fusidic acid	*Fusidium coccineus*	Fungus	Gram-positive, including MRSA	Inhibition of protein synthesis	Medicine	[116]
Gentamicin	*Micromonospora purpurea*	Actinomycete	Gram-negative	Inhibition of protein synthesis	Medicine	[117]
Gramicidin S	*B. subtilis*	Bacillales	Gram-positive and Gram-negative	Delocalizes peripheral membrane proteins involved in cell division and cell envelope synthesis	Medicine	[118]
Hc-CATH	*Hydrophis cyanocinctus*	Reptile	Gram-positive and Gram-negative	Damage in microbial cytoplasmic membrane	Research	[119]
Hygromycin	*Streptomyces hygroscopicus*	Actinomycete	Gram-positive	Inhibition of protein synthesis	Veterinary and research	[120]
Josamycin	*Streptomyces narbonensis*	Actinomycete	Gram-positive, certain Gram-negative and *mycoplasma*	Inhibition of protein synthesis	Medicine	[121]
Kanamycin	*Streptomyces kanamyceticus*	Actinomycete	Mainly Gram-negative and certain Gram-positive	Inhibition of protein synthesis	Medicine	[122]
Kirromycin	*Streptomyces collinus*	Actinomycete	Anaerobes, *neisseriae* and *streptococci*	Inhibition of protein synthesis	Research	[123,124]
Lincomycin	*Streptomyces lincolnensis*	Actinomycete	Gram-positive	Inhibition of protein synthesis	Medicine	[125]
Lipiaramycin	*Dactosporangium aurantiacum*	Actinomycete	Gram-positive and *Mycobacterium*, including MDR strains	Inhibition of early transcription	Medicine	[126]
Melittin	*A. mellifera*	Insect	Gram-positive and Gram-negative, including MDR strains	Damage in microbial cytoplasmic membrane	Medicine	[36]
Mirandamycin	Endophytic fungus isolated from the twig of *Neomirandea angularis*	Fungus	Gram-negative and Gram-positive, including MRSA	Inhibition of bacterial quinol oxidase/ROS production	In research for medical use	[61]
Moenomycin	*Streptomyces ghanaensis*	Actinomycete	Gram-positive	Inhibition of cell wall synthesis	Veterinary	[127]
Morin	*Moraceae* family	Plant	Gram-positive and Gram-negative	Inhibition of adhesion to host tissue and DNA helicase	Food technology	[79]
Mucroporin	*Lychas mucronatus*	Arachnid	Gram-positive and Gram-negative, including MDR strains	Damage in microbial cytoplasmic membrane	Research	[128]
Neomycin	*S. fradiae*	Actinomycete	Gram-positive and Gram-negative	Inhibition of ribonuclease P	Medicine	[129]
Orthoformimycin	*S. griseus*	Actinomycete	Gram-positive and Gram-negative	Inhibition of protein synthesis	In research for medical use	[49]
Oxytetracycline	*Streptomyces rimosus*	Actinomycete	Gram-positive and Gram-negative	Inhibition of protein synthesis	Aquaculture	[130]

Table 1. Cont.

Natural Product	Productor Organism	Type of Organism	Activity Against	Mechanism of Action	Main Use	Reference
Penicillins	*Penicillium crysogenum*	Fungus	Gram-positive and Gram-negative	Inhibition of cell wall synthesis and activation of the endogenous autolytic system	Medicine	[131]
Pleuromutalin	*Clitopilus scyphoides*	Fungus	Gram-positive, Gram-negative and *Mycoplasma*	Inhibition of translation	Veterinary	[132]
Polymycin	*Paenibacillus polymyxa*	Bacillales	Mainly Gram-negative (including MDR) and certain Gram-positive	Disruption of the cytoplasmic membrane	Medicine	[133]
Pristinamycin	*Streptomyces pristinaespiralis*	Actinomycete	Gram-positive, including MRSA	Inhibition of protein synthesis	Medicine	[134]
Punicalagin	Abundant in *Punica granatum*	Plant	Gram-positive and Gram-negative	Damage in microbial cytoplasmic membrane	Food technology	[80,84]
Quercetin	Ubiquitous in plants	Plant	Gram-positive and Gram-negative	Damage in the structure of the bacterial cell wall and cell membrane	In research for medical use	[135]
Ramoplanin	*Actinoplanes sp.* ATCC 33076	Actinomycete	Gram-positive, including MDR strains	Inhibition of cell wall synthesis	Medicine	[136]
Resveratrol	Abundant in grapes, berries and legumes	Plant	Gram-positive and Gram-negative, including MDR strains	Inhibition of motility, adhesion, quorum sensing, biofilm formation, flagellar gene expression and hemolytic activity	Medicine	[75]
Rifamycin	*Amycolatopsis mediterranei*	Actinomycete	Gram-positive and certain Gram-negative	Inhibition of DNA-dependent RNA synthesis	Medicine	[137]
Ristocetin A	*A. orientalis*	Actinomycete	Gram-positive, including MRSA	Inhibition of cell wall synthesis	Medicine	[138]
Royalisin	*Apis melifera*	Insect	Mainly gram-positive	Damage in the structure of the bacterial cell wall and cell membrane	Research	[37]
Skyllamycins	*Streptomyces sp.* KY 11784	Actinomycete	Gram-positive	Inhibition of biofilm formation	In research for medical use	[139]
SlLebocin1	*Spodoptera litura*	Insect	Gram-positive and Gram-negative	Damage in microbial cytoplasmic membrane or cell division inhibition	Research	[140]
Spectinomycin	*Streptomyces spectabilis*	Actinomycete	Gram-positive and Gram-negative	Inhibition of protein synthesis	Medicine	[141]
Spiramycin	*Streptomyces ambofaciens*	Actinomycete	Gram-positive and Gram-negative	Inhibition of protein synthesis	Medicine	[142]
Streptothricin	*Streptomyces* (multiple species)	Actinomycete	Gram-positive and Gram-negative	Inhibition of protein synthesis	Veterinary and plant production	[143]

Table 1. Cont.

Natural Product	Producer Organism	Type of Organism	Activity Against	Mechanism of Action	Main Use	Reference
Teicoplanin	*Actinoplanes teichomyceticus*	Actinomycete	Gram-positive, including MRSA	Inhibition of bacterial cell wall synthesis	Medicine	[144]
Teixobactin	*Eleftheria terrae*	Betaproteobacteria	Gram-positive, including MRSA	Causes digestion of the cell wall by autolysins	Medicine	[35]
Tetracycline	*Streptomyces rimosus*	Actinomycete	Gram-positive and Gram-negative	Inhibition of protein synthesis	Medicine	[145]
Thienamycin	*Streptomyces cattleya*	Actinomycete	Gram-positive and Gram-negative	Inhibition of bacterial cell wall synthesis	Derivates used in medicine	[146]
Thiostrepton	*Streptomyces azureus*	Actinomycete	Gram-positive and Gram-negative	Inhibition of protein synthesis	Veterinary and research	[147]
Tobramycin	*Streptoalloteicus hindustanus*	Actinomycete	Gram-negative	Inhibition of protein synthesis and membrane destabilization	Medicine	[148]
Tunicamycin	*Streptomyces chartreusis*	Actinomycete	Gram-positive	Inhibition of peptidoglycan and lipopolysaccharide synthesis	Research	[149]
Tylosin	*S. fradiae*	Actinomycete	Gram-positive and *Mycoplasma*	Inhibition of protein synthesis	Veterinary	[150]
Vancomycin	*S. orientalis*	Actinomycete	Gram-positive, including MRSA	Inhibition of bacterial cell wall synthesis	Medicine	[45]
Vejovine	*V. mexicanus*	Arachnid	Gram-negative, including MDR	Damage in microbial cytoplasmic membrane	Research	[44]
Viomycin	*Streptomyces sp.* 11861	Actinomycete	MDR *Mycobacterium*	Inhibition of protein synthesis	Medicine	[151]
Virginiamycin	*Streptomyces virginiae*	Actinomycete	Gram-positive	Inhibition of protein synthesis	Agriculture and industry	[152]

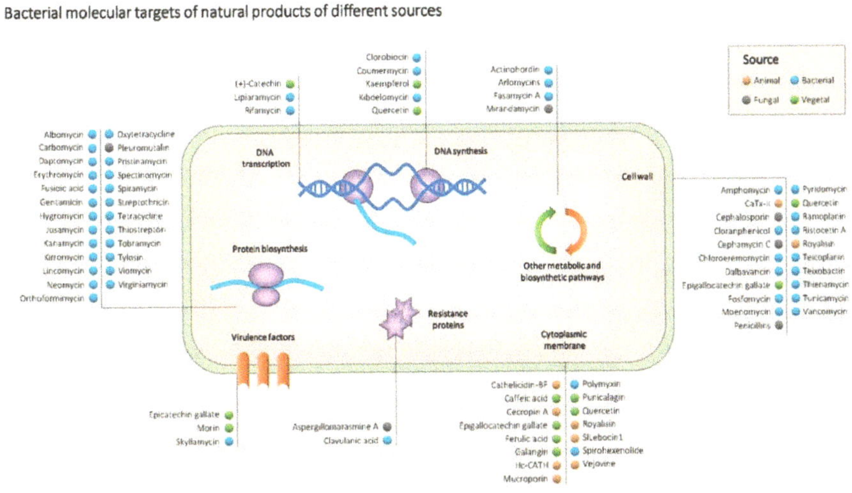

Figure 4. Main known molecular targets of antimicrobial NPs described in this review.

3.3. Antibiotics and Plant Compounds Combinations to Get around AMR

The synergic combination of antibiotics and phytochemicals represents a promising strategy with numerous clinical and developmental benefits. Some plant compounds have direct antimicrobial activity against antibiotic-resistant bacteria, while others can sensitize resistant bacteria against antibiotics, reversing the resistance as mentioned and exemplified in the previous section. Some of these NPs can enhance the effect of antibiotics in different ways, such as facilitating their entry into the cell by destabilizing the cytoplasmic membrane [153,154], inhibiting efflux pumps (EPs) [155] or dispersing biofilms [156] among other mechanisms of action (Figure 4). Some of the synergistic interactions between phytochemicals and antibiotics include increased efficiency, lower antibiotic doses, reduced side effects, increased bioavailability and increased stability [157]. The multidimensional and multifactorial activity of phytochemicals studied by network pharmacology is crucial for synergy with clinical antibiotics, opening the door to many different potential combinations. Moreover, the use of molecules that have already passed the relevant clinical controls, as in the case of antibiotics, in combination with innocuous natural compounds facilitates the process of research and development of new potential therapies [158].

There is clear evidence of NPs capable of inhibiting efflux pumps of AMR bacteria, specifically, phytochemicals. These molecules can inhibit various efflux pumps in different pathogenic bacterial species, both Gram-positive and Gram-negative. As an example, the NorA efflux pump of *S. aureus* SA-1199-B has been effectively inhibited using baicalein plant molecules [159], capsaicin [160], indirubin [161], kaempferol rhamnoside [162] and olympicin A [163]. NorA of *S. aureus* NCTC 8325-4 was inhibited using sarothrin [164]. Cumin demonstrated antimicrobial activity on its own and also resistance modulation properties against MRSA by inhibiting LmrS efflux pump [155]. Plant molecules inhibiting the ethidium bromide efflux pump (EtBr) have also been found: 1′-S-1′-acetoxyeugenol acetate inhibits it in *Mycobacterium smegmatis* [165], catechol and catharanthine inhibits it in *P. aeruginosa* [166,167] and galotannins inhibit it in MDR uropathogenic *E. coli* [168]. The YojI efflux pump of MDR *E. coli* has been shown to be inhibited by molecules such as 4-hydroxy—tetralone, ursolic acid and its derivatives [169] and lysergol [170]. Berberine and palmatine inhibit MexAB-OprM from clinical isolates of MDR *P. aeruginosa* [171]. There are also complete extracts of plants with EPs inhibitory activity with clear synergistic effects with antibiotics in the treatment of MDR bacterial infections. The extract made from *Rhus coriaria* seeds have shown an obvious synergistic effect with oxytetracycline, penicillin G, cephalexin, sulfadimethoxine and enrofloxacin against MDR clinical isolates of *P. aeruginosa*. This effect is mainly attributed to the inhibitory capacity of EPs of the phytochemicals present in the extract [172]. The activity of these plant molecules as inhibitors of microbial efflux pumps can act as restorers of antimicrobial susceptibility and open the door to combined antibiotic treatments, since these could exert their action more easily by not being expelled from the bacterial interior, allowing relive obsolete or discarded therapies due to this resistance mechanism [173]. A catechin, (-)-epigallocatechin gallate (EGCg), has shown sensitizing activity in *S. aureus* against tetracycline by inhibiting EPs such as Tet (K), increasing intracellular retention of the antibiotic and enhancing its effect [174]. Stilbenes also act as EPs inhibitors against antibiotic-resistant *Arcobacter butzleri*, reducing its resistance. Resveratrol and pinosylvin have also shown activity as resistance modulators being able to even reverse the resistance completely [175].

There are studies that state that certain polyphenols, such as catechins, can enter deeply into the structure of the lipid bilayer of bacterial membranes, causing significant thermotropic changes. Lipophilic hydrocarbons present in plant extracts are known to destabilize the cellular structure of the cytoplasmic membrane, increase its permeability and interact with hydrophobic portions of proteins [176]. This could explain the potentiation in the effect of certain antibiotics against resistant bacteria, as these compounds could increase antibiotic intake and interact with resistance proteins, hindering their activity. Specifically, (-)-epicatechin gallate (ECg) has a great affinity for the staphylococcal wall and its binding to it produces biophysical changes in it that are capable of dispersing the biosynthetic machinery responsible for resistance to β-lactam antibiotics [177]. This activity would explain the restoration of the sensitivity of bacteria resistant to traditional antibiotics through the use of polyphenolic compounds capable of interacting with bacterial membranes, as in the case of catechins capable of sensitizing MRSA against oxacillin and other β-lactam antibiotics thanks to its ability to integrate and interact with the cell membrane [178,179].

Plant extracts are also capable of exert antimicrobial activity against AMR bacteria and synergize with antibiotics. For instance, extracts of *Duabanga grandiflora* can restore MRSA's sensitivity to ampicillin. The mechanism proposed by the researchers is that the components of this extract can decrease the expression of the mecA gene that gives rise to the resistance protein PBP2a [180]. Extracts of *Acacia nilotica*, *Syzygium aromaticum* and *Cinnamum zeylanicum* exhibited antimicrobial capacity against a panel of AMR bacteria including clinical isolates and ATCC strains. Extract of *A. nilotica* showed MIC values as low as 9.75 µg/mL against *K. pneumoniae* ATCC-700803, *Salmonella typhimurium* ATCC-13311 and *E. faecalis* ATCC-29212 [181]. Extracts of *Salvia spp.* and *Matricaria recutita* have shown great synergy with the antibiotic oxacillin [182]. The multifactorial and multi-target character of the compounds that make up plant extracts can hinder the development of resistance by bacteria [80]. The molecular promiscuity of polyphenols, their multarget activity, the possibility of obtaining complex extracts containing multiple different polyphenols, and their synergistic effect in combined use with clinical antibiotics make natural antimicrobial compounds of plant origin ideal tools to be studied from the point of view of network pharmacology in the future. The evidence found in the combination studies between plant extracts and clinical antibiotics shows a synergistic enhancement that may be key to the fight against AMR bacteria. Although the development of new synthetic antibiotics is essential to continue the fight, the sensitization of resistant bacteria by phytochemicals is also crucial to achieving effective and long-lasting therapies [158].

Infections caused by bacteria forming biofilms are extremely difficult to treat and are much less susceptible to antibiotics [183,184]. One way to enhance the effect of an antimicrobial agent is to disrupt the biofilm that certain resistant bacteria form. Studies on *P. aeruginosa* showed that many natural products can inhibit biofilm formation or disrupt the previously formed biofilm: alginate lyase [185], ursolic acid [186], zingerone [187], cranberry proanthocyanidins [188], casbane diterpene [189], manoalide [190], solenopsin A [191], catechin [192], naringenin [193], ajoene [194], rosmarinic acid [195], eugenol [196], bergamottin [197], emodin [198] and baicalein [199] among others. These natural biofilm disrupting compounds could be a very valuable tool to be incorporated into joint therapies with traditional antibiotics when treating infections caused by AMR bacteria. For example, cranberry proanthocyanidins enhanced the activity of gentamicin in an in vivo model of infection using *Galleria mellonella* [188]. In addition, some of these compounds have intrinsic antimicrobial activity on its own, which could further increase the potency of the treatment.

3.4. Development of Resistance to Natural Products

Historically, bacteria have managed to develop resistance to a greater or lesser extent against most antimicrobial agents used in medicine. Nevertheless, the ability of bacteria to develop a resistance mechanism against natural products is not well documented [200]. Due to the huge chemical and structural diversity among antimicrobial products of natural origin, it is often stated the difficulty for bacteria to avoid the action of NPs [201,202]. However, there are some recent studies that suggest that bacteria can develop certain levels of resistance against plant compounds, especially enteric bacteria [203]. The mechanisms of resistance behind these observations remain unknown and literature on the subject is scarce.

There are multiple mechanisms by which a bacterium can get rid of the action of an antimicrobial molecule: target alterations, expulsion or modification of the antibiotic, inactivation, reduced permeability and biofilm formation among others [204]. These resistant mechanisms can be spontaneously developed (mutations) or acquired (by transduction, transfection or conjugation processes) as shown in Figure 5. Understanding the mechanism by which bacteria can circumvent the action of antibiotics and how they acquire these capabilities is crucial to developing effective and lasting therapies.

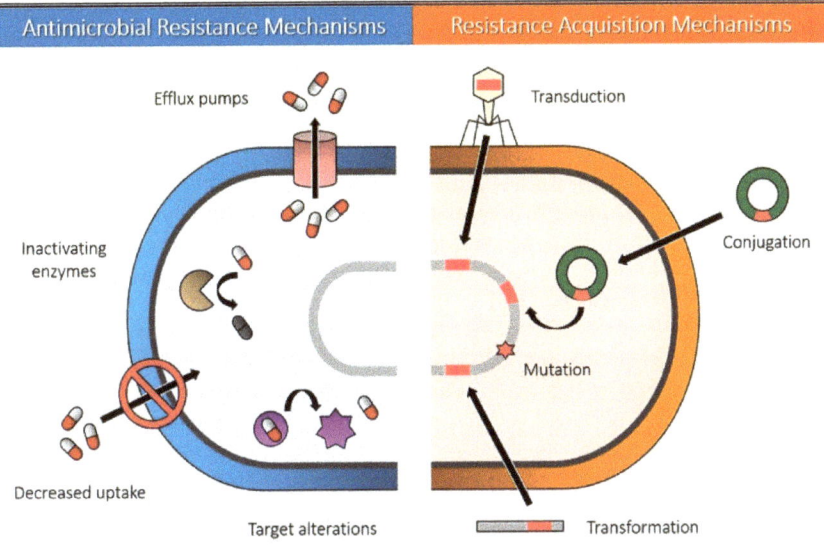

Figure 5. Antimicrobial resistance mechanisms and acquisition mechanisms in bacteria.

Depending on their properties, some products are more susceptible than others to the appearance of bacteria resistant to them. Molecules that attack highly conserved targets are less conducive to the appearance of bacteria with mutations in said targets that confer resistance to the antimicrobial in question, since modifying one or more fundamental routes or targets can imply an unbearable fitness cost for the bacteria [205].

On the other hand, molecules against less conserved molecular targets are more likely to promote the development of resistance mechanisms against them. Modification of less evolutionarily conserved or non-essential targets is easier for bacteria to assimilate since they have greater flexibility to modify the molecular target or adapt their metabolism without paying a high fitness cost. Although the acquisition of antimicrobial resistance mechanisms is often accompanied by reduced fitness in the absence of a selective environment, this loss of adaptive efficacy can be counteracted by compensatory mutations or modifications in epistasis [206].

Thanks to the multifactorial nature of the molecular promiscuity of naturally occurring antimicrobial compounds, bacteria experience difficulties in changing several molecular targets simultaneously [80]. Multiple simultaneous molecular changes in a bacterium to overcome the action of a multifactorial antimicrobial agent would very negatively affect its metabolism, that is, it would have a high fitness cost potentially unacceptable for its development. Likewise, mutations that carry a high fitness cost are less likely to persist in bacterial populations once the selective pressure disappears [207]. This cost would be higher if the molecular targets of the antimicrobial were highly evolutionary conserved molecules or routes, since they would be more difficult to change while maintaining the metabolic efficiency necessary for survival and competition with other living beings. Furthermore, there are studies that affirm that many of the natural antimicrobial compounds attack macromolecular structures such as the membrane or the bacterial wall and that this fact could hinder the appearance of resistance, given that they are very difficult targets to vary as a whole [208,209].

Despite the multiple possible mechanisms for acquiring existing resistances, the use of new technologies in NPs can help prevent their development. Based on new laboratory bacterial culture techniques, it has been possible to identify and isolate interesting natural compounds such as teixobactin. This molecule displays a mechanism of action that is capable of using the bacteria's own machinery to kill itself, in a similar way to how vancomycin, a really successful antibiotic, works. No resistant mutants have been found against teixobactin. Theoretically, the generation of resistant mutants to this compound is difficult, since its target is very conserved among the eubacteria, in addition to being exposed in the outermost part of Gram-positive bacteria. In addition, as teixobactin is produced by a Gram-negative bacterium, the molecule cannot re-enter the cell and exert its action due to the presence of the outer envelope characteristic of Gram-negative bacteria. This fact is crucial in the process of the eventual development of resistance, since the producing microorganism does not use a different metabolic route to avoid the action of the antibiotic it produces. Thus, in the absence of an intrinsic resistance mechanism in the producer, horizontal transfer of resistance genes to other species susceptible to teixobactin cannot occur [55].

Vancomycin, discovered in 1958, enjoyed a period of 30 years in which no bacterium resistant to its antibiotic action was identified, thanks to its potent and unusual mechanism of action. However, during the last 20 years, *S. aureus* strains resistant to this antibiotic have been detected [210]. One of the resistance mechanisms identified is the incorporation of D-Ala-D-lactate instead of the usual D-Ala-D-Ala at the dipeptide termini of nascent peptidoglycan, considerably reducing its binding affinity and formation disruption capacity of the bacterial wall. Other resistant strains identified have a thicker cell wall with free D-Ala-D-Ala ends that can sequester vancomycin and removing it from the place where the biosynthesis of the wall occurs [211]. Despite the emergence of these and other resistance mechanisms, researchers are currently working on vancomycin derivatives that have promising qualities that allow them to circumvent these resistance mechanisms and exert their antibiotic action. An example of this is the discovery of a new vancomycin resistance mechanism mediated by the activity of Atl amidase. This inhibition produces cellular morphological changes that reduce the action of vancomycin on the main target in the biosynthesis of the wall, increasing the tolerance of the pathogen against the antibiotic without any changes at the genetic level. The discovery of this target opens the door to the design of derivatives of vancomycin with a reduced affinity for Atl, resulting in greater efficacy against MRSA [46]. Another resistance mechanism found in *S. aureus* against vancomycin is based on the thickening of the bacterial wall, which slows the penetration of vancomycin into the bacteria [212].

A possible strategy to prevent or slow the appearance of antimicrobial-resistant bacteria is the combined use of various agents that act against different molecular targets. In this way, the bacteria will have to adopt different resistance mechanisms, which would imply a greater and less likely adaptive cost. This hypothesis could support the use of plant extracts and essential oils in traditional medicine used for millennia, since these may be composed of dozens of different phytochemicals with different mechanisms of action. The combined activity of these molecules would hinder bacterial adaptation and extend the therapeutic shelf life of antimicrobial plant extracts.

Although the idea of the difficulty of acquiring resistance against complex plant extracts is widespread, some studies go in the opposite direction. It has been observed that certain antimicrobial extracts used against enterobacteria isolated from geckos from various environments in India have reduced effectiveness. The authors attribute this resistance to the variability and changing environment that has shaped the isolates collected and used in the assay. They suggest that exposure of geckos to medicinal plants may have caused a process of selecting the bacteria present in them, resulting in strains more resistant to plant compounds [203]. Mechanisms of possible resistance are not mentioned.

3.5. New Methodologies to Find Antimicrobial Compounds against AMR Bacteria

Currently, there are many methodologies capable of having a very positive impact on the discovery of new natural molecules with antimicrobial capacity against AMR bacteria. Some of these methodologies are the use of -omics technologies, network pharmacology, synergy studies and in silico trials.

Thanks to the -omics technologies, today it is known that genomes of bacteria such as actinomycetes are much more complex than previously thought in the mid-twentieth century and that there are multiple secondary metabolite gene clusters (SMGCs) that could produce new NPs. It is estimated that under the conditions of the classic fermentation studies for NP isolation, less than 10% of the SMGCs are active, which could be activated using genetic techniques and varying the culture conditions to reveal potential new NPs hidden inside of the "biosynthetic dark matter" [213]. By combining the progressive lowering of the massive sequencing of bacterial genomes and the advancement of the analysis and prediction software it will be possible to identify new SMGCs and their products [214,215]. The discovery and deepening of knowledge of NP-producing modular macroenzymes such as non-ribosomal peptide synthetases and polyketide synthetases open the door to new NPs production strategies based on combinatorial biosynthesis [15]. Scientists now have greater access to soil samples and other potential sources of NPs, which significantly increases the likelihood of finding new compounds. The use of non-laboratory-dependent metagenomic techniques and the heterologous expression of DNA extracted directly from complex samples will allow the identification and production of new NPs hitherto unknown or impossible to produce [216].

Other new technologies such as molecular docking or virtual simulations open the door to the effective discovery of new natural antimicrobial compounds unknown so far using computers [76,217]. In silico assays allow hundreds of thousands of molecules to be screened to efficiently select leaders, greatly reducing the cost of new drug development processes. Prediction via molecular docking or virtual simulation makes it possible to predict the interactions of a molecule with its target, obtaining huge amounts of valuable information and allowing the screening of drug libraries in a short time if the necessary computing capacity is available [218,219].

Emerging studies based on network pharmacology that expand the classic single-ligand-target viewpoint provide excellent opportunities for the development of new antimicrobial compounds. The study of the network pharmacology of phytochemicals based on their molecular promiscuity and multi-target capacity can help to better understand their antimicrobial mechanisms of action and to develop more effective therapies [220]. In turn, this point also has a positive impact on synergy studies between antibiotics and phytochemicals such as those described in the previous sections, and they are currently showing such good results.

4. Conclusions and Future Perspectives

In conclusion, most NPs do not have sufficient therapeutic power to perform monotherapies based on them against antibiotic resistant bacteria, however, their joint application in combination therapy with traditional antibiotics could contribute to enhance their effect, reduce their dosage, side effects and improve its pharmacokinetics and pharmacodynamics properties. Natural antimicrobial products offer a promising avenue of study in the field of antibiotic development thanks to their unique properties, natural availability and enormous chemical diversity. The prospects in the discovery of new NPs with antibiotic activity are very positive. There is a tendency to revise the traditional sources of NPs that offered such good results during the "Golden Age" [221]. The use of new technologies and applications of non-existent knowledge during that age opens the door to the second era of massive discovery of molecules with remarkable and novel biological activity against AMR bacteria.

Author Contributions: Conceptualization, F.J.Á.-M., E.B.-C. and V.M.; methodology, F.J.Á.-M.; investigation, F.J.Á.-M.; data curation, F.J.Á.-M., E.B.-C. and V.M.; writing—original draft preparation, F.J.Á.-M.; writing—review and editing, F.J.Á.-M., E.B.-C. and V.M.; visualization, F.J.Á.-M., E.B.-C. and V.M.; supervision, E.B.-C. and V.M.; project administration, E.B.-C. and V.M.; funding acquisition, E.B.-C. and V.M. All authors have read and agreed to the published version of the manuscript.

Funding: We thank grants RTI2018-096724-B-C21 from the Spanish Ministry of Economy and Competitiveness (MINECO); PROMETEO/2016/006, from Generalitat Valenciana; CIBER (CB12/03/30038, Fisiopatologia de la Obesidad y la Nutricion, CIBERobn, Instituto de Salud Carlos III) and the "Aid for the support to the training of research staff" of the Miguel Hernández University of Elche (resolution 0236/17).

Conflicts of Interest: The authors declare no conflict of interest.

References

1. IHME; GBD. The Review on Antimicrobial Resistance. Available online: https://amr-review.org/ (accessed on 20 May 2020).
2. Goossens, H. The chennai declaration on antimicrobial resistance in india. *Lancet Infect. Dis.* **2013**, *13*, 105–106. [CrossRef]
3. Sultan, I.; Rahman, S.; Jan, A.T.; Siddiqui, M.T.; Mondal, A.H.; Haq, Q.M.R. Antibiotics, resistome and resistance mechanisms: A bacterial perspective. *Front. Microbiol.* **2018**, *9*, 2066. [CrossRef] [PubMed]
4. Daubin, V.; Szollosi, G.J. Horizontal gene transfer and the history of life. *Cold Spring Harb Perspect. Biol.* **2016**, *8*, a018036. [CrossRef] [PubMed]
5. Munita, J.M.; Arias, C.A. Mechanisms of antibiotic resistance. *Microbiol. Spectr.* **2016**, *4*, 481–511. [CrossRef]
6. Wong, A. Epistasis and the evolution of antimicrobial resistance. *Front. Microbiol.* **2017**, *8*, 246. [CrossRef]
7. Clarke, L.; Pelin, A.; Phan, M.; Wong, A. The effect of environmental heterogeneity on the fitness of antibiotic resistance mutations in *Escherichia coli*. *Evol. Ecol.* **2020**, *34*, 379–390. [CrossRef]
8. Davies, J.; Davies, D. Origins and evolution of antibiotic resistance. *Microbiol. Mol. Biol. Rev.* **2010**, *74*, 417–433. [CrossRef]
9. Hiltunen, T.; Virta, M.; Laine, A.L. Antibiotic resistance in the wild: An eco-evolutionary perspective. *Philos. Trans. R. Soc. B Biol. Sci.* **2017**, *372*, 20160039. [CrossRef]
10. Wong, A. Unknown risk on the farm: Does agricultural use of ionophores contribute to the burden of antimicrobial resistance? *mSphere* **2019**, *4*, e00433-19. [CrossRef]
11. Machowska, A.; Stalsby Lundborg, C. Drivers of irrational use of antibiotics in Europe. *Int. J. Environ. Res. Public Health* **2018**, *16*, 27. [CrossRef]
12. Towse, A.; Hoyle, C.K.; Goodall, J.; Hirsch, M.; Mestre-Ferrandiz, J.; Rex, J.H. Time for a change in how new antibiotics are reimbursed: Development of an insurance framework for funding new antibiotics based on a policy of risk mitigation. *Health Policy* **2017**, *121*, 1025–1030. [CrossRef] [PubMed]
13. Sabtu, N.; Enoch, D.A.; Brown, N.M. Antibiotic resistance: What, why, where, when and how? *Br. Med. Bull.* **2015**, *116*, 105–113. [CrossRef] [PubMed]

14. EUCAST. Determination of minimum inhibitory concentrations (mics) of antibacterial agents by broth dilution. *Clin. Microbiol. Infect.* **2003**, *9*, 1–7.
15. Katz, L.; Baltz, R.H. Natural product discovery: Past, present, and future. *J. Ind. Microbiol. Biotechnol.* **2016**, *43*, 155–176. [CrossRef] [PubMed]
16. Berdy, J. Thoughts and facts about antibiotics: Where we are now and where we are heading. *J. Antibiot.* **2012**, *65*, 385–395. [CrossRef] [PubMed]
17. Bar-On, Y.M.; Phillips, R.; Milo, R. The biomass distribution on earth. *Proc. Natl. Acad. Sci. USA* **2018**, *115*, 6506–6511. [CrossRef]
18. Muthamilarasan, M.; Prasad, M. Plant innate immunity: An updated insight into defense mechanism. *J. Biosci.* **2013**, *38*, 433–449. [CrossRef]
19. Tapsell, C.L.; Hemphill, I.; Cobiac, L. Health benefits of herbs and spices: The past, the present, the future. *MJA* **2006**, *185*, S1–S24. [CrossRef]
20. Leja, K.B.; Czaczyk, K. The industrial potential of herbs and spices—A mini review. *Acta Sci. Pol. Technol. Aliment.* **2016**, *15*, 353–365. [CrossRef]
21. Franke, H.; Scholl, R.; Aigner, A. Ricin and ricinus communis in pharmacology and toxicology-from ancient use and "papyrus ebers" to modern perspectives and "poisonous plant of the year 2018". *Naunyn Schmiedebergs Arch. Pharm.* **2019**, *392*, 1181–1208. [CrossRef]
22. Dwivedi, G.; Shridhar, D. Sushruta—The clinician—Teacher par excellence. *Indian J. Chest Dis. Allied Sci.* **2007**, *49*, 243–244.
23. Aggarwal, B.B.; Sundaram, C.; Malani, N.; Ichikawa, H. Curcumin: The indian solid gold. In *The Molecular Targets and Therapeutic Uses of Curcumin in Health and Disease*; Aggarwal, B.B., Surh, Y.-J., Shishodia, S., Eds.; Springer: Boston, MA, USA, 2007; Volume 595.
24. Woodruff, H.B. Selman A. Waksman, winner of the 1952 nobel prize for physiology or medicine. *Appl. Environ. Microbiol.* **2014**, *80*, 2–8. [CrossRef] [PubMed]
25. Kurt, E.L. Small World Initiative. Available online: http://www.smallworldinitiative.org/ (accessed on 5 August 2020).
26. Gould, K. Antibiotics: From prehistory to the present day. *J. Antimicrob. Chemother.* **2016**, *71*, 572–575. [CrossRef] [PubMed]
27. Silver, L. Natural products as a source of drug leads to overcome drug resistance. *Future Microbiol.* **2015**, *10*, 1711–1718. [CrossRef] [PubMed]
28. Barrajon-Catalan, E.; Menendez-Gutierrez, M.P.; Falco, A.; Carrato, A.; Saceda, M.; Micol, V. Selective death of human breast cancer cells by lytic immunoliposomes: Correlation with their her2 expression level. *Cancer Lett.* **2010**, *290*, 192–203. [CrossRef] [PubMed]
29. Falco, A.; Barrajón-Catalán, E.; Menéndez-Gutiérrez, M.P.; Coll, J.; Micol, V.; Estepa, A. Melittin-loaded immunoliposomes against viral surface proteins, a new approach to antiviral therapy. *Antivir. Res.* **2013**, *97*, 218–221. [CrossRef] [PubMed]
30. Yi, H.Y.; Chowdhury, M.; Huang, Y.D.; Yu, X.Q. Insect antimicrobial peptides and their applications. *Appl. Microbiol. Biotechnol.* **2014**, *98*, 5807–5822. [CrossRef]
31. Lee, M.; Bang, K.; Kwon, H.; Cho, S. Enhanced antibacterial activity of an attacin-coleoptericin hybrid protein fused with a helical linker. *Mol. Biol. Rep.* **2013**, *40*, 3953–3960. [CrossRef]
32. Ali, S.M.; Siddiqui, R.; Ong, S.K.; Shah, M.R.; Anwar, A.; Heard, P.J.; Khan, N.A. Identification and characterization of antibacterial compound(s) of cockroaches (*Periplaneta americana*). *Appl. Microbiol. Biotechnol.* **2017**, *101*, 253–286. [CrossRef]
33. Arora, S.; Baptista, C.; Lim, C.S. Maggot metabolites and their combinatory effects with antibiotic on *Staphylococcus aureus*. *Ann. Clin. Microbiol. Antimicrob.* **2011**, *10*, 6. [CrossRef]
34. Kwakman, P.H.; Te Velde, A.A.; de Boer, L.; Vandenbroucke-Grauls, C.M.; Zaat, S.A. Two major medicinal honeys have different mechanisms of bactericidal activity. *PLoS ONE* **2011**, *6*, e17709. [CrossRef] [PubMed]
35. Zabaiou, N.; Fouache, A.; Trousson, A.; Baron, S.; Zellagui, A.; Lahouel, M.; Lobaccaro, J.A. Biological properties of propolis extracts: Something new from an ancient product. *Chem. Phys. Lipids* **2017**, *207*, 214–222. [CrossRef] [PubMed]
36. Rahman, M.M.; Richardson, A.; Sofian-Azirun, M. Antibacterial activity of propolis and honey against *Staphylococcus aureus* and *Escherichia coli*. *Afr. J. Microbiol. Res.* **2010**, *4*, 1872–1878.

37. Bilikova, K.; Huang, S.C.; Lin, I.P.; Simuth, J.; Peng, C.C. Structure and antimicrobial activity relationship of royalisin, an antimicrobial peptide from royal jelly of *Apis mellifera*. *Peptides* **2015**, *68*, 190–196. [CrossRef]
38. Fratini, F.; Cilia, G.; Mancini, S.; Felicioli, A. Royal jelly: An ancient remedy with remarkable antibacterial properties. *Microbiol. Res.* **2016**, *192*, 130–141. [CrossRef]
39. Memariani, H.; Memariani, M.; Shahidi-Dadras, M.; Nasiri, S.; Akhavan, M.M.; Moravvej, H. Melittin: From honeybees to superbugs. *Appl. Microbiol. Biotechnol.* **2019**, *103*, 3265–3276. [CrossRef]
40. Sagheer, M.; Siddiqui, R.; Iqbal, J.; Khan, N.A. Black cobra (*Naja naja karachiensis*) lysates exhibit broad-spectrum antimicrobial activities. *Pathog. Glob. Health* **2014**, *108*, 129–136. [CrossRef]
41. Wang, Y.; Hong, J.; Liu, X.; Yang, H.; Liu, R.; Wu, J.; Wang, A.; Lin, D.; Lai, R. Snake cathelicidin from *Bungarus fasciatus* is a potent peptide antibiotics. *PLoS ONE* **2008**, *3*, e3217. [CrossRef]
42. Samy, R.P.; Kandasamy, M.; Gopalakrishnakone, P.; Stiles, B.G.; Rowan, E.G.; Becker, D.; Shanmugam, M.K.; Sethi, G.; Chow, V.T. Wound healing activity and mechanisms of action of an antibacterial protein from the venom of the eastern diamondback rattlesnake (*Crotalus adamanteus*). *PLoS ONE* **2014**, *9*, e80199. [CrossRef]
43. Lin, F.Y.; Gao, Y.; Wang, H.; Zhang, Q.X.; Zeng, C.L.; Liu, H.P. Identification of an anti-lipopolysacchride factor possessing both antiviral and antibacterial activity from the red claw crayfish cherax quadricarinatus. *Fish Shellfish Immunol.* **2016**, *57*, 213–221. [CrossRef]
44. Hernandez-Aponte, C.A.; Silva-Sanchez, J.; Quintero-Hernandez, V.; Rodriguez-Romero, A.; Balderas, C.; Possani, L.D.; Gurrola, G.B. Vejovine, a new antibiotic from the scorpion venom of vaejovis mexicanus. *Toxicon* **2011**, *57*, 84–92. [CrossRef] [PubMed]
45. Bruniera, F.R.; Ferreira, F.M.; Saviolli, L.R.M.; Bacci, M.R.; Feder, D.; Pedreira, M.; Peterlini, M.A.; Azzalis, L.A.; Junqueira, V.B.; Fonseca, F.L.A. The use of vancomycin with its therapeutic and adverse effects: A review. *Eur. Rev. Med. Pharm. Sci.* **2015**, *19*, 694–700.
46. Eirich, J.; Orth, R.; Sieber, S.A. Unraveling the protein targets of vancomycin in living *S. aureus* and *E. faecalis* cells. *J. Am. Chem. Soc.* **2011**, *133*, 12144–12153. [CrossRef] [PubMed]
47. Tripathi, A.; Schofield, M.M.; Chlipala, G.E.; Schultz, P.J.; Yim, I.; Newmister, S.A.; Nusca, T.D.; Scaglione, J.B.; Hanna, P.C.; Tamayo-Castillo, G.; et al. Baulamycins a and b, broad-spectrum antibiotics identified as inhibitors of siderophore biosynthesis in *Staphylococcus aureus* and *Bacillus anthracis*. *J. Am. Chem. Soc.* **2014**, *136*, 1579–1586. [CrossRef] [PubMed]
48. Feng, Z.; Chakraborty, D.; Dewell, S.B.; Reddy, B.V.; Brady, S.F. Environmental DNA-encoded antibiotics fasamycins a and b inhibit fabf in type ii fatty acid biosynthesis. *J. Am. Chem. Soc.* **2012**, *134*, 2981–2987. [CrossRef]
49. Maffioli, S.I.; Fabbretti, A.; Brandi, L.; Savelsbergh, A.; Monciardini, P.; Abbondi, M.; Rossi, R.; Donadio, S.; Gualerzi, C.O. Orthoformimycin, a selective inhibitor of bacterial translation elongation from streptomyces containing an unusual orthoformate. *ACS Chem. Biol.* **2013**, *8*, 1939–1946. [CrossRef]
50. Phillips, J.W.; Goetz, M.A.; Smith, S.K.; Zink, D.L.; Polishook, J.; Onishi, R.; Salowe, S.; Wiltsie, J.; Allocco, J.; Sigmund, J.; et al. Discovery of kibdelomycin, a potent new class of bacterial type ii topoisomerase inhibitor by chemical-genetic profiling in *Staphylococcus aureus*. *Chem. Biol.* **2011**, *18*, 955–965. [CrossRef]
51. Singh, S.B. Discovery and development of kibdelomycin, a new class of broad-spectrum antibiotics targeting the clinically proven bacterial type ii topoisomerase. *Bioorg. Med. Chem.* **2016**, *24*, 6291–6297. [CrossRef]
52. Wright, G.D. Back to the future: A new 'old' lead for tuberculosis. *EMBO Mol. Med.* **2012**, *4*, 1029–1031. [CrossRef]
53. Xiao, Y.; Gerth, K.; Muller, R.; Wall, D. Myxobacterium-produced antibiotic ta (myxovirescin) inhibits type ii signal peptidase. *Antimicrob. Agents Chemother.* **2012**, *56*, 2014–2021. [CrossRef]
54. Nonejuie, P.; Burkart, M.; Pogliano, K.; Pogliano, J. Bacterial cytological profiling rapidly identifies the cellular pathways targeted by antibacterial molecules. *Proc. Natl. Acad. Sci. USA* **2013**, *110*, 16169–16174. [CrossRef] [PubMed]
55. Ling, L.L.; Schneider, T.; Peoples, A.J.; Spoering, A.L.; Engels, I.; Conlon, B.P.; Mueller, A.; Schaberle, T.F.; Hughes, D.E.; Epstein, S.; et al. A new antibiotic kills pathogens without detectable resistance. *Nature* **2015**, *517*, 455–459. [CrossRef] [PubMed]
56. Therien, A.G.; Huber, J.L.; Wilson, K.E.; Beaulieu, P.; Caron, A.; Claveau, D.; Deschamps, K.; Donald, R.G.; Galgoci, A.M.; Gallant, M.; et al. Broadening the spectrum of beta-lactam antibiotics through inhibition of signal peptidase type i. *Antimicrob. Agents Chemother.* **2012**, *56*, 4662–4670. [CrossRef] [PubMed]

57. Navarro, G.; Cheng, A.T.; Peach, K.C.; Bray, W.M.; Bernan, V.S.; Yildiz, F.H.; Linington, R.G. Image-based 384-well high-throughput screening method for the discovery of skyllamycins a to c as biofilm inhibitors and inducers of biofilm detachment in pseudomonas aeruginosa. *Antimicrob. Agents Chemother.* **2014**, *58*, 1092–1099. [CrossRef]
58. Hawksworth, D.L.; Lücking, R. Fungal diversity revisited: 2.2 to 3.8 million species. *Microbiol. Spectr.* **2017**, *5*, 79–95.
59. King, A.M.; Reid-Yu, S.A.; Wang, W.; King, D.T.; De Pascale, G.; Strynadka, N.C.; Walsh, T.R.; Coombes, B.K.; Wright, G.D. Aspergillomarasmine a overcomes metallo-beta-lactamase antibiotic resistance. *Nature* **2014**, *510*, 503–506. [CrossRef]
60. Ymele-Leki, P.; Cao, S.; Sharp, J.; Lambert, K.G.; McAdam, A.J.; Husson, R.N.; Tamayo, G.; Clardy, J.; Watnick, P.I. A high-throughput screen identifies a new natural product with broad-spectrum antibacterial activity. *PLoS ONE* **2012**, *7*, e31307. [CrossRef]
61. Karaman, M.; Jovin, E.; Malbasa, R.; Matavuly, M.; Popovic, M. Medicinal and edible lignicolous fungi as natural sources of antioxidative and antibacterial agents. *Phytother. Res.* **2010**, *24*, 1473–1481. [CrossRef]
62. Wu, B.; Wiese, J.; Labes, A.; Kramer, A.; Schmaljohann, R.; Imhoff, J.F. Lindgomycin, an unusual antibiotic polyketide from a marine fungus of the lindgomycetaceae. *Mar. Drugs* **2015**, *13*, 4617–4632. [CrossRef]
63. Wei, M.Y.; Li, D.; Shao, C.L.; Deng, D.S.; Wang, C.Y. (+/−)-pestalachloride d, an antibacterial racemate of chlorinated benzophenone derivative from a soft coral-derived fungus *Pestalotiopsis* sp. *Mar. Drugs* **2013**, *11*, 1050–1060. [CrossRef]
64. Pruksakorn, P.; Arai, M.; Kotoku, N.; Vilcheze, C.; Baughn, A.D.; Moodley, P.; Jacobs, W.R., Jr.; Kobayashi, M. Trichoderins, novel aminolipopeptides from a marine sponge-derived *Trichoderma* sp., are active against dormant mycobacteria. *Bioorg. Med. Chem. Lett.* **2010**, *20*, 3658–3663. [CrossRef] [PubMed]
65. Chandra, H.; Bishnoi, P.; Yadav, A.; Patni, B.; Mishra, A.P.; Nautiyal, A.R. Antimicrobial resistance and the alternative resources with special emphasis on plant-based antimicrobials—A review. *Plants* **2017**, *6*, 16. [CrossRef] [PubMed]
66. Quideau, S.; Deffieux, D.; Douat-Casassus, C.; Pouysegu, L. Plant polyphenols: Chemical properties, biological activities, and synthesis. *Angew. Chem. Int. Ed. Engl.* **2011**, *50*, 586–621. [CrossRef] [PubMed]
67. Harvey, A.L.; Edrada-Abel, R.; Quinn, R.J. The re-emergence of natural products for drug discovery in the genomics era. *Nat. Rev. Drug Discov.* **2015**, *14*, 111–129. [CrossRef]
68. Radulovic, N.S.B.; Blagojevic, P.D.; Stojanovic-Radic, Z.Z.; Stojanovic, N.M. Antimicrobial plant metabolites: Structural diversity and mechanism of action. *Curr. Med. Chem.* **2013**, *20*, 932–952.
69. Coban, I.; Toplan, G.G.; Ozbek, B.; Gurer, C.U.; Sariyar, G. Variation of alkaloid contents and antimicrobial activities of papaver rhoeas l. Growing in turkey and northern cyprus. *Pharm. Biol.* **2017**, *55*, 1894–1898. [CrossRef]
70. Nugraha, A.S.; Damayanti, Y.D.; Wangchuk, P.; Keller, P.A. Anti-infective and anti-cancer properties of the annona species: Their ethnomedicinal uses, alkaloid diversity, and pharmacological activities. *Molecules* **2019**, *24*, 4419. [CrossRef]
71. Tian, J.; Ban, X.; Zeng, H.; He, J.; Huang, B.; Wang, Y. Chemical composition and antifungal activity of essential oil from *Cicuta virosa* L. Var. Latisecta celak. *Int. J. Food Microbiol.* **2011**, *145*, 464–470. [CrossRef]
72. Tariq, S.; Wani, S.; Rasool, W.; Shafi, K.; Bhat, M.A.; Prabhakar, A.; Shalla, A.H.; Rather, M.A. A comprehensive review of the antibacterial, antifungal and antiviral potential of *Essential oils* and their chemical constituents against drug-resistant microbial pathogens. *Microb. Pathog.* **2019**, *134*, 103580. [CrossRef]
73. Yang, Y.; Zhang, T. Antimicrobial activities of tea polyphenol on phytopathogens: A review. *Molecules* **2019**, *24*, 816. [CrossRef]
74. Bouarab Chibane, L.; Degraeve, P.; Ferhout, H.; Bouajila, J.; Oulahal, N. Plant antimicrobial polyphenols as potential natural food preservatives. *J. Sci. Food Agric.* **2019**, *99*, 1457–1474. [CrossRef] [PubMed]
75. Bostanghadiri, N.; Pormohammad, A.; Chirani, A.S.; Pouriran, R.; Erfanimanesh, S.; Hashemi, A. Comprehensive review on the antimicrobial potency of the plant polyphenol resveratrol. *Biomed. Pharm.* **2017**, *95*, 1588–1595. [CrossRef] [PubMed]
76. Alvarez-Martinez, F.J.; Barrajon-Catalan, E.; Encinar, J.A.; Rodriguez-Diaz, J.C.; Micol, V. Antimicrobial capacity of plant polyphenols against gram-positive bacteria: A comprehensive review. *Curr. Med. Chem.* **2018**, *27*, 2576–2606. [CrossRef] [PubMed]

77. Su, Y.; Ma, L.; Wen, Y.; Wang, H.; Zhang, S. Studies of the in vitro antibacterial activities of several polyphenols against clinical isolates of methicillin-resistant *Staphylococcus aureus*. *Molecules* **2014**, *19*, 12630–12639. [CrossRef]
78. Mokhtar, M.; Ginestra, G.; Youcefi, F.; Filocamo, A.; Bisignano, C.; Riazi, A. Antimicrobial activity of selected polyphenols and capsaicinoids identified in pepper (*Capsicum annuum* L.) and their possible mode of interactio. *Curr. Microbiol.* **2017**, *74*, 1253–1260. [CrossRef]
79. Caselli, A.; Cirri, P.; Santi, A.; Paoli, P. Morin: A promising natural drug. *Curr. Med. Chem.* **2016**, *23*, 774–791. [CrossRef]
80. Tomas-Menor, L.; Barrajon-Catalan, E.; Segura-Carretero, A.; Marti, N.; Saura, D.; Menendez, J.A.; Joven, J.; Micol, V. The promiscuous and synergic molecular interaction of polyphenols in bactericidal activity: An opportunity to improve the performance of antibiotics? *Phytother. Res.* **2015**, *29*, 466–473. [CrossRef]
81. Bai, L.; Takagi, S.; Ando, T.; Yoneyama, H.; Ito, K.; Mizugai, H.; Isogai, E. Antimicrobial activity of tea catechin against canine oral bacteria and the functional mechanisms. *J. Vet. Med. Sci.* **2016**, *78*, 1439–1445. [CrossRef]
82. Cushnie, T.P.; Hamilton, V.E.; Lamb, A.J. Assessment of the antibacterial activity of selected flavonoids and consideration of discrepancies between previous reports. *Microbiol. Res.* **2003**, *158*, 281–289. [CrossRef]
83. Cushnie, T.P.; Lamb, A.J. Antimicrobial activity of flavonoids. *Int. J. Antimicrob. Agents* **2005**, *26*, 343–356. [CrossRef]
84. Xu, Y.; Shi, C.; Wu, Q.; Zheng, Z.; Liu, P.; Li, G.; Peng, X.; Xia, X. Antimicrobial activity of punicalagin against *Staphylococcus aureus* and its effect on biofilm formation. *Foodborne Pathog. Dis.* **2017**, *14*, 282–287. [CrossRef] [PubMed]
85. Daglia, M. Polyphenols as antimicrobial agents. *Curr. Opin. Biotechnol.* **2012**, *23*, 174–181. [CrossRef] [PubMed]
86. Bernal, P.; Lemaire, S.; Pinho, M.G.; Mobashery, S.; Hinds, J.; Taylor, P.W. Insertion of epicatechin gallate into the cytoplasmic membrane of methicillin-resistant *Staphylococcus aureus* disrupts penicillin-binding protein (pbp) 2a-mediated beta-lactam resistance by delocalizing pbp2. *J. Biol. Chem.* **2010**, *285*, 24055–24065. [CrossRef] [PubMed]
87. Miklasinska-Majdanik, M.; Kepa, M.; Wojtyczka, R.D.; Idzik, D.; Wasik, T.J. Phenolic compounds diminish antibiotic resistance of *Staphylococcus aureus* clinical strains. *Int. J. Environ. Res. Public Health* **2018**, *15*, 2321. [CrossRef] [PubMed]
88. Qin, R.; Xiao, K.; Li, B.; Jiang, W.; Peng, W.; Zheng, J.; Zhou, H. The combination of catechin and epicatechin callate from fructus crataegi potentiates beta-lactam antibiotics against methicillin-resistant staphylococcus aureus (mrsa) in vitro and in vivo. *Int. J. Mol. Sci.* **2013**, *14*, 1802–1821. [CrossRef] [PubMed]
89. Betts, J.W.; Sharili, A.S.; Phee, L.M.; Wareham, D.W. In vitro activity of epigallocatechin gallate and quercetin alone and in combination versus clinical isolates of methicillin-resistant *Staphylococcus aureus*. *J. Nat. Prod.* **2015**, *78*, 2145–2148. [CrossRef]
90. Zwingelstein, M.; Draye, M.; Besombes, J.L.; Piot, C.; Chatel, G. Viticultural wood waste as a source of polyphenols of interest: Opportunities and perspectives through conventional and emerging extraction methods. *Waste Manag.* **2020**, *102*, 782–794. [CrossRef]
91. Tomas-Menor, L.; Morales-Soto, A.; Barrajon-Catalan, E.; Roldan-Segura, C.; Segura-Carretero, A.; Micol, V. Correlation between the antibacterial activity and the composition of extracts derived from various spanish cistus species. *Food Chem. Toxicol.* **2013**, *55*, 313–322. [CrossRef]
92. Dubey, D.; Padhy, R.N. Antibacterial activity of *Lantana camara* L. Against multidrug resistant pathogens from icu patients of a teaching hospital. *J. Herb. Med.* **2013**, *3*, 65–75. [CrossRef]
93. Dubey, D.; Sahu, M.C.; Rath, S.; Paty, B.P.; Debata, N.K.; Padhy, R.N. Antimicrobial activity of medicinal plants used by aborigines of kalahandi, orissa, india against multidrug resistant bacteria. *Asian Pac. J. Trop. Biomed.* **2012**, *2*, S846–S854. [CrossRef]
94. Sahu, M.C.; Padhy, R.N. In vitro antibacterial potency of *Butea monosperma* Lam. Against 12 clinically isolated multidrug resistant bacteria. *Asian Pac. J. Trop. Dis.* **2013**, *3*, 217–226. [CrossRef]
95. Mak, S.; Nodwell, J.R. Actinorhodin is a redox-active antibiotic with a complex mode of action against gram-positive cells. *Mol. Microbiol.* **2017**, *106*, 597–613. [CrossRef] [PubMed]
96. Lin, Z.; Xu, X.; Zhao, S.; Yang, X.; Guo, J.; Zhang, Q.; Jing, C.; Chen, S.; He, Y. Total synthesis and antimicrobial evaluation of natural albomycins against clinical pathogens. *Nat. Commun.* **2018**, *9*, 3445. [CrossRef] [PubMed]

97. Pramanik, A.; Stroeher, U.H.; Krejci, J.; Standish, A.J.; Bohn, E.; Paton, J.C.; Autenrieth, I.B.; Braun, V. Albomycin is an effective antibiotic, as exemplified with *Yersinia enterocolitica* and *Streptococcus pneumoniae*. *Int. J. Med. Microbiol.* **2007**, *297*, 459–469. [CrossRef]
98. Singh, M.; Chang, J.; Coffman, L.; Kim, S.J. Solid-state nmr characterization of amphomycin effects on peptidoglycan and wall teichoic acid biosyntheses in *Staphylococcus aureus*. *Sci. Rep.* **2016**, *6*, 31757. [CrossRef]
99. Kang, A.D.; Smith, K.P.; Eliopoulos, G.M.; Berg, A.H.; McCoy, C.; Kirby, J.E. Invitro apramycin activity against multidrug-resistant *Acinetobacter baumannii* and *Pseudomonas aeruginosa*. *Diagn. Microbiol. Infect. Dis.* **2017**, *88*, 188–191. [CrossRef]
100. Liu, J.; Smith, P.A.; Steed, D.B.; Romesberg, F. Efforts toward broadening the spectrum of arylomycin antibiotic activity. *Bioorg. Med. Chem. Lett.* **2013**, *23*, 5654–5659. [CrossRef]
101. Zhong, J.; Lu, Z.; Dai, J.; He, W. Identification of two regulatory genes involved in carbomycin biosynthesis in streptomyces thermotolerans. *Arch. Microbiol.* **2017**, *199*, 1023–1033. [CrossRef]
102. Zheng, Z.; Tharmalingam, N.; Liu, Q.; Jayamani, E.; Kim, W.; Fuchs, B.B.; Zhang, R.; Vilcinskas, A.; Mylonakis, E. Synergistic efficacy of aedes aegypti antimicrobial peptide cecropin a2 and tetracycline against *Pseudomonas aeruginosa*. *Antimicrob. Agents* **2017**, *61*, e00617–e00686. [CrossRef]
103. Gustaferro, C.A.; Steckelberg, J.M. Cephalosporin antimicrobial agents and related compounds. *Mayo Clin. Proc.* **1991**, *66*, 1064–1073. [CrossRef]
104. Brites, L.M.; Oliveira, L.M.; Barboza, M. Kinetic study on cephamycin c degradation. *Appl. Biochem. Biotechnol.* **2013**, *171*, 2121–2128. [CrossRef] [PubMed]
105. Schwarz, S.; Kehrenberg, C.; Doublet, B.; Cloeckaert, A. Molecular basis of bacterial resistance to chloramphenicol and florfenicol. *FEMS Microbiol. Rev.* **2004**, *28*, 519–542. [CrossRef] [PubMed]
106. Allen, N.E.; Nicas, T.I. Mechanism of action of oritavancin and related glycopeptide antibiotics. *FEMS Microbiol. Rev.* **2003**, *26*, 511–532. [CrossRef] [PubMed]
107. Hakami, A.Y.; Sari, Y. Beta-lactamase inhibitor, clavulanic acid, attenuates ethanol intake and increases glial glutamate transporters expression in alcohol preferring rats. *Neurosci. Lett.* **2017**, *657*, 140–145. [CrossRef]
108. Eustáquio, A.S.; Gust, B.; Luft, T.; Li, S.-M.; Chater, K.F.; Heide, L. Clorobiocin biosynthesis in streptomyces. *Chem. Biol.* **2003**, *10*, 279–288. [CrossRef]
109. Samuels, D.S.; Garon, C.F. Coumermycin a1 inhibits growth and induces relaxation of supercoiled plasmids in borrelia burgdorferi, the lyme disease agent. *Antimicrob. Agents Chemother.* **1993**, *37*, 46–50. [CrossRef]
110. Fedorko, J.; Katz, S.; Allnoch, H. In vitro activity of coumermycin a. *Appl. Microbiol.* **1969**, *18*, 869–873. [CrossRef]
111. Cercenado, E. Espectro antimicrobiano de dalbavancina. Mecanismo de acción y actividad in vitro frente a microorganismos gram positivos. *Enferm. Infecc. Y Microbiol. Clín.* **2017**, *35*, 9–14. [CrossRef]
112. Heidary, M.; Khosravi, A.D.; Khoshnood, S.; Nasiri, M.J.; Soleimani, S.; Goudarzi, M. Daptomycin. *J. Antimicrob. Chemother.* **2018**, *73*, 1–11. [CrossRef]
113. Chu, C.; Deng, J.; Man, Y.; Qu, Y. Green tea extracts epigallocatechin-3-gallate for different treatments. *BioMed Res. Int.* **2017**, *2017*, 5615647. [CrossRef]
114. Li, Z.; He, M.; Dong, X.; Lin, H.; Ge, H.; Shen, S.; Li, J.; Ye, R.D.; Chen, D. New erythromycin derivatives enhance beta-lactam antibiotics against methicillin-resistant *Staphylococcus aureus*. *Lett. Appl. Microbiol.* **2015**, *60*, 352–358. [CrossRef] [PubMed]
115. Falagas, M.E.; Vouloumanou, E.K.; Samonis, G.; Vardakas, K.Z. Fosfomycin. *Clin. Microbiol. Rev.* **2016**, *29*, 321–347. [CrossRef] [PubMed]
116. Curbete, M.M.; Salgado, H.R. A critical review of the properties of fusidic acid and analytical methods for its determination. *Crit. Rev. Anal. Chem.* **2016**, *46*, 352–360. [CrossRef] [PubMed]
117. Wargo, K.A.; Edwards, J.D. Aminoglycoside-induced nephrotoxicity. *J. Pharm. Pr.* **2014**, *27*, 573–577. [CrossRef] [PubMed]
118. Wenzel, M.; Rautenbach, M.; Vosloo, J.A.; Siersma, T.; Aisenbrey, C.H.; Zaitseva, E.; Laubscher, W.E.; Rensburg, W.; Behrends, J.C.; Bechinger, B.; et al. The multifaceted antibacterial mechanisms of the pioneering peptide antibiotics tyrocidine and gramicidin s. *mBio* **2018**, *9*, e00802-18. [CrossRef]
119. Wei, L.; Gao, J.; Zhang, S.; Wu, S.; Xie, Z.; Ling, G.; Kuang, Y.Q.; Yang, Y.; Yu, H.; Wang, Y. Identification and characterization of the first cathelicidin from sea snakes with potent antimicrobial and anti-inflammatory activity and special mechanism. *J. Biol. Chem.* **2015**, *290*, 16633–16652. [CrossRef]

120. Guerrero, M.C.; Modolell, J. Hygromycin a, a novel inhibitor of ribosomal peptidyltransferase. *Eur. J. Biochem.* **1980**, *107*, 409–414. [CrossRef]
121. Arsic, B.; Barber, J.; Cikos, A.; Mladenovic, M.; Stankovic, N.; Novak, P. 16-membered macrolide antibiotics: A review. *Int. J. Antimicrob. Agents* **2018**, *51*, 283–298. [CrossRef]
122. Hoerr, V.; Duggan, G.E.; Zbytnuik, L.; Poon, K.K.; Grosse, C.; Neugebauer, U.; Methling, K.; Loffler, B.; Vogel, H.J. Characterization and prediction of the mechanism of action of antibiotics through nmr metabolomics. *BMC Microbiol.* **2016**, *16*, 82. [CrossRef]
123. Beretta, G. Novel producer of the antibiotic kirromycin belonging to the genus actinoplanes. *J. Antibiot.* **1993**, *46*, 1175–1177. [CrossRef]
124. Wolf, H.; Chinali, G.; Parmeggiani, A. Kirromycin, an inhibitor of protein biosynthesis that acts on elongation factor tu. *Proc. Natl. Acad. Sci. USA* **1974**, *71*, 4910–4914. [CrossRef] [PubMed]
125. Spizek, J.; Rezanka, T. Lincomycin, clindamycin and their applications. *Appl. Microbiol. Biotechnol.* **2004**, *64*, 455–464. [CrossRef] [PubMed]
126. Kurabachew, M.; Lu, S.H.; Krastel, P.; Schmitt, E.K.; Suresh, B.L.; Goh, A.; Knox, J.E.; Ma, N.L.; Jiricek, J.; Beer, D.; et al. Lipiarmycin targets rna polymerase and has good activity against multidrug-resistant strains of mycobacterium tuberculosis. *J. Antimicrob. Chemother.* **2008**, *62*, 713–719. [CrossRef] [PubMed]
127. Rebets, Y.; Lupoli, T.; Qiao, Y.; Schirner, K.; Villet, R.; Hooper, D.; Kahne, D.; Walker, S. Moenomycin resistance mutations in *Staphylococcus aureus* reduce peptidoglycan chain length and cause aberrant cell division. *ACS Chem. Biol.* **2014**, *9*, 459–467. [CrossRef]
128. Dai, C.; Ma, Y.; Zhao, Z.; Zhao, R.; Wang, Q.; Wu, Y.; Cao, Z.; Li, W. Mucroporin, the first cationic host defense peptide from the venom of *Lychas mucronatus*. *Antimicrob. Agents Chemother.* **2008**, *52*, 3967–3972. [CrossRef]
129. Blanchard, C.; Brooks, L.; Beckley, A.; Colquhoun, J.; Dewhurst, S.; Dunman, P.M. Neomycin sulfate improves the antimicrobial activity of mupirocin-based antibacterial ointments. *Antimicrob. Agents Chemother.* **2016**, *60*, 862–872. [CrossRef]
130. Leal, J.F.; Henriques, I.S.; Correia, A.; Santos, E.B.H.; Esteves, V.I. Antibacterial activity of oxytetracycline photoproducts in marine aquaculture's water. *Environ. Pollut.* **2017**, *220*, 644–649. [CrossRef]
131. Wright, A.J. The penicillins. *Mayo Clin. Proc.* **1999**, *74*, 290–307. [CrossRef]
132. Paukner, S.; Riedl, R. Pleuromutilins: Potent drugs for resistant bugs-mode of action and resistance. *Cold Spring Harb. Perspect. Med.* **2017**, *7*, a027110. [CrossRef]
133. Trimble, M.J.; Mlynarcik, P.; Kolar, M.; Hancock, R.E. Polymyxin: Alternative mechanisms of action and resistance. *Cold Spring Harb. Perspect. Med.* **2016**, *6*, a025288. [CrossRef]
134. Cooper, E.C.; Curtis, N.; Cranswick, N.; Gwee, A. Pristinamycin: Old drug, new tricks? *J. Antimicrob. Chemother.* **2014**, *69*, 2319–2325. [CrossRef] [PubMed]
135. Wang, S.; Yao, J.; Zhou, B.; Yang, J.; Chaudry, M.T.; Wang, M.; Xiao, F.; Li, Y.; Yin, W. Bacteriostatic effect of quercetin as an antibiotic alternative in vivo and its antibacterial mechanism in vitro. *J. Food. Prot.* **2018**, *81*, 68–78. [CrossRef] [PubMed]
136. de la Cruz, M.; Gonzalez, I.; Parish, C.A.; Onishi, R.; Tormo, J.R.; Martin, J.; Pelaez, F.; Zink, D.; El Aouad, N.; Reyes, F.; et al. Production of ramoplanin and ramoplanin analogs by actinomycetes. *Front. Microbiol.* **2017**, *8*, 343. [CrossRef] [PubMed]
137. Floss, H.G.; Yu, T.W. Rifamycins mode of action, resistance, and biosynthesis. *Chem. Rev.* **2005**, *105*, 621–632. [CrossRef]
138. Nahoum, V.; Spector, S.; Loll, P.J. Structure of ristocetin a in complex with a bacterial cell-wall mimetic. *Acta Cryst. D Biol. Cryst.* **2009**, *65*, 832–838. [CrossRef]
139. Sweeney, P.; Murphy, C.D.; Caffrey, P. Exploiting the genome sequence of streptomyces nodosus for enhanced antibiotic production. *Appl. Microbiol. Biotechnol.* **2016**, *100*, 1285–1295. [CrossRef]
140. Yang, L.L.; Zhan, M.Y.; Zhuo, Y.L.; Pan, Y.M.; Xu, Y.; Zhou, X.H.; Yang, P.J.; Liu, H.L.; Liang, Z.H.; Huang, X.D.; et al. Antimicrobial activities of a proline-rich proprotein from *Spodoptera litura*. *Dev. Comp. Immunol.* **2018**, *87*, 137–146. [CrossRef]
141. Holloway, W.J. Spectinomyein. *Med. Clin. N. Am.* **1982**, *66*, 169–173. [CrossRef]
142. Rubinstein, E.; Keller, N. Spiramycin renaissance. *J. Antimicrob. Chemother.* **1998**, *42*, 572–576. [CrossRef]
143. Webb, H.E.; Angulo, F.J.; Granier, S.A.; Scott, H.M.; Loneragan, G.H. Illustrative examples of probable transfer of resistance determinants from food animals to humans: Streptothricins, glycopeptides, and colistin. *F1000Research* **2017**, *6*, 1805. [CrossRef]

144. Ramos-Martin, V.; Johnson, A.; McEntee, L.; Farrington, N.; Padmore, K.; Cojutti, P.; Pea, F.; Neely, M.N.; Hope, W.W. Pharmacodynamics of teicoplanin against mrsa. *J. Antimicrob. Chemother.* **2017**, *72*, 3382–3389. [CrossRef] [PubMed]
145. Nguyen, F.; Starosta, A.L.; Arenz, S.; Sohmen, D.; Dönhöfer, A.; Wilson, D.N. Tetracycline antibiotics and resistance mechanisms. *Biol. Chem.* **2014**, *395*, 559–575. [CrossRef] [PubMed]
146. Papp-Wallace, K.M.; Endimiani, A.; Taracila, M.A.; Bonomo, R.A. Carbapenems: Past, present, and future. *Antimicrob. Agents Chemother.* **2011**, *55*, 4943–4960. [CrossRef] [PubMed]
147. Nicolaou, K.C. How thiostrepton was made in the laboratory. *Angew. Chem. Int. Ed. Engl.* **2012**, *51*, 12414–12436. [CrossRef] [PubMed]
148. Bothra, M.; Lodha, R.; Kabra, S.K. Tobramycin for the treatment of bacterial pneumonia in children. *Expert Opin. Pharm.* **2012**, *13*, 565–571. [CrossRef]
149. Yamamoto, K.; Ichikawa, S. Tunicamycin: Chemical synthesis and biosynthesis. *J. Antibiot.* **2019**, *72*, 924–933. [CrossRef]
150. Huang, L.; Zhang, H.; Li, M.; Ahmad, I.; Wang, Y.; Yuan, Z. Pharmacokinetic-pharmacodynamic modeling of tylosin against *Streptococcus suis* in pigs. *BMC Vet. Res.* **2018**, *14*, 319. [CrossRef]
151. Holm, M.; Borg, A.; Ehrenberg, M.; Sanyal, S. Molecular mechanism of viomycin inhibition of peptide elongation in bacteria. *Proc. Natl. Acad. Sci. USA* **2016**, *113*, 978–983. [CrossRef]
152. Bischoff, K.M.; Zhang, Y.; Rich, J.O. Fate of virginiamycin through the fuel ethanol production process. *World J. Microbiol. Biotechnol.* **2016**, *32*, 76. [CrossRef]
153. Lee, T.H.; Hall, K.N.; Aguilar, M.I. Antimicrobial peptide structure and mechanism of action: A focus on the role of membrane structure. *Curr. Top. Med. Chem.* **2016**, *16*, 25–39. [CrossRef]
154. Bhattacharya, D.; Ghosh, D.; Bhattacharya, S.; Sarkar, S.; Karmakar, P.; Koley, H.; Gachhui, R. Antibacterial activity of polyphenolic fraction of kombucha against *Vibrio cholerae*: Targeting cell membrane. *Lett. Appl. Microbiol.* **2018**, *66*, 145–152. [CrossRef]
155. Kakarla, P.; Floyd, J.; Mukherjee, M.; Devireddy, A.R.; Inupakutika, M.A.; Ranweera, I.; Kc, R.; Shrestha, U.; Cheeti, U.R.; Willmon, T.M.; et al. Inhibition of the multidrug efflux pump lmrs from *Staphylococcus aureus* by cumin spice *Cuminum cyminum*. *Arch. Microbiol.* **2017**, *199*, 465–474. [CrossRef] [PubMed]
156. Skariyachan, S.; Sridhar, V.S.; Packirisamy, S.; Kumargowda, S.T.; Challapilli, S.B. Recent perspectives on the molecular basis of biofilm formation by *Pseudomonas aeruginosa* and approaches for treatment and biofilm dispersal. *Folia Microbiol.* **2018**, *63*, 413–432. [CrossRef] [PubMed]
157. Inui, T.; Wang, Y.; Deng, S.; Smith, D.C.; Franzblau, S.G.; Pauli, G.F. Counter-current chromatography based analysis of synergy in an anti-tuberculosis ethnobotanical. *J. Chromatogr. A* **2007**, *1151*, 211–215. [CrossRef]
158. Cheesman, J.M.; Ilanko, A.; Blonk, B.; Cock, I.E. Developing new antimicrobial therapies: Are synergistic combinations of plant extracts/compounds with conventional antibiotics the solution? *Pharm. Rev.* **2017**, *11*, 57–72.
159. Chan, B.C.; Ip, M.; Lau, C.B.; Lui, S.L.; Jolivalt, C.; Ganem-Elbaz, C.; Litaudon, M.; Reiner, N.E.; Gong, H.; See, R.H.; et al. Synergistic effects of baicalein with ciprofloxacin against nora over-expressed methicillin-resistant *Staphylococcus aureus* (mrsa) and inhibition of mrsa pyruvate kinase. *J. Ethnopharmacol.* **2011**, *137*, 767–773. [CrossRef]
160. Kalia, N.P.; Mahajan, P.; Mehra, R.; Nargotra, A.; Sharma, J.P.; Koul, S.; Khan, I.A. Capsaicin, a novel inhibitor of the nora efflux pump, reduces the intracellular invasion of *Staphylococcus aureus*. *J. Antimicrob. Chemother.* **2012**, *67*, 2401–2408. [CrossRef]
161. Ponnusamy, K.; Ramasamy, M.; Savarimuthu, I.; Paulraj, M.G. Indirubin potentiates ciprofloxacin activity in the nora efflux pump of *Staphylococcus aureus*. *Scand. J. Infect. Dis.* **2010**, *42*, 500–505. [CrossRef]
162. Holler, J.G.; Christensen, S.B.; Slotved, H.C.; Rasmussen, H.B.; Guzman, A.; Olsen, C.E.; Petersen, B.; Molgaard, P. Novel inhibitory activity of the *Staphylococcus aureus* nora efflux pump by a kaempferol rhamnoside isolated from *Persea lingue* nees. *J. Antimicrob. Chemother.* **2012**, *67*, 1138–1144. [CrossRef]
163. Shiu, W.K.; Malkinson, J.P.; Rahman, M.M.; Curry, J.; Stapleton, P.; Gunaratnam, M.; Neidle, S.; Mushtaq, S.; Warner, M.; Livermore, D.M.; et al. A new plant-derived antibacterial is an inhibitor of efflux pumps in *Staphylococcus aureus*. *Int. J. Antimicrob. Agents* **2013**, *42*, 513–518. [CrossRef]
164. Bame, J.R.; Graf, T.N.; Junio, H.A.; Bussey, R.O., III; Jarmusch, S.A.; El-Elimat, T.; Falkinham, J.O., III; Oberlies, N.H.; Cech, R.A.; Cech, N.B. Sarothrin from *Alkanna orientalis* is an antimicrobial agent and efflux pump inhibitor. *Planta Med.* **2013**, *79*, 327–329. [CrossRef] [PubMed]

165. Roy, S.K.; Pahwa, S.; Nandanwar, H.; Jachak, S.M. Phenylpropanoids of *Alpinia galanga* as efflux pump inhibitors in *Mycobacterium smegmatis* mc(2) 155. *Fitoterapia* **2012**, *83*, 1248–1255. [CrossRef] [PubMed]
166. Dwivedi, G.R.; Tyagi, R.; Sanchita; Tripathi, S.; Pati, S.; Srivastava, S.K.; Darokar, M.P.; Sharma, A. Antibiotics potentiating potential of catharanthine against superbug *Pseudomonas aeruginosa*. *J. Biomol. Struct. Dyn.* **2018**, *36*, 4270–4284. [CrossRef] [PubMed]
167. Maisuria, V.B.; Hosseinidoust, Z.; Tufenkji, N. Polyphenolic extract from maple syrup potentiates antibiotic susceptibility and reduces biofilm formation of pathogenic bacteria. *Appl. Environ. Microbiol.* **2015**, *81*, 3782–3792. [CrossRef]
168. Bag, A.; Chattopadhyay, R.R. Efflux-pump inhibitory activity of a gallotannin from *Terminalia chebula* fruit against multidrug-resistant uropathogenic *Escherichia coli*. *Nat. Prod. Res.* **2014**, *28*, 1280–1283. [CrossRef]
169. Dwivedi, G.R.; Maurya, A.; Yadav, D.K.; Khan, F.; Darokar, M.P.; Srivastava, S.K. Drug resistance reversal potential of ursolic acid derivatives against nalidixic acid- and multidrug-resistant *Escherichia coli*. *Chem. Biol. Drug Des.* **2015**, *86*, 272–283. [CrossRef]
170. Maurya, A.; Dwivedi, G.R.; Darokar, M.P.; Srivastava, S.K. Antibacterial and synergy of clavine alkaloid lysergol and its derivatives against nalidixic acid-resistant *Escherichia coli*. *Chem. Biol. Drug Des.* **2013**, *81*, 484–490. [CrossRef]
171. Aghayan, S.S.; Mogadam, H.K.; Fazli, M.; Darban-Sarokhalil, D.; Khoramrooz, S.S.; Jabalameli, F.; Yaslianifard, S.; Mirzaii, M. The effects of berberine and palmatine on efflux pumps inhibition with different gene patterns in *Pseudomonas aeruginosa* isolated from burn infections. *Avicenna J. Med. Biotechnol.* **2017**, *9*, 2–7.
172. Adwan, G.; Abu-Shanab, B.; Adwan, K. Antibacterial activities of some plant extracts alone and in combination with different antimicrobials against multidrug-resistant *Pseudomonas aeruginosa* strains. *Asian Pac. J. Trop. Biomed.* **2010**, *3*, 266–269. [CrossRef]
173. Shriram, V.; Khare, T.; Bhagwat, R.; Shukla, R.; Kumar, V. Inhibiting bacterial drug efflux pumps via phyto-therapeutics to combat threatening antimicrobial resistance. *Front. Microbiol.* **2018**, *9*, 2990. [CrossRef]
174. Sudano Roccaro, A.; Blanco, A.R.; Giuliano, F.; Rusciano, D.; Enea, V. Epigallocatechin-gallate enhances the activity of tetracycline in staphylococci by inhibiting its efflux from bacterial cells. *Antimicrob. Agents Chemother.* **2004**, *48*, 1968–1973. [CrossRef] [PubMed]
175. Sousa, V.; Luis, A.; Oleastro, M.; Domingues, F.; Ferreira, S. Polyphenols as resistance modulators in *Arcobacter butzleri*. *Folia Microbiol.* **2019**, *64*, 547–554. [CrossRef] [PubMed]
176. Fazly Bazzaz, B.S.; Sarabandi, S.; Khameneh, B.; Hosseinzadeh, H. Effect of catechins, green tea extract and methylxanthines in combination with gentamicin against *Staphylococcus aureus* and *Pseudomonas aeruginosa*: -combination therapy against resistant bacteria. *J. Pharmacopunct.* **2016**, *19*, 312–318. [CrossRef] [PubMed]
177. Palacios, L.; Rosado, H.; Micol, V.; Rosato, A.E.; Bernal, P.; Arroyo, R.; Grounds, H.; Anderson, J.C.; Stabler, R.A.; Taylor, P.W. Staphylococcal phenotypes induced by naturally occurring and synthetic membrane-interactive polyphenolic beta-lactam resistance modifiers. *PLoS ONE* **2014**, *9*, e93830. [CrossRef] [PubMed]
178. Stapleton, P.D.; Shah, S.; Anderson, J.C.; Hara, Y.; Hamilton-Miller, J.M.; Taylor, P.W. Modulation of beta-lactam resistance in *Staphylococcus aureus* by catechins and gallates. *Int. J. Antimicrob. Agents* **2004**, *23*, 462–467. [CrossRef]
179. Stapleton, P.D.; Shah, S.; Hara, Y.; Taylor, P.W. Potentiation of catechin gallate-mediated sensitization of *Staphylococcus aureus* to oxacillin by nongalloylated catechins. *Antimicrob. Agents Chemother.* **2006**, *50*, 752–755. [CrossRef]
180. Santiago, C.; Pang, E.L.; Lim, K.H.; Loh, H.S.; Ting, K.N. Inhibition of penicillin-binding protein 2a (pbp2a) in methicillin resistant *Staphylococcus aureus* (mrsa) by combination of ampicillin and a bioactive fraction from *Duabanga grandiflora*. *BMC Complement. Altern. Med.* **2015**, *15*, 178. [CrossRef]
181. Khan, R.; Islam, B.; Akram, M.; Shakil, S.; Ahmad, A.; Ali, S.M.; Siddiqui, M.; Khan, A.U. Antimicrobial activity of five herbal extracts against multi drug resistant (mdr) strains of bacteria and fungus of clinical origin. *Molecules* **2009**, *14*, 586–597. [CrossRef]
182. Chovanova, R.; Mikulasova, M.; Vaverkova, S. In vitro antibacterial and antibiotic resistance modifying effect of bioactive plant extracts on methicillin-resistant *Staphylococcus epidermidis*. *Int. J. Microbiol.* **2013**, *2013*, 760969. [CrossRef]

183. Hall, C.W.; Mah, T.F. Molecular mechanisms of biofilm-based antibiotic resistance and tolerance in pathogenic bacteria. *FEMS Microbiol. Rev.* **2017**, *41*, 276–301. [CrossRef]
184. Rasamiravaka, T.; Labtani, Q.; Duez, P.; El Jaziri, M. The formation of biofilms by *Pseudomonas aeruginosa*: A review of the natural and synthetic compounds interfering with control mechanisms. *BioMed Res. Int.* **2015**, *2015*, 759348. [CrossRef] [PubMed]
185. Alkawash, M.A.; Soothill, J.S.; Schiller, N.L. Alginate lyase enhances antibiotic killing of mucoid *Pseudomonas aeruginosa* in biofilms. *APMIS* **2006**, *114*, 131–138. [CrossRef]
186. Ren, D.; Zuo, R.; Gonzalez Barrios, A.F.; Bedzyk, L.A.; Eldridge, G.R.; Pasmore, M.E.; Wood, T.K. Differential gene expression for investigation of *Escherichia coli* biofilm inhibition by plant extract ursolic acid. *Appl. Environ. Microbiol.* **2005**, *71*, 4022–4034. [CrossRef] [PubMed]
187. Kim, H.S.; Park, H.D. Ginger extract inhibits biofilm formation by *Pseudomonas aeruginosa* pa14. *PLoS ONE* **2013**, *8*, e76106. [CrossRef] [PubMed]
188. Ulrey, R.K.; Barksdale, S.M.; Zhou, W.; van Hoek, M.L. Cranberry proanthocyanidins have anti biofilm properties against *Pseudomonas aeruginosa*. *BMC Complement. Altern. Med.* **2014**, *14*, 1–12. [CrossRef] [PubMed]
189. Carneiro, V.A.; Santos, H.S.; Arruda, F.V.; Bandeira, P.N.; Albuquerque, M.R.; Pereira, M.O.; Henriques, M.; Cavada, B.S.; Teixeira, E.H. Casbane diterpene as a promising natural antimicrobial agent against biofilm-associated infections. *Molecules* **2010**, *16*, 190–201. [CrossRef] [PubMed]
190. Skindersoe, M.E.; Ettinger-Epstein, P.; Rasmussen, T.B.; Bjarnsholt, T.; de Nys, R.; Givskov, M. Quorum sensing antagonism from marine organisms. *Mar. Biotechnol.* **2008**, *10*, 56–63. [CrossRef]
191. Park, J.; Kaufmann, G.F.; Bowen, J.P.; Arbiser, J.L.; Janda, K.D. Solenopsin a, a venom alkaloid from the fire ant *Solenopsis invicta*, inhibits quorum-sensing signaling in *Pseudomonas aeruginosa*. *J. Infect. Dis.* **2008**, *198*, 1198–1201. [CrossRef]
192. Vandeputte, O.M.; Kiendrebeogo, M.; Rajaonson, S.; Diallo, B.; Mol, A.; El Jaziri, M.; Baucher, M. Identification of catechin as one of the flavonoids from *Combretum albiflorum* bark extract that reduces the production of quorum-sensing-controlled virulence factors in *Pseudomonas aeruginosa* pao1. *Appl. Environ. Microbiol.* **2010**, *76*, 243–253. [CrossRef]
193. Vandeputte, O.M.; Kiendrebeogo, M.; Rasamiravaka, T.; Stevigny, C.; Duez, P.; Rajaonson, S.; Diallo, B.; Mol, A.; Baucher, M.; El Jaziri, M. The flavanone naringenin reduces the production of quorum sensing-controlled virulence factors in *Pseudomonas aeruginosa* pao1. *Microbiology* **2011**, *157*, 2120–2132. [CrossRef]
194. Jakobsen, T.H.; van Gennip, M.; Phipps, R.K.; Shanmugham, M.S.; Christensen, L.D.; Alhede, M.; Skindersoe, M.E.; Rasmussen, T.B.; Friedrich, K.; Uthe, F.; et al. Ajoene, a sulfur-rich molecule from garlic, inhibits genes controlled by quorum sensing. *Antimicrob. Agents Chemother.* **2012**, *56*, 2314–2325. [CrossRef] [PubMed]
195. Walker, T.S.; Bais, H.P.; Deziel, E.; Schweizer, H.P.; Rahme, L.G.; Fall, R.; Vivanco, J.M. *Pseudomonas aeruginosa*-plant root interactions. Pathogenicity, biofilm formation, and root exudation. *Plant. Physiol.* **2004**, *134*, 320–331. [CrossRef] [PubMed]
196. Zhou, L.; Zheng, H.; Tang, Y.; Yu, W.; Gong, Q. Eugenol inhibits quorum sensing at sub-inhibitory concentrations. *Biotechnol. Lett.* **2013**, *35*, 631–637. [CrossRef]
197. Girennavar, B.; Cepeda, M.L.; Soni, K.A.; Vikram, A.; Jesudhasan, P.; Jayaprakasha, G.K.; Pillai, S.D.; Patil, B.S. Grapefruit juice and its furocoumarins inhibits autoinducer signaling and biofilm formation in bacteria. *Int. J. Food Microbiol.* **2008**, *125*, 204–208. [CrossRef] [PubMed]
198. Ding, X.; Yin, B.; Qian, L.; Zeng, Z.; Yang, Z.; Li, H.; Lu, Y.; Zhou, S. Screening for novel quorum-sensing inhibitors to interfere with the formation of *Pseudomonas aeruginosa* biofilm. *J. Med. Microbiol.* **2011**, *60*, 1827–1834. [CrossRef]
199. Zeng, Z.; Qian, L.; Cao, L.; Tan, H.; Huang, Y.; Xue, X.; Shen, Y.; Zhou, S. Virtual screening for novel quorum sensing inhibitors to eradicate biofilm formation of *Pseudomonas aeruginosa*. *Appl. Microbiol. Biotechnol.* **2008**, *79*, 119–126. [CrossRef]
200. Vadhana, P.; Singh, B.R.; Bharadwaj, M.; Singh, S.V. Emergence of herbal antimicrobial drug resistance in clinical bacterial isolates. *Pharm. Anal. Acta* **2015**, *6*, 1–7. [CrossRef]

201. Warnke, P.H.; Becker, S.T.; Podschun, R.; Sivananthan, S.; Springer, I.N.; Russo, P.A.; Wiltfang, J.; Fickenscher, H.; Sherry, E. The battle against multi-resistant strains: Renaissance of antimicrobial essential oils as a promising force to fight hospital-acquired infections. *J. Cranio Maxillofac Surg.* **2009**, *37*, 392–397. [CrossRef]
202. Pisoschi, A.M.; Pop, A.; Georgescu, C.; Turcus, V.; Olah, N.K.; Mathe, E. An overview of natural antimicrobials role in food. *Eur. J. Med. Chem.* **2018**, *143*, 922–935. [CrossRef]
203. Singh, B.R.; Singh, V.; Ebibeni, N.; Singh, R.K. Antimicrobial and herbal drug resistance in enteric bacteria isolated from faecal droppings of common house lizard/gecko (*Hemidactylus frenatus*). *Int. J. Microbiol.* **2013**, *2013*, 340848. [CrossRef]
204. Gupta, P.D.; Birdi, T.J. Development of botanicals to combat antibiotic resistance. *J. Ayurveda Integr. Med.* **2017**, *8*, 266–275. [CrossRef] [PubMed]
205. San Millan, A.; MacLean, R.C. Fitness costs of plasmids: A limit to plasmid transmission. *Microbiol. Spectr.* **2017**, *5*, 65–79.
206. Durão, P.; Balbontín, R.; Gordo, I. Evolutionary mechanisms shaping the maintenance of antibiotic resistance. *Trends Microbiol.* **2018**, *26*, 677–691. [CrossRef] [PubMed]
207. Melnyk, A.H.; Wong, A.; Kassen, R. The fitness costs of antibiotic resistance mutations. *Evol. Appl.* **2015**, *8*, 273–283. [CrossRef]
208. Sang, Y.; Blecha, F. Antimicrobial peptides and bacteriocins: Alternatives to traditional antibiotics. *Anim. Health Res. Rev.* **2008**, *9*, 227–235. [CrossRef]
209. Hintz, T.; Matthews, K.K.; Di, R. The use of plant antimicrobial compounds for food preservation. *BioMed Res. Int.* **2015**, *2015*, 246264. [CrossRef]
210. McGuiness, W.A.; Malachowa, N.; DeLeo, F.R. Vancomycin resistance in *Staphylococcus aureus*. *Yale J. Biol. Med.* **2017**, *90*, 269–281.
211. Nannini, E.; Murray, B.E.; Arias, C.A. Resistance or decreased susceptibility to glycopeptides, daptomycin, and linezolid in methicillin-resistant *Staphylococcus aureus*. *Curr. Opin. Pharm.* **2010**, *10*, 516–521. [CrossRef]
212. Cui, L.; Iwamoto, A.; Lian, J.Q.; Neoh, H.M.; Maruyama, T.; Horikawa, Y.; Hiramatsu, K. Novel mechanism of antibiotic resistance originating in vancomycin-intermediate *Staphylococcus aureus*. *Antimicrob. Agents Chemother.* **2006**, *50*, 428–438. [CrossRef]
213. Baltz, R.H. Genetic manipulation of secondary metabolite biosynthesis for improved production in *Streptomyces* and other actinomycetes. *J. Ind. Microbiol. Biotechnol.* **2016**, *43*, 343–370. [CrossRef]
214. Johnston, C.W.; Connaty, A.D.; Skinnider, M.A.; Li, Y.; Grunwald, A.; Wyatt, M.A.; Kerr, R.G.; Magarvey, N.A. Informatic search strategies to discover analogues and variants of natural product archetypes. *J. Ind. Microbiol. Biotechnol.* **2016**, *43*, 293–298. [CrossRef] [PubMed]
215. Medema, M.H.; Fischbach, M.A. Computational approaches to natural product discovery. *Nat. Chem. Biol.* **2015**, *11*, 639–648. [CrossRef]
216. Katz, M.; Hover, B.M.; Brady, S.F. Culture-independent discovery of natural products from soil metagenomes. *J. Ind. Microbiol. Biotechnol.* **2016**, *43*, 129–141. [CrossRef] [PubMed]
217. Zakeri, B.; Lu, T.K. Synthetic biology of antimicrobial discovery. *ACS Synth. Biol.* **2013**, *2*, 358–372. [CrossRef] [PubMed]
218. Morris, G.M.; Lim-Wilby, M. *Molecular Modeling of Proteins*; Humana Press: Totowa, NJ, USA, 2008; Volume 443.
219. Saikia, S.; Bordoloi, M. Molecular docking: Challenges, advances and its use in drug discovery perspective. *Curr. Drug Targets* **2019**, *20*, 501–521. [CrossRef] [PubMed]
220. Gertsch, J. Botanical drugs, synergy, and network pharmacology: Forth and back to intelligent mixtures. *Planta Med.* **2011**, *77*, 1086–1098. [CrossRef] [PubMed]
221. Moore, B.S.; Carter, G.T.; Bronstrup, M. Editorial: Are natural products the solution to antimicrobial resistance? *Nat. Prod. Rep.* **2017**, *34*, 685–686. [CrossRef] [PubMed]

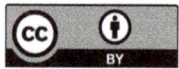

© 2020 by the authors. Licensee MDPI, Basel, Switzerland. This article is an open access article distributed under the terms and conditions of the Creative Commons Attribution (CC BY) license (http://creativecommons.org/licenses/by/4.0/).

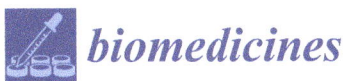

Article

Treatment with Luteolin Improves Lipopolysaccharide-Induced Periodontal Diseases in Rats

Giovanna Casili [1], Alessio Ardizzone [1], Marika Lanza [1], Enrico Gugliandolo [1], Marco Portelli [2], Angela Militi [2], Salvatore Cuzzocrea [1], Emanuela Esposito [1] and Irene Paterniti [1,*]

[1] Department of Chemical, Biological, Pharmaceutical and Environmental Sciences, University of Messina, Viale Ferdinando Stagno D'Alcontres, 31-98166 Messina, Italy; gcasili@unime.it (G.C.); aleardizzone@unime.it (A.A.); mlanza@unime.it (M.L.); egugliandolo@unime.it (E.G.); salvator@unime.it (S.C.); eesposito@unime.it (E.E.)
[2] Department of Biomedical and Dental Science, Morphological and Functional Images, University of Messina, Via Consolare Valeria, 98125 Messina, Italy; mportelli@unime.it (M.P.); amiliti@unime.it (A.M.)
* Correspondence: ipaterniti@unime.it; Tel.: +39-090-676-5208

Received: 2 September 2020; Accepted: 20 October 2020; Published: 21 October 2020

Abstract: Periodontitis is a dental disease that produces the progressive destruction of the bone surrounding the tooth. Especially, lipopolysaccharide (LPS) is involved in the deterioration of the alveolar bone, inducing the release of pro-inflammatory mediators, which cause periodontal tissue inflammation. Luteolin (Lut), a molecule of natural origin present in a large variety of fruits and vegetables, possess beneficial properties for human health. On this basis, we investigated the anti-inflammatory properties of Lut in a model of periodontitis induced by LPS in rats. Animal model predicted a single intragingival injection of LPS (10 µg/µL) derived from *Salmonella typhimurium*. Lut administration, was performed daily at different doses (10, 30, and 100 mg/kg, orally), starting from 1 h after the injection of LPS. After 14 days, the animals were sacrificed, and their gums were processed for biochemical analysis and histological examinations. Results showed that Lut (30 and 100 mg/kg) was equally able to reduce alveolar bone loss, tissue damage, and neutrophilic infiltration. Moreover, Lut treatment reduced the concentration of collagen fibers, mast cells degranulation, and NF-κB activation, as well as the presence of pro-inflammatory enzymes and cytokines. Therefore, Lut implementation could represent valid support in the pharmacological strategy for periodontitis, thus improving the well-being of the oral cavity.

Keywords: dental diseases; periodontitis; luteolin; flavonoids; lipopolysaccharide; anti-inflammatory

1. Introduction

Periodontal disease can be defined as an infectious–inflammatory process that affects anatomical structures supporting the tooth: gums, periodontal ligament, cement, and alveolar bone [1,2]. Periodontitis is the leading cause of tooth loss in the adult population of industrialized countries; thus, it represents a serious health problem that affects a great portion of the world's population (more than 50%). It is generally more frequent in adults and the elderly, but some forms can also affect children and adolescents [3]. Predisposing factors are incorrect nutrition [4], cigarette smoking [5], and certainly poor oral hygiene [6], as well as a possible hereditary component [7]. However, the process of altering periodontal structures is always the consequence of the concurrent action of immunological and microbial factors [2]. The oral cavity is colonized by more than 600 species of bacteria [8]. Some of them are beneficial to the health; however, when the balance in the microbial flora of the oral cavity is altered, this can establish conditions that favor the onset of infection [9]. Specifically, bacteria responsible for periodontitis hold lipopolysaccharides (LPS).

LPS is one of the most important molecules involved in the development of periapical inflammation and deterioration of the alveolar bone; the increase in its concentration causes the release of a variety of pro-inflammatory mediators, including prostaglandins and cytokines, which cause periodontal tissues inflammation through the activation of multiple pathways [10]. Inflammatory condition implicates the stimulation of fibroblasts, the increase of collagen breakdown, and the rise of osteoclast activity [11,12].

Given the severity of the disease, it is certainly important to act promptly with effective therapy. Currently, the most suitable drugs in the case of periodontitis are anti-inflammatory drugs of both steroid and non-steroidal origin (NSAIDs) [13], as well as antibiotics [14] and antibacterial mouthwashes containing chlorhexidine [15]; all of this should be combined with proper oral hygiene.

In the most advanced forms of periodontitis, surgical techniques are also required.

In addition to conventional drugs, natural compounds can also be a valuable aid, providing additional support in the management of many inflammatory diseases.

Luteolin (Lut; 3′,4′,5′,7′-tetrahydroxyflavone) is a polyphenolic compound that belongs to flavones [16]. It was originally isolated from thyme, dandelion, and sage leaves but is also present in numerous foods, such as carrots, fennel, peppers, celery, and in officinal herbs like chamomile tea [17]. The attention to this compound is due to its multiple biological properties, especially to its antioxidant and anti-inflammatory effects, as evidenced by numerous scientific studies [18,19]; in many in vitro and in vivo models, Lut has been shown to inhibit several pro-inflammatory cytokines, including tumor necrosis factor-alpha (TNF-α), and to modulate nuclear factor kappa-light-chain-enhancer of activated B cells (NF-κB) pathway, thus demonstrating the ability of flavonoids to inhibit inflammatory processes [20–22].

On these bases, the purpose of this work was to investigate the anti-inflammatory properties of Lut on an animal model of periodontitis induced by LPS in rats.

2. Results

2.1. Effects of Lut Administration on Bone Destruction Induced by LPS in Gingival Tissues

In the LPS-induced periodontitis group (Figure 1B,F), the radiographic distance from the cement–enamel junction (CEJ) to the bone was considerably larger than the sham group (Figure 1A,F). Treatment with Lut at a dose of 10 mg/kg (Figure 1C,F) has proved to be ineffective for decreasing this distance, whereas the treatment with Lut at a dose of 30 (Figure 1D,F) and 100 mg/kg (Figure 1E,F) has proved to be equally effective in decreasing the alveolar bone distance.

2.2. Effects of Lut Administration on Histological Damage and Neutrophilic Infiltration

Trough H/E staining the tissue integrity of each section was analyzed. No histopathological alteration was found in sham-group rats (Figure 2A, and see histological score 2F). While, histological examination of the LPS group revealed a significant increase in edema and tissue damage (Figure 2B, and see histological score 2F) that was significantly reduced after Lut 30 mg/kg and Lut 100 mg/kg administrations (Figure 2D,E, and see histological score 2F). Contrarily, rats treated with Lut 10 mg/kg still showed considerable tissue damage (Figure 2C, and see histological score 2F).

Similar results were obtained from the myeloperoxidase (MPO) analysis, a marker for neutrophil infiltration. In the LPS group were revealed increased levels of MPO, whereas the two higher doses of Lut were able to markedly decrease the MPO expression; meanwhile rats treated with Lut 10 mg/kg showed MPO levels almost equivalent to the LPS group. The sham group instead revealed minimal expressions of neutrophilic infiltration (Figure 3).

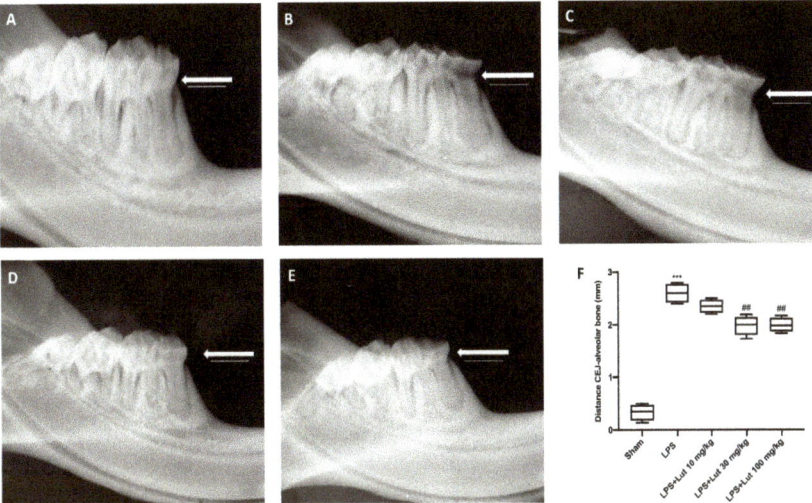

Figure 1. Luteolin (Lut) administration decreased the alveolar bone distance. Fourteen days after the lipopolysaccharide (LPS) injection, the X-rays of the rats LPS-induce periodontitis showed a greater distance from the cement–enamel junction (CEJ) to the bone (**B,F**), compared to the sham group rats (**A,F**). Lut 30 mg/kg (**D,F**) and 100 mg/kg (**E,F**) were effective in reducing this distance, as opposed to treatment with Lut 10 mg/kg which proved ineffective (**C,F**). Values reported in the box plot are expressed as mean ± SEM of 10 rats for each group. *** $p < 0.001$ vs. sham; ## $p < 0.01$ vs. LPS group.

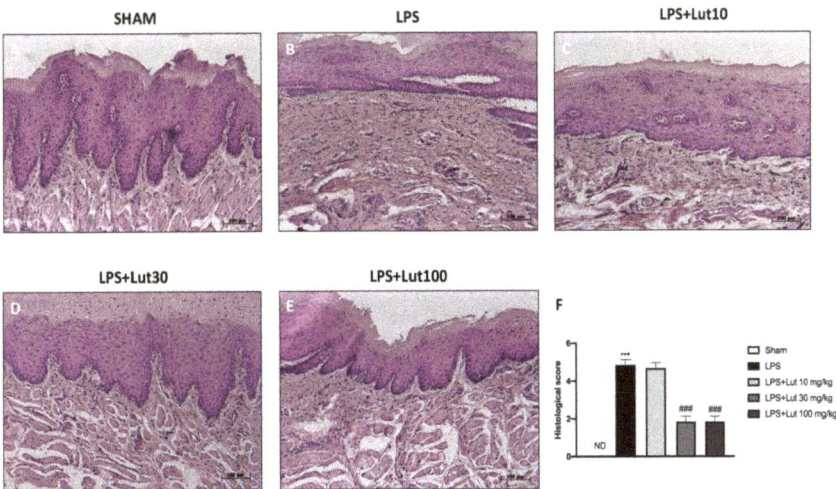

Figure 2. Lut administration reduced histological damage LPS-induced periodontitis. No histological damage was found in the gingivomucosal tissues from sham-group rats (**A**), see histological score (**F**). Extensive damage, accompanied by edema, tissue injury, and inflammatory cells infiltration, was assessed in LPS rats (**B**), see histological score (**F**). The administration of Lut 30 mg/kg (**D**), see histological score (**F**) and 100 mg/kg (**E**), see histological score (**F**), reduced LPS tissue damage as opposed to treatment with Lut 10 mg/kg which proved ineffective (**C**), see histological score (**F**). Data are representative of at least three independent experiments; One-Way ANOVA test.*** $p < 0.001$ vs. sham; ### $p < 0.001$ vs. LPS group. ND = not detectable.

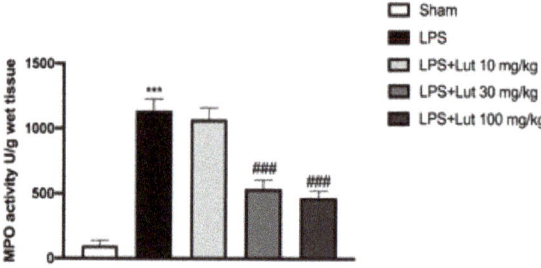

Figure 3. Lut treatment moderated neutrophilic infiltration. An increase in MPO levels was found in LPS-induced periodontitis rats, compared to the sham group. Only the 30 and 100 mg/kg dosages proved to be equally effective in reducing MPO levels. One-Way ANOVA test.*** $p < 0.001$ vs. sham; ### $p < 0.001$ vs. LPS group.

Based on these results, we decided to continue our experiments with the dose of 30 mg/kg of Lut that possesses the same efficacy as the highest dose, 100 mg/kg, but with less toxicity.

2.3. Effects of Lut Treatment on Collagen Fibers

Masson's staining allowed us to evaluate the development of fibrous connective tissue as a repairing response to injury or damage. LPS injected rats (Figure 4B, and see fibrosis score 4D) presented an increase of collagen formation in gingivomucosal tissue sections in comparison with the sham group (Figure 4A, and see fibrosis score 4D). The increase in collagen fibers was considerably decreased by Lut 30 mg/kg treatment (Figure 4C, and see fibrosis score 4D).

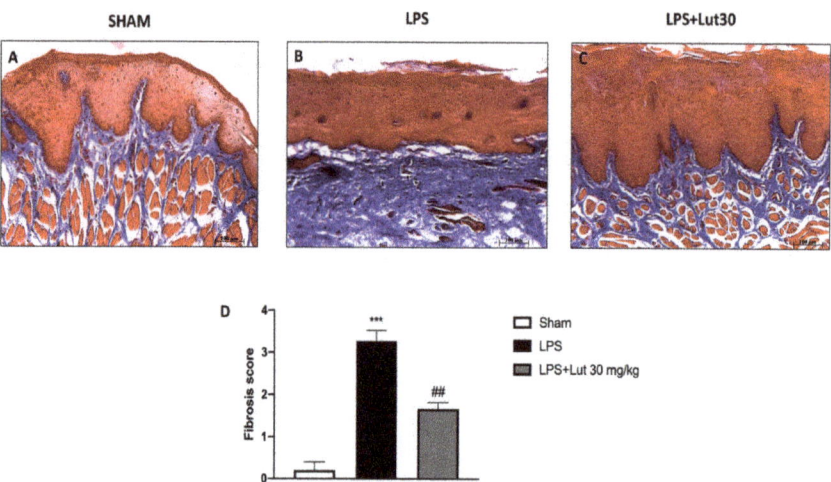

Figure 4. Lut treatment reduced collagen formation. Masson's trichrome stain presented an increase in the concentration of collagen fibers in gingivomucosal tissues in the LPS group (**B,D**), compared to the control group (**A,D**). Lut 30 mg/kg significantly attenuated collagen formation (**C,D**). One-Way ANOVA test.*** $p < 0.001$ vs. sham; ## $p < 0.01$ vs. LPS group.

2.4. Effects of Lut Treatment on Mast Cell Degranulation

We investigated mast cell infiltration and their degranulation through toluidine blue staining. There was no full-blown inflammatory state in the gingivomucosal tissues of the sham group, as confirmed by the minimal presence of mast cells (Figure 5A,D). The group treated with LPS instead showed high levels of mast cell infiltration (as shown in Figure 5B,D); these elevated levels were extensively reduced by Lut 30 mg/kg treatment (Figure 5C,D).

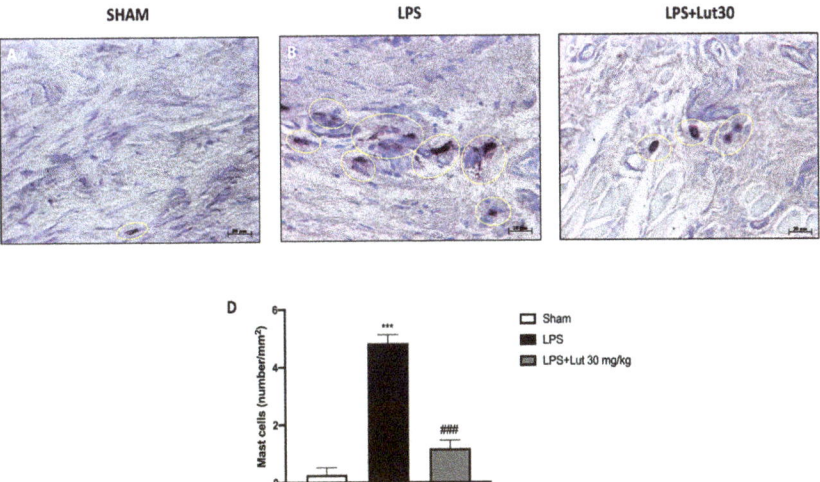

Figure 5. Effects of Lut treatment on mast cell degranulation. Toluidine blue staining allowed mast cell count. In gingivomucosal tissues of rats belonging to the LPS group, an increased number of mast cells was identified (**B,D**), as compared to control group (**A,D**). Lut 30 mg/kg considerably reduced mast cell infiltration (**C,D**). Yellow circles indicate the mast cells degranulated appeared in the tissue. One-Way ANOVA test.*** $p < 0.001$ vs. sham; ### $p < 0.001$ vs. LPS group.

2.5. Lut Treatment Modulated NF-κB Pathway and Pro-Inflammatory Cytokines Production

To prove the anti-inflammatory effect of Lut, we investigated, through Western blot analysis, its action on NF-κB pathway. The expression of NF-κB was found at basal levels in the sham group (Figure 6B and densitometric analysis 6B1), elevated in the LPS group (Figure 6B and densitometric analysis 6B1) and appreciably reduced by treatment with Lut 30 mg/kg (Figure 6B and densitometric analysis 6B1). In relation to this, the protein levels of IκB-α (cytosolic protein associated with NF-κB) confirmed the action of Lut in the NF-κB pathway. In fact, these levels appeared high in the sham group (Figure 6A and densitometric analysis 6A1), significantly downregulated in rats injected with LPS (Figure 6A and densitometric analysis 6A1) and remarkably restored in rats administered with Lut 30 mg/kg (Figure 6A and densitometric analysis 6A1).

Furthermore, TNF-α, together with IL-6, plays a crucial role in establishing the inflammatory state in periodontitis; therefore, they can be considered specific markers of the disease [23]. All of these considerations led us to investigate the levels of cytokines previously mentioned. Samples from the sham group exhibited minimal levels of both cytokines (Figure 6C,D, respectively); on the other hand, such expressions were significantly increased in LPS-induced periodontitis rats (Figure 6C,D, respectively). In contrast, treatment with Lut 30 mg/kg significantly reduced TNF-α and IL-6 levels (Figure 6C,D, respectively).

2.6. Lut Treatment Decreased Pro-Inflammatory Enzymes Following LPS-Induced Periodontitis

The degradation of IκB-α, accompanied, consequently, by the translocation of NF-κB in the nucleus, involves the transcription of numerous proinflammatory genes, including the inducible enzymes COX-2 and iNOS, which play a fundamental role in the inflammatory response.

Lut 30 mg/kg treatment had the ability to modulate the expression of both COX-2 (Figure 7B and densitometric analysis 7B1) and iNOS (Figure 7A and densitometric analysis 7A1), compared to the damage induced by LPS (Figure 6A and densitometric analysis 6A1; Figure 7A and densitometric analysis 7A1). However, the sham-operated group shown minimal expression of both pro-inflammatory enzymes (Figure 6A and densitometric analysis 6A1; Figure 7A and densitometric analysis 7A1).

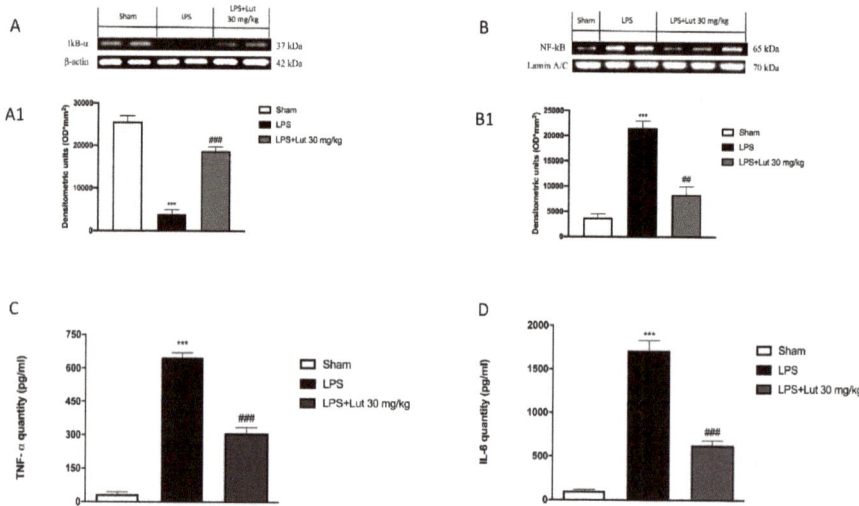

Figure 6. Effects of Lut treatment on NF-κB pathway and pro-inflammatory cytokines. Western blot analysis demonstrated an increase in the degradation of IκB-α in the LPS group (**A**) and densitometric analysis (**A1**) compared to the sham group (**A**) and densitometric analysis (**A1**). Lut 30 mg/kg has proven to be truly effective in restoring these levels (**A**) and densitometric analysis (**A1**). NF-κB was significantly increased in the LPS group (**B**) and densitometric analysis (**B1**), as compared to the sham group (**B**) and densitometric analysis (**B1**); Lut 30 mg/kg effectively decreased the levels of NF-κB (**B**) and densitometric analysis (**B1**). The levels of TNF-α (**C**) and IL-6 (**D**) were significantly increased in rats injected with LPS. The increases in levels of TNF-α and IL-6 were significantly attenuated in rats administrated with Lut 30 mg/kg. Data are representative of at least three independent experiments. One-Way ANOVA test. *** $p < 0.001$ vs. sham; ### $p < 0.001$ vs. LPS group. ## $p < 0.01$ vs. LPS group.

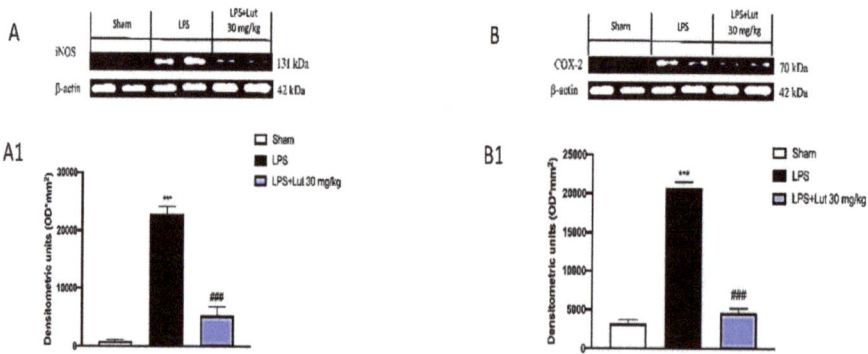

Figure 7. Effects of Lut treatment on pro-inflammatory enzymes. Western blot analysis of iNOS (**A**) and densitometric analysis (**A1**) and COX-2 (**B**) and densitometric analysis (**B1**) revealed minimal levels in the sham group that conversely were increased in the LPS group. Treatment with Lut 30 mg/kg proved effective to reduce COX-2 and iNOS expressions. Data are representative of at least three independent experiments. One-Way ANOVA test. *** $p < 0.001$ vs. sham; ### $p < 0.001$ vs. LPS group.

3. Discussion

Periodontitis is one of the most common and most serious dental diseases that causes progressive destruction of the bone surrounding the tooth; this condition, due to inflammatory processes of the marginal gingiva, is debilitating for the patient, hence the need to intervene as soon as possible through pharmacological therapy [24]. In recent years, the appreciation of natural compounds as a potential innovative treatment for human health has grown considerably [25].

Lut is a molecule of natural origin that is present in a large variety of fruits and vegetables and also in medicinal herbs; it has been shown to have great beneficial properties on human health [26–28]. Specifically, its anticancer properties are known, as shown by several studies [27,29], but it also has anti-inflammatory [20] and antioxidant effects [30].

Previous evidence led us to investigate the properties of this compound in an experimental model of periodontitis induced by LPS, in order to evaluate its potentiality.

One of the hallmarks of periodontitis is alveolar bone loss; this bone destruction is due to a process, both immune and inflammatory, with which our body tries to counteract oral bacterial dysbiosis [31]. As demonstrated by our results, Lut had the ability to reduce alveolar bone loss caused by LPS injection. The most significant results were obtained exclusively at the doses of 30 and 100 mg/kg of Lut, while, at the dose of 10 mg/kg, alveolar bone loss was comparable to the LPS group.

The pathogenic developments of inflammatory periodontal diseases are originated by subgingival plaque microflora and factors such as LPS derived from specific pathogens [31]. Locally, this inflammatory condition promotes tissue damage, thus causing the morphological alteration of the periodontium [32]. In particular, tissue damage is associated with the formation of edema and inflammatory cell infiltration with clear damage to gingivomucosal architecture [12,33].

Lut administration at the two highest doses (30 and 100 mg/kg) was equally able to mitigate tissue damage caused by LPS injection, as is visible from our histological analyses.

Neutrophils constitute the primary defense system in periodontal tissues [34]; in fact, in a healthy oral cavity, populations of neutrophils tend to be para-inflammatory. On the contrary, the phenotypes of pro-inflammatory neutrophils are present in periodontal disease [35]. Lut treatment, as demonstrated by the MPO analysis, significantly reduced the presence of neutrophilic infiltration; this reduction was equally significant at the doses of 30 and 100 mg/kg, while it was ineffective, once again, at the dose of 10 mg/kg.

Given the effectiveness of Lut 30 mg/kg in counteracting tissue damage, as already highlighted by the H&E staining, we also assessed the effect of Lut treatment on collagen fibers through Masson's trichrome stain. In periodontitis, in fact, prolonged inflammation causes apical migration of junctional epithelium on the root surface and activates collagen destruction; specifically, degradation of type I collagen occurs in the connective tissue and periodontal ligament [33].

Our results clearly demonstrated that Lut 30 mg/kg was able to decrease the concentration of collagen fibers in gingivomucosal tissues.

There is also a probable cross-talk between the increase in collagen fibers and the presence of mast cell infiltration in periodontitis [36]. Mast cells are immune cells that stimulate the inflammatory process [37] and therefore play a primary role in inflammation disease like periodontitis. Lut 30 mg/kg, as evidenced by our results, significantly reduced the degranulation of mast cells in the inflamed gingivomucosal tissues.

The intense inflammatory condition that characterizes periodontitis includes the involvement of several pathways; in particular, the correlation between NF-κB and periodontitis is widely known, as demonstrated by several clinical studies [38,39]. Lut 30 mg/kg decreased the levels of NF-κB and increased the expression of the cytosolic protein IκB-α, as shown from Western blot analysis performed. Furthermore, it is known that the translocation of NF-κB in the nucleus promotes the transcription of pro-inflammatory genes, upregulating the expression of pro-inflammatory proteins. Western blot analysis showed that Lut administration also moderated the expression of two key enzymes of the inflammatory cascade, namely iNOS and COX-2.

Furthermore, the production of pro-inflammatory cytokines has also been related to periodontal disease. Particularly, many clinical studies [33,40,41] have demonstrated the correlation between high TNF-α and IL-6 expressions and periodontal disease, highlighting their involvement and crucial role in the evolution of gingival inflammation. As shown by our results, treatment with Lut 30 mg/kg decreased the expressions of both cytokines.

Persistent gingivitis in young patients represents, in fact, a risk factor for periodontal attachment loss and for tooth loss in adulthood; inflammation of the gingival tissues represents not only the precursor of periodontitis but also a clinically relevant risk factor for disease progression and tooth loss [42].

Given the results obtained from this study through several methodological approaches, it is possible to affirm that Lut has good anti-inflammatory capacities in counteracting the inflammatory state caused by LPS-induced periodontitis. Therefore, Lut implementation could represent a valid natural support in the pharmacological strategy for periodontitis, thus improving the well-being of the oral cavity. Furthermore, Lut's anti-inflammatory capabilities could open new perspectives in the field of applicability of this natural compound also in products used for the prevention of inflammatory processes of the oral cavity, like toothpaste and mouthwash; further experiments need to be carried out in more in-depth studies, to confirm this preventive applicability.

4. Materials and Methods

4.1. Materials

Unless otherwise indicated, all materials were acquired from Sigma-Aldrich Company Ltd. (St. Louis, Missouri, USA). All stock solutions were made in non-pyrogenic saline (0.9 % NaCl, Baxter, Milan, Italy). All other chemicals were of the highest commercial grade available.

4.2. Animals

The study was performed on Sprague-Dawley male rats (Envigo, Milan, Italy), weighing 200–230 g. They were housed in a controlled environment (22 ± 2 °C, 55 ± 15 % relative humidity, 12 h light/dark cycle), with food and water ad libitum, minimizing stress conditions.

Animal experiments complied with Italian regulations on the protection of animals used for experimental and other scientific purposes (DM 116192), as well as EU regulations (OJ of EC L 358/1, 18th December 1986).

4.3. LPS-Induced Periodontitis

Periodontitis was induced as described by Reference [43] and reported below. After slightly anesthetizing the animals with sodium pentobarbital (35 mg/kg), periodontitis was induced by a single 1 μL LPS (10 μg/μL) intragingival injection derived from *Salmonella typhimurium* (Sigma-Aldrich) in sterile saline solution. The inoculation was made in the mesolateral side at the interdental papilla between the first and the second molar. It was performed slowly, and the needle was kept in place for some seconds after the injection, to guarantee that LPS was not lost through needle extraction. In addition, the animals were weighed daily, in order to control regular food intake and their masticatory behavior.

4.4. Experimental Groups

Rats were randomly divided into several groups (n = 10 for each), as reported below:

Group 1: sham + saline: animals received a single intragingival injection of saline solution instead of LPS (N = 10);

Group 2: LPS + saline: rats were subjected to LPS-induced periodontitis (N = 10);

Group 3: LPS + Lut 10 mg/kg: rats were subjected to LPS-induced periodontitis plus daily administration of Lut (10 mg/kg) for 14 days, starting from 1 h after the injection of LPS (N = 10);

Group 4: LPS + Lut 30 mg/kg: rats were subjected to LPS-induced periodontitis plus daily administration of Lut (30 mg/kg) for 14 days, starting from 1 h after the injection of LPS ($N = 10$);

Group 5: LPS + Lut 100 mg/kg: rats were subjected to LPS-induced periodontitis plus daily administration of Lut (100 mg/kg) for 14 days, starting from 1 h after the injection of LPS ($N = 10$).

For oral administration, Lut was dissolved in 0.5 mL ethanol (50% purity) and given to the rats by oral gavage; the dosages of Lut were chosen on the basis of previous studies [44,45].

At the end of the experiment, 14 days after LPS injection, the animals were sacrificed, and the gums removed by surgical procedure and processed for biochemical analysis and histological examinations.

4.5. Radiography

For each rat belonging to the five experimental groups, radiographic analyses were performed, using an X-ray machine (Bruker MS FX Pro, Billerica, MA, USA). The X-ray tube was operated at 30 kW, with a current of 6 mA, for 0.01 s, and the source-to-sensor distance was 50 cm. At the end of the experiment, through the radiographs, we estimated the dental alveolar bone level expressed as the distance from the cement–enamel junction (CEJ) to the maximum coronal level of the alveolar bone crest (CEJ bone distance), using IMAGE J processing software (Image J software, National Institutes of Health, Bethesda, MD, USA).

4.6. Histological Examination

Histological procedures were performed as previously reported by Reference [46] and described below. Samples were fixed in 10% (*w/v*) PBS-buffered formaldehyde solution at 25 °C for 24 h, after which they were dehydrated via an increasing scale of alcohols and xylene, included in paraffin, and cut under the microtome to obtain sections of 7 micrometers. After being hydrated, tissue sections were stained with Hematoxylin/Eosin (H&E, Bio-Optica, Milano, Italy). A histological injury score for gingivomucosal tissue was determined, using a semiquantitative scale that measures the subsequent morphological criteria: 0, normal gingivomucosal tissue; grade 1, minimal edema or infiltration; grade 2, moderate edema and inflammatory cell infiltration without obvious damage to gingivomucosal architecture; and grade 3, severe inflammatory cell infiltration with obvious damage to gingivomucosal architecture. For H&E staining, the results were shown at 10x magnification (100 μm scale bar). All the histological studies were performed in a blinded fashion.

4.7. Myeloperoxidase Activity

Myeloperoxidase (MPO) is an enzyme contained in the azurophilic granules of polymorphonuclear neutrophils and macrophages and is released in the extracellular liquid in the presence of inflammatory states. Various studies have highlighted how MPO is related to oxidative stress and inflammatory processes; its determination is, therefore, a useful biomarker for diagnostic purposes.

MPO activity was determined in gingivomucosal tissues as previously described by Reference [47]. Samples were homogenized in a buffer containing 0.5% hexadecyl-trimethyl-ammonium bromide dissolved in 10 mM potassium phosphate buffer, pH 7, and centrifuged for 30 min, at 20,000 rpm at 4 °C. Subsequently, the fraction "supernatant" was reacted with a solution of 1.6 vmM tetramethylbenzidine and 0.1 mM H_2O_2. The rate of change in absorbance was measured spectrophotometrically at 650 nm. MPO activity was measured as the quantity of enzyme degrading 1 mM of peroxide 1 min at 37 °C and was expressed in units per gram weight of wet tissue.

4.8. Masson Trichrome Stain

Masson's trichrome is a coloring particularly useful for highlighting connective tissue, collagen, reticular fibers, and muscle fibers. Thus, to assess fibrosis degree, gingivomucosal sections were stained with the Masson trichrome stain, according to the manufacturer's instructions (Bio-Optica, Milan, Italy). For Masson trichrome staining, the results were shown at 10x magnification (100 μm scale bar).

4.9. Blue Toluidine Staining

To evaluate mast cell amount and their degranulation, gingivomucosal sections were stained with toluidine blue (Bio-Optica, Milano, Italy). This basic dye colors the sections blue, highlighting the mast cells that appear purple. The number of metachromatic stained mast cells was obtained by counting five high-power fields for the section, using an Axiovision Zeiss (Milan, Italy) microscope and the correlated AxioVision software (Carl Zeiss Vision, Jena, Germany). Data were reported as the mean with standard deviation (SD). For toluidine blue staining, results were shown at 40× magnification (20 µm scale bar).

4.10. Western Blot Analysis for IκB-α, NF-κB, COX-2, and iNOS

Cytosolic and nuclear extracts of gingivomucosal tissues were prepared as previously described by Reference [48].

In the cytosolic fraction, the expressions of kappa light polypeptide gene enhancer in B cells inhibitor alpha (IκB-α), iNOS, and cyclooxygenase 2 (COX-2) were quantified.

In the nuclear fraction, the expression of NF-κB was quantified. Filters were blocked with 1× PBS, 5% (*w/v*) nonfat dried milk (PM), for 40 min, at room temperature, and then probed with following antibodies: anti-IkB-α (1:500, Santa Cruz Biotechnology, Dallas, Texas, USA #sc1643), anti-NF-κB (1:500, Santa Cruz Biotechnology, #sc8008), anti-Cox2 (1:500, Santa Cruz Biotechnology, #sc-1746), anti-iNOS (1:500, Santa Cruz Biotechnology, #sc8310) in 1× PBS, and 0.1% Tween-20, 5% *w/v* nonfat dried milk (PMT) at 4 °C, overnight. After that, the membranes were incubated with peroxidase-conjugated bovine anti-mouse IgG secondary antibody or peroxidase-conjugated goat anti-rabbit IgG (1:2000, Jackson ImmunoResearch, West Grove, Pennsylvania, USA) for 1 h, at room temperature. To ascertain that blots were loaded with equal amounts of proteins, they were also incubated in the presence of the antibody against GAPDH (cytosolic fraction 1:500; Santa Cruz Biotechnology) or lamin A/C (nuclear fraction 1:500 Sigma-Aldrich Corp.), as described by Reference [49].

4.11. ELISA Assay for TNF- α and IL-6

ELISA assay was performed as described by Campolo M. et al. [50].

Gingivomucosal tissues were thawed on ice and homogenized in 300 µL lysis buffer (750 µL, Pierce #87787, Thermo Fisher Scientific, Waltham, MA, USA) and then complemented with a protease inhibitor cocktail (Sigma-Aldrich, Rehovot, Israel). Subsequently, the samples were homogenized and centrifuged at 14,000× *g* for 10 min at 4 °C; supernatants were collected, aliquoted, and deposited at −20 °C. Cytokines levels were measured by ELISA, according to the manufacturer's instructions.

4.12. Statistical Analysis

All values are showed as mean ± standard error of the mean (SEM) of N observations. N denotes the number of animals employed. The experiment is representative of at least three experiments performed on different days on tissue sections collected from all animals in each group. Data were analyzed by one-way ANOVA, followed by a Bonferroni post hoc test for multiple comparisons. A *P*-value of less than 0.05 was considered significant.

Author Contributions: Conceptualization, I.P. and E.E.; methodology, A.A., M.L. and E.G.; validation, M.P. and A.M.; formal analysis, G.C. and M.L.; investigation, G.C. and A.A.; resources, E.E. and S.C.; data curation, E.G. and M.L.; writing—original draft preparation, A.A. and G.C.; writing—review and editing, I.P. and E.E.; supervision, M.P., A.M., I.P. and S.C. All authors have read and agreed to the published version of the manuscript.

Funding: This research received no external funding.

Conflicts of Interest: The authors declare no conflict of interest.

References

1. Gasner, N.S.; Schure, R.S. *Periodontal Disease*; StatPearls: Treasure Island, FL, USA, 2020.
2. Van Dyke, T.E.; Sima, C. Understanding resolution of inflammation in periodontal diseases: Is chronic inflammatory periodontitis a failure to resolve? *Periodontol. 2000* **2020**, *82*, 205–213. [CrossRef] [PubMed]
3. Nazir, M.A. Prevalence of periodontal disease, its association with systemic diseases and prevention. *Int. J. Health Sci. (Qassim)* **2017**, *11*, 72–80.
4. Riley, M. Incorrect nutrition as a risk factor for periodontal disease. *Alpha Omegan* **2007**, *100*, 85–88. [CrossRef] [PubMed]
5. Leite, F.R.M.; Nascimento, G.G.; Scheutz, F.; Lopez, R. Effect of Smoking on Periodontitis: A Systematic Review and Meta-regression. *Am. J. Prev. Med.* **2018**, *54*, 831–841. [CrossRef]
6. Lertpimonchai, A.; Rattanasiri, S.; Arj-Ong Vallibhakara, S.; Attia, J.; Thakkinstian, A. The association between oral hygiene and periodontitis: A systematic review and meta-analysis. *Int. Dent. J.* **2017**, *67*, 332–343. [CrossRef]
7. Hassell, T.M.; Harris, E.L. Genetic influences in caries and periodontal diseases. *Crit. Rev. Oral Biol. Med.* **1995**, *6*, 319–342. [CrossRef]
8. Duran-Pinedo, A.E.; Chen, T.; Teles, R.; Starr, J.R.; Wang, X.; Krishnan, K.; Frias-Lopez, J. Community-wide transcriptome of the oral microbiome in subjects with and without periodontitis. *ISME J.* **2014**, *8*, 1659–1672. [CrossRef]
9. Sbordone, L.; Bortolaia, C. Oral microbial biofilms and plaque-related diseases: Microbial communities and their role in the shift from oral health to disease. *Clin. Oral Investig.* **2003**, *7*, 181–188. [CrossRef]
10. Barksby, H.E.; Nile, C.J.; Jaedicke, K.M.; Taylor, J.J.; Preshaw, P.M. Differential expression of immunoregulatory genes in monocytes in response to Porphyromonas gingivalis and Escherichia coli lipopolysaccharide. *Clin. Exp. Immunol.* **2009**, *156*, 479–487. [CrossRef]
11. Kinney, J.S.; Ramseier, C.A.; Giannobile, W.V. Oral fluid-based biomarkers of alveolar bone loss in periodontitis. *Ann. N. Y. Acad. Sci.* **2007**, *1098*, 230–251. [CrossRef]
12. Gugliandolo, E.; Fusco, R.; D'Amico, R.; Peditto, M.; Oteri, G.; Di Paola, R.; Cuzzocrea, S.; Navarra, M. Treatment With a Flavonoid-Rich Fraction of Bergamot Juice Improved Lipopolysaccharide-Induced Periodontitis in Rats. *Front. Pharmacol.* **2018**, *9*, 1563. [CrossRef] [PubMed]
13. Hughes, F.J.; Bartold, P.M. Periodontal complications of prescription and recreational drugs. *Periodontol. 2000* **2018**, *78*, 47–58. [CrossRef] [PubMed]
14. Feres, M.; Figueiredo, L.C.; Soares, G.M.; Faveri, M. Systemic antibiotics in the treatment of periodontitis. *Periodontol. 2000* **2015**, *67*, 131–186. [CrossRef] [PubMed]
15. Szulc, M.; Zakrzewska, A.; Zborowski, J. Local drug delivery in periodontitis treatment: A review of contemporary literature. *Dent. Med. Probl.* **2018**, *55*, 333–342. [CrossRef] [PubMed]
16. Fan, X.; Du, K.; Li, N.; Zheng, Z.; Qin, Y.; Liu, J.; Sun, R.; Su, Y. Evaluation of Anti-Nociceptive and Anti-Inflammatory Effect of Luteolin in Mice. *J. Environ. Pathol. Toxicol. Oncol.* **2018**, *37*, 351–364. [CrossRef]
17. Lopez-Lazaro, M. Distribution and biological activities of the flavonoid luteolin. *Mini Rev. Med. Chem.* **2009**, *9*, 31–59. [CrossRef]
18. Palombo, R.; Caporali, S.; Falconi, M.; Iacovelli, F.; Morozzo Della Rocca, B.; Lo Surdo, A.; Campione, E.; Candi, E.; Melino, G.; Bernardini, S.; et al. Luteolin-7-O-beta-d-Glucoside Inhibits Cellular Energy Production Interacting with HEK2 in Keratinocytes. *Int. J. Mol. Sci.* **2019**, *20*, 2689. [CrossRef]
19. Zhang, T.; Kimura, Y.; Jiang, S.; Harada, K.; Yamashita, Y.; Ashida, H. Luteolin modulates expression of drug-metabolizing enzymes through the AhR and Nrf2 pathways in hepatic cells. *Arch. Biochem. Biophys.* **2014**, *557*, 36–46. [CrossRef]
20. Aziz, N.; Kim, M.Y.; Cho, J.Y. Anti-inflammatory effects of luteolin: A review of in vitro, in vivo, and in silico studies. *J. Ethnopharmacol.* **2018**, *225*, 342–358. [CrossRef]
21. Ruiz, P.A.; Haller, D. Functional diversity of flavonoids in the inhibition of the proinflammatory NF-kappaB, IRF, and Akt signaling pathways in murine intestinal epithelial cells. *J. Nutr.* **2006**, *136*, 664–671. [CrossRef]
22. Seelinger, G.; Merfort, I.; Schempp, C.M. Anti-oxidant, anti-inflammatory and anti-allergic activities of luteolin. *Planta Med.* **2008**, *74*, 1667–1677. [CrossRef] [PubMed]

23. Zheng, X.Y.; Mao, C.Y.; Qiao, H.; Zhang, X.; Yu, L.; Wang, T.Y.; Lu, E.Y. Plumbagin suppresses chronic periodontitis in rats via down-regulation of TNF-alpha, IL-1beta and IL-6 expression. *Acta Pharmacol. Sin.* **2017**, *38*, 1150–1160. [CrossRef] [PubMed]
24. Golub, L.M.; Lee, H.M. Periodontal therapeutics: Current host-modulation agents and future directions. *Periodontol. 2000* **2020**, *82*, 186–204. [CrossRef] [PubMed]
25. Thomford, N.E.; Senthebane, D.A.; Rowe, A.; Munro, D.; Seele, P.; Maroyi, A.; Dzobo, K. Natural Products for Drug Discovery in the 21st Century: Innovations for Novel Drug Discovery. *Int. J. Mol. Sci.* **2018**, *19*, 1578. [CrossRef]
26. Imran, M.; Rauf, A.; Abu-Izneid, T.; Nadeem, M.; Shariati, M.A.; Khan, I.A.; Imran, A.; Orhan, I.E.; Rizwan, M.; Atif, M.; et al. Luteolin, a flavonoid, as an anticancer agent: A review. *Biomed. Pharmacother.* **2019**, *112*, 108612. [CrossRef]
27. Lin, Y.; Shi, R.; Wang, X.; Shen, H.M. Luteolin, a flavonoid with potential for cancer prevention and therapy. *Curr. Cancer Drug Targets* **2008**, *8*, 634–646. [CrossRef]
28. Nabavi, S.F.; Braidy, N.; Gortzi, O.; Sobarzo-Sanchez, E.; Daglia, M.; Skalicka-Wozniak, K.; Nabavi, S.M. Luteolin as an anti-inflammatory and neuroprotective agent: A brief review. *Brain Res. Bull.* **2015**, *119*, 1–11. [CrossRef] [PubMed]
29. Franco, Y.E.M.; de Lima, C.A.; Rosa, M.N.; Silva, V.A.O.; Reis, R.M.; Priolli, D.G.; Carvalho, P.O.; do Nascimento, J.R.; da Rocha, C.Q.; Longato, G.B. Investigation of U-251 cell death triggered by flavonoid luteolin: Towards a better understanding on its anticancer property against glioblastomas. *Nat. Prod. Res.* **2020**. [CrossRef]
30. Ahmadi, S.M.; Farhoosh, R.; Sharif, A.; Rezaie, M. Structure-Antioxidant Activity Relationships of Luteolin and Catechin. *J. Food Sci.* **2020**, *85*, 298–305. [CrossRef]
31. Hienz, S.A.; Paliwal, S.; Ivanovski, S. Mechanisms of Bone Resorption in Periodontitis. *J. Immunol. Res.* **2015**, *2015*, 615486. [CrossRef]
32. Hoare, A.; Soto, C.; Rojas-Celis, V.; Bravo, D. Chronic Inflammation as a Link between Periodontitis and Carcinogenesis. *Mediat. Inflamm.* **2019**, *2019*, 1029857. [CrossRef] [PubMed]
33. Kononen, E.; Gursoy, M.; Gursoy, U.K. Periodontitis: A Multifaceted Disease of Tooth-Supporting Tissues. *J. Clin. Med.* **2019**, *8*, 1135. [CrossRef] [PubMed]
34. Parkos, C.A. Neutrophil-Epithelial Interactions: A Double-Edged Sword. *Am. J. Pathol.* **2016**, *186*, 1404–1416. [CrossRef] [PubMed]
35. Fine, N.; Hassanpour, S.; Borenstein, A.; Sima, C.; Oveisi, M.; Scholey, J.; Cherney, D.; Glogauer, M. Distinct Oral Neutrophil Subsets Define Health and Periodontal Disease States. *J. Dent. Res.* **2016**, *95*, 931–938. [CrossRef]
36. LSF, E.R.; Dos Santos, J.N.; Rocha, C.A.G.; Cury, P.R. Association Between Mast Cells and Collagen Maturation in Chronic Periodontitis in Humans. *J. Histochem. Cytochem.* **2018**, *66*, 467–475. [CrossRef]
37. Gonzalez-de-Olano, D.; Alvarez-Twose, I. Mast Cells as Key Players in Allergy and Inflammation. *J. Investig. Allergol. Clin. Immunol.* **2018**, *28*, 365–378. [CrossRef]
38. Diomede, F.; Zingariello, M.; Cavalcanti, M.; Merciaro, I.; Pizzicannella, J.; De Isla, N.; Caputi, S.; Ballerini, P.; Trubiani, O. MyD88/ERK/NFkB pathways and pro-inflammatory cytokines release in periodontal ligament stem cells stimulated by Porphyromonas gingivalis. *Eur. J. Histochem.* **2017**, *61*, 2791. [CrossRef]
39. Venugopal, P.; Koshy, T.; Lavu, V.; Ranga Rao, S.; Ramasamy, S.; Hariharan, S.; Venkatesan, V. Differential expression of microRNAs let-7a, miR-125b, miR-100, and miR-21 and interaction with NF-kB pathway genes in periodontitis pathogenesis. *J. Cell Physiol.* **2018**, *233*, 5877–5884. [CrossRef]
40. Dessaune Neto, N.; Porpino, M.T.M.; Antunes, H.D.S.; Rodrigues, R.C.V.; Perez, A.R.; Pires, F.R.; Siqueira, J.F., Jr.; Armada, L. Pro-inflammatory and anti-inflammatory cytokine expression in post-treatment apical periodontitis. *J. Appl. Oral Sci.* **2018**, *26*, e20170455. [CrossRef]
41. Wang, Y.Y.; Lin, X.P. Detection and significance of IL-6 and TNF-alpha in patients with Graves disease and periodontitis. *Shanghai Kou Qiang Yi Xue* **2018**, *27*, 43–47.
42. Lang, N.P.; Schatzle, M.A.; Loe, H. Gingivitis as a risk factor in periodontal disease. *J. Clin. Periodontol.* **2009**, *36* (Suppl. 10), 3–8. [CrossRef] [PubMed]
43. Gugliandolo, E.; Fusco, R.; D'Amico, R.; Militi, A.; Oteri, G.; Wallace, J.L.; Di Paola, R.; Cuzzocrea, S. Anti-inflammatory effect of ATB-352, a H2S -releasing ketoprofen derivative, on lipopolysaccharide-induced periodontitis in rats. *Pharmacol. Res.* **2018**, *132*, 220–231. [CrossRef]

44. Boeing, T.; de Souza, P.; Speca, S.; Somensi, L.B.; Mariano, L.N.B.; Cury, B.J.; Ferreira Dos Anjos, M.; Quintao, N.L.M.; Dubuqoy, L.; Desreumax, P.; et al. Luteolin prevents irinotecan-induced intestinal mucositis in mice through antioxidant and anti-inflammatory properties. *Br. J. Pharmacol.* **2020**, *177*, 2393–2408. [CrossRef] [PubMed]
45. Ding, X.; Zheng, L.; Yang, B.; Wang, X.; Ying, Y. Luteolin Attenuates Atherosclerosis Via Modulating Signal Transducer And Activator Of Transcription 3-Mediated Inflammatory Response. *Drug Des. Devel. Ther.* **2019**, *13*, 3899–3911. [CrossRef] [PubMed]
46. Esposito, E.; Campolo, M.; Casili, G.; Lanza, M.; Franco, D.; Filippone, A.; Peritore, A.F.; Cuzzocrea, S. Protective Effects of Xyloglucan in Association with the Polysaccharide Gelose in an Experimental Model of Gastroenteritis and Urinary Tract Infections. *Int. J. Mol. Sci.* **2018**, *19*, 1844. [CrossRef]
47. Casili, G.; Cordaro, M.; Impellizzeri, D.; Bruschetta, G.; Paterniti, I.; Cuzzocrea, S.; Esposito, E. Dimethyl Fumarate Reduces Inflammatory Responses in Experimental Colitis. *J. Crohns Colitis* **2016**, *10*, 472–483. [CrossRef]
48. Campolo, M.; Ahmad, A.; Crupi, R.; Impellizzeri, D.; Morabito, R.; Esposito, E.; Cuzzocrea, S. Combination therapy with melatonin and dexamethasone in a mouse model of traumatic brain injury. *J. Endocrinol.* **2013**, *217*, 291–301. [CrossRef]
49. Casili, G.; Campolo, M.; Paterniti, I.; Lanza, M.; Filippone, A.; Cuzzocrea, S.; Esposito, E. Dimethyl Fumarate Attenuates Neuroinflammation and Neurobehavioral Deficits Induced by Experimental Traumatic Brain Injury. *J. Neurotrauma* **2018**, *35*, 1437–1451. [CrossRef]
50. Campolo, M.; Casili, G.; Paterniti, I.; Filippone, A.; Lanza, M.; Ardizzone, A.; Scuderi, S.A.; Cuzzocrea, S.; Esposito, E. Effect of a Product Containing Xyloglucan and Pea Protein on a Murine Model of Atopic Dermatitis. *Int. J. Mol. Sci.* **2020**, *21*, 3596. [CrossRef]

Publisher's Note: MDPI stays neutral with regard to jurisdictional claims in published maps and institutional affiliations.

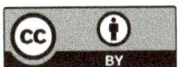

© 2020 by the authors. Licensee MDPI, Basel, Switzerland. This article is an open access article distributed under the terms and conditions of the Creative Commons Attribution (CC BY) license (http://creativecommons.org/licenses/by/4.0/).

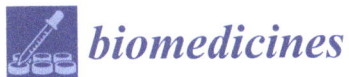

Review

Molecular Insights into the Multifunctional Role of Natural Compounds: Autophagy Modulation and Cancer Prevention

Md. Ataur Rahman [1,2,3,*], **MD. Hasanur Rahman** [3,4], **Md. Shahadat Hossain** [3,5], **Partha Biswas** [3,6], **Rokibul Islam** [2,7], **Md Jamal Uddin** [3,8], **Md. Habibur Rahman** [9] and **Hyewhon Rhim** [1,10,*]

1. Center for Neuroscience, Korea Institute of Science and Technology (KIST), 5 Hwarang-ro 14-gil, Seoul 02792, Korea
2. Global Biotechnology & Biomedical Research Network (GBBRN), Department of Biotechnology and Genetic Engineering, Faculty of Biological Sciences, Islamic University, Kushtia 7003, Bangladesh; mrislam@btge.iu.ac.bd
3. ABEx Bio-Research Center, East Azampur, Dhaka 1230, Bangladesh; hasanurrahman.bge@gmail.com (M.H.R.); shahadat4099@gmail.com (M.S.H.); parthabiswas2025@gmail.com (P.B.); hasan800920@gmail.com (M.J.U.)
4. Department of Biotechnology and Genetic Engineering, Bangabandhu Sheikh Mujibur Rahman Science and Technology University, Gopalganj 8100, Bangladesh
5. Department of Biotechnology and Genetic Engineering, Noakhali Science and Technology University, Noakhali 3814, Bangladesh
6. Department of Genetic Engineering and Biotechnology, Jashore University of Science and Technology, Jashore 7408, Bangladesh
7. Department of Biotechnology and Genetic Engineering, Faculty of Biological Sciences, Islamic University, Kushtia 7003, Bangladesh
8. Graduate School of Pharmaceutical Sciences, College of Pharmacy, Ewha Womans University, Seoul 03760, Korea
9. Department of Global Medical Science, Wonju College of Medicine, Yonsei University, Seoul 03722, Korea; pharmacisthabib@gmail.com
10. Division of Bio-Medical Science and Technology, KIST School, Korea University of Science and Technology (UST), Seoul 02792, Korea
* Correspondence: mar13bge@gmail.com (M.A.R.); hrhim@kist.re.kr (H.R.); Tel.: +82-2-958-5923 (H.R.); Fax: +82-2-958-6937 (H.R.)

Received: 15 October 2020; Accepted: 12 November 2020; Published: 19 November 2020

Abstract: Autophagy is a vacuolar, lysosomal degradation pathway for injured and damaged protein molecules and organelles in eukaryotic cells, which is controlled by nutrients and stress responses. Dysregulation of cellular autophagy may lead to various diseases such as neurodegenerative disease, obesity, cardiovascular disease, diabetes, and malignancies. Recently, natural compounds have come to attention for being able to modulate the autophagy pathway in cancer prevention, although the prospective role of autophagy in cancer treatment is very complex and not yet clearly elucidated. Numerous synthetic chemicals have been identified that modulate autophagy and are favorable candidates for cancer treatment, but they have adverse side effects. Therefore, different phytochemicals, which include natural compounds and their derivatives, have attracted significant attention for use as autophagy modulators in cancer treatment with minimal side effects. In the current review, we discuss the promising role of natural compounds in modulating the autophagy pathway to control and prevent cancer, and provide possible therapeutic options.

Keywords: autophagy; cancer; phytochemical; natural compound; treatment

1. Introduction

Autophagy is triggered by the entrapment of abnormal intracellular proteins, invading microorganisms, and damaged organelles with the formation of double-layer autophagosomes, in the presence of nutrient stress, injury, and fasting [1,2]. Along with cellular energy stability, autophagy contributes to the control of cellular quality, and destruction of abnormal proteins and damaged organelles [3]. As a result, the origin and development of many diseases, such as neurodegenerative disorders, cancer, and autoimmune diseases, can be explained by defective autophagy [4]. Multiple data states a connection between the variety of diet and feedback to cancer medication [5]. It has been established that sufficient consumption of dietary and medicinal plant-derived biochemical compounds lowers the frequency of cancer mortality. This occurs due to the activation or balancing of various cellular oncogenes. In different human disorders, including cancer, there is documented evidence of reduction of autophagic regulation. Several lines of evidence have shown that cancer plays a critical role in inhibiting or augmenting autophagic pathways [6]. In addition, this dual role of autophagy has a significant therapeutic benefit against cancer [7]. The present report has established that natural product-derived bioactive molecules, along with lysosomal inhibitors, including chloroquine (CQ) and hydroxychloroquine (HCQ) are important regulators of autophagy signaling [8]. In addition, these proactive molecules can regulate the process of autophagy both in vitro and in vivo by involving the enzymes, transcription factors, and various intracellular communication pathways [9]. The autophagy stimulation or prohibition process is vastly complicated and regulated, so it needs to be extensively explored. However, emerging evidence has implicated that extreme or damaged autophagy might lead to a unique type of cell death known as autophagic cell death [10]. Conversely, the proposal of using natural compounds as anti-cancer and autophagy-modulating agents requires a better understanding of their cellular and molecular mechanisms. The mechanism of action needs to be further addressed.

In this review, we compiled the cellular and molecular mechanisms involved in the dual role of autophagy, as a tumor-suppressing as well as a tumor-augmenting phenomenon in cancer. Current improvements in the use of natural bioactive compounds for cancer treatment by targeting autophagic action have been consistently analyzed [11]. Given the vital role of autophagy in cancer prevention and treatment, we closely reviewed different plant-derived biomolecules that may play a role in modulating the autophagy-linked signaling pathways as well as contribute towards competent treatment strategies against specific molecular aspects in cancer. In particular, administration of naturally derived compounds have been considered to regulate autophagy modulation, which might help improve our understanding of the mechanisms of natural compounds in the management and treatment of autophagy-linked diseases and cancers.

2. Mechanisms of Autophagy Signaling Pathway

Autophagy is a sensitive and tightly mannered process that has multiple steps [12]. Proteins crucial for autophagy were first reported in yeast and are termed as autophagy-related (Atg) proteins [1,13]. Multiple sequential molecular events take place to initiate the autophagy signaling cascade. First, an Atg1/unc51-like kinase (ULK) complex kinase regulates the induction, and the BECN1/class III PI3K complex initiates the nucleation of vesicles [14]. In addition, ubiquitin-like conjugation systems (Atg12 and Atg8/LC3B) control vesicle elongation as well as retrieval of lipids mediated by transmembrane Atg9 and associated proteins, which involve other Atg proteins [15]. Lysosome-associated membrane protein 2 (LAMP2) and RAS-related protein-7 (RAB7A) participate in the fusion between lysosomes and autophagosome formation [16]. Finally, vesicle breakdown and degradation by lysosomal hydrolases produce recyclable products [17] (Figure 1). Microtubule-associated protein 1 light chain 3-beta (MAP1LC3B) and Atg5-Atg12 complex pathways, which are ubiquitin-like pathways, are regulatory for vesicle elongation and are encoded by the yeast Atg8 pathway, which has a human homologue [18]. Following the autophagy response, human Atg4 cysteine protease cleaves LC3B protein and thereby produces the LC3B-I isoform [19]. Activated LC3B-I isoform causes the activation of Atg7 protein through LC3B-I and is transported to the Atg3 before formation of the LC3B-II isoform by the phosphatidylethanolamine (PE) conjugation with the carboxyl glycine of LC3B-I protein [20]. As a consequence, elevated synthesis and processing of LC3B shows promise and has been mentioned as a key marker of autophagy [20]. In the degradation of matured autophagosomes through the enzymatic action of lysosomal enzymes, small molecules are produced that are used for de novo protein synthesis, helping in survival and maintenance of homeostasis [21].

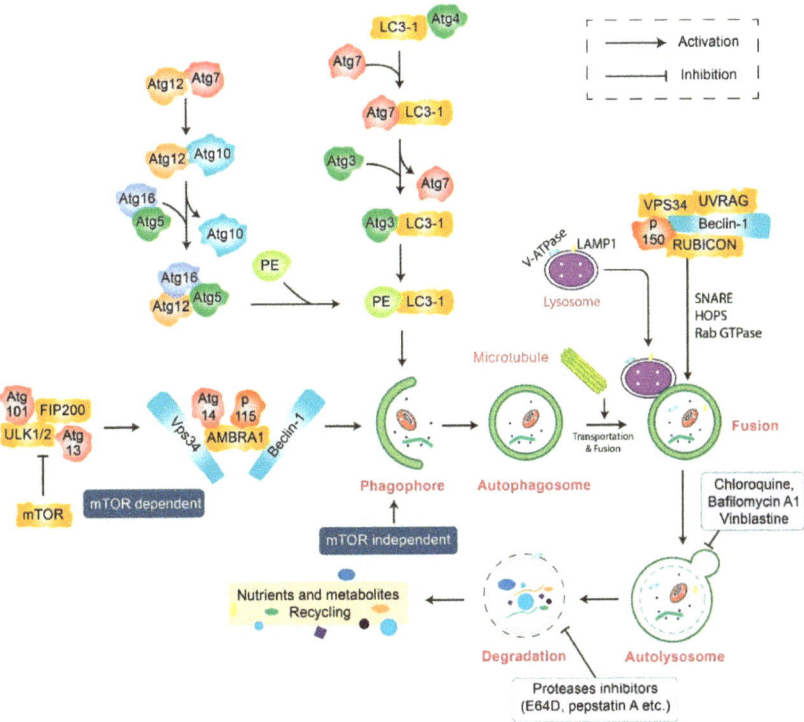

Figure 1. Molecular mechanism of autophagy signaling. Autophagy is generally initiated by a deficiency of growth factors or nutrients that trigger AMPK or mTOR inhibition. This stimulates FIP200 and Atg13 associated ULK complex. After that phosphorylation of Beclin-1, it leads to the activation of VPS34, which further initiates the formation of phagophore. Conjugation of Atg5-Atg12 encompasses Atg7 as well as Atg10 to form an Atg12-Atg5-Atg16 complex that also stimulates phagophores formation. Atg5, in addition to Atg12, makes an Atg16 complex, which acts as an E3-function concerning LC3-PE assembly (LC3-II). This complex likewise initiates the formation of a phagophore. Specifically, LC3-II is an autophagy marker that is ultimately interrupted via autolysosomes. Maturation of autophagosome leads to fusion with lysosomes in association with several lysosomal proteins, finally leading to degradation of cargo in addition to recycling of metabolites and nutrients.

3. Molecular Mechanism of Autophagy Signaling in Cancer Pathogenesis

Under healthy conditions, cells have an innate ability for autophagy mechanisms to defend against malignant transformation [22]. Generally, autophagy is initiated by the induction of tumor-suppressing proteins, and oncoproteins are reported to inhibit this action [23]. Therefore, autophagy can act in both pro-survival and pro-death stages of tumor initiation and development [23]. The disturbed autophagy pathway can contribute to tumor development, as it leads to accumulation of damaged organelles and protein aggregates, which ultimately produce reactive oxygen species (ROS) and lead to genome instability [24]. Several researchers have reported that chemotherapeutics and avenues for cancer treatment can be accelerated by altering autophagic signaling that result in tumor cell death by inhibition of pro-survival and tissue specific apoptosis inducing factors [25]. Additionally, autophagy has been described as having a dual function in the promotion as well as inhibition of metastasis [26]. In the early stages, autophagy prevents metastasis, whereas in later stages it favors metastatic activity [26]. However, poorly vascularized tumor cells may survive at low nutrient and low oxygen levels through TGF-β, and other signals that trigger autophagy [27]. Furthermore, autophagy has directly regulated the metastatic cascade mainly through migration, invasion, and epithelial to mesenchymal transition (EMT) of cancer cells [26,28]. The importance of autophagy at diverse stages of tumorigenesis and metastasis is illustrated in Figure 2. It has been found that many cells within the tumors such as immune cells, fibroblasts, and endothelial cells are surrounded by the tumor microenvironment and have been acknowledged as an attractive target to reduce resistance to anticancer treatment. Natural compounds from vegetables, spices, marine organisms, herbs, and fruits have been reported to prevent or reverse multistage carcinogenesis as well as to prevent cancerous cell proliferation [29]. Additionally, microRNAs (miRNAs), which control the expression of genes, play an important role in diverse biological processes. It has been found that miRNA expression dysregulation is highly related to cancer development [30]. Recently, several studies have shown that natural compounds, such as paclitaxel (PTX), genistein, curcumin, epigallocatechin-3-gallate (EGCG), and resveratrol exhibit pro-apoptotic or anti-proliferative properties that are controlled by miRNAs, and lead to inhibition of cancer cell growth and proliferation, apoptosis induction, and improvement of conventional cancer treatment and therapeutic efficiency [30]. However, these naturally occurring compounds could be modulated by different signal transduction pathways through their connection via cancer cells, tumor microenvironment, and miRNA. These are described later in this study.

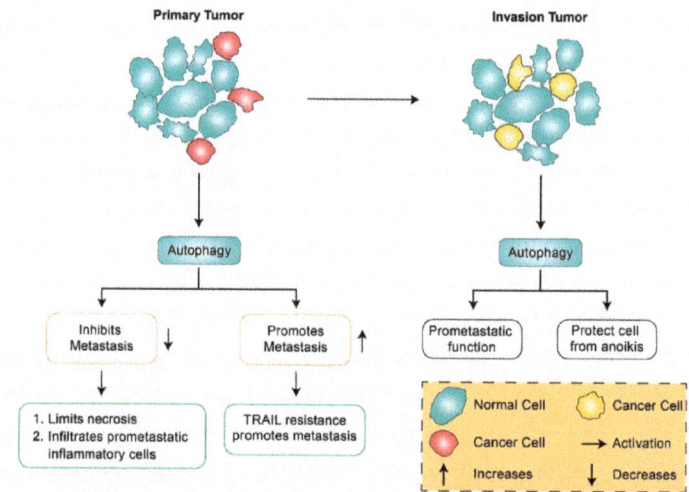

Figure 2. In cancer cells, autophagy exhibits a dual role in metastasis and invasion. Depending on the stage and type of tumor cell, autophagy can prevent or stimulate cancer cell maintenance. In the early stages of autophagy in primary tumors, metastasis has been suppressed via anti-metastatic elements in addition to stimulation of tumor conservation along with progression by inducing cellular resistance against TRAIL, a tumor necrosis factor-related apoptosis-inducing ligand, to induce apoptosis. Later, in the course of invasion, tumor cells spread and enter lymphatic or blood vessels. Here, autophagy shows a pro-metastatic function through cell protection from anoikis triggered via extracellular matrix detachment.

3.1. Autophagy Signaling Roles in Cancer Inhibition

Several studies have reported that autophagy inhibition via manipulated pharmacological or genetic tools can be a possible chemotherapeutic option. Recently, scientists have focused on the combined treatment of chemically synthesized autophagy inhibitors and traditional chemotherapeutics [31]. Cancer cell sensitization with 3-methyladenine (3-MA), wortmannin, CQ, LY294002, bafilomycin A1 (Baf A1), and HCQ-like inhibitors of autophagy to chemotherapeutic drugs have been reported to accelerate cell death pathway action [32,33]. In the abovementioned inhibitors, some of them are preliminary stage inhibitors of autophagy, like wortmannin, LY294002, and 3-MA, which block the autophagosomes formation, while others act on the basis of lysosomal action at late stages [34]. Table 1 shows several valuable effects of natural compounds combined with some autophagy inhibitors in different cellular cancer models. In breast cancer cells, the pro-survival nature of cancer cells can be downregulated by LC3 via shRNA blocking and sensitization of the carcinoma cells to apoptotic factors such as trastuzumab [35]. In leukemia, pro-survival function with pharmacological inhibitors or RNAi can also block accelerated induced cell death by imatinib mesylate [36]. Autophagy can sensitize and make cells susceptible to radiotherapy, such as HBL-100 cells, for radiotherapy treatment, and 3-MA leads to the inhibition of autophagy by imposing the pro-death effects of therapy [37]. In BIF-1 knockout mice, there is impairment of autophagy in addition to an increase in the rate of tumor formation, while mutations in UVRAG decrease autophagy along with increased proliferation of colorectal cancer cells [38]. These reports propose that Beclin-1 acts as an insufficient tumor-suppressor gene and fully incorporates the theory of tumor-suppressive autophagy induction at early stages [39]. In the livers of mice, Atg gene deletion can lead to the formation of multiple benign tumors. In systematic mosaic Atg5 and Atg7 deletion mice, these specific deletions magnify the chance of tumor induction and lead to tumor development [40]. At early stages of cancer formation, Atg4 suppresses tumor developing activity and Atg4c deficiency is proven to be more easily identifiable in chemical carcinogen-induced fibrosarcoma. These reports help to understand the suppressive roles of autophagy in cancer with genetic deletion of specific regions [41].

Table 1. Mechanism of action of combination of natural compounds and autophagy blockers, 3-methyladenine (3-MA), chloroquine (CQ), and bafilomycin A1 (Baf A1) in modulating autophagy and apoptosis in various cancer cell models.

Natural Compound/Chemical	Cell Model	Molecular Mechanisms	Combination with Autophagy Inhibitors	References
18α-Glycyrrhetinic acid	Neuroblastoma	Autophagy and apoptosis induction	CQ combination induces cell death	[42]
Resveratrol	Glioblastomas	Induction of apoptosis and autophagy via reduction of ROS/MAPK pathway	Baf A1 combination augments apoptotic cell death	[43]
Curcumin	Glioblastomas	Induction of autophagy and apoptosis	CQ combination rises apoptotic cell death	[44]
Gintonin	Cortical astrocytes and glioblastoma cells	Induction of autophagy	CQ and Baf A1 combination stimulates autophagy	[45]
Quercetin	U373MG cells	PI3K/Akt inhibition and causes apoptosis and autophagy	CQ combination increases apoptotic cell death	[46]
Paclitaxel	Human lung carcinoma A549 cells	Induction of autophagy and apoptosis	3-MA combination enhances apoptotic cell death	[47]

Table 1. Cont.

Natural Compound/Chemical	Cell Model	Molecular Mechanisms	Combination with Autophagy Inhibitors	References
Genistein	MIA PaCa-2 human pancreatic cancer cell	Autophagy and apoptosis induction	CQ combination stimulates apoptotic cell death	[48]
Honokiol	Non-small cell lung cancer A549 and H460 cells	p62 and LC3 induces autophagy induction	Combination of CQ triggered apoptosis	[49]
Ginsenoside Compound K	Neuroblastoma SK-N-BE(2) and SH-SY5Y cells	ROS-mediated autophagy inhibition and apoptosis induction	Combination of CQ inhibit autophagy and induces apoptosis	[50]
Oxyresveratrol	Neuroblastoma SK-N-BE(2) and SH-SY5Y cells	PI3K/AKT/mTOR pathway independent autophagy and apoptosis	3-MA combination enhances apoptotic cell death	[51]

3.2. Autophagy Signaling Roles in Cancer Promotion

Autophagy induction is a possible anti-cancer mechanism in which cancer cells have a faulty or altered apoptotic cell death pathway [52]. Consequently, autophagy induction along with autophagy inhibition can induce apoptosis and exert anti-cancer effects [53]. Several inhibitors, such as Bcl-2, EGFR, and mTOR, are currently used in cancer treatment [54]. Inhibitory molecules are known to be effective against a variety of cancers, and some induce autophagy in breast cancers, gliomas, and lung cancers through rapamycin, an inhibitor of mTORC2 [54]. Another known inhibitor of the mTOR, deforolimus (AP23573, MK-8669), is proposed to treat patients with relapsed or refractory hematologic malignancies [55]. Another antibody against epidermal growth factor, cetuximab, can regulate autophagic cell death in cancer cells by disrupting the interaction between Bcl-2 and Beclin-1 [56]. Several reports explain that the expression of the viral oncogenes Kirsten and Harvey RAS virus is capable of autophagy induction in certain cells [22]. In pancreatic and colorectal cancer cells, elevated levels of RAS mutations are reported to be correlated with higher autophagy rates, where increased levels maintain cell proliferation in RAS-activated tumors and inhibition of autophagy results in reduced cell proliferation, ultimately leading to tumor regression [57]. Lung cancers are also dependent on autophagy, which is similar to the mechanism of RAS-driven cancers regulated by valine-to-glutamic acid substitution at BRAF position 600 (BRAFV600E) [58]. In vivo studies have reported that deletion of subunit FIP200 related to the ULK1 complex in autophagy initiation blocks the growth of breast cancer and extends the life cycle of mice [59]. In addition, activated AMPK generated by ATP can also trigger an autophagic event [60].

4. Natural Compound Triggers in Autophagy Modulation

A single therapeutic strategy and a combination modality can both be favorable for cancer treatment. The various strategies include radiation therapy, immune or genetic therapy, and chemotherapy, all of which create new diversions and avenues in the field of cancer treatment with adequate levels of safety and accuracy [15,61,62]. Natural compounds are effective in the positive regulation of anticancer activity, as they inhibit cellular proliferation, adjust the oxidative stress response, and manipulate autophagic signaling and response [15,63]. This entire response of natural compounds is dependent on the cell type. The role of several natural compounds that modulate different pathways of autophagy signaling is illustrated in Figure 3.

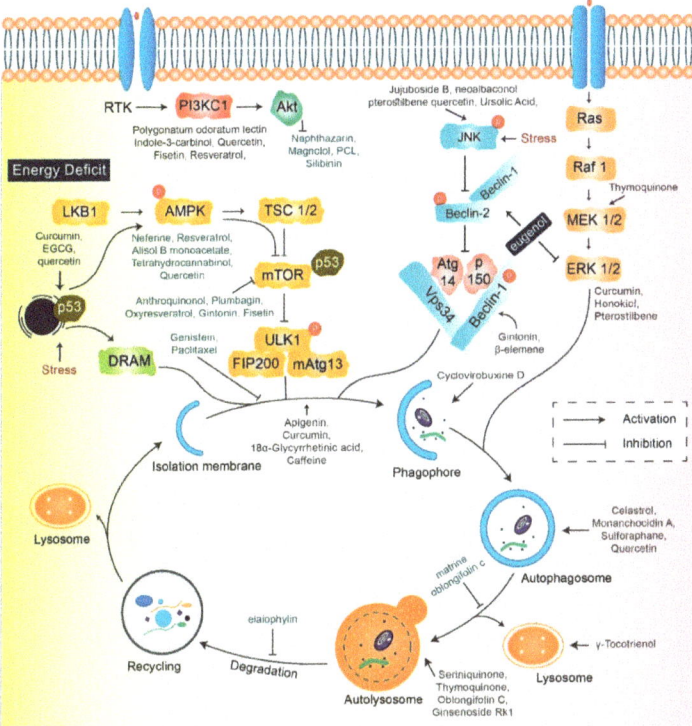

Figure 3. Key autophagy pathway and its regulators (natural compounds) for treating diverse cancers. This figure is modified from Wang et al. [64]. Natural compounds activate autophagy by several autophagic signaling targets and show a close relationship with cancer development and control. Multiple signaling pathways are activated or inhibited by natural compounds to modulate cancer cells.

4.1. Inhibition of Autophagy by Natural Compounds for Cancer Therapy

Apigenin: Apigenin, a flavonoid found in vegetables and fruits, can initiate tumor cell death through autophagy and apoptosis [65]. In combination with retinamide, N-(4-hydroxyphenyl), apigenin suppresses autophagy and increases apoptosis in human neuroblastoma (NB) cells [66].

Genistein: Genistein, a nutritive natural compound, has been documented to repress autophagy and induce apoptosis of human colon cancer HT-29 cells alone with downregulation of the PI3K/Akt signaling pathway [67]. Another mechanism of action of genistein is that it also exerts an antiproliferative effect on ovarian cancer cells through autophagy as well as apoptosis [67]. Genistein augments miR-451 expression and improves isoproterenol-mediated cardiac hypertrophy [68]. Furthermore, genistein increases miR-1469 expression and prevents Mcl-1 expression in laryngeal cancer [69].

Indole-3-carbinol: Indole-3-carbinol, a natural compound collected from cruciferous vegetables, usually inhibits the PI3K/Akt pathway along with blockage of autophagy signaling in human colon cancer HT-29 cells [67].

Plumbagin: Plumbagin is obtained from *Plumbago zeylandica* L. root and has a prompt antiproliferative activity through autophagic cell death, mediated via inhibition of AKT/mTOR pathway in human cervical cancer cells [70].

4.2. Induction of Autophagy by Natural Compounds as Potential Cancer Therapy

Antroquinonol: Antroquinonol, produced from *Antrodia Camphorata*, shows anti-tumor activity in various cancer cells [71]. Antroquinonol has been demonstrated to exhibit inhibitory effects on non-small cell lung cancer (NSCLC), as well as human pancreatic cancer, PANC-1 and ASPC-1, via the PI3K/Akt/mTOR pathway [72]. The anti-proliferative effect of antroquinonol is related to apoptosis, autophagic cell death, and rapid senescence of the pancreatic cells [72]. Several studies have demonstrated that antroquinonol can be introduced for the treatment of neoplasms [73]. A proposed clinical trial in metastatic pancreatic carcinoma is aimed at evaluating the anticancer activity of antroquinonol in combination with nab-PTX and gemcitabine [74].

18α-Glycyrrhetinic acid: 18α-Glycyrrhetinic acid (18-GA), a known gap-junction inhibitor, has been shown to demonstrate anticancer properties in human NB cells [42]. 18-GA has been shown to induce autophagy as well as apoptosis. Autophagy increases Atg5, Atg7, and LC3II along with degradation of p62 (Figure 4). Furthermore, 18-GA, along with the autophagy inhibitor CQ, induces significant cell death in NB cells. Moreover, the Bcl-2/Beclin-1 interaction in addition to the cleavage of Beclin-1 has been revealed by 18-GA in autophagy and apoptosis induced cell death. Caspase-3 siRNA and pan-caspase inhibitor treatment have been demonstrated to prevent 18-GA-induced cellular cytotoxicity, indicating that caspase-mediated apoptosis induction was observed in human NB cells [42].

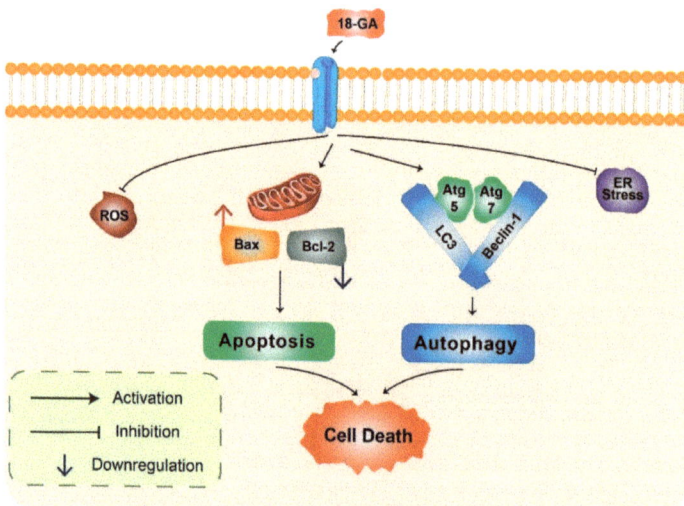

Figure 4. 18α-Glycyrrhetinic acid-mediated cell death in human neuroblastoma cells. 18-GA induces mitochondria-mediated apoptosis to alter mitochondrial membrane potential in a significant change in with Bax/Bcl-2 ratio. Autophagy-related proteins Atg5/7, Beclin-1, LC3, and p62 were activated during 18-GA-mediated autophagic cell death. Beclin-1 contributes to autophagy in addition to apoptosis induction in 18-GA-mediated cell death. Additionally, ROS and ER stress showed no changes during 18-GA treatment in SH-SY5Y and B103.

Celastrol: Celastrol, a popular natural medicinal compound triperine secreted from *Tripterygium wilfordii* Hook, is a polyubiquitinated aggregate that degrades the autophagy substrate p62 in the human glioblastoma (GBM) cancer cells [75]. Celastrol-mediated cytotoxicity was not sensitized by adjustment with autophagy inhibitors. Paraptosis-like cytoplasmic vacuolization can be induced by celastrol and has been associated with autophagy and the initiation of apoptosis in PC-3, A549, and HeLa cancer cells [76]. Celastrol can be used to treat fever, joint pain, and edema without causing any side effects [77]. Recently, many research studies have identified celastrol as a neuroprotective agent via a collaborative drug screen that can be used for the treatment of many neurodegenerative diseases.

Monanchocidin A: An active novel alkaloid, monanchocidin A, has been recently isolated from *Monanchora pulchra*, a marine sponge [78]. Monanchocidin can initiate autophagy and lysosomal membrane permeabilization in tumor cells [78]. Many studies have demonstrated that monanchocidin A can inhibit human urogenital cancers, including germ cell tumors, through autophagy signaling [79].

Paclitaxel: PTX, a natural medicinal compound isolated from *Taxus brevifolia* Nutt, shows a vast range of effect against various types of cancer such as breast, endometrial, bladder, and cervical cancer, by influencing the autophagy pathway [80]. The US Food and Drug Administration (FDA) has approved PTX for the treatment of ovarian cancer and early stage breast cancer. The anticancer activity of PTX is increased when PTX is combined with cisplatin or carboplatin, and the combined compound can be used for the early treatment of advanced ovarian cancer [81]. It has been shown that PTX can inhibit the initial stage of autophagy, along with apoptosis, under normoxic and hypoxic conditions in human breast cancer cells [82]. PTX-initiated apoptosis was combined with the initiation of autophagy in A549 lung cancer cells [47]. Treatment with PTX also initiated acidic vesicular organelle formation, Beclin-1, Atg5, and LC3 expression, and the prevention of autophagy proceeds via PTX-mediated cell death [83,84]. Autophagy can promote PTX-mediated cell death. In human breast cancer cells, PTX prevents autophagy via an individual mechanism based on the cell-cycle phase [84].

Gintonin: Gintonin (GT), a novel ginseng-derived exogenous ligand of lysophosphatidic acid (LPA) receptors, has shown to induce autophagy in cortical astrocytes [45]. GT intensely augmented the autophagy marker LC3 via the G protein-coupled LPA receptor-mediated pathway. However, GT-mediated autophagy was considerably decreased via autophagy inhibition 3-MA as well as Beclin-1, Atg5, and Atg7 gene knockdown [15,45]. Notably, pretreatment with a lysosomotropic agent, Baf A1 and E-64d/peps A, GT significantly improved LC3-II levels in addition to the formation of LC3 puncta (Figure 5). Furthermore, GT treatment improved autophagic flux, which influenced lysosome-associated membrane protein 1 (LAMP1) in addition to degradation of the autophagy substrate ubiquitinated p62/SQSTM1 protein in mouse cortical astrocytes [45].

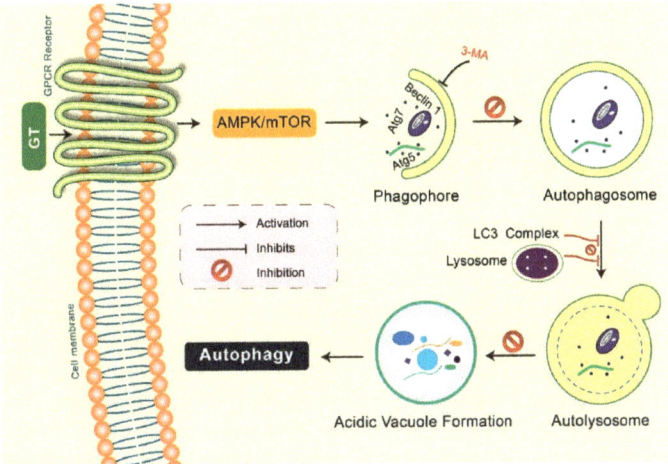

Figure 5. Gintonin (GT) activates autophagy in mouse cortical astrocytes. GT-mediated autophagy was dependent on GPCR-LPA receptors. Pretreatment with an LPA receptor antagonist, Ki16425, considerably decreased GT-mediated autophagy, while LPA agonist pretreatment, LPA 18:1, augmented autophagy in astrocytes. Autophagy initiation proteins Atg5, Atg7, and Beclin-1 were found to be activated in GT-mediated autophagy in astrocytes. Inhibition of autophagy by 3-MA, GT-mediated autophagy was prevented. Pretreated with E-64d/pepstatin A and bafilomycin A1, GT additionally improved LC3 puncta formation indicating enhanced autophagic flux in cortical astrocytes. GT treatment increased acidic vacuole formation along with p62 protein accumulation during this autophagy process.

β-elemene: β-elemene, derived from *Rhizoma Curcumae*, is a natural terpenoid bioactive compound that shows strong activity against various types of cancers [40]. In the human body, β-elemene works against the PI3K/Akt/mTOR/p70S6K pathway that induces autophagy and apoptosis of human NSCLCA549 cells [85]. As β-elemene increases the antitumor effect, autophagy is prevented by the interception with chlorochine [85]. In human renal-cell carcinoma 786-0 cells, β-elemene is used for the inhibition of the MAPK/ERK and PI3K/Akt/mTOR signaling pathways to initiate defensive autophagy and apoptosis [86].

Caffeine: In HeLa cells, the Akt/mTOR/p70S6K pathway initiates autophagy and apoptotic cell death under the influence of caffeine that is routinely consumed in beverages [87].

Curcumin: Curcumin is a non-toxic toxic polyphenol with yellow pigment isolated from the rhizome of *Curcuma longa* L. [88]. Curcumin-associated autophagy is considered to be a signal for cellular death in various types of cancer cells in the human body. Nevertheless, in the human body, curcumin can induce cellular differentiation and cellular survival by regulating the activities of AKT-AMPK-mediated autophagy induction [89]. Thus, it prevents the growth of malignant glioma cells in vitro and in vivo. Curcumin is used to induce non-apoptotic autophagy cell death in U87-MG and U373-MG malignant glioma cells [90]. This activity is related to the G2/M phase cell cycle attack, the prevention of the ribosomal S6 protein kinase pathway with the ERK1/ERK2 activation pathway [90]. Curcumin is responsible for Atg apoptosis in mesothelioma and k562 long-standing myelogenous leukemia cells by AKT/mTOR and NF-κB signaling pathways [91]. Curcumin can be used as an effective therapeutic compound in cancer management and is well endured, as confirmed by preclinical data in clinical experiments [88]. Curcumin has been found to suppress TGF-β expression, such as p-SMAD2, TGF-β3, MMP-13, and NF-κB tumor-promoting factors as well as metastatic active adhesion molecules, such as intercellular adhesion molecule 1 (ICAM-1) and β1-integrin in stromal fibroblasts and colorectal cancer cells [92]. In addition, MiR-1246 has been shown to be involved in curcumin-induced radiosensitizing actions on bladder cancer cells by targeting p53 translation [93].

Tetrahydrocurcumin: Tetrahydrocurcumin (THC) is one of the strongest bioactive natural metabolite derived from curcumin. THC effectively shows strong antioxidant, anticancer, and cardioprotective properties [94]. The action of THC on autophagy was assessed by the decrease in the PI3K/Akt-mTOR and MAPK signaling pathways and initiation of caspase-7 mediated apoptosis [95].

Oxyresveratrol: Oxyresveratrol (Oxy R), 4-[(E)-2-(3,5-dihydroxyphenyl) ethenyl] benzene-1,3-diol/ 2,3,4,5-tetrahydroxy-trans-stilbene found in *Morus alba*, has been shown to activate autophagy and apoptotic cell death in NB cells [51] (Figure 6). Oxy R-mediated autophagic cells were independent of apoptotic cell death. The PI3K/AKT/mTOR and p38 MAPK pathways control Oxy R-induced cell death in SH-SY5Y human NB cells [51].

Epigallocatechin-3-gallate: The activity of cisplatin and oxaliplatin-initiated autophagy was promoted by EGCG in HT-29 and DLD-1 colorectal cancer cells, as identified by the multiplication of LC3B-II protein and autophagosome organization [96]. EGCG initiated autophagy as well as apoptosis in SSC-4 squamous cell carcinoma in combination with the upregulation of FAS, BAK, BAD, IGF-IR, WNT1l, and ZEB1 proteins along with downregulation of MYC, TP53, and CASP8 proteins [97]. The formation of autophagosomes is increased by EGCG. In hepatic cells, the processes of lysosomal acidification and autophagic flux are also increased by EGCG in vitro, as well as in vivo [98]. Remarkably, luteolin and EGCG combination repressed TGF-β-mediated demonstration of myofibroblast phenotypes by reducing RhoA as well as ERK activation [99]. EGCG suggestively repressed rat hepatic stellate cells proliferation through hindering expression of PDGF-β receptor and tyrosine phosphorylation [100]. Furthermore, it has been found that EGCG attenuates uric acid-mediated NRK-49 F cell injury by up-regulating miR-9, and successively by JAK-STAT as well as NF-κB signaling pathway activation [101]. EGCG reduces carcinoma cell growth probably by regulating miRNA expression, and may be a potential beneficial target for the prevention of cancers.

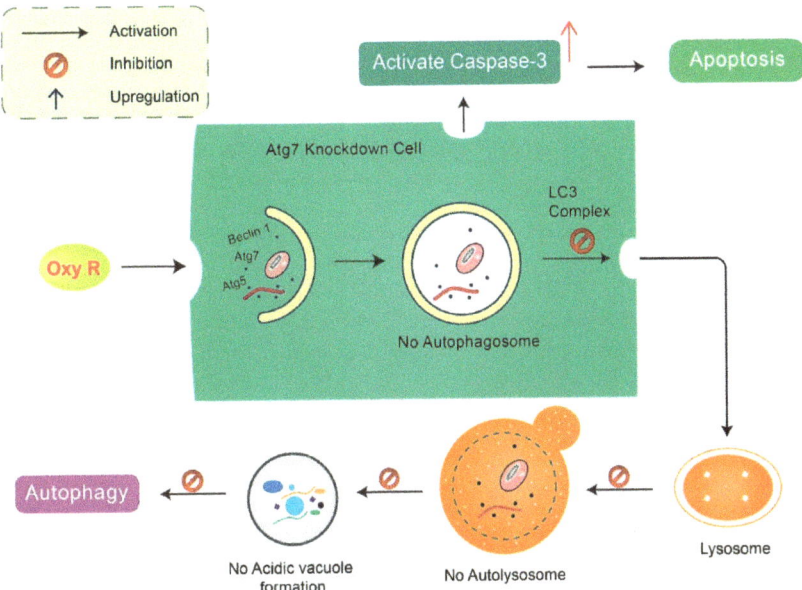

Figure 6. Natural compound oxyresveratrol (Oxy R) stimulates apoptosis and autophagy-dependent cell death. Oxy R activates autophagy through autophagy initiation Atg7 and Beclin 1 dependent pathways. Atg7 knockdown prevents autophagy, but activates apoptotic cell death in SH-SY5Y cells. Blockage of autophagy via 3-MA, Oxy R inhibits autophagic cell death. When apoptosis signaling is inhibited by Z-DEVD-FMK caspase-3 inhibitor, Oxy R exhibits autophagic cell death.

Fisetin: Fisetin (3,7,3′,4′-tetrahydroxyflavone), a flavonol and a member of flavonoid polyphenols [102], is usually isolated from many vegetables and fruits [102]. Fisetin can function as an inhibitor of the expression of PI3K/Akt/mTOR pathways and regulate autophagy in prostate cancer and human NSCLC cells [103,104]. Fisetin has been found to inhibit the mTOR pathway and induce autophagy in human prostate cancer cells [105]. In addition, the effects of fisetin on autophagy are cell-type specific because fisetin inhibits autophagy in MCF-7 breast cancer cells and induces caspase-7-mediated apoptosis [106].

γ-Tocotrienol: Tocotrienols and the isoforms of vitamin E are differentiated on the basis of their antioxidant, anti-inflammatory, and anticancer properties. γ-tocotrienol induces endoplasmic inflammation and autophagy-associated cell death [107]. Pretreatment with the autophagy inhibitors 3-MA or Baf1 prevented the γ-tocotrienol-initiated cytotoxicity [108]. Many other studies have demonstrated that in mouse mammary cancer cells, the attachment of γ-tocotrienol with oridonin effectively initiated both autophagic and apoptotic effects [109]. The potency of autophagy cellular markers was significantly enhanced by the attachment of γ-tocotrienol with oridonin [110]. Simultaneously, this potency also improved the transformation of LC3-I to LC3-II, Atg3, Atg7, Beclin-1, Atg5-Atg12, LAMP-1, and cathepsin-D.

Geraniol: Fruits, vegetables, and cereal grains contain geraniol, a secondary metabolite, that in human PC-3 prostate cancer cells was shown to induce apoptosis and Atg cell death [111].

Seriniquinone: Seriniquinone is a medicinal compound derived from a marine bacterium of the genus Serinicoccus. It exhibits effective anti-proliferative activity against melanoma cell lines by activation of autophagocytosis [112].

Thymoquinone: Thymoquinone (TQ) is a key bioactive natural product isolated from black cumin, *Nigella sativa* L. TQ is related to increased volumes of autophagic vacuoles, as well as LC3 proteins, and enhances the combination of autophagosomes in the head and neck squamous carcinoma cells [113]. TQ effectively reduced the growth rate of GBM cells in association with the lysosomal inhibitor CQ, mostly causing apoptosis, and initiating autophagy [114]. LC3-II and p62 proteins are enhanced by the expression of TQ [114]. It was also shown that TQ prevented the growth of irinotecan-inhibited LoVo colon cancer cells by primarily activating apoptosis before autophagy [115]. Activation of the p38 and JNK MAP kinase pathways is related to TQ, which causes autophagic cell death [115]. TQ-induced caspase and autophagic cell death were also related to mitochondrial outward membrane penetrability [114].

Magnolol: Magnolol, isolated from *Magnolia officinalis*, exhibited anti-cancer and anti-tumor activity by directing autophagy and apoptosis signaling pathways [116]. However, magnolol promotes autophagy-mediated cell death in human non-small lung cancer H460 cells at high concentrations [117]. Additionally, in SGC-7901 human gastric adenocarcinoma cells, magnolol has been shown to repress PI3K/Akt pathway and encourage death by inducing autophagy [118].

Polyphenol mulberry extract: Mulberry is derived from *Morus Alba* leaf, which modulates the autophagy AMPK/PI3K/Akt pathway [119]. In Hep3B human hepatocellular carcinoma cells, mulberry extract modulates autophagic or apoptotic cell death by the activation of the p53-dependent pathway [120]. It has been found that in NB cells, *Morus alba* root extract initiates apoptosis through FOXO-Caspase-3 dependent pathway [121].

Oblongifolin C: Oblongifolin C (OC), isolated from *Garcinia yunnanensis* Hu, is a strong autophagy inhibitor [122]. Treatment with OC resulted in an augmented number of autophagosomes as well as reduced SQSTM1/p62 and degradation [123]. OC showed anticancer effectiveness by improved staining of LC3 puncta, SQSTM1, and cleaved CASP-3, along with decreased expression levels of lysosomal cathepsins in an in vivo xenograft mouse model [122].

Naphthazarin: Naphthazarin repressed the Akt/PI3K pathway by activating autophagy and apoptosis pathways and by inducing A549 lung cancer cell death [124].

Sulforaphane: Sulforaphane is derived from cruciferous vegetables, such as cauliflower, cabbage, broccoli, and hoary weed [125]. In human prostate cancer PC-3 cells, sulforaphane has been shown to prompt autophagosome formation as well as acidic vesicular organelle formation [126]. Sulforaphane augmented the protein levels of LC3B-I in addition to encouraging LC3B-II processing. Exposure to sulforaphane in tumor cells displayed LC3B-II puncta related to autophagosome formation [127]. It also disrupted BECN1/BCL-2 interaction, causing autophagy initiation through the release of BECN1. Phosphorylated AKT-Ser473 levels decreased by sulforaphane in addition to simultaneous treatment with autophagy inhibitors, 3-MA or CQ, and inhibited tumor cell growth and proliferation [128]. Sulforaphane initiation decreases oxidative stress in addition to misfolded protein accumulation [129].

Mollugin: A bioactive phytochemical, mollugin, sequestered from *Rubia cordifolia* L., showed anticancer potential against numerous cancer cells [130]. Additional studies confirmed that the mTOR and ERK pathways are involved in mollugin-prompted autophagy in addition to apoptosis [131].

Jujuboside B: Jujuboside B is a saponin found in the seeds of *Zizyphus jujubavar* Spinose. It increased autophagy and apoptosis in human HCT-116 and AGS gastric adenocarcinoma cells in vitro and successfully repressed tumor growth in a xenograft model of nude mice in vivo [132]. Furthermore, jujuboside B activated p38/JNK-mediated autophagy induction through cytoplasmic vacuole formation in addition to LC3-I/II conversion [132].

Cyclovirobuxine D: Cyclovirobuxine D (CVB-D) has been shown to activate autophagy in the human MCF-7 breast cancer cell line through the addition of autophagosomes as well as raised LC3 puncta, along with augmented conversion of LC3-I to LC3-II [133]. However, CVB-D-mediated autophagy induction and cell viability were blocked by 3-MA [133].

Polygonatum odoratum lectin: Polygonatum odoratum lectin (POL) has been shown to reveal apoptosis-inducing and anti-proliferative properties in a wide range of cancer cells [134]. In human breast cancer NSCLC A549 and MCF-7 cells, POL prompted both autophagy and apoptosis [135].

POL stimulated apoptosis by preventing the AKT/NF-κB pathway, whereas augmented autophagy through AKT-mTOR pathway suppression [135].

Resveratrol: Resveratrol, a polyphenol compound derived from berries, red grapes, and peanuts, has been shown to facilitate cell death in a diverse variety of cancer cells through autophagy, apoptosis, and necrosis [136,137]. In ovarian cancer cells, resveratrol has been found to activate autophagic cell death [138]. However, resveratrol inhibited NF-κB stimulation in association with augmented permeability of lysosomal in cervical cancer cells, demonstrating autophagic cell death [139]. Additionally, in HL-60 promyelocytic leukemia cells, it has been described that resveratrol-prompted apoptosis increased LC3-II levels in addition to dependency on mTOR pathway [140]. Meanwhile, resveratrol-mediated apoptosis was related to reduced p53 and AMPK/mTOR autophagy signaling pathways in renal carcinoma cells [141]. The antiproliferative action of resveratrol has been found in liver myofibroblasts by preventing PDGF signaling and decreasing EGF-dependent DNA synthesis [142]. Additionally, in retinal endothelial cells, resveratrol has been found to increase miR15a expression under conditions of high glucose levels and decreased insulin signaling [143].

Quercetin: Quercetin, a bioflavonoid, is generally found in fruits, beverages, and vegetables. In vitro and in vivo studies have shown that it exhibits antiproliferative activities in numerous tumors conventionally related to its antioxidant properties [144].

Rottlerin: Rottlerin, a natural product sequestered from *Mallotus philippinensis*, repressed PI3K/mTOR signaling in human pancreatic cancer stem cells, and activated autophagy-mediated apoptotic cell death [145].

Angelicin: Angelicin, a psoralen, is derived from *Angelica polymorpha* and has been shown to induce apoptosis [146,147] and autophagy [148]. Angelicin increased autophagy-related proteins Atg3, Atg7 and Atg12-5 with phosphorylation of mTOR [148,149].

Ursolic acid: A triterpenoid phytochemical, ursolic acid (UA), has been found to activate autophagy by inducing LC3 in addition to p62 protein accumulation [150]. In HCT15 cells, UA repressed growth by modulating autophagy in the JNK pathway [151]. However, UA induced cytotoxicity in addition to repressing concentration-dependent TC-1 cervical cancer cells by controlling Atg5 and LC3-II, which demonstrated its anticancer activity [150]. Furthermore, in MCF7 breast cancer cells, UA activated autophagy under ER stress [152]. In PC3 prostate cancer cells, UA-induced autophagy was facilitated by the Akt/mTOR and Beclin-1 pathways [153].

Polygonatum Cyrtonema Lectin: Polygonatum Cyrtonema Lectin (PCL) inhibits the PI3K-Akt pathway in addition to prompting autophagy and apoptosis in cancer cells [154]. Although PCL significantly prevented the growth of A375 human melanoma cells, normal melanocytes were not affected [155]. Additionally, PCL has been found to stimulate both autophagy and apoptosis in A375 cells [156].

Silibinin: Silibinin, derived from *Silybum marianum*, has been shown to induce autophagic HT1080 cell death in human fibrosarcoma through diverse mechanisms, including inhibition of MEK/ERK and PI3K/Akt pathways [157].

Plant extract induces autophagy: Several plant-derived extracts from *Dioscorea nipponica* Makino, *Melandrium firmum*, marine algae, and natural flavonoids have been found to induce apoptosis and autophagic properties [158–161]. *Saussurea lappa* ethanol extract has been investigated to activate apoptosis in NB [162] and autophagy in LNCaP prostate cancer cells [163].

Ginsenoside Rk1: Ginsenoside Rk1, an NMDA receptor inhibitor [164], exhibited antitumor and autophagy modulation activities in HepG2 cells. Rk1-prompted autophagy was recognized through LC3-I to LC3-II conversion, which incorporated lysosomes into the autolysosome process [165]. However, the autophagy inhibitor, Beclin 1 siRNA or bafilomycin A1, and Rk1 combination boosted autophagic activities in HepG2 [165].

Climacostol: In mouse B16-F10 melanoma cells, autophagosomes accumulate with dysfunctional autophagic degradation. However, climacostol provides mechanistic insights and promotes autophagosome turnover through the p53-AMPK pathway and activated p53 protein levels [166].

5. Role of Natural Compounds in Autophagy Modulation of Neurodegenerative Diseases

Natural plant-derived compounds are able to modulate autophagy and can be used to develop treatments for neurodegenerative diseases such as Alzheimer's disease (AD), Parkinson's disease (PD), Huntington's disease (HD), Amyotrophic lateral sclerosis (ALS), Spinocerebellar ataxia (SCA), and NB [167]. Oleuropein aglycone (OLE), a natural phenol, can protect the Aβ-driven cytotoxicity of neuronal cells by stimulating autophagy found in in vitro and in vivo examinations, thereby easing Aβ toxicity clearance of AD. [168,169]. Arctigenin, derived from *Arctium lappa* (L.), inhibits Aβ production by decreasing BACE1 and boosts Aβ clearance by increasing autophagy via AKT/mTOR inhibition [170]. Another polyphenol, resveratrol, significantly represses Aβ aggregation via autophagy and shows antioxidant effects in AD [171–173]. Kaempferol, a flavone, increases autophagy and encourages mitochondrial damage repair, protecting neuronal cells against death via rotenone-induced toxicity in PD models [174]. *Uncaria rhynchophylla* contains alkaloids of oxindole and was found to prompt Beclin-1-dependent as well as mTOR-independent autophagy, which stimulated α-synuclein clearance in the *Drosophila* model of A53T, both wild-type and mutant [175]. Conophylline, *Tavertaemontana divaricate*-derived vinca alkaloid, has been shown to promote α-synuclein degradation via the mTOR-independent pathway in MPP^+-mediated neurotoxin [176]. Curcumin, a polyphenol from *Curcuma longa* turmeric plant, has been shown to exhibit neuroprotective properties against PD models via mTOR-dependent autophagy and preventing oxidative stress, inflammation, and α-synuclein aggregation. [177]. Trehalose, resveratrol, and onjisaponin B improve autophagic degradation of α-synuclein when treating MPTP-induced mice, in addition to stimulating AMPK and sirtuin 1 protein [178,179]. A natural alkaloid, harmine, has been found to stimulate α-synuclein removal by PKA-mediated PD pathogenesis of UPS activation [180]. Distinct AD, PD, and HD neurodegenerative syndromes might be treated via natural compounds through modulation of autophagy [1]. *Nelumbo nucifera* contains neferine, which has been shown to protect Htt mutant proteins via autophagy triggering with the AMPK/mTOR pathway [181]. Aggregate-prone mutant Htt protein has been removed by trehalose through an mTOR-independent autophagy pathway [182]. Berberine, an isoquinoline alkaloid, has been shown to prevent mutant Htt protein accumulation and activate autophagy in mouse and cell models of HD [183]. In particular, trehalose has been found to stimulate mTOR-independent autophagy in superoxide dismutase mutant mice in the management of ALS in vivo [184]. Trehalose and its analogs, such as lactulose and melibiose, have been determined to substantially reduce the aggregation of abnormal ataxin-3 by stimulation of autophagy, which reduces free radical production [185], indicating that natural compounds might be used as a therapeutic approach to control SCA.

6. Effect of Natural Compounds on Solid Tumors and Lymphomas

Neuroblastoma, the most common extracranial solid malignant tumor of childhood, is the third most common form of pediatric malignancy worldwide. Didymin, a dietary flavonoid glycoside, has been found to be effective in NB treatment [186]. A *Morus alba* root extract compound, Oxy R, has been shown to accumulate ROS as well as inducing autophagic and apoptotic cell death in NB cells via the FOXO and caspase-3 induction pathways [51,121]. A psoralen compound angelicin derived from *Angelica polymorpha* increases cytotoxicity in addition to inducing apoptosis through anti-apoptotic proteins (Bcl-xL, Bcl-2, and Mcl-1) downregulation in SH-SY5Y human NB cells [146,147]. However, *Saussurea lappa* Clarke, *Dioscorea nipponica* Makino, and *Melandrium firmum* extracts have been shown to have apoptotic and anti-proliferative effects in NB cells [158,162,187]. Additionally, curcumin, propolis, quercetin, icariin, withaferin A, tetrandrine, and resveratrol have been used for the treatment of aggressive GBM [188]. In addition, a combination therapy with temozolomide and resveratrol substantially diminished the growth of GBM cells in a xenograft model [189]. Natural compounds such as PTX, wortmannin, and beta-lapachone have been found to be involved in the ARF/MDM2-MDMX/p53 signaling pathway in the human retinoblastoma (RB) Y79 cell line [190].

Lymphoma is the most common type of blood cancer, and various natural compounds have been used to treat lymphomas. Several natural compounds have shown anticancer effects on lymphomas (Table 2). *Nigella sativa* Linn. containing TQ has been shown to induce apoptosis and ROS production at 5 and 10 mM concentrations of 24 h treatment in ABC-DLBCL activated B cell lymphoma cell lines [191]. It has been stated that fuxocanthinol induces apoptosis in addition to arrest in cell cycle progression in lymphoma cells [192].

Table 2. Anticancer effects of natural cancers in the management of lymphomas.

Natural Compounds	Cellular/Animal Models	Concentrations/Doses	Effects and Mechanisms	References
Thymoquinone from *Nigella sativa*	Activated B cell lymphoma cell lines	5–10 mM	ROS production and apoptosis	[191]
Resveratrol	Neuroblastoma	30 µM	Apoptosis induction and antiproliferation	[137]
Fuxocanthinol	Primary effusion lymphomas BCBL-1 and TY-1	1.3–5 µM	Apoptosis induction and cell cycle arrest	[192]
Curcumin	CH12F3 lymphoma cells	5 µM	Caspase-3 dependent apoptosis and DNA damage	[193]
Peperobtusin A	Lymphoma U937 cells	25, 50, 100 µM	Caspase-3, 8, 9 dependent apoptosis and p38 MAPK activation	[194]
11(13)-dehydroivaxillin (DHI)	Lymphoid malignancies of NHL cells xenografts	5, 7, 10 µM	Induction of NF-κB and apoptosis	[195]
Psilostachyin C	Murine lymphoma cell line BW5147	0.01–50 µg/mL	Induction of apoptosis, necrosis, and ROS generation	[196]

Curcumin has been reported to induce antitumor effects on CH12F3 cell lines through DNA breaks and apoptosis [193]. An extract from *Peperomia tetraphylla*, Peperobtusin A, has been found to induce S phase cell cycle arrest and p38 MAPK-dependent apoptosis in U937 cells [194]. However, induction of apoptosis, necrosis, and cell cycle arrest by psilostachyin C has been found in lymphoma BW5147 cell lines [196]. In a xenograft mouse model, 11(13)-dehydroivaxillin (DHI) has shown antitumor activity via the apoptosis pathway [195].

7. Therapeutic View of Autophagy in Heart/Cardiovascular Diseases

Autophagy has been shown to play a major regulatory role in cellular longevity [197] and in heart/cardiovascular diseases towards maintaining homeostasis by conserving cardiac function and structure [198] and determining a potential connection between ventricular fibrillation and autophagy [199]. There is evidence suggesting that mitochondrial autophagy downregulation plays a vital role in mitochondrial dysfunction, as well as heart failure, while re-establishment of mitochondrial autophagy mitigates this heart dysfunction [200]. It has been revealed that cardiac myocytes are reduced through autophagy inhibitor, 3-MA, with AMP-activated protein kinase (AMPK) activation via inactivation of mTOR under glucose deprivation [201]. In addition, the autophagy-related gene, Beclin-1, protected the heart in LPS-induced sepsis in a mouse model and targeted autophagy induction, and therefore has an important role with therapeutic potential for treating cardiovascular diseases [202]. Under high glucose conditions, it has been found that heme-oxygenase-1 (HO-1) overexpression via human HO-1 recombinant plasmid inhibited dysfunction of cardiac arrest, improving autophagy levels. Numerous hemin concentrations induce HO-1, which affects endothelial cell mitochondrial dysfunction. Likewise, exposure to hemin further prompts mitophagy, although it is not adequate to inhibit cell death [203]. It has been found that regulating Sirt3 concentration in myocytes via proper autophagy expression in diverse stages of myocardial ischemia-reperfusion might effectively decrease the morbidity of patients with myocardial infarction in the future [204]. Metformin has been used to treat cardiotoxicity induced by doxorubicin via the autophagy pathway [205]. In contrast, a non-selective β-adrenergic agonist, isoproterenol, has been investigated for the treatment of autophagy as well as cell death pathway induced cardiac injury such as necrosis or apoptosis induced cardiac injury [206]. Currently, it is accepted that pharmacological approaches targeting autophagy and apoptosis are useful in the treatment of coronary heart disease, therefore providing new favorable therapeutic interventions in the future [207]. Hence, consideration of emerging molecular mechanisms towards the understanding of autophagy has recently gained importance for regulating cellular systems that can be used to prevent and treat cardiovascular disease [208].

8. Perspectives of Naturally Occurring Autophagy Modulators in Cancer Therapy

Despite anti-cancer drug development, natural compounds contribute to cancer and cancer stem cell [209] suppressive action without any severe complications, and thus it is an emerging topic with respect to autophagy. Natural compounds have also appeared as unique therapeutic agents for cancer and drug repositioning via their impact on autophagy [210]. It is remarkable that the study of cell fate by natural stimulators should be the focal point, although technological dissimilarities in autophagy detection may affect the outcome. In addition, in vivo examination of natural stimulators of autophagy in cancer therapy or prevention will be an emerging field of research in the future. Moreover, studies on the effects of natural product-derived molecules on autophagy should be highlighted at the translational level.

9. Conclusions and Future Directions

Cancer cells can convert and reuse necessary amino acids by imposing autophagic signaling pathways, thereby ensuring their consistent growth and longevity. Accordingly, autophagy serves a dual role in cancer—augmentation or hindrance—and can either boost or down-regulate cancer cell proliferation. As a result, autophagy moderators can play the role of a promising novel therapeutic approach towards cancer inhibition by helping overcome resistance against chemotherapy and radiotherapy. Potential targets of autophagic progress and autophagosome formation in the initial phase and lysosomal deterioration in the late phase have been considered. However, mTOR and AMPK are the leading regulatory molecules of autophagy in upstream signaling pathways. These are also known targets for natural compound derived modulators of autophagy. Therefore, using plant-derived and semisynthetic components to target the regulation of the entire pathway can provide an opportunity to design a powerful remedy for cancer patients.

Author Contributions: Conceptualization by M.A.R. Writing and original draft preparation by M.S.H., P.B., R.I., M.H.R. (Md. Habibur Rahman) Figures are drawing by M.H.R. (MD. Hasanur Rahman). Review and editing by M.J.U. Visualization and supervision by H.R. All authors have read and agreed to the published version of the manuscript.

Funding: This work was supported by NRF Research Program (2016M3C7A1913845) and the Korea Research Fellowship (KRF) Program (M.A.R. 2016H1D3A1908615; R.I. 2020H1D3A1A04104782) funded by the Ministry of Science and ICT, Republic of Korea, and also supported by (M.J.U. 2020R1I1A1A01072879 and 2020H1D3A2A02110924), Republic of Korea.

Conflicts of Interest: The authors declare no conflict of interest.

References

1. Rahman, M.A.; Rhim, H. Therapeutic implication of autophagy in neurodegenerative diseases. *BMB Rep.* **2017**, *50*, 345–354. [CrossRef] [PubMed]
2. Corti, O.; Blomgren, K.; Poletti, A.; Beart, P.M. Autophagy in neurodegeneration: New insights underpinning therapy for neurological diseases. *J. Neurochem.* **2020**, e15002. [CrossRef] [PubMed]
3. Uddin, M.S.; Stachowiak, A.; Al Mamun, A.; Tzvetkov, N.T.; Takeda, S.; Atanasov, A.G.; Bergantin, L.B.; Abdel-Daim, M.M.; Stankiewicz, A.M. Autophagy and Alzheimer's Disease: From Molecular Mechanisms to Therapeutic Implications. *Front. Aging Neurosci.* **2018**, *10*. [CrossRef] [PubMed]
4. Arroyo, D.S.; Gaviglio, E.A.; Ramos, J.M.P.; Bussi, C.; Rodriguez-Galan, M.C.; Iribarren, P. Autophagy in inflammation, infection, neurodegeneration and cancer. *Int. Immunopharmacol.* **2014**, *18*, 55–65. [CrossRef]
5. Perry, R.J.; Shulman, G.I. Mechanistic Links between Obesity, Insulin, and Cancer. *Trends Cancer* **2020**, *6*, 75–78. [CrossRef]
6. Ling, Y.; Perez-Soler, R. Disruption of autophagic and autolysosomal signaling pathways leads to synergistic augmentation of erlotinib-induced apoptosis in wild type EGFR human non-small cell lung cancer cell lines. *EJC Suppl.* **2010**, *8*, 183. [CrossRef]
7. Towers, C.G.; Wodetzki, D.; Thorburn, A. Autophagy and cancer: Modulation of cell death pathways and cancer cell adaptations. *J. Cell Biol.* **2020**, *219*. [CrossRef]
8. Manic, G.; Obrist, F.; Kroemer, G.; Vitale, I.; Galluzzi, L. Chloroquine and hydroxychloroquine for cancer therapy. *Mol. Cell. Oncol.* **2014**, *1*, e29911. [CrossRef]
9. Khandia, R.; Dadar, M.; Munjal, A.; Dhama, K.; Karthik, K.; Tiwari, R.; Yatoo, M.I.; Iqbal, H.M.N.; Singh, K.P.; Joshi, S.K.; et al. A Comprehensive Review of Autophagy and Its Various Roles in Infectious, Non-Infectious, and Lifestyle Diseases: Current Knowledge and Prospects for Disease Prevention, Novel Drug Design, and Therapy. *Cells* **2019**, *8*. [CrossRef] [PubMed]
10. Bialik, S.; Dasari, S.K.; Kimchi, A. Autophagy-dependent cell death—Where, how and why a cell eats itself to death. *J. Cell Sci.* **2018**, *131*. [CrossRef]
11. Lagoa, R.; Silva, J.; Rodrigues, J.R.; Bishayee, A. Advances in phytochemical delivery systems for improved anticancer activity. *Biotechnol. Adv.* **2020**, *38*. [CrossRef]
12. Tavakol, S.; Ashrafizadeh, M.; Deng, S.; Azarian, M.; Abdoli, A.; Motavaf, M.; Poormoghadam, D.; Khanbabaei, H.; Afshar, E.G.; Mandegary, A.; et al. Autophagy Modulators: Mechanistic Aspects and Drug Delivery Systems. *Biomolecules* **2019**, *9*. [CrossRef] [PubMed]
13. Hirata, E.; Ohya, Y.; Suzuki, K. Atg4 plays an important role in efficient expansion of autophagic isolation membranes by cleaving lipidated Atg8 in Saccharomyces cerevisiae. *PLoS ONE* **2017**, *12*. [CrossRef] [PubMed]
14. Chen, Y.; He, J.; Tian, M.; Zhang, S.Y.; Guo, M.R.; Kasimu, R.; Wang, J.H.; Ouyang, L. UNC51-like kinase 1, autophagic regulator and cancer therapeutic target. *Cell Proliferat.* **2014**, *47*, 494–505. [CrossRef] [PubMed]
15. Rahman, M.A.; Rahman, M.R.; Zaman, T.; Uddin, M.S.; Islam, R.; Abdel-Daim, M.M.; Rhim, H. Emerging Potential of Naturally Occurring Autophagy Modulators Against Neurodegeneration. *Curr. Pharm. Des.* **2020**, *26*, 772–779. [CrossRef]
16. Nakamura, S.; Yoshimori, T. New insights into autophagosome-lysosome fusion. *J. Cell Sci.* **2017**, *130*, 1209–1216. [CrossRef]
17. Schulze, H.; Kolter, T.; Sandhoff, K. Principles of lysosomal membrane degradation Cellular topology and biochemistry of lysosomal lipid degradation. *BBA-Mol. Cell Res.* **2009**, *1793*, 674–683. [CrossRef]
18. Shpilka, T.; Weidberg, H.; Pietrokovski, S.; Elazar, Z. Atg8: An autophagy-related ubiquitin-like protein family. *Genome Biol.* **2011**, *12*. [CrossRef]
19. Agrotis, A.; von Chamier, L.; Oliver, H.; Kiso, K.; Singh, T.; Ketteler, R. Human ATG4 autophagy proteases counteract attachment of ubiquitin-like LC3/GABARAP proteins to other cellular proteins. *J. Biol. Chem.* **2019**, *294*, 12610–12621. [CrossRef]
20. Lystad, A.H.; Simonsen, A. Mechanisms and Pathophysiological Roles of the ATG8 Conjugation Machinery. *Cells* **2019**, *8*. [CrossRef]
21. Ward, C.; Martinez-Lopez, N.; Otten, E.G.; Carroll, B.; Maetzel, D.; Singh, R.; Sarkar, S.; Korolchuk, V.I. Autophagy, lipophagy and lysosomal lipid storage disorders. *BBA-Mol. Cell Biol. Lipids* **2016**, *1861*, 269–284. [CrossRef] [PubMed]

22. Galluzzi, L.; Pietrocola, F.; Bravo-San Pedro, J.M.; Amaravadi, R.K.; Baehrecke, E.H.; Cecconi, F.; Codogno, P.; Debnath, J.; Gewirtz, D.A.; Karantza, V.; et al. Autophagy in malignant transformation and cancer progression. *Embo J.* **2015**, *34*, 856–880. [CrossRef]
23. Desantis, V.; Saltarella, I.; Lamanuzzi, A.; Mariggio, M.A.; Racanelli, V.; Vacca, A.; Frassanito, M.A. Autophagy: A New Mechanism of Prosurvival and Drug Resistance in Multiple Myeloma. *Transl. Oncol.* **2018**, *11*, 1350–1357. [CrossRef] [PubMed]
24. Yang, Z.N.J.; Chee, C.E.; Huang, S.B.; Sinicrope, F.A. The Role of Autophagy in Cancer: Therapeutic Implications. *Mol. Cancer Ther.* **2011**, *10*, 1533–1541. [CrossRef]
25. Ricci, M.S.; Zong, W.X. Chemotherapeutic approaches for targeting cell death pathways. *Oncologist* **2006**, *11*, 342–357. [CrossRef] [PubMed]
26. Mowers, E.E.; Sharifi, M.N.; Macleod, K.F. Autophagy in cancer metastasis. *Oncogene* **2017**, *36*, 1619–1630. [CrossRef] [PubMed]
27. Altman, B.J.; Rathmell, J.C. Metabolic Stress in Autophagy and Cell Death Pathways. *CSH Perspect. Biol.* **2012**, *4*. [CrossRef] [PubMed]
28. Mowers, E.E.; Sharifi, M.N.; Macleod, K.F. Functions of autophagy in the tumor microenvironment and cancer metastasis. *FEBS J.* **2018**, *285*, 1751–1766. [CrossRef]
29. Park, S.A.; Surh, Y.J. Modulation of tumor microenvironment by chemopreventive natural products. *Ann. N. Y. Acad. Sci.* **2017**, *1401*, 65–74. [CrossRef]
30. Zhang, B.; Tian, L.; Xie, J.; Chen, G.; Wang, F. Targeting miRNAs by natural products: A new way for cancer therapy. *Biomed. Pharmacother.* **2020**, *130*, 110546. [CrossRef]
31. Jiang, J.W.; Zhang, L.; Chen, H.N.; Lei, Y.L.; Zhang, T.; Wang, Y.L.; Jin, P.; Lan, J.; Zhou, L.; Huang, Z.; et al. Regorafenib induces lethal autophagy arrest by stabilizing PSAT1 in glioblastoma. *Autophagy* **2020**, *16*, 106–122. [CrossRef] [PubMed]
32. Cuomo, F.; Altucci, L.; Cobellis, G. Autophagy Function and Dysfunction: Potential Drugs as Anti-Cancer Therapy. *Cancers* **2019**, *11*. [CrossRef] [PubMed]
33. Livesey, K.M.; Tang, D.L.; Zeh, H.J.; Lotze, M.T. Autophagy inhibition in combination cancer treatment. *Curr. Opin. Investig. Drugs* **2009**, *10*, 1269–1279. [PubMed]
34. Wu, Y.T.; Tan, H.L.; Shui, G.H.; Bauvy, C.; Huang, Q.; Wenk, M.R.; Ong, C.N.; Codogno, P.; Shen, H.M. Dual Role of 3-Methyladenine in Modulation of Autophagy via Different Temporal Patterns of Inhibition on Class I and III Phosphoinositide 3-Kinase. *J. Biol. Chem.* **2010**, *285*, 10850–10861. [CrossRef] [PubMed]
35. Vazquez-Martin, A.; Oliveras-Ferraros, C.; Menendez, J.A. Autophagy Facilitates the Development of Breast Cancer Resistance to the Anti-HER2 Monoclonal Antibody Trastuzumab. *PLoS ONE* **2009**, *4*. [CrossRef]
36. Rothe, K.; Porter, V.; Jiang, X.Y. Current Outlook on Autophagy in Human Leukemia: Foe in Cancer Stem Cells and Drug Resistance, Friend in New Therapeutic Interventions. *Int. J. Mol. Sci.* **2019**, *20*. [CrossRef]
37. Jo, G.H.; Bogler, O.; Chwae, Y.J.; Yoo, H.; Lee, S.H.; Park, J.B.; Kim, Y.J.; Kim, J.H.; Gwak, H.S. Radiation-Induced Autophagy Contributes to Cell Death and Induces Apoptosis Partly in Malignant Glioma Cells. *Cancer Res. Treat.* **2015**, *47*, 221–241. [CrossRef]
38. He, S.S.; Zhao, Z.; Yang, Y.F.; O'Connell, D.; Zhang, X.W.; Oh, S.; Ma, B.Y.; Lee, J.H.; Zhang, T.; Varghese, B.; et al. Truncating mutation in the autophagy gene UVRAG confers oncogenic properties and chemosensitivity in colorectal cancers. *Nat. Commun.* **2015**, *6*. [CrossRef]
39. Yue, Z.Y.; Jin, S.K.; Yang, C.W.; Levine, A.J.; Heintz, N. Beclin 1, an autophagy gene essential for early embryonic development, is a haploinsufficient tumor suppressor. *Proc. Natl. Acad. Sci. USA* **2003**, *100*, 15077–15082. [CrossRef]
40. Takamura, A.; Komatsu, M.; Hara, T.; Sakamoto, A.; Kishi, C.; Waguri, S.; Eishi, Y.; Hino, O.; Tanaka, K.; Mizushima, N. Autophagy-deficient mice develop multiple liver tumors. *Genes Dev.* **2011**, *25*, 795–800. [CrossRef] [PubMed]
41. Yang, X.; Yu, D.D.; Yan, F.; Jing, Y.Y.; Han, Z.P.; Sun, K.; Liang, L.; Hou, J.; Wei, L.X. The role of autophagy induced by tumor microenvironment in different cells and stages of cancer. *Cell Biosci.* **2015**, *5*. [CrossRef] [PubMed]
42. Rahman, M.A.; Bishayee, K.; Habib, K.; Sadra, A.; Huh, S.O. 18alpha-Glycyrrhetinic acid lethality for neuroblastoma cells via de-regulating the Beclin-1/Bcl-2 complex and inducing apoptosis. *Biochem. Pharmacol.* **2016**, *117*, 97–112. [CrossRef] [PubMed]

43. Lin, C.J.; Lee, C.C.; Shih, Y.L.; Lin, T.Y.; Wang, S.H.; Lin, Y.F.; Shih, C.M. Resveratrol enhances the therapeutic effect of temozolomide against malignant glioma in vitro and in vivo by inhibiting autophagy. *Free Radic. Biol. Med.* **2012**, *52*, 377–391. [CrossRef] [PubMed]
44. Zanotto-Filho, A.; Braganhol, E.; Klafke, K.; Figueiro, F.; Terra, S.R.; Paludo, F.J.; Morrone, M.; Bristot, I.J.; Battastini, A.M.; Forcelini, C.M.; et al. Autophagy inhibition improves the efficacy of curcumin/temozolomide combination therapy in glioblastomas. *Cancer Lett.* **2015**, *358*, 220–231. [CrossRef]
45. Rahman, M.A.; Hwang, H.; Nah, S.Y.; Rhim, H. Gintonin stimulates autophagic flux in primary cortical astrocytes. *J. Ginseng Res.* **2020**, *44*, 67–78. [CrossRef]
46. Kim, H.; Moon, J.Y.; Ahn, K.S.; Cho, S.K. Quercetin induces mitochondrial mediated apoptosis and protective autophagy in human glioblastoma U373MG cells. *Oxid. Med. Cell. Longev.* **2013**, *2013*, 596496. [CrossRef]
47. Xi, G.; Hu, X.; Wu, B.; Jiang, H.; Young, C.Y.; Pang, Y.; Yuan, H. Autophagy inhibition promotes paclitaxel-induced apoptosis in cancer cells. *Cancer Lett.* **2011**, *307*, 141–148. [CrossRef]
48. Suzuki, R.; Kang, Y.; Li, X.; Roife, D.; Zhang, R.; Fleming, J.B. Genistein potentiates the antitumor effect of 5-Fluorouracil by inducing apoptosis and autophagy in human pancreatic cancer cells. *Anticancer Res.* **2014**, *34*, 4685–4692.
49. Lv, X.Q.; Liu, F.; Shang, Y.; Chen, S.Z. Honokiol exhibits enhanced antitumor effects with chloroquine by inducing cell death and inhibiting autophagy in human non-small cell lung cancer cells. *Oncol. Rep.* **2015**, *34*, 1289–1300. [CrossRef]
50. Oh, J.M.; Kim, E.; Chun, S. Ginsenoside Compound K Induces Ros-Mediated Apoptosis and Autophagic Inhibition in Human Neuroblastoma Cells In Vitro and In Vivo. *Int. J. Mol. Sci.* **2019**, *20*. [CrossRef]
51. Rahman, M.A.; Bishayee, K.; Sadra, A.; Huh, S.O. Oxyresveratrol activates parallel apoptotic and autophagic cell death pathways in neuroblastoma cells. *Biochim. Biophys. Acta Gen Subj.* **2017**, *1861*, 23–36. [CrossRef] [PubMed]
52. Russo, M.; Russo, G.L. Autophagy inducers in cancer. *Biochem. Pharmacol.* **2018**, *153*, 51–61. [CrossRef] [PubMed]
53. Nunez-Olvera, S.I.; Gallardo-Rincon, D.; Puente-Rivera, J.; Salinas-Vera, Y.M.; Marchat, L.A.; Morales-Villegas, R.; Lopez-Camarillo, C. Autophagy Machinery as a Promising Therapeutic Target in Endometrial Cancer. *Front. Oncol.* **2019**, *9*. [CrossRef] [PubMed]
54. Wu, Y.Y.; Wu, H.C.; Wu, J.E.; Huang, K.Y.; Yang, S.C.; Chen, S.X.; Tsao, C.J.; Hsu, K.F.; Chen, Y.L.; Hong, T.M. The dual PI3K/mTOR inhibitor BEZ235 restricts the growth of lung cancer tumors regardless of EGFR status, as a potent accompaniment in combined therapeutic regimens. *J. Exp. Clin. Cancer Res.* **2019**, *38*. [CrossRef] [PubMed]
55. Rizzieri, D.A.; Feldman, E.; DiPersio, J.F.; Gabrail, N.; Stock, W.; Strair, R.; Rivera, V.M.; Albitar, M.; Bedrosian, C.L.; Giles, F.J. A phase 2 clinical trial of deforolimus (AP23573, MK-8669), a novel mammalian target of rapamycin inhibitor, in patients with relapsed or refractory hematologic malignancies. *Clin. Cancer Res.* **2008**, *14*, 2756–2762. [CrossRef] [PubMed]
56. Li, X.; Lu, Y.; Pan, T.; Fan, Z. Roles of autophagy in cetuximab-mediated cancer therapy against EGFR. *Autophagy* **2010**, *6*, 1066–1077. [CrossRef]
57. Lauzier, A.; Normandeau-Guimond, J.; Vaillancourt-Lavigueur, V.; Boivin, V.; Charbonneau, M.; Rivard, N.; Scott, M.S.; Dubois, C.M.; Jean, S. Colorectal cancer cells respond differentially to autophagy inhibition in vivo. *Sci. Rep.* **2019**, *9*, 11316. [CrossRef]
58. Strohecker, A.M.; White, E. Autophagy promotes BrafV600E-driven lung tumorigenesis by preserving mitochondrial metabolism. *Autophagy* **2014**, *10*, 384–385. [CrossRef]
59. Avalos, Y.; Canales, J.; Bravo-Sagua, R.; Criollo, A.; Lavandero, S.; Quest, A.F. Tumor suppression and promotion by autophagy. *BioMed Res. Int.* **2014**, *2014*, 603980. [CrossRef]
60. Shteingauz, A.; Porat, Y.; Voloshin, T.; Schneiderman, R.S.; Munster, M.; Zeevi, E.; Kaynan, N.; Gotlib, K.; Giladi, M.; Kirson, E.D.; et al. AMPK-dependent autophagy upregulation serves as a survival mechanism in response to Tumor Treating Fields (TTFields). *Cell. Death Dis.* **2018**, *9*. [CrossRef]
61. Rahman, M.A.; Rahman, M.S.; Uddin, M.J.; Mamum-Or-Rashid, A.N.M.; Pang, M.G.; Rhim, H. Emerging risk of environmental factors: Insight mechanisms of Alzheimer's diseases. *Environ. Sci. Pollut. Res.* **2020**. [CrossRef] [PubMed]
62. Chen, H.H.W.; Kuo, M.T. Improving radiotherapy in cancer treatment: Promises and challenges. *Oncotarget* **2017**, *8*, 62742–62758. [CrossRef] [PubMed]

63. Luo, H.; Vong, C.T.; Chen, H.B.; Gao, Y.; Lyu, P.; Qiu, L.; Zhao, M.M.; Liu, Q.; Cheng, Z.H.; Zou, J.; et al. Naturally occurring anti-cancer compounds: Shining from Chinese herbal medicine. *Chin. Med.* **2019**, *14*. [CrossRef] [PubMed]
64. Wang, P.Q.; Zhu, L.J.; Sun, D.J.; Gan, F.H.; Gao, S.Y.; Yin, Y.Y.; Chen, L.X. Natural products as modulator of autophagy with potential clinical prospects. *Apoptosis* **2017**, *22*, 325–356. [CrossRef]
65. Choi, E.J.; Kim, G.H. Apigenin Induces Apoptosis through a Mitochondria/Caspase-Pathway in Human Breast Cancer MDA-MB-453 Cells. *J. Clin. Biochem. Nutr.* **2009**, *44*, 260–265. [CrossRef]
66. Mohan, N.; Banik, N.L.; Ray, S.K. Combination of N-(4-hydroxyphenyl) retinamide and apigenin suppressed starvation-induced autophagy and promoted apoptosis in malignant neuroblastoma cells. *Neurosci. Lett.* **2011**, *502*, 24–29. [CrossRef]
67. Nakamura, Y.; Yogosawa, S.; Izutani, Y.; Watanabe, H.; Otsuji, E.; Sakai, T. A combination of indol-3-carbinol and genistein synergistically induces apoptosis in human colon cancer HT-29 cells by inhibiting Akt phosphorylation and progression of autophagy. *Mol. Cancer* **2009**, *8*, 100. [CrossRef]
68. Gan, M.L.; Zheng, T.; Shen, L.Y.; Tan, Y.; Fan, Y.; Shuai, S.R.; Bai, L.; Li, X.W.; Wang, J.Y.; Zhang, S.H.; et al. Genistein reverses isoproterenol-induced cardiac hypertrophy by regulating miR-451/TIMP2. *Biomed. Pharmacother.* **2019**, *112*. [CrossRef]
69. Ma, C.H.; Zhang, Y.X.; Tang, L.H.; Yang, X.J.; Cui, W.M.; Han, C.C.; Ji, W.Y. MicroRNA-1469, a p53-responsive microRNA promotes Genistein induced apoptosis by targeting Mcl1 in human laryngeal cancer cells. *Biomed. Pharmacother.* **2018**, *106*, 665–671. [CrossRef]
70. Kuo, P.L.; Hsu, Y.L.; Cho, C.Y. Plumbagin induces G2-M arrest and autophagy by inhibiting the AKT/mammalian target of rapamycin pathway in breast cancer cells. *Mol. Cancer Ther.* **2006**, *5*, 3209–3221. [CrossRef]
71. Thiyagarajan, V.; Tsai, M.J.; Weng, C.F. Antroquinonol Targets FAK-Signaling Pathway Suppressed Cell Migration, Invasion, and Tumor Growth of C6 Glioma. *PLoS ONE* **2015**, *10*, e0141285. [CrossRef] [PubMed]
72. Yu, C.C.; Chiang, P.C.; Lu, P.H.; Kuo, M.T.; Wen, W.C.; Chen, P.N.; Guh, J.H. Antroquinonol, a natural ubiquinone derivative, induces a cross talk between apoptosis, autophagy and senescence in human pancreatic carcinoma cells. *J. Nutr. Biochem.* **2012**, *23*, 900–907. [CrossRef] [PubMed]
73. Chiang, P.C.; Lin, S.C.; Pan, S.L.; Kuo, C.H.; Tsai, I.L.; Kuo, M.T.; Wen, W.C.; Chen, P.; Guh, J.H. Antroquinonol displays anticancer potential against human hepatocellular carcinoma cells: A crucial role of AMPK and mTOR pathways. *Biochem. Pharmacol.* **2010**, *79*, 162–171. [CrossRef] [PubMed]
74. Chiou, J.F.; Wu, A.T.H.; Wang, W.T.; Kuo, T.H.; Gelovani, J.G.; Lin, I.H.; Wu, C.H.; Chiu, W.T.; Deng, W.P. A Preclinical Evaluation of Antrodia camphorata Alcohol Extracts in the Treatment of Non-Small Cell Lung Cancer Using Non-Invasive Molecular Imaging. *Evid.-Based Complement. Altern. Med.* **2011**, 1–12. [CrossRef]
75. Kannaiyan, R.; Manu, K.A.; Chen, L.X.; Li, F.; Rajendran, P.; Subramaniam, A.; Lam, P.; Kumar, A.P.; Sethi, G. Celastrol inhibits tumor cell proliferation and promotes apoptosis through the activation of c-Jun N-terminal kinase and suppression of PI3 K/Akt signaling pathways. *Apoptosis* **2011**, *16*, 1028–1041. [CrossRef]
76. Wang, W.B.; Feng, L.X.; Yue, Q.X.; Wu, W.Y.; Guan, S.H.; Jiang, B.H.; Yang, M.; Liu, X.; Guo, D.A. Paraptosis accompanied by autophagy and apoptosis was induced by celastrol, a natural compound with influence on proteasome, ER stress and Hsp90. *J. Cell. Physiol.* **2012**, *227*, 2196–2206. [CrossRef]
77. Li, H.; Zhang, Y.Y.; Tan, H.W.; Jia, Y.F.; Li, D. Therapeutic effect of tripterine on adjuvant arthritis in rats. *J. Ethnopharmacol.* **2008**, *118*, 479–484. [CrossRef]
78. Dyshlovoy, S.A.; Hauschild, J.; Amann, K.; Tabakmakher, K.M.; Venz, S.; Walther, R.; Guzii, A.G.; Makarieva, T.N.; Shubina, L.K.; Fedorov, S.N.; et al. Marine alkaloid Monanchocidin a overcomes drug resistance by induction of autophagy and lysosomal membrane permeabilization. *Oncotarget* **2015**, *6*, 17328–17341. [CrossRef]
79. Dyshlovoy, S.A.; Venz, S.; Hauschild, J.; Tabakmakher, K.M.; Otte, K.; Madanchi, R.; Walther, R.; Guzii, A.G.; Makarieva, T.N.; Shubina, L.K.; et al. Anti-migratory activity of marine alkaloid monanchocidin A—Proteomics-based discovery and confirmation. *Proteomics* **2016**, *16*, 1590–1603. [CrossRef]
80. McGuire, W.P.; Blessing, J.A.; Moore, D.; Lentz, S.S.; Photopulos, G. Paclitaxel has moderate activity in squamous cervix cancer: A gynecologic oncology group study. *J. Clin. Oncol.* **1996**, *14*, 792–795. [CrossRef]
81. Kampan, N.C.; Madondo, M.T.; McNally, O.M.; Quinn, M.; Plebanski, M. Paclitaxel and Its Evolving Role in the Management of Ovarian Cancer. *Biomed. Res. Int.* **2015**, *2015*, 413076. [CrossRef] [PubMed]

82. Qiu, Y.; Li, P.; Ji, C.Y. Cell Death Conversion under Hypoxic Condition in Tumor Development and Therapy. *Int. J. Mol. Sci.* **2015**, *16*, 25536–25551. [CrossRef] [PubMed]
83. Lee, Y.; Na, J.; Lee, M.S.; Cha, E.Y.; Sul, J.Y.; Park, J.B.; Lee, J.S. Combination of pristimerin and paclitaxel additively induces autophagy in human breast cancer cells via ERK1/2 regulation. *Mol. Med. Rep.* **2018**, *18*, 4281–4288. [CrossRef] [PubMed]
84. Veldhoen, R.A.; Banman, S.L.; Hemmerling, D.R.; Odsen, R.; Simmen, T.; Simmonds, A.J.; Underhill, D.A.; Goping, I.S. The chemotherapeutic agent paclitaxel inhibits autophagy through two distinct mechanisms that regulate apoptosis. *Oncogene* **2013**, *32*, 736–746. [CrossRef] [PubMed]
85. Liu, J.; Hu, X.J.; Jin, B.; Qu, X.J.; Hou, K.Z.; Liu, Y.P. ss-Elemene induces apoptosis as well as protective autophagy in human non-small-cell lung cancer A549 cells. *J. Pharm. Pharmacol.* **2012**, *64*, 146–153. [CrossRef]
86. Zhan, Y.H.; Liu, J.; Qu, X.J.; Hou, K.Z.; Wang, K.F.; Liu, Y.P.; Wu, B. beta-Elemene Induces Apoptosis in Human Renal-cell Carcinoma 786-0 Cells through Inhibition of MAPK/ERK and PI3K/Akt/mTOR Signalling Pathways. *Asian Pac. J. Cancer P* **2012**, *13*, 2739–2744. [CrossRef]
87. Saiki, S.; Sasazawa, Y.; Imamichi, Y.; Kawajiri, S.; Fujimaki, T.; Tanida, I.; Kobayashi, H.; Sato, F.; Sato, S.; Ishikawa, K.I.; et al. Caffeine induces apoptosis by enhancement of autophagy via PI3K/Akt/mTOR/p70S6K inhibition. *Autophagy* **2011**, *7*, 176–187. [CrossRef]
88. Lopez-Lazaro, M. Anticancer and carcinogenic properties of curcumin: Considerations for its clinical development as a cancer chemopreventive and chemotherapeutic agent. *Mol. Nutr. Food Res.* **2008**, *52*, S103–S127. [CrossRef]
89. Aoki, H.; Takada, Y.; Kondo, S.; Sawaya, R.; Aggarwal, B.B.; Kondo, Y. Evidence that curcumin suppresses the growth of malignant gliomas in vitro and in vivo through induction of autophagy: Role of Akt and extracellular signal-regulated kinase signaling pathways. *Mol. Pharmacol.* **2007**, *72*, 29–39. [CrossRef]
90. Klinger, N.V.; Mittal, S. Therapeutic Potential of Curcumin for the Treatment of Brain Tumors. *Oxid. Med. Cell. Longev.* **2016**, *2016*, 9324085. [CrossRef]
91. Masuelli, L.; Benvenuto, M.; Di Stefano, E.; Mattera, R.; Fantini, M.; De Feudis, G.; De Smaele, E.; Tresoldi, I.; Giganti, M.G.; Modesti, A.; et al. Curcumin blocks autophagy and activates apoptosis of malignant mesothelioma cell lines and increases the survival of mice intraperitoneally transplanted with a malignant mesothelioma cell line. *Oncotarget* **2017**, *8*, 34405–34422. [CrossRef] [PubMed]
92. Buhrmann, C.; Kraehe, P.; Lueders, C.; Shayan, P.; Goel, A.; Shakibaei, M. Curcumin Suppresses Crosstalk between Colon Cancer Stem Cells and Stromal Fibroblasts in the Tumor Microenvironment: Potential Role of EMT. *PLoS ONE* **2014**, *9*. [CrossRef] [PubMed]
93. Xu, R.; Li, H.B.; Wu, S.Q.; Qu, J.; Yuan, H.Y.; Zhou, Y.G.; Lu, Q. MicroRNA-1246 regulates the radio-sensitizing effect of curcumin in bladder cancer cells via activating P53. *Int. Urol. Nephrol.* **2019**, *51*, 1771–1779. [CrossRef] [PubMed]
94. Aggarwal, B.B.; Deb, L.; Prasad, S. Curcumin Differs from Tetrahydrocurcumin for Molecular Targets, Signaling Pathways and Cellular Responses. *Molecules* **2015**, *20*, 185–205. [CrossRef]
95. Wu, J.C.; Lai, C.S.; Badmaev, V.; Nagabhushanam, K.; Ho, C.T.; Pan, M.H. Tetrahydrocurcumin, a major metabolite of curcumin, induced autophagic cell death through coordinative modulation of PI3K/Akt-mTOR and MAPK signaling pathways in human leukemia HL-60 cells. *Mol. Nutr. Food Res.* **2011**, *55*, 1646–1654. [CrossRef] [PubMed]
96. Hu, F.; Wei, F.; Wang, Y.L.; Wu, B.B.; Fang, Y.; Xiong, B. EGCG synergizes the therapeutic effect of cisplatin and oxaliplatin through autophagic pathway in human colorectal cancer cells. *J. Pharmacol. Sci.* **2015**, *128*, 27–34. [CrossRef] [PubMed]
97. Irimie, A.I.; Braicu, C.; Zanoaga, O.; Pileczki, V.; Gherman, C.; Berindan-Neagoe, I.; Campian, R.S. Epigallocatechin-3-gallate suppresses cell proliferation and promotes apoptosis and autophagy in oral cancer SSC-4 cells. *Oncotargets Ther.* **2015**, *8*, 461–470. [CrossRef]
98. Zhou, J.; Farah, B.L.; Sinha, R.A.; Wu, Y.; Singh, B.K. Epigallocatechin-3-Gallate (EGCG), a Green Tea Polyphenol, Stimulates Hepatic Autophagy and Lipid Clearance (vol 9, e87161, 2014). *PLoS ONE* **2014**, *9*. [CrossRef]
99. Gray, A.L.; Stephens, C.A.; Bigelow, R.L.H.; Coleman, D.T.; Cardelli, J.A. The Polyphenols (-)-Epigallocatechin-3-Gallate and Luteolin Synergistically Inhibit TGF-beta-Induced Myofibroblast Phenotypes through RhoA and ERK Inhibition. *PLoS ONE* **2014**, *9*, e109208. [CrossRef]

100. Chen, A.P.; Zhang, L. The antioxidant (-)-epigallocatechin-3-gallate inhibits rat hepatic stellate cell proliferation in vitro by blocking the tyrosine phosphorylation and reducing the gene expression of platelet-derived growth factor-beta receptor. *J. Biol. Chem.* **2003**, *278*, 23381–23389. [CrossRef]

101. Chen, L.L.; Xu, Y. Epigallocatechin gallate attenuates uric acid-induced injury in rat renal interstitial fibroblasts NRK-49F by up-regulation of miR-9. *Eur. Rev. Med. Pharmacol.* **2018**, *22*, 7458–7469.

102. Adhami, V.M.; Syed, D.N.; Khan, N.; Mukhtar, H. Dietary flavonoid fisetin: A novel dual inhibitor of PI3K/Akt and mTOR for prostate cancer management. *Biochem. Pharmacol.* **2012**, *84*, 1277–1281. [CrossRef] [PubMed]

103. Sun, X.; Ma, X.M.; Li, Q.W.; Yang, Y.; Xu, X.L.; Sun, J.Q.; Yu, M.W.; Cao, K.X.; Yang, L.; Yang, G.W.; et al. Anti-cancer effects of fisetin on mammary carcinoma cells via regulation of the PI3K/Akt/mTOR pathway: In vitro and in vivo studies. *Int. J. Mol. Med.* **2018**, *42*, 811–820. [CrossRef] [PubMed]

104. Khan, N.; Afaq, F.; Khusro, F.H.; Adhami, V.M.; Suh, Y.; Mukhtar, H. Dual inhibition of phosphatidylinositol 3-kinase/Akt and mammalian target of rapamycin signaling in human nonsmall cell lung cancer cells by a dietary flavonoid fisetin. *Int. J. Cancer* **2012**, *130*, 1695–1705. [CrossRef] [PubMed]

105. Suh, Y.; Afaq, F.; Khan, N.; Johnson, J.J.; Khusro, F.H.; Mukhtar, H. Fisetin induces autophagic cell death through suppression of mTOR signaling pathway in prostate cancer cells. *Carcinogenesis* **2010**, *31*, 1424–1433. [CrossRef]

106. Yang, P.M.; Tseng, H.H.; Peng, C.W.; Chen, W.S.; Chiu, S.J. Dietary flavonoid fisetin targets caspase-3-deficient human breast cancer MCF-7 cells by induction of caspase-7-associated apoptosis and inhibition of autophagy. *Int. J. Oncol.* **2012**, *40*, 469–478. [CrossRef]

107. Tiwari, R.V.; Parajuli, P.; Sylvester, P.W. gamma-Tocotrienol-induced endoplasmic reticulum stress and autophagy act concurrently to promote breast cancer cell death. *Biochem. Cell. Biol.* **2015**, *93*, 306–320. [CrossRef]

108. Deng, S.; Shanmugam, M.K.; Kumar, A.P.; Yap, C.T.; Sethi, G.; Bishayee, A. Targeting autophagy using natural compounds for cancer prevention and therapy. *Cancer-Am. Cancer Soc.* **2019**, *125*, 1228–1246. [CrossRef]

109. Jiang, Q.; Rao, X.Y.; Kim, C.Y.; Freiser, H.; Zhang, Q.B.; Jiang, Z.Y.; Li, G.L. Gamma-tocotrienol induces apoptosis and autophagy in prostate cancer cells by increasing intracellular dihydrosphingosine and dihydroceramide. *Int. J. Cancer* **2012**, *130*, 685–693. [CrossRef]

110. Tiwari, R.V.; Parajuli, P.; Sylvester, P.W. gamma-Tocotrienol-induced autophagy in malignant mammary cancer cells. *Exp. Biol. Med.* **2014**, *239*, 33–44. [CrossRef]

111. Kim, S.H.; Park, E.J.; Lee, C.R.; Chun, J.N.; Cho, N.H.; Kim, I.G.; Lee, S.; Kim, T.W.; Park, H.H.; So, I.; et al. Geraniol induces cooperative interaction of apoptosis and autophagy to elicit cell death in PC-3 prostate cancer cells. *Int. J. Oncol.* **2012**, *40*, 1683–1690. [CrossRef] [PubMed]

112. Trzoss, L.; Fukuda, T.; Costa-Lotufo, L.V.; Jimenez, P.; La Clair, J.J.; Fenical, W. Seriniquinone, a selective anticancer agent, induces cell death by autophagocytosis, targeting the cancer-protective protein dermcidin. *Proc. Natl. Acad. Sci. USA* **2014**, *111*, 14687–14692. [CrossRef] [PubMed]

113. Chu, S.C.; Hsieh, Y.S.; Yu, C.C.; Lai, Y.Y.; Chen, P.N. Thymoquinone Induces Cell Death in Human Squamous Carcinoma Cells via Caspase Activation-Dependent Apoptosis and LC3-II Activation-Dependent Autophagy. *PLoS ONE* **2014**, *9*. [CrossRef] [PubMed]

114. Racoma, I.O.; Meisen, W.H.; Wang, Q.E.; Kaur, B.; Wani, A.A. Thymoquinone Inhibits Autophagy and Induces Cathepsin-Mediated, Caspase-Independent Cell Death in Glioblastoma Cells. *PLoS ONE* **2013**, *8*. [CrossRef] [PubMed]

115. Chen, M.C.; Lee, N.H.; Hsu, H.H.; Ho, T.J.; Tu, C.C.; Hsieh, D.J.Y.; Lin, Y.M.; Chen, L.M.; Kuo, W.W.; Huang, C.Y. Thymoquinone Induces Caspase-Independent, Autophagic Cell Death in CPT-11-Resistant LoVo Colon Cancer via Mitochondrial Dysfunction and Activation of JNK and p38. *J. Agric. Food Chem.* **2015**, *63*, 1540–1546. [CrossRef] [PubMed]

116. Xu, H.L.; Tang, W.; Du, G.H.; Kokudo, N. Targeting apoptosis pathways in cancer with magnolol and honokiol, bioactive constituents of the bark of Magnolia officinalis. *Drug Discov. Ther.* **2011**, *5*, 202–210. [CrossRef] [PubMed]

117. Li, H.B.; Yi, X.; Gao, J.M.; Ying, X.X.; Guan, H.Q.; Li, J.C. Magnolol-induced H460 cells death via autophagy but not apoptosis. *Arch. Pharm. Res.* **2007**, *30*, 1566–1574. [CrossRef]

118. Rasul, A.; Yu, B.; Khan, M.; Zhang, K.; Iqbal, F.; Ma, T.H.; Yang, H. Magnolol, a natural compound, induces apoptosis of SGC-7901 human gastric adenocarcinoma cells via the mitochondrial and PI3K/Akt signaling pathways. *Int. J. Oncol.* **2012**, *40*, 1153–1161. [CrossRef]
119. Bae, U.J.; Jung, E.S.; Jung, S.J.; Chae, S.W.; Park, B.H. Mulberry leaf extract displays antidiabetic activity in db/db mice via Akt and AMP-activated protein kinase phosphorylation. *Food Nutr. Res.* **2018**, *62*. [CrossRef]
120. Cheng, K.C.; Wang, C.J.; Chang, Y.C.; Hung, T.W.; Lai, C.J.; Kuo, C.W.; Huang, H.P. Mulberry fruits extracts induce apoptosis and autophagy of liver cancer cell and prevent hepatocarcinogenesis in vivo. *J. Food Drug Anal.* **2020**, *28*, 84–93. [CrossRef]
121. Kwon, Y.H.; Bishayee, K.; Rahman, M.A.; Hong, J.S.; Lim, S.S.; Huh, S.O. Morus alba Accumulates Reactive Oxygen Species to Initiate Apoptosis via FOXO-Caspase 3-Dependent Pathway in Neuroblastoma Cells. *Mol. Cells* **2015**, *38*, 630–637. [CrossRef] [PubMed]
122. Lao, Y.Z.; Wan, G.; Liu, Z.Y.; Wang, X.Y.; Ruan, P.; Xu, W.; Xu, D.Q.; Xie, W.D.; Zhang, Y.; Xu, H.X.; et al. The natural compound oblongifolin C inhibits autophagic flux and enhances antitumor efficacy of nutrient deprivation. *Autophagy* **2014**, *10*, 736–749. [CrossRef] [PubMed]
123. Wu, M.; Lao, Y.Z.; Tan, H.S.; Lu, G.; Ren, Y.; Zheng, Z.Q.; Yi, J.; Fu, W.W.; Shen, H.M.; Xu, H.X. Oblongifolin C suppresses lysosomal function independently of TFEB nuclear translocation. *Acta Pharmacol. Sin.* **2019**, *40*, 929–937. [CrossRef] [PubMed]
124. Acharya, B.R.; Bhattacharyya, S.; Choudhury, D.; Chakrabarti, G. The microtubule depolymerizing agent naphthazarin induces both apoptosis and autophagy in A549 lung cancer cells. *Apoptosis* **2011**, *16*, 924–939. [CrossRef]
125. Herr, I.; Lozanovski, V.; Houben, P.; Schemmer, P.; Buchler, M.W. Sulforaphane and related mustard oils in focus of cancer prevention and therapy. *Wien. Med. Wochenschr.* **2013**, *163*, 80–88. [CrossRef]
126. Herman-Antosiewicz, A.; Johnson, D.E.; Singh, S.V. Sulforaphane causes autophagy to inhibit release of cytochrome C and apoptosis in human prostate cancer cells. *Cancer Res.* **2006**, *66*, 5828–5835. [CrossRef]
127. Zheng, Z.; Lin, K.; Hu, Y.; Zhou, Y.; Ding, X.; Wang, Y.; Wu, W. Sulforaphane metabolites inhibit migration and invasion via microtubule-mediated Claudins dysfunction or inhibition of autolysosome formation in human non-small cell lung cancer cells. *Cell Death Dis.* **2019**, *10*, 259. [CrossRef]
128. Chaudhuri, D.; Orsulic, S.; Ashok, B.T. Antiproliferative activity of sulforaphane in Akt-overexpressing ovarian cancer cells. *Mol. Cancer Ther.* **2007**, *6*, 334–345. [CrossRef]
129. Uddin, M.S.; Mamun, A.A.; Jakaria, M.; Thangapandiyan, S.; Ahmad, J.; Rahman, M.A.; Mathew, B.; Abdel-Daim, M.M.; Aleya, L. Emerging promise of sulforaphane-mediated Nrf2 signaling cascade against neurological disorders. *Sci. Total Environ.* **2020**, *707*, 135624. [CrossRef]
130. Kim, S.M.; Park, H.S.; Jun, D.Y.; Woo, H.J.; Woo, M.H.; Yang, C.H.; Kim, Y.H. Mollugin induces apoptosis in human Jurkat T cells through endoplasmic reticulum stress-mediated activation of JNK and caspase-12 and subsequent activation of mitochondria-dependent caspase cascade regulated by Bcl-xL. *Toxicol. Appl. Pharm.* **2009**, *241*, 210–220. [CrossRef]
131. Zhang, L.; Wang, H.D.; Zhu, J.H.; Xu, J.G.; Ding, K. Mollugin induces tumor cell apoptosis and autophagy via the PI3K/AKT/mTOR/p70S6K and ERK signaling pathways. *Biochem. Biophys Res. Commun.* **2014**, *450*, 247–254. [CrossRef] [PubMed]
132. Xu, M.Y.; Lee, S.Y.; Kang, S.S.; Kim, Y.S. Antitumor Activity of Jujuboside B and the Underlying Mechanism via Induction of Apoptosis and Autophagy. *J. Nat. Prod.* **2014**, *77*, 370–376. [CrossRef] [PubMed]
133. Lu, J.; Sun, D.P.; Gao, S.; Gao, Y.; Ye, J.T.; Liu, P.Q. Cyclovirobuxine D Induces Autophagy-Associated Cell Death via the Akt/mTOR Pathway in MCF-7 Human Breast Cancer Cells. *J. Pharmacol. Sci.* **2014**, *125*, 74–82. [CrossRef] [PubMed]
134. Ouyang, L.; Chen, Y.; Wang, X.Y.; Lu, R.F.; Zhang, S.Y.; Tian, M.; Xie, T.; Liu, B.; He, G. Polygonatum odoratum lectin induces apoptosis and autophagy via targeting EGFR-mediated Ras-Raf-MEK-ERK pathway in human MCF-7 breast cancer cells. *Phytomedicine* **2014**, *21*, 1658–1665. [CrossRef]
135. Li, C.Y.; Chen, J.; Lu, B.M.; Shi, Z.; Wang, H.L.; Zhang, B.; Zhao, K.L.; Qi, W.; Bao, J.K.; Wang, Y. Molecular Switch Role of Akt in Polygonatum odoratum Lectin-Induced Apoptosis and Autophagy in Human Non-Small Cell Lung Cancer A549 Cells. *PLoS ONE* **2014**, *9*, e101526. [CrossRef]
136. Jiang, H.; Zhang, L.; Kuo, J.; Kuo, K.; Gautam, S.C.; Groc, L.; Rodriguez, A.I.; Koubi, D.; Hunter, T.J.; Corcoran, G.B.; et al. Resveratrol-induced apoptotic death in human U251 glioma cells. *Mol. Cancer Ther.* **2005**, *4*, 554–561. [CrossRef]

137. Rahman, M.A.; Kim, N.H.; Kim, S.H.; Oh, S.M.; Huh, S.O. Antiproliferative and Cytotoxic Effects of Resveratrol in Mitochondria-Mediated Apoptosis in Rat B103 Neuroblastoma Cells. *Korean J. Physiol. Pharm.* **2012**, *16*, 321–326. [CrossRef]
138. Lang, F.F.; Qin, Z.Y.; Li, F.; Zhang, H.L.; Fang, Z.H.; Hao, E.K. Apoptotic Cell Death Induced by Resveratrol Is Partially Mediated by the Autophagy Pathway in Human Ovarian Cancer Cells. *PLoS ONE* **2015**, *10*. [CrossRef]
139. Garg, T.; Yadav, V.K. Effects of Resveratrol as an anticancer agent. A Systematic Review and Meta-Analysis. *Indian J. Pharmacol.* **2013**, *45*, S206.
140. Gong, C.H.; Xia, H.L. Resveratrol suppresses melanoma growth by promoting autophagy through inhibiting the PI3K/AKT/mTOR signaling pathway. *Exp. Ther. Med.* **2020**, *19*, 1878–1886. [CrossRef]
141. Liu, Q.J.; Fang, Q.; Ji, S.Q.; Han, Z.X.; Cheng, W.L.; Zhang, H.J. Resveratrol-mediated apoptosis in renal cell carcinoma via the p53/AMP-activated protein kinase/mammalian target of rapamycin autophagy signaling pathway. *Mol. Med. Rep.* **2018**, *17*, 502–508. [CrossRef] [PubMed]
142. Godichaud, S.; Si-Tayeb, K.; Auge, N.; Desmouliere, A.; Balabaud, C.; Payrastre, B.; Negre-Salvayre, A.; Rosenbaum, J. The grape-derived polyphenol resveratrol differentially affects epidermal and platelet-derived growth factor signaling in human liver myofibroblasts. *Int. J. Biochem. Cell Biol.* **2006**, *38*, 629–637. [CrossRef] [PubMed]
143. Jiang, Y.D.; Liu, L.; Steinle, J.J. miRNA15a regulates insulin signal transduction in the retinal vasculature. *Cell. Signal.* **2018**, *44*, 28–32. [CrossRef]
144. Anand David, A.V.; Arulmoli, R.; Parasuraman, S. Overviews of Biological Importance of Quercetin: A Bioactive Flavonoid. *Pharmacogn. Rev.* **2016**, *10*, 84–89. [CrossRef] [PubMed]
145. Singh, B.N.; Kumar, D.; Shankar, S.; Srivastava, R.K. Rottlerin induces autophagy which leads to apoptotic cell death through inhibition of PI3K/Akt/mTOR pathway in human pancreatic cancer stem cells. *Biochem. Pharmacol.* **2012**, *84*, 1154–1163. [CrossRef]
146. Rahman, M.A.; Kim, N.H.; Yang, H.; Huh, S.O. Angelicin induces apoptosis through intrinsic caspase-dependent pathway in human SH-SY5Y neuroblastoma cells. *Mol. Cell. Biochem.* **2012**, *369*, 95–104. [CrossRef]
147. Rahman, M.A.; Bishayee, K.; Huh, S.O. Angelica polymorpha Maxim Induces Apoptosis of Human SH-SY5Y Neuroblastoma Cells by Regulating an Intrinsic Caspase Pathway. *Mol. Cells* **2016**, *39*, 119–128. [CrossRef]
148. Wang, Y.R.; Chen, Y.Q.; Chen, X.D.; Liang, Y.; Yang, D.P.; Dong, J.; Yang, N.; Liang, Z.Q. Angelicin inhibits the malignant behaviours of human cervical cancer potentially via inhibiting autophagy. *Exp. Ther. Med.* **2019**, *18*, 3365–3374. [CrossRef]
149. Uddin, M.S.; Rahman, M.A.; Kabir, M.T.; Behl, T.; Mathew, B.; Perveen, A.; Barreto, G.E.; Bin-Jumah, M.N.; Abdel-Daim, M.M.; Ashraf, G.M. Multifarious roles of mTOR signaling in cognitive aging and cerebrovascular dysfunction of Alzheimer's disease. *IUBMB Life* **2020**. [CrossRef]
150. Leng, S.; Hao, Y.; Du, D.; Xie, S.; Hong, L.; Gu, H.; Zhu, X.; Zhang, J.; Fan, D.; Kung, H.F. Ursolic acid promotes cancer cell death by inducing Atg5-dependent autophagy. *Int. J. Cancer* **2013**, *133*, 2781–2790. [CrossRef]
151. Xavier, C.P.R.; Lima, C.F.; Pedro, D.F.N.; Wilson, J.M.; Kristiansen, K.; Pereira-Wilson, C. Ursolic acid induces cell death and modulates autophagy through JNK pathway in apoptosis-resistant colorectal cancer cells. *J. Nutr. Biochem.* **2013**, *24*, 706–712. [CrossRef] [PubMed]
152. Zhao, C.; Yin, S.T.; Dong, Y.H.; Guo, X.; Fan, L.H.; Ye, M.; Hu, H.B. Autophagy-dependent EIF2AK3 activation compromises ursolic acid-induced apoptosis through upregulation of MCL1 in MCF-7 human breast cancer cells. *Autophagy* **2013**, *9*, 196–207. [CrossRef] [PubMed]
153. Shin, S.W.; Park, J.W. Autophagy inhibition enhances ursolic acid-induced apoptosis in PC3 cells. *Free Radic. Biol. Med.* **2012**, *53*, S116. [CrossRef]
154. Wang, S.Y.; Yu, Q.J.; Bao, J.K.; Liu, B. Polygonatum cyrtonema lectin, a potential antineoplastic drug targeting programmed cell death pathways. *Biochem. Biophys. Res. Commun.* **2011**, *406*, 497–500. [CrossRef]
155. Liu, B.; Cheng, Y.; Bian, H.J.; Bao, J.K. Molecular mechanisms of Polygonatum cyrtonema lectin-induced apoptosis and autophagy in cancer cells. *Autophagy* **2009**, *5*, 253–255. [CrossRef]
156. Liu, B.; Cheng, Y.; Zhang, B.; Bian, H.J.; Bao, J.K. Polygonatum cyrtonema lectin induces apoptosis and autophagy in human melanoma A375 cells through a mitochondria-mediated ROS-p38-p53 pathway. *Cancer Lett.* **2009**, *275*, 54–60. [CrossRef]

157. Duan, W.J.; Li, Q.S.; Xia, M.Y.; Tashiro, S.I.; Onodera, S.; Ikejima, T. Silibinin Activated p53 and Induced Autophagic Death in Human Fibrosarcoma HT1080 Cells via Reactive Oxygen Species-p38 and c-Jun N-Terminal Kinase Pathways. *Biol. Pharm. Bull.* **2011**, *34*, 47–53. [CrossRef]
158. Rahman, M.A.; Yang, H.; Kim, N.H.; Huh, S.O. Induction of apoptosis by Dioscorea nipponica Makino extracts in human SH-SY5Y neuroblastoma cells via mitochondria-mediated pathway. *Anim. Cells Syst.* **2014**, *18*, 41–51. [CrossRef]
159. Rahman, M.A.; Yang, H.; Lim, S.S.; Huh, S.O. Apoptotic Effects of Melandryum firmum Root Extracts in Human SH-SY5Y Neuroblastoma Cells. *Exp. Neurobiol.* **2013**, *22*, 208–213. [CrossRef]
160. Bassham, D.C.; Crespo, J.L. Autophagy in plants and algae. *Front. Plant Sci.* **2014**, *5*. [CrossRef]
161. Uddin, M.S.; Mamun, A.A.; Rahman, M.A.; Kabir, M.T.; Alkahtani, S.; Alanazi, I.S.; Perveen, A.; Ashraf, G.M.; Bin-Jumah, M.N.; Abdel-Daim, M.M. Exploring the Promise of Flavonoids to Combat Neuropathic Pain: From Molecular Mechanisms to Therapeutic Implications. *Front. Neurosci.* **2020**, *14*, 478. [CrossRef]
162. Rahman, M.A.; Hong, J.S.; Huh, S.O. Antiproliferative properties of Saussurea lappa Clarke root extract in SH-SY5Y neuroblastoma cells via intrinsic apoptotic pathway. *Anim. Cells Syst.* **2015**, *19*, 119–126. [CrossRef]
163. Tian, X.; Song, H.S.; Cho, Y.M.; Park, B.; Song, Y.J.; Jang, S.; Kang, S.C. Anticancer effect of Saussurea lappa extract via dual control of apoptosis and autophagy in prostate cancer cells. *Medicine* **2017**, *96*. [CrossRef]
164. Ryoo, N.; Rahman, M.A.; Hwang, H.; Ko, S.K.; Nah, S.Y.; Kim, H.C.; Rhim, H. Ginsenoside Rk1 is a novel inhibitor of NMDA receptors in cultured rat hippocampal neurons. *J. Ginseng Res.* **2020**, *44*, 490–495. [CrossRef]
165. Ko, H.; Kim, Y.J.; Park, J.S.; Park, J.H.; Yang, H.O. Autophagy Inhibition Enhances Apoptosis Induced by Ginsenoside Rk1 in Hepatocellular Carcinoma Cells. *Biosci. Biotechnol. Biochem.* **2009**, *73*, 2183–2189. [CrossRef]
166. Zecchini, S.; Serafini, F.P.; Catalani, E.; Giovarelli, M.; Coazzoli, M.; Di Renzo, I.; De Palma, C.; Perrotta, C.; Clementi, E.; Buonanno, F.; et al. Dysfunctional autophagy induced by the pro-apoptotic natural compound climacostol in tumour cells. *Cell Death Dis.* **2018**, *10*. [CrossRef]
167. Saha, S.; Panigrahi, D.P.; Patil, S.; Bhutia, S.K. Autophagy in health and disease: A comprehensive review. *Biomed. Pharmacother.* **2018**, *104*, 485–495. [CrossRef]
168. Grossi, C.; Rigacci, S.; Ambrosini, S.; Ed Dami, T.; Luccarini, I.; Traini, C.; Failli, P.; Berti, A.; Casamenti, F.; Stefani, M. The polyphenol oleuropein aglycone protects TgCRND8 mice against Ass plaque pathology. *PLoS ONE* **2013**, *8*, e71702. [CrossRef]
169. Luccarini, I.; Grossi, C.; Rigacci, S.; Coppi, E.; Pugliese, A.M.; Pantano, D.; la Marca, G.; Ed Dami, T.; Berti, A.; Stefani, M.; et al. Oleuropein aglycone protects against pyroglutamylated-3 amyloid-ss toxicity: Biochemical, epigenetic and functional correlates. *Neurobiol. Aging* **2015**, *36*, 648–663. [CrossRef]
170. Zhu, Z.; Yan, J.; Jiang, W.; Yao, X.G.; Chen, J.; Chen, L.; Li, C.; Hu, L.; Jiang, H.; Shen, X. Arctigenin effectively ameliorates memory impairment in Alzheimer's disease model mice targeting both beta-amyloid production and clearance. *J. Neurosci.* **2013**, *33*, 13138–13149. [CrossRef]
171. Lu, C.; Guo, Y.; Yan, J.; Luo, Z.; Luo, H.B.; Yan, M.; Huang, L.; Li, X. Design, synthesis, and evaluation of multitarget-directed resveratrol derivatives for the treatment of Alzheimer's disease. *J. Med. Chem.* **2013**, *56*, 5843–5859. [CrossRef] [PubMed]
172. de Oliveira, M.R.; Nabavi, S.F.; Manayi, A.; Daglia, M.; Hajheydari, Z.; Nabavi, S.M. Resveratrol and the mitochondria: From triggering the intrinsic apoptotic pathway to inducing mitochondrial biogenesis, a mechanistic view. *BBA-Gen. Subj.* **2016**, *1860*, 727–745. [CrossRef] [PubMed]
173. Juhasz, B.; Varga, B.; Gesztelyi, R.; Kemeny-Beke, A.; Zsuga, J.; Tosaki, A. Resveratrol: A Multifunctional Cytoprotective Molecule. *Curr. Pharm. Biotechnol.* **2010**, *11*, 810–818. [CrossRef] [PubMed]
174. Filomeni, G.; Graziani, I.; De Zio, D.; Dini, L.; Centonze, D.; Rotilio, G.; Ciriolo, M.R. Neuroprotection of kaempferol by autophagy in models of rotenone-mediated acute toxicity: Possible implications for Parkinson's disease. *Neurobiol. Aging* **2012**, *33*, 767–785. [CrossRef]
175. Lu, J.H.; Tan, J.Q.; Durairajan, S.S.; Liu, L.F.; Zhang, Z.H.; Ma, L.; Shen, H.M.; Chan, H.Y.; Li, M. Isorhynchophylline, a natural alkaloid, promotes the degradation of alpha-synuclein in neuronal cells via inducing autophagy. *Autophagy* **2012**, *8*, 98–108. [CrossRef]
176. Sasazawa, Y.; Sato, N.; Umezawa, K.; Simizu, S. Conophylline protects cells in cellular models of neurodegenerative diseases by inducing mammalian target of rapamycin (mTOR)-independent autophagy. *J. Biol. Chem.* **2015**, *290*, 6168–6178. [CrossRef]

177. Jiang, T.F.; Zhang, Y.J.; Zhou, H.Y.; Wang, H.M.; Tian, L.P.; Liu, J.; Ding, J.Q.; Chen, S.D. Curcumin ameliorates the neurodegenerative pathology in A53T alpha-synuclein cell model of Parkinson's disease through the downregulation of mTOR/p70S6K signaling and the recovery of macroautophagy. *J. Neuroimmune Pharmacol.* **2013**, *8*, 356–369. [CrossRef]
178. Guo, Y.J.; Dong, S.Y.; Cui, X.X.; Feng, Y.; Liu, T.; Yin, M.; Kuo, S.H.; Tan, E.K.; Zhao, W.J.; Wu, Y.C. Resveratrol alleviates MPTP-induced motor impairments and pathological changes by autophagic degradation of alpha-synuclein via SIRT1-deacetylated LC3. *Mol. Nutr. Food Res.* **2016**, *60*, 2161–2175. [CrossRef]
179. Ferretta, A.; Gaballo, A.; Tanzarella, P.; Piccoli, C.; Capitanio, N.; Nico, B.; Annese, T.; Di Paola, M.; Dell'aquila, C.; De Mari, M.; et al. Effect of resveratrol on mitochondrial function: Implications in parkin-associated familiar Parkinson's disease. *Biochim. Biophys. Acta* **2014**, *1842*, 902–915. [CrossRef]
180. Cai, C.Z.; Zhou, H.F.; Yuan, N.N.; Wu, M.Y.; Lee, S.M.; Ren, J.Y.; Su, H.X.; Lu, J.J.; Chen, X.P.; Li, M.; et al. Natural alkaloid harmine promotes degradation of alpha-synuclein via PKA-mediated ubiquitin-proteasome system activation. *Phytomedicine* **2019**, *61*, 152842. [CrossRef]
181. Wong, V.K.; Wu, A.G.; Wang, J.R.; Liu, L.; Law, B.Y. Neferine attenuates the protein level and toxicity of mutant huntingtin in PC-12 cells via induction of autophagy. *Molecules* **2015**, *20*, 3496–3514. [CrossRef] [PubMed]
182. Sarkar, S.; Davies, J.E.; Huang, Z.; Tunnacliffe, A.; Rubinsztein, D.C. Trehalose, a novel mTOR-independent autophagy enhancer, accelerates the clearance of mutant huntingtin and alpha-synuclein. *J. Biol. Chem.* **2007**, *282*, 5641–5652. [CrossRef] [PubMed]
183. Jiang, W.; Wei, W.; Gaertig, M.A.; Li, S.; Li, X.J. Therapeutic Effect of Berberine on Huntington's Disease Transgenic Mouse Model. *PLoS ONE* **2015**, *10*, e0134142. [CrossRef] [PubMed]
184. Castillo, K.; Nassif, M.; Valenzuela, V.; Rojas, F.; Matus, S.; Mercado, G.; Court, F.A.; van Zundert, B.; Hetz, C. Trehalose delays the progression of amyotrophic lateral sclerosis by enhancing autophagy in motoneurons. *Autophagy* **2013**, *9*, 1308–1320. [CrossRef]
185. Menzies, F.M.; Huebener, J.; Renna, M.; Bonin, M.; Riess, O.; Rubinsztein, D.C. Autophagy induction reduces mutant ataxin-3 levels and toxicity in a mouse model of spinocerebellar ataxia type 3. *Brain* **2010**, *133*, 93–104. [CrossRef]
186. Singhal, J.; Nagaprashantha, L.D.; Vatsyayan, R.; Awasthi, S.; Singhal, S.S. Didymin induces apoptosis by inhibiting N-Myc and upregulating RKIP in neuroblastoma. *Cancer Prev. Res.* **2012**, *5*, 473–483. [CrossRef]
187. Rahman, M.A.; Kim, N.H.; Huh, S.O. Cytotoxic effect of gambogic acid on SH-SY5Y neuroblastoma cells is mediated by intrinsic caspase-dependent signaling pathway. *Mol. Cell. Biochem.* **2013**, *377*, 187–196. [CrossRef]
188. Vengoji, R.; Macha, M.A.; Batra, S.K.; Shonka, N.A. Natural products: A hope for glioblastoma patients. *Oncotarget* **2018**, *9*, 22194–22219. [CrossRef]
189. Yuan, Y.; Xue, X.; Guo, R.B.; Sun, X.L.; Hu, G. Resveratrol Enhances the Antitumor Effects of Temozolomide in Glioblastoma via ROS-dependent AMPK-TSC-mTOR Signaling Pathway. *CNS. Neurosci. Ther.* **2012**, *18*, 536–546. [CrossRef]
190. Shah, S.H. Carbonic anhydrase, net photosynthetic rate and yield of black cumin (*Nigella sativa*) plants sprayed with kinetin. *Acta Bot. Croat.* **2008**, *67*, 63–68.
191. Hussain, A.R.; Uddin, S.; Ahmed, M.; Al-Dayel, F.; Bavi, P.P.; Al-Kuraya, K.S. Phosphorylated IkappaBalpha predicts poor prognosis in activated B-cell lymphoma and its inhibition with thymoquinone induces apoptosis via ROS release. *PLoS ONE* **2013**, *8*, e60540. [CrossRef] [PubMed]
192. Yamamoto, K.; Ishikawa, C.; Katano, H.; Yasumoto, T.; Mori, N. Fucoxanthin and its deacetylated product, fucoxanthinol, induce apoptosis of primary effusion lymphomas. *Cancer Lett.* **2011**, *300*, 225–234. [CrossRef] [PubMed]
193. Zhao, Q.; Guan, J.W.; Qin, Y.H.; Ren, P.; Zhang, Z.W.; Lv, J.; Sun, S.J.; Zhang, C.L.; Mao, W.F. Curcumin sensitizes lymphoma cells to DNA damage agents through regulating Rad51-dependent homologous recombination. *Biomed. Pharmacother.* **2018**, *97*, 115–119. [CrossRef] [PubMed]
194. Shi, L.Y.; Qin, H.H.; Jin, X.D.; Yang, X.X.; Lu, X.; Wang, H.G.; Wang, R.Y.; Yu, D.Y.; Feng, B.M. The natural phenolic peperobtusin A induces apoptosis of lymphoma U937 cells via the Caspase dependent and p38 MAPK signaling pathways. *Biomed. Pharmacother.* **2018**, *102*, 772–781. [CrossRef] [PubMed]

195. Xiao, X.H.; Li, H.L.; Jin, H.Z.; Jin, J.; Yu, M.; Ma, C.M.; Tong, Y.; Zhou, L.; Lei, H.; Xu, H.Z.; et al. Identification of 11(13)-dehydroivaxillin as a potent therapeutic agent against non-Hodgkin's lymphoma. *Cell Death Dis.* **2017**, *8*. [CrossRef] [PubMed]
196. Martino, R.; Beer, M.F.; Elso, O.; Donadel, O.; Sulsen, V.; Anesini, C. Sesquiterpene lactones from Ambrosia spp. are active against a murine lymphoma cell line by inducing apoptosis and cell cycle arrest. *Toxicol. In Vitro* **2015**, *29*, 1529–1536. [CrossRef]
197. Leidal, A.M.; Levine, B.; Debnath, J. Autophagy and the cell biology of age-related disease. *Nat. Cell Biol.* **2018**, *20*, 1338–1348. [CrossRef]
198. Sciarretta, S.; Maejima, Y.; Zablocki, D.; Sadoshima, J. The Role of Autophagy in the Heart. *Annu. Rev. Physiol.* **2018**, *80*, 1–26. [CrossRef]
199. Meyer, G.; Czompa, A.; Reboul, C.; Csepanyi, E.; Czegledi, A.; Bak, I.; Balla, G.; Balla, J.; Tosaki, A.; Lekli, I. The cellular autophagy markers Beclin-1 and LC3B-II are increased during reperfusion in fibrillated mouse hearts. *Curr. Pharm. Des.* **2013**, *19*, 6912–6918. [CrossRef]
200. Shirakabe, A.; Zhai, P.; Ikeda, Y.; Saito, T.; Maejima, Y.; Hsu, C.P.; Nomura, M.; Egashira, K.; Levine, B.; Sadoshima, J. Drp1-Dependent Mitochondrial Autophagy Plays a Protective Role Against Pressure Overload-Induced Mitochondrial Dysfunction and Heart Failure. *Circulation* **2016**, *133*, 1249–1263. [CrossRef]
201. Matsui, Y.; Takagi, H.; Qu, X.P.; Abdellatif, M.; Sakoda, H.; Asano, T.; Levine, B.; Sadoshima, J. Distinct roles of autophagy in the heart during ischemia and reperfusion—Roles of AMP-activated protein kinase and Beclin 1 in mediating autophagy. *Circ. Res.* **2007**, *100*, 914–922. [CrossRef] [PubMed]
202. Sun, Y.; Yao, X.; Zhang, Q.J.; Zhu, M.; Liu, Z.P.; Ci, B.; Xie, Y.; Carlson, D.; Rothermel, B.A.; Sun, Y.; et al. Beclin-1-Dependent Autophagy Protects the Heart During Sepsis. *Circulation* **2018**, *138*, 2247–2262. [CrossRef] [PubMed]
203. Gyongyosi, A.; Szoke, K.; Fenyvesi, F.; Fejes, Z.; Debreceni, I.B.; Nagy, B.; Tosaki, A.; Lekli, I. Inhibited autophagy may contribute to heme toxicity in cardiomyoblast cells. *Biochem. Biophys Res. Commun.* **2019**, *511*, 732–738. [CrossRef] [PubMed]
204. Zheng, Y.T.; Shi, B.H.; Ma, M.Q.; Wu, X.Q.; Lin, X.H. The novel relationship between Sirt3 and autophagy in myocardial ischemia-reperfusion. *J. Cell Physiol.* **2019**, *234*, 5488–5495. [CrossRef] [PubMed]
205. Zilinyi, R.; Czompa, A.; Czegledi, A.; Gajtko, A.; Pituk, D.; Lekli, I.; Tosaki, A. The Cardioprotective Effect of Metformin in Doxorubicin-Induced Cardiotoxicity: The Role of Autophagy. *Molecules* **2018**, *23*. [CrossRef] [PubMed]
206. Gyongyosi, A.; Zilinyi, R.; Czegledi, A.; Tosaki, A.; Tosaki, A.; Lekli, I. The Role of Autophagy and Death Pathways in Dose-dependent Isoproterenolinduced Cardiotoxicity. *Curr. Pharm. Des.* **2019**, *25*, 2192–2198. [CrossRef]
207. Dong, Y.; Chen, H.W.; Gao, J.L.; Liu, Y.M.; Li, J.; Wang, J. Molecular machinery and interplay of apoptosis and autophagy in coronary heart disease. *J. Mol. Cell. Cardiol.* **2019**, *136*, 27–41. [CrossRef]
208. Lekli, I.; Haines, D.D.; Balla, G.; Tosaki, A. Autophagy: An adaptive physiological countermeasure to cellular senescence and ischaemia/reperfusion-associated cardiac arrhythmias. *J. Cell. Mol. Med.* **2017**, *21*, 1058–1072. [CrossRef]
209. Rahman, M.A.; Saha, S.K.; Rahman, M.S.; Uddin, M.J.; Uddin, M.S.; Pang, M.G.; Rhim, H.; Cho, S.G. Molecular Insights Into Therapeutic Potential of Autophagy Modulation by Natural Products for Cancer Stem Cells. *Front. Cell Dev. Biol.* **2020**, *8*. [CrossRef]
210. Sohn, E.J.; Park, H.T. Natural agents mediated autophagic signal networks in cancer. *Cancer Cell Int.* **2017**, *17*. [CrossRef]

Publisher's Note: MDPI stays neutral with regard to jurisdictional claims in published maps and institutional affiliations.

© 2020 by the authors. Licensee MDPI, Basel, Switzerland. This article is an open access article distributed under the terms and conditions of the Creative Commons Attribution (CC BY) license (http://creativecommons.org/licenses/by/4.0/).

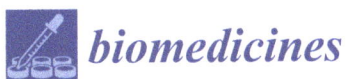

Article

Chronic Treatment with a Phytosomal Preparation Containing *Centella asiatica* L. and *Curcuma longa* L. Affects Local Protein Synthesis by Modulating the BDNF-mTOR-S6 Pathway

Giulia Sbrini, Paola Brivio, Enrico Sangiovanni, Marco Fumagalli, Giorgio Racagni, Mario Dell'Agli and Francesca Calabrese *

Department of Pharmacological and Biomolecular Sciences, Università degli Studi di Milano, 20133 Milan, Italy; giulia.sbrini@unimi.it (G.S.); paola.brivio@unimi.it (P.B.); enrico.sangiovanni@unimi.it (E.S.); marco.fumagalli3@unimi.it (M.F.); giorgio.racagni@unimi.it (G.R.); mario.dellagli@unimi.it (M.D.)
* Correspondence: francesca.calabrese@unimi.it; Tel.: +39-02-50318277

Received: 20 October 2020; Accepted: 24 November 2020; Published: 26 November 2020

Abstract: Brain derived neurotrophic factor (Bdnf) is the most diffuse neurotrophin in the central nervous system and it is crucial for the proper brain development and maintenance. Indeed, through the binding to its high affinity receptor TRKB and the activation of different intracellular cascades, it boosts cell survival, neurite growth and spine maturations mechanisms. Here, we evaluated if the chronic oral treatment for 10 days with a phytosomal preparation containing *Centella asiatica* L. and *Curcuma longa* L. could improve Bdnf levels in the prefrontal cortex of adult rats. Interestingly we found an increased expression of Bdnf with main effect of the treatment on the mTOR-S6 downstream signaling pathway. Accordingly, we found an increase in the expression of eukaryotic elongation factor (eEF2) with a shift towards the phosphorylated form thus increasing the transcription of Oligophrenin-1, a protein carrying the upstream Open Reading Frame (uORF) which reduction is paralleled by memory dysfunctions. These results show the ability of the phytosome to enhance mTOR-S6 regulated transcription and suggest the possibility to use this preparation in subjects with impairments in neuroplastic mechanisms, memory and cognitive abilities.

Keywords: *Centella asiatica* L.; *Curcuma longa* L.; Bdnf; mTOR; protein synthesis; neuroplasticity; botanicals

1. Introduction

Brain-Derived Neurotrophic Factor (Bdnf) is the most diffuse neurotrophin, involved in several positive functions both during the development and at adulthood [1,2]. Indeed, it stimulates a plethora of mechanisms involved in cell survival, neurite growth and spine maturations through the activation of the high affinity receptor Tropomyosin Sensitive Receptor Kinase B (TRKB) that in turn activates different downstream pathways [3].

Among these intracellular mechanisms, Bdnf can stimulate protein translation by triggering the mammalian target of rapamycin (mTOR)-ribosomal protein (S6) signaling pathway thus boosting the activity of several translation-related proteins such as the initiation and the elongation factors [3,4]. Interestingly, although protein synthesis mainly occurs close to the nucleus, it can also happen at synaptic level improving neuroplasticity, memory and cognitive functions [5,6].

Protein synthesis is a complex process consisting of at least 3 steps: initiation, elongation and termination [7]. The ratio between the total and the phosphorylated form of the elements involved in the first two steps, namely eukaryotic initiation factors (eIF2) and eukaryotic elongation factors (eEF2), determines the set of proteins to be translated. In particular, when the total form is more abundant than the phosphorylated one, the general translation is preferred while it has been demonstrated that an increase of the phosphorylated form enhances the translation of peptides whose genes carry the upstream Open Reading Frame (uORF) [8–10].

Considering the positive effects of Bdnf, it is not surprising that its alterations are associated with different pathological conditions [11,12]. Hence, it has been demonstrated that different drugs and phytochemicals lead to beneficial effects at molecular levels and improve memory and cognitive functions by targeting Bdnf machinery [13–19].

However, the downstream mechanisms activated by Bdnf that may be responsible for the outcomes of both chemical and natural compounds are not completely defined.

On these bases, the aim of this study was to determine the effect of the chronic administration for 10 days of a phytosomal preparation containing *Centella asiatica* L. (Gotu kola, Asiatic pennywort) and *Curcuma longa* L. (Turmeric) (50 mg/kg or 250 mg/kg) on Bdnf expression and on its high affinity receptor TRKB. Furthermore, we assessed whether the increase in Bdnf signaling was paralleled by an upregulation of de novo protein synthesis by focusing on the prefrontal cortex (PFC), a brain region affected by the phytosome ingredients [15,16].

2. Material and Methods

2.1. Plant Material

The Phytosome® was provided by Indena S.p.A. and contained a purified and standardized dry extract from leaves of *Centella asiatica* L. (*C. asiatica*) (19.6%) and *Curcuma longa* L. (*C. longa*) rhizome extract (29.1% as total curcuminoid content). The percentage of *C. asiatica* L. asiaticoside in the phytosome formulation, analyzed by HPLC, was 3.8% according to ARM/79-8031. Phytosome is an innovative vesicular delivery system, where extracts are complexed with phosphatidylcholine, aimed at improving the absorption and the bioavailability of the active compounds.

2.2. Animals

Adult male Sprague Dawley rats (Charles River, Calco, Italy) (10 weeks; 320–340 grams) were habituated to the laboratory conditions for one week before starting the experiment, and they were housed with food and water *ad libitum* with a 12 h light/dark cycle at constant temperature (22 ± 2 °C) and humidity (50 ± 5%) conditions.

All animal procedures were conducted according to the authorization n 977/2017-PR (approved on 11 December 2017) from the Italian Health Ministry in full accordance with the Italian legislation in animal experimentation (DL 26/2014) and conformed to EU recommendations (EEC Council Directive 2010/63). All efforts were made to minimize animal suffering and to reduce the number of animals.

2.3. Treatment

After the habituation, rats were chronically treated by oral gavage (os) once a day for 10 consecutive days with water (vehicle) or phytosomal preparation at 50 mg/kg or 250 mg/kg; composed by 20 mg/kg or 100 mg/kg of *C. asiatica* L. extract plus 30 mg/kg or 150 mg/kg of *C. longa* L., respectively.

Two hours after the last administration, animals were anesthetized with isoflurane and then suppressed with CO_2. After decapitation, the PFC, defined as cingulate cortex (Cg) 1–3 and infralimbic sub-regions (plates 6–10), was immediately dissected from 2 mm thick slices, according to the atlas of Paxinos and Watson [20] and then stored at −80 °C for the subsequent molecular analyses.

2.4. Quantification of Triterpenes and Curcuminoids in Plasma by LC-MS/MS Analysis

Curcumin and *C. asiatica* triterpenes were simultaneously quantified, in the plasma of rats treated with the phytosomal preparation containing *C. longa* and *C. asiatica*, by the LC–MS/MS method reported in Sbrini et al., 2020 [15]. Resveratrol was used as internal standard. Curcumin glucuronide, which is considered the most abundant curcumin metabolite in the blood, was also quantified. The analytes and the internal standard were quantified by using the following mass transitions: 367/149 (curcumin), 543/367 (curcumin glucuronide), 533/487 (asiatic acid), 549/503 (madecassic acid), 1003.8/958 (asiaticoside), and 1019.9/973 (madecassoside), 227/185 (resveratrol).

2.5. RNA Preparation and Gene Expression Analysis by Quantitative Real-Time PCR

Total RNA was isolated by a single step of guanidinium isothiocyanate/phenol extraction by using a PureZol RNA isolation reagent (Bio-Rad Laboratories, Segrate, Italy) according to the manufacturer's instructions and quantified by spectrophotometric analysis.

The samples were then processed for real-time polymerase chain reaction (RT-PCR) to assess total *Bdnf* and of *Bdnf* long 3′ untranslated region (UTR), (primer and probes sequences are listed in the Table 1). An aliquot of each sample was treated with DNase (Thermoscientific, Rodano, Italy) to avoid DNA contamination. RNA was analyzed by TaqMan qRT-PCR one-step RT-PCR kit for probes (Bio-Rad laboratories, Italy). Samples were run in 384 well formats in triplicate as multiplexed reactions with a normalizing internal control (*36b4*).

Table 1. sequence of forward and reverse primers and probes used in the real-time polymerase chain reaction analyses and purchased from Eurofins MWG-Operon (Germany) (**a**) and from Life technologies, which does not disclose the sequences (**b**).

(a) Gene	Forward Primer	Reverse Primer	Probe
36b4	TTCCCACTGGCTGAAAAGGT	CGCAGCCGCAAATGC	AAGGCCTTCCTGGCCGATCCATC
Total *Bdnf*	AAGTCTGCATTACATTCCTCGA	GTTTTCTGAAAGAGGGACAGTTTAT	TGTGGTTTGTTGCCGTTGCCAAG
(b) Gene		**Accession Number**	**Assay ID**
Bdnf long 3′UTR		EF125675	Rn02531967_s1

Thermal cycling was started with an incubation at 50 °C for 10 min (RNA retrotranscription) and then at 95 °C for 5 min (TaqMan polymerase activation). After this initial step, 39 cycles of PCR were performed. Each PCR cycle consisted of heating the samples at 95 °C for 10 s to enable the melting process and then for 30 s at 60 °C for the annealing and extension reactions. A comparative cycle threshold (Ct) method was used to calculate the relative target gene expression.

2.6. Protein Extraction and Western Blot Analysis

Western blot was employed to measure mature BDNF (mBDNF), TRKB (pTRKB Tyr816 and full-length), mammalian target of rapamycin (pmTOR Ser2448 and mTOR), ribosomal protein (pS6 Ser240/244 and S6), PLC (pPLC Tyr783 and PLC), AKT (pAKT Ser473 and AKT), ERK1 (pERK1 Thr202 and ERK1), ERK2 (pERK2 Tyr204 and ERK2), CAMP Responsive Element Binding Protein (pCREB Ser133 and CREB), eukaryotic initiation factor 2 (peIF2 Ser51and eIF2), eukaryotic elongation factor 2 (peEF2 Thr56 and eEF2) and Oligophrenin-1 (OPHN-1) protein levels in the crude synaptosomal fraction and in the whole homogenate (representative western blot bands of the proteins measured are showed in Figure S1).

Tissues were homogenized, and proteins were extracted as previously described [21]. The protein concentration of each sample was assessed according to the Bradford protein assay procedure (Bio-Rad Laboratories) with albumin (Sigma Aldrich, Milano, Italy) as the calibration standard. The purity of fraction was previously reported [22].

Western blot was run in reducing conditions by using Tris-Glycine eXtended (TGX) precast gel criterion (Bio-Rad Laboratories). All blots were blocked with 5% nonfat dried milk and incubated with the appropriate primary and secondary antibodies, as specified in Table 2.

Immunocomplexes were visualized with Western Lightning Clarity ECL (Bio-Rad Laboratories) and the Chemidoc MP imaging system (Bio-Rad Laboratories). Protein levels were quantified with ImageLab (Bio-Rad Laboratories) and normalized versus β-ACTIN.

Table 2. antibodies condition used in the western blot analyses. Over/Night (O/N); Room Temperature (RT); Milk (M); Bovine serum albumin (BSA).

Protein	Primary Antibody	Secondary Antibody
mBDNF (14 KDa)	1:1000 M 3% (Icosagen) 4° O/N	Anti-mouse 1:2000 M 3% 1 h RT
pTRKB Y816 (145 KDa)	1:1000 BSA 5% (Cell Signalling) 4°O/N	Anti-rabbit 1:1000 M 3% 1 h RT
TRKB full length (145 KDa)	1:750 BSA 5% (Cell Signalling) 4° O/N	Anti-rabbit 1:1000 M 3% 1 h RT
pmTOR Ser2448 (289 KDa)	1:1000 BSA 5% (Cell Signalling) 4° O/N	Anti-rabbit 1:5000 M 3% 1 h RT
mTOR (289 KDa)	1:1000 BSA 5% (Cell Signalling) 4° O/N	Anti-rabbit 1:5000 M 3% 1 h RT
pS6 Ser240/244 (32 KDa)	1:1000 BSA 5% (Cell Signalling) 4° O/N	Anti-rabbit 1:2000 M 3% 1 h RT
S6 (32 KDa)	1:1000 BSA 5% (Cell Signalling) 4° O/N	Anti-rabbit 1:1000 M 3% 1 h RT
pPLC Tyr783 (155 KDa)	1:1000 BSA 5% (Cell Signalling) 4° O/N	Anti-rabbit 1:1000 M 5%, 1 h RT
PLC (155 KDa)	1:1000 BSA 5% (Cell Signalling) 4° O/N	Anti-rabbit 1:1000 M 3% 1 h RT
pAKT Ser473 (60 KDa)	1:1000 BSA 5% (Cell Signalling) 4° O/N	Anti-rabbit 1:1000 M 3% 1 h RT
AKT (60 KDa)	1:1000 BSA 5% (Cell Signalling) 4° O/N	Anti-rabbit 1:1000 M 3% 1 h RT
pERK1 Thr202 (44 KDa)	1:1000 BSA 5% (Cell Signalling) 4° O/N	Anti-rabbit 1:2000 M 3% 1 h RT
ERK1 (44 KDa)	1:1000 BSA 5% (Santa Cruz Biotechnology) 4° O/N	Anti-rabbit 1:5000 M 3% 1 h RT
pERK2 Tyr204 (44 KDa)	1:1000 BSA 5% (Cell Signalling) 4° O/N	Anti-rabbit 1:2000 M 3% 1 h RT
ERK2 (44 KDa)	1:1000 BSA 5% (Santa Cruz Biotechnology) 4° O/N	Anti-rabbit 1:5000 M 3% 1 h RT
pCREB Ser133 (43 KDa)	1:1000 BSA 5% (Cell Signalling) 4° O/N	Anti-rabbit 1:5000 M 3% 1 h RT
CREB (43 KDa)	1:1000 BSA 5% (Cell Signalling) 4° O/N	Anti-rabbit 1:5000 M 3% 1 h RT
peIF2 Ser51 (38 kDa)	1:1000 BSA 5% (Cell Signalling) 4° O/N	Anti-rabbit 1:1000 M 3% 1 h RT
eIF2 (38 kDa)	1:1000 BSA 5% (Cell Signalling) 4° O/N	Anti-rabbit 1:1000 M 3% 1 h RT
peEF2 Thr56(95 KDa)	1:1000 BSA 5% (Cell Signalling) 4° O/N	Anti-rabbit 1:1000 M 3% 1 h RT
eEF2 (95 KDa)	1:1000 BSA 5% (Cell Signalling) 4° O/N	Anti-rabbit 1:1000 M 3% 1 h RT
OPHN-1 (91 KDa)	1:1000 BSA 5% (Santa Cruz) 4° O/N	Anti-mouse 1:1000 M 3% 1 h RT
β-ACTIN (43 KDa)	1:10,000 M 3% (Sigma-Aldrich) 45 min RT	Anti-mouse 1:10,000 M 3% 45 min RT

2.7. Statistical Analysis

All the data were checked for normality using the Kolmogorov-Smirnov test and the Shapiro-Wilk tests and for homoscedasticity with the Brown-Forsythe test and Bartlett's test. Normally distributed and homoscedastic data were further analyzed using "IBM SPSS Statistics, version 26" with the one-way analysis of variance (ANOVA). When appropriate, further differences were analyzed by the Fisher's protected least significance difference (PLSD) method. Moreover, non-parametric datasets, belonging to Figure 1, were analyzed with Mann-Whitney nonparametric test. Significance for all tests was assumed for $p < 0.05$.

Each experimental group consisted of 5–6 rats, and data are presented as mean ± standard error (SEM).

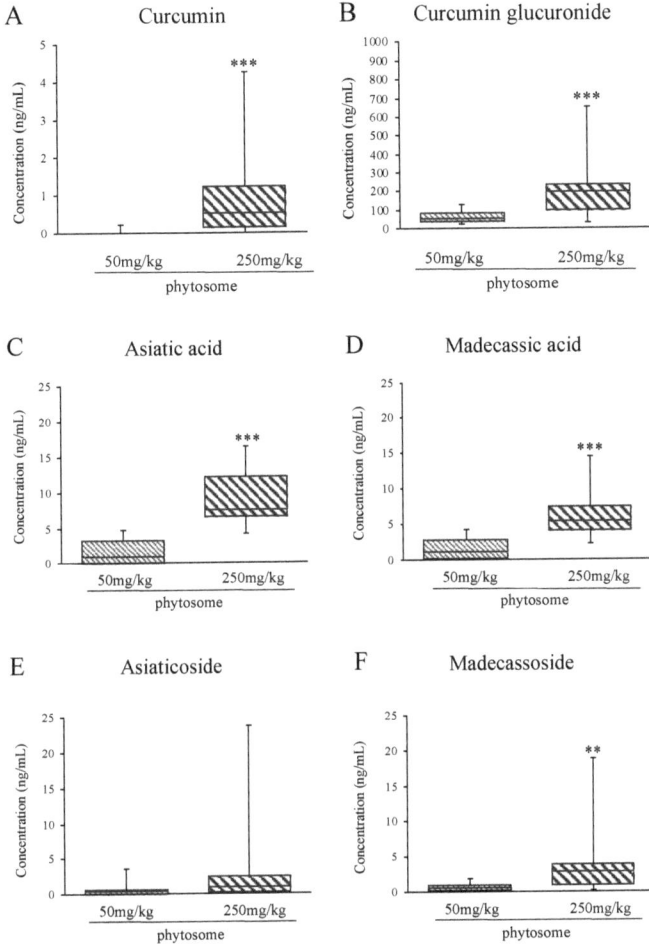

Figure 1. Concentration of Curcumin (**A**), Curcumin glucuronide (**B**), Asiatic acid (**C**), Madecassic acid (**D**), Asiaticoside (**E**) and Madecassoside (**F**) in the plasma of rats following the repeated oral administration of the phytosomal preparation. Data are expressed in ng/mL as are represented as boxes and whiskers graphs. ** $p < 0.01$, *** $p < 0.001$ vs. vehicle; Mann-Whitney nonparametric test.

3. Results

3.1. Quantification of Terpenes and Curcuminoids in Plasma by LC-MS/MS Analysis

To assess the plasmatic concentrations of the main compounds or their metabolites following repeated oral administration, an analytical method to quantify simultaneously terpenes and curcuminoids was set up. All compounds quantified reached concentrations in the ng/mL order and, as expected, were more abundant in the plasma of rats treated with the higher dose (250 mg/kg).

Curcumin was present mostly as glucuronide, reaching concentrations 200-fold higher than the corresponding free form (192 vs. 0.93 ng/mL, respectively) in rats treated with 250 mg/kg phytosome (Figure 1A,B).

Terpenes quantification showed that the acid forms (Figure 1C,D) were found to be more abundant than the corresponding glucosides (Figure 1E,F); asiatic acid reached the highest concentration (9.2 ng/mL, corresponding to 19 nM).

3.2. Phytosome Administration Increased Bdnf Levels in the PFC

Phytosome administration for 10 consecutive days significantly affected the expression of the neurotrophin *Bdnf* in the rat prefrontal cortex. As shown in Figure 2A, we observed a significant effect of the treatment ($F_{2-14} = 4.085\ p < 0.05$, one-way ANOVA) on the total form of *Bdnf* with the lower dosage of phytosome that increased its mRNA levels (+38% $p < 0.05$ vs. vehicle, Fisher's PLSD). Similarly, also the pool of the long transcripts of *Bdnf* was significantly modulated by the treatment ($F_{2-15} = 11.245\ p < 0.01$, one-way ANOVA). Indeed, the administration of phytosome at both 50 and 250 mg/kg significantly up regulated its mRNA levels (+58% $p < 0.01$ vs. vehicle; +53% $p < 0.01$ vs. vehicle respectively; Fisher's PLSD) (Figure 2B).

On the basis of the transcriptional results, we measured also the protein levels of the neurotrophin and accordingly we found that both the dosages induced a significant increase (50 mg/kg: +183% $p < 0.001$ vs. vehicle; 250 mg/kg: +87% $p < 0.05$ vs. vehicle; Fisher's PLSD) in mBDNF protein levels in the crude synaptosomal fraction ($F_{2-14} = 15.740\ p < 0.001$, one-way ANOVA) (Figure 2D). On the contrary, we did not observe any changes of mBDNF levels in the whole homogenate (Figure 2C).

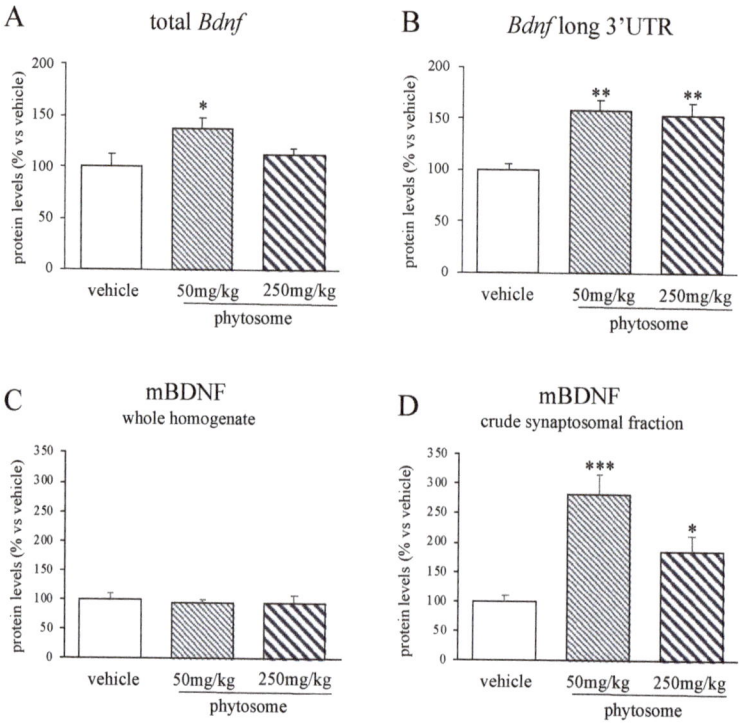

Figure 2. Analyses of total *Bdnf*, (**A**) *Bdnf* long 3'UTR (**B**) mRNA levels and mBDNF protein levels in the whole homogenate (**C**) and crude synaptosomal fraction (**D**) of the PFC of rats treated with phytosome 50 mg/kg or 250 mg/kg. Data are expressed as percent change of vehicle treated rats and are represented in the histograms graphs as mean ± SEM of 5–6 independent determinations. * $p < 0.05$, ** $p < 0.01$, *** $p < 0.001$ vs. vehicle; one-way ANOVA with Fisher's PLSD.

3.3. The Increase of mBDNF Protein Levels Was Paralleled by an Increased Activity of Its Receptor TRKB

In the whole homogenate, in line with our findings on mBDNF protein levels, we did not observe any changes neither in the phosphorylated form nor in the total levels of the receptor TRKB (Figure 3A,B), whereas in the crude synaptosomal fraction, phytosome administration positively affected both pTRKB Tyr816 and TRKB full length protein levels. Indeed, as revealed by the significant effect of the treatment ($F_{2-14} = 5.873$ $p < 0.05$, one-way ANOVA), the phosphorylated form was increased in the crude synaptosomal fraction of rats treated with the lower dose of phytosome (+103% vs. vehicle $p < 0.01$; Fisher's PLSD), while we observed only a not significant increase with the higher dosage (+45% $p > 0.05$ vs. vehicle; Fisher's PLSD) (Figure 3C). Similarly, we found a significant effect of the treatment on TRKB full length protein levels ($F_{2-12} = 6.284$ $p < 0.05$, one-way ANOVA), that were increased at both the dosages tested (50 mg/kg: +173% $p < 0.01$; 250 mg/kg: +135% $p < 0.05$ vs. vehicle; Fisher's PLSD) (Figure 3D).

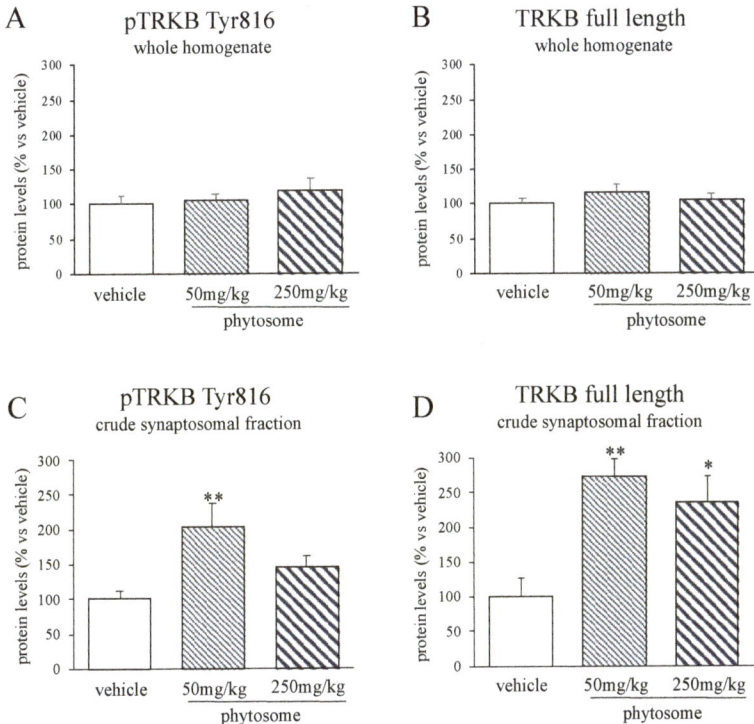

Figure 3. Analyses of pTRKB Tyr816 (**A–C**) and TRKB full length (**B–D**) protein levels in the whole homogenate (**A,B**) and crude synaptosomal fraction (**C,D**) of the PFC of rats treated with phytosome 50 mg/kg or 250 mg/kg. Data are expressed as percent change of vehicle treated rats and are represented in the histograms graphs as mean ± SEM of 4–6 independent determinations. * $p < 0.05$, ** $p < 0.01$ vs. vehicle; one-way ANOVA with Fisher's PLSD.

3.4. TRKB Phosphorylation in Phytosome-Treated Animals Specifically Activated mTOR-S6 Intracellular Signaling Pathway

The phosphorylation of the high affinity receptor TRKB produces the activation of different intracellular signaling cascades as result of several stimuli thus producing a specific outcome in term of brain plasticity [3].

In this study, we investigated some of these pathways uncovering that our experimental conditions specifically affected the mTOR-S6 signaling, which is well-known to control protein synthesis and cell growth [23]. In particular, the phosphorylated form of mTOR in Ser2448 was upregulated by the higher dose of phytosome (+79% $p < 0.05$ vs. vehicle; Fisher's PLSD) (treatment effect: $F_{2-11} = 3.016$ $p < 0.05$, one-way ANOVA) whereas we did not found changes in total mTOR protein levels (Figure 4A,B). Therefore, as shown in Figure 4C, we observed a significant effect of the treatment on the ratio pmTOR/mTOR ($F_{2-11} = 4.865$ $p < 0.05$, one-way ANOVA), specifically in the animals treated with phytosome 250 mg/kg (+27% $p < 0.05$ vs. vehicle; Fisher's PLSD).

Similarly, the active form of S6 (pS6 Ser240/244) was affected (Figure 4D), as indicated by the significant effect of the treatment ($F_{2-13} = 5.202$ $p < 0.05$, one-way ANOVA) with the lower dose, which significantly increased pS6 Ser240/244 protein levels (+97% $p < 0.05$ vs. vehicle; Fisher's PLSD). On the contrary, no changes were found on the total form of S6 (Figure 4E).

Accordingly, we observed a significant increase of the ratio between the activated form of S6 and its total protein ($F_{2-13} = 5.650$ $p < 0.05$, one-way ANOVA) due to the treatments (phytosome 50 mg/kg: +97% $p < 0.05$; phytosome 250 mg/kg: +68% $p > 0.05$ vs. vehicle; Fisher's PLSD) (Figure 4F).

Finally, the other pathways investigated were only partially modulated with changes restricted to pAKT Ser473 (treatment effect: $F_{2-13} = 3.998$ $p < 0.05$, one-way ANOVA), pAKT Ser473 and AKT ratio (treatment effect: $F_{2-14} = 5.705$ $p < 0.05$, one-way ANOVA) and pERK2 Tyr204 (treatment effect: $F_{2-14} = 3.301$ $p > 0.05$, one-way ANOVA) protein levels (results summarized in Table 3).

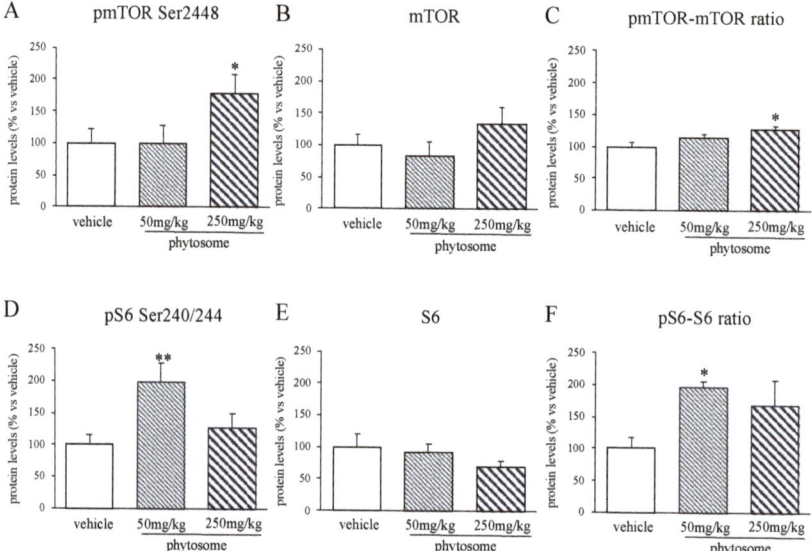

Figure 4. Analyses of mTOR (**A–C**) and S6 (**D–F**) protein levels in the PFC of rats treated with phytosome 50 mg/kg or 250 mg/kg. Data are expressed as percent change of vehicle treated rats and are represented in the histograms graphs as mean ± SEM of 3–6 independent determinations. * $p < 0.05$, ** $p < 0.01$ vs. vehicle; one-way ANOVA with Fisher's PLSD.

Table 3. Analyses of PLC, AKT, ERK1, ERK2, CREB, eIF2 (phosphorylated and total) protein levels in the PFC of rats treated with phytosome 50 mg/kg or 250 mg/kg. Data are expressed as percent change of vehicle treated rats and are expressed as mean ± SEM of 3–6 independent determinations. * $p < 0.05$ vs. vehicle; one-way ANOVA with Fisher's PLSD.

Protein	Vehicle	Phytosome 50 mg/kg	Phytosome 250 mg/kg
pPLC Tyr783	100 ± 10	76 ± 7	104 ± 17
PLC	100 ± 13	97 ± 9	114 ± 15
pPLC–PLC ratio	100 ± 5	94 ± 7	92 ± 10
pAKT Ser473	100 ± 13	200 ± 35 *	203 ± 34 *
AKT	100 ± 28	115 ± 20	85 ± 5
pAKT–AKT ratio	100 ± 16	165 ± 64	204 ± 31 *
pERK1 Thr202	100 ± 21	96 ± 15	106 ± 24
ERK1	100 ± 15	101 ± 13	81 ± 11
pERK1–ERK1 ratio	100 ± 8	127 ± 22	131 ± 29
pERK2 Tyr204	100 ± 20	142 ± 21	202 ± 37 *
ERK2	100 ± 13	97 ± 7	80 ± 9
pERK2–ERK2 ratio	100 ± 46	110 ± 18	187 ± 49
pCREB Ser133	100 ± 18	115 ± 27	87 ± 15
CREB	100 ± 14	107 ± 19	114 ± 38
pCREB–CREB ratio	100 ± 10	131 ± 24	118 ± 21
peIF2 Ser51	100 ± 11	123 ± 23	118 ± 15
eIF2	100 ± 6	116 ± 15	111 ± 10
peIF2–eIF2 ratio	100 ± 10	104 ± 11	105 ± 9

3.5. Local Protein Synthesis Is Boosted by Phytosome Administration

mTOR together with S6 contributes to the control of the translational machinery [24]. In particular, the phosphorylation of these two factors can trigger the translational initiation and the peptide elongation thus increasing the protein synthesis and contributing to neuronal plasticity [25,26].

Here, we observed no effect of the treatment on the initiation process with unchanged eIF2 protein levels (Table 3).

On the contrary, protein elongation process was modulated by phytosome administration. In particular, we observed a significant effect of the treatment on peEF2 Thr56 protein levels ($F_{2-14} = 7.044$ $p < 0.01$, one-way ANOVA) with both doses increasing its protein levels (50 mg/kg: +259% $p < 0.01$ vs. vehicle; 250 mg/kg: +194% $p < 0.05$ vs. vehicle; Fisher's PLSD) (Figure 5A); however, no changes were observed for the total form of eEF2 (Figure 5B). Accordingly, the ratio peEF2/eEF2 (Figure 5C) was significantly increased in treated rats (50 mg/kg: +207% $p < 0.05$ vs. vehicle; 250 mg/kg: +123% $p > 0.05$ vs. vehicle; Fisher's PLSD) (treatment effect: $F_{2-13} = 4.944$ $p < 0.05$, one-way ANOVA).

It has been demonstrated that a shift of the balance between the phosphorylated and the total form of eEF2 towards the phosphorylated form leads to an increased translation of specific mRNA containing the uORF sequence [10]; our results suggest that phytosome administration may enhance the synthesis of new proteins containing the uORF in their sequence.

On this bases, we measured the expression of OPHN-1 that contains 2 uORF and, as shown in Figure 5D, we observed an increase in the protein levels in rats treated with the lower dose (+81% $p > 0.05$ vs. vehicle; Fisher's PLSD) and a significant up-regulation due to the higher dose administration (+143% $p < 0.05$ vs. vehicle; Fisher's PLSD), despite the effect of the treatment was not statistically significant ($F_{2-11} = 2.730$ $p > 0.05$, one-way ANOVA).

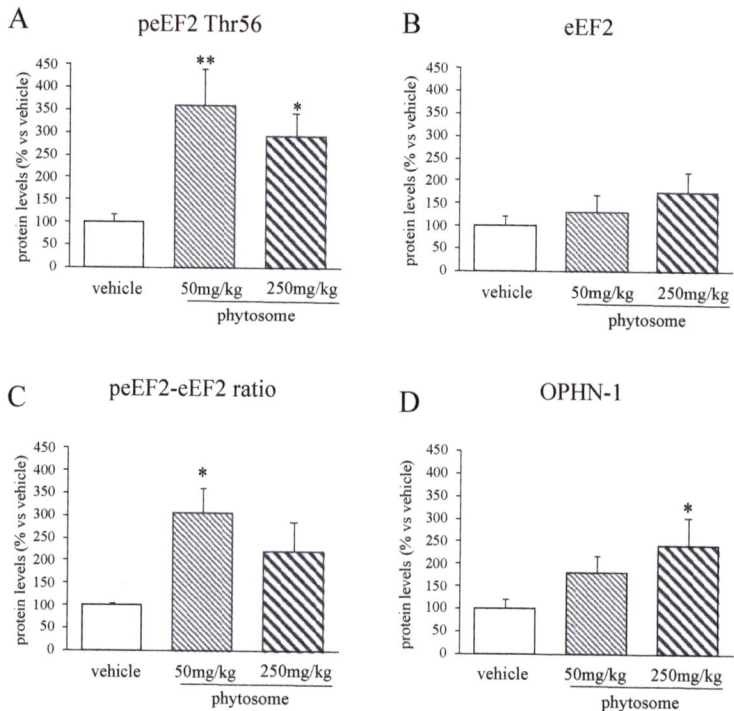

Figure 5. Analyses of eEF2 (**A–C**) and OPHN-1 (**D**) protein levels in the PFC of rats treated with phytosome 50 mg/kg or 250 mg/kg. Data are expressed as percent change of vehicle treated rats and are represented in the histograms graphs as mean ± SEM of 4–6 independent determinations. * $p < 0.05$, ** $p < 0.01$ vs. vehicle; one-way ANOVA with Fisher's PLSD.

4. Discussion

In the present study, we provide evidence that the chronic administration of the phytosomal preparation containing *C. asiatica* and *C. longa* positively affects neuroplastic mechanisms by increasing the expression of Bdnf and the activation of the downstream pathways via TRKB receptor. Moreover, we observed that the increase of the neurotrophin induced changes in the translation machinery with an enhanced activation of proteins involved in cognitive and memory processes.

In particular, we measured the neurotrophin expression in the PFC of phytosome-treated rats finding an increase of the total form of *Bdnf* and of the long 3'UTR pool of transcripts. Moreover, in line with the preferential localization of *Bdnf* mRNAs carrying the long 3'UTR in the dendrites where they are translated in case of demand [27], we observed an upregulation of mBDNF protein levels in the synaptic fraction. These findings suggest that 10 days of phytosome administration may promote neuroplastic mechanisms by increasing the production of trophic factors as, for example, mBDNF. Accordingly, a similar effect was observed after the administration of a wide range of botanicals as well as pharmacological pure compounds [14–19,28–30]. Interestingly, both the active principles contained in the phytosome (terpenes from *C. asiatica* and curcumin from *C. longa*) may contribute to the effects described in the present paper. Indeed, it has been previously reported that *C. asiatica* extract up-regulates Bdnf thus improving memory performance [15,17]. Moreover, Wang R. and colleagues showed in vitro protective effects of curcumin against glutamate excitotoxicity in rat cortical neurons, the effect was accompanied by an increase in the Bdnf level and activation of TRKB [18]. Similarly, in the same cell model, curcumin produced neuroprotective effects via mBDNF/TRKB-dependent MAPK and PI-3K cascades [19]; however, this is the first study investigating in vivo a combination of the two botanicals in a phytosomal formulation.

Furthermore, we demonstrated that the increase of mBDNF protein levels induced by the treatment was reflected by an increase of the phosphorylated and active form of TRKB receptor suggesting that the higher amount of mBDNF produced is released from the synapses, being able to activate its downstream pathways.

Notably, TRKB activation may set in motion different intracellular cascades [3,31] that can be specifically modulated by several compounds [32,33].

To deeper investigate the mechanism of action of the phytosomal preparation, we analyzed the activation of some pathways activated by an increased phosphorylation of the TRKB receptor finding the most relevant effect on mTOR-S6 signaling via AKT and ERK phosphorylation. Interestingly, ketamine, *Glycyrrhiza glabra* root extract as well as zinc administration induce a similar modulation on this pathway that is accompanied by an antidepressant-like effect [34,35], thus suggesting a possible antidepressant effect of the phytosomal preparation.

Finally, since protein translation is also controlled by mTOR complex [7] that in turn can be boosted by increased levels of the neurotrophin [3], we measured the initiation and the elongation factors protein levels, and we found an increase of peEF2 Thr56 with respect to the total form of the protein due to phytosome administration. Interestingly, this shift toward the phosphorylated form, able to increase the translation of specific proteins carrying the uORF sequence [36], was paralleled by increased levels of OPHN-1. Notably, memory and cognitive alterations not only in animal models of depression but also in humans with X-linked mental retardation are characterized by impairments in OPHN-1 transduction and translation [6,37] supporting the possibility that chronic phytosome administration, by increasing OPHN-1 translation, could induce an enhancement in brain mechanisms crucially involved in cognitive processes.

5. Conclusions

In conclusion, our data support the use of phytosome preparation in ameliorating brain plasticity through the activation of mBDNF-mTOR-S6 intracellular cascade and the transcription of specific proteins involved in memory processes in the PFC. Hence, despite the necessity of further experiments focused on evaluation of the animal behavior following phytosomal administration, this phytosomal preparation could be used as supporting therapy in subjects characterized by memory and cognitive disfunctions mainly related to alterations in frontal brain regions.

Supplementary Materials: The following are available online at http://www.mdpi.com/2227-9059/8/12/544/s1, Figure S1: Representative western blot bands of the proteins measured.

Author Contributions: Conceptualization, F.C. and M.D.; Methodology, G.S., P.B.; Formal Analysis, G.S.; Data Curation, G.S.; Writing—Original Draft Preparation, F.C. and G.S.; Writing—Review and Editing, P.B., E.S., M.F., G.R., M.D. and F.C.; Funding Acquisition, F.C. and M.D. All authors have read and agreed to the published version of the manuscript.

Funding: This research was funded by MIUR Progetto di Eccellenza and Regione Lombardia.

Acknowledgments: G.S. was supported by the doctorate in Experimental and Clinical Pharmacological Sciences (cycle XXXIV), University of Milan, Italy. We thank Indena S.p.A. for providing the phytosome.

Conflicts of Interest: The authors declare no conflict of interest.

References

1. Lu, B.; Pang, P.T.; Woo, N.H. The yin and yang of neurotrophin action. *Nat. Rev. Neurosci.* **2005**, *6*, 603–613. [CrossRef] [PubMed]
2. Monteggia, L.M.; Tamminga, C.A. Elucidating the role of brain-derived neurotrophic factor in the brain. *Am. J. Psychiatry* **2007**, *164*, 1790. [CrossRef] [PubMed]
3. Yoshii, A.; Constantine-Paton, M. Postsynaptic BDNF-TrkB signaling in synapse maturation, plasticity, and disease. *Dev. Neurobiol.* **2010**, *70*, 304–322. [CrossRef] [PubMed]

4. Manadas, B.; Santos, A.R.; Szabadfi, K.; Gomes, J.R.; Garbis, S.D.; Fountoulakis, M.; Duarte, C.B. BDNF-induced changes in the expression of the translation machinery in hippocampal neurons: Protein levels and dendritic mRNA. *J. Proteome Res.* **2009**, *8*, 4536–4552. [CrossRef]
5. Buffington, S.A.; Huang, W.; Costa-Mattioli, M. Translational Control in Synaptic Plasticity and Cognitive Dysfunction. *Annu. Rev. Neurosci.* **2014**, *37*, 17–38. [CrossRef]
6. Calabrese, F.; Brivio, P.; Gruca, P.; Lason-Tyburkiewicz, M.; Papp, M.; Riva, M.A. Chronic Mild Stress-Induced Alterations of Local Protein Synthesis: A Role for Cognitive Impairment. *ACS Chem. Neurosci.* **2017**, *8*, 817–825. [CrossRef]
7. Sonenberg, N.; Hinnebusch, A.G. Regulation of Translation Initiation in Eukaryotes: Mechanisms and Biological Targets. *Cell* **2009**, *136*, 731–745. [CrossRef]
8. Costa-Mattioli, M.; Gobert, D.; Harding, H.; Herdy, B.; Azzi, M.; Bruno, M.; Bidinosti, M.; Ben Mamou, C.; Marcinkiewicz, E.; Yoshida, M.; et al. Translational control of hippocampal synaptic plasticity and memory by the eIF2α kinase GCN2. *Nature* **2005**, *436*, 1166–1173. [CrossRef]
9. Takei, N.; Kawamura, M.; Hara, K.; Yonezawa, K.; Nawa, H. Brain-derived Neurotrophic Factor Enhances Neuronal Translation by Activating Multiple Initiation Processes. *J. Biol. Chem.* **2001**, *276*, 42818–42825. [CrossRef]
10. Klann, E.; Dever, T.E. Biochemical mechanisms for translational regulation in synaptic plasticity. *Nat. Rev. Neurosci.* **2004**, *5*, 931–942. [CrossRef]
11. Duman, R.S.; Monteggia, L.M. A Neurotrophic Model for Stress-Related Mood Disorders. *Biol. Psychiatry* **2006**, *59*, 1116–1127. [CrossRef] [PubMed]
12. Tanila, H. The role of BDNF in Alzheimer's disease. *Neurobiol. Dis.* **2017**, *97 Pt B*, 114–118. [CrossRef]
13. Björkholm, C.; Monteggia, L.M. BDNF—A key transducer of antidepressant effects. *Neuropharmacology* **2016**, *102*, 72–79. [CrossRef] [PubMed]
14. Sangiovanni, E.; Brivio, P.; Dell'Agli, M.; Calabrese, F. Botanicals as Modulators of Neuroplasticity: Focus on BDNF. *Neural Plast.* **2017**. [CrossRef] [PubMed]
15. Sbrini, G.; Brivio, P.; Fumagalli, M.; Giavarini, F.; Caruso, D.; Racagni, G.; Dell'agli, M.; Sangiovanni, E.; Calabrese, F. *Centella asiatica* l. Phytosome improves cognitive performance by promoting bdnf expression in rat prefrontal cortex. *Nutrients* **2020**, *12*, 355. [CrossRef] [PubMed]
16. Xu, Y.; Ku, B.; Tie, L.; Yao, H.; Jiang, W.; Ma, X.; Li, X. Curcumin reverses the effects of chronic stress on behavior, the HPA axis, BDNF expression and phosphorylation of CREB. *Brain Res.* **2006**, *1122*, 56–64. [CrossRef] [PubMed]
17. Sari, D.C.R.; Arfian, N.; Tranggono, U.; Setyaningsih, W.A.W.; Romi, M.M.; Emoto, N. *Centella asiatica* (Gotu kola) ethanol extract up-regulates hippocampal brain-derived neurotrophic factor (BDNF), tyrosine kinase B (TrkB) and extracellular signal-regulated protein kinase 1/2 (ERK1/2) signaling in chronic electrical stress model in rats. *Iran. J. Basic Med. Sci.* **2019**, *22*, 1218–1224. [CrossRef] [PubMed]
18. Wang, R.; Li, Y.B.; Li, Y.H.; Xu, Y.; Wu, H.L.; Li, X.J. Curcumin protects against glutamate excitotoxicity in rat cerebral cortical neurons by increasing brain-derived neurotrophic factor level and activating TrkB. *Brain Res.* **2008**. [CrossRef]
19. Wang, R.; Li, Y.H.; Xu, Y.; Li, Y.B.; Wu, H.L.; Guo, H.; Zhang, J.Z.; Zhang, J.J.; Pan, X.Y.; Li, X.J. Curcumin produces neuroprotective effects via activating brain-derived neurotrophic factor/TrkB-dependent MAPK and PI-3K cascades in rodent cortical neurons. *Prog. Neuro-Psychopharmacol. Biol. Psychiatry* **2010**. [CrossRef]
20. Paxinos, G.; Watson, C. *The Rat Brain in Stereotaxic Coordinates*, 6th ed.; Academic Press: Cambridge, MA, USA, 2007.
21. Brivio, P.; Sbrini, G.; Peeva, P.; Todiras, M.; Bader, M.; Alenina, N.; Calabrese, F. TPH2 deficiency influences neuroplastic mechanisms and alters the response to an acute stress in a sex specific manner. *Front. Mol. Neurosci.* **2018**, *11*, 389. [CrossRef]
22. Brivio, P.; Corsini, G.; Riva, M.A.; Calabrese, F. Chronic vortioxetine treatment improves the responsiveness to an acute stress acting through the ventral hippocampus in a glucocorticoid-dependent way. *Pharmacol. Res.* **2019**. [CrossRef] [PubMed]
23. Hall, M.N. mTOR-What Does It Do? *Transplant. Proc.* **2008**, *40*, S5–S8. [CrossRef] [PubMed]
24. Wang, X.; Proud, C.G. The mTOR Pathway in the Control of Protein Synthesis. *Physiology* **2006**, *21*, 362–369. [CrossRef] [PubMed]

25. Browne, G.J.; Proud, C.G. A Novel mTOR-Regulated Phosphorylation Site in Elongation Factor 2 Kinase Modulates the Activity of the Kinase and Its Binding to Calmodulin. *Mol. Cell. Biol.* **2004**, *24*, 2986–2997. [CrossRef] [PubMed]
26. Taha, E.; Gildish, I.; Gal-Ben-Ari, S.; Rosenblum, K. The role of eEF2 pathway in learning and synaptic plasticity. *Neurobiol. Learn. Mem.* **2013**, *105*, 100–106. [CrossRef] [PubMed]
27. An, J.J.; Gharami, K.; Liao, G.Y.; Woo, N.H.; Lau, A.G.; Vanevski, F.; Torre, E.R.; Jones, K.R.; Feng, Y.; Lu, B.; et al. Distinct Role of Long 3′ UTR BDNF mRNA in Spine Morphology and Synaptic Plasticity in Hippocampal Neurons. *Cell* **2008**, *134*, 175–187. [CrossRef] [PubMed]
28. Calabrese, F.; Molteni, R.; Maj, P.F.; Cattaneo, A.; Gennarelli, M.; Racagni, G.; Riva, M.A. Chronic duloxetine treatment induces specific changes in the expression of BDNF transcripts and in the subcellular localization of the neurotrophin protein. *Neuropsychopharmacology* **2007**, *32*, 2351–2359. [CrossRef]
29. Calabrese, F.; Molteni, R.; Gabriel, C.; Mocaer, E.; Racagni, G.; Riva, M.A. Modulation of neuroplastic molecules in selected brain regions after chronic administration of the novel antidepressant agomelatine. *Psychopharmacology* **2011**, *215*, 267–275. [CrossRef]
30. Calabrese, F.; Luoni, A.; Guidotti, G.; Racagni, G.; Fumagalli, F.; Riva, M.A. Modulation of neuronal plasticity following chronic concomitant administration of the novel antipsychotic lurasidone with the mood stabilizer valproic acid. *Psychopharmacology* **2013**, *226*, 101–112. [CrossRef]
31. Brivio, P.; Sbrini, G.; Corsini, G.; Paladini, M.S.; Racagni, G.; Molteni, R.; Calabrese, F. Chronic Restraint Stress Inhibits the Response to a Second Hit in Adult Male Rats: A Role for BDNF Signaling. *Int. J. Mol. Sci.* **2020**, *21*, 6261. [CrossRef]
32. Rantamäki, T.; Hendolin, P.; Kankaanpää, A.; Mijatovic, J.; Piepponen, P.; Domenici, E.; Chao, M.V.; Männistö, P.T.; Castrén, E. Pharmacologically diverse antidepressants rapidly activate brain-derived neurotrophic factor receptor TrkB and induce phospholipase-Cγ signaling pathways in mouse brain. *Neuropsychopharmacology* **2007**, *32*, 2152–2162. [CrossRef] [PubMed]
33. Moghbelinejad, S.; Nassiri-Asl, M.; Naserpour Farivar, T.; Abbasi, E.; Sheikhi, M.; Taghiloo, M.; Farsad, F.; Samimi, A.; Hajiali, F. Rutin activates the MAPK pathway and BDNF gene expression on beta-amyloid induced neurotoxicity in rats. *Toxicol. Lett.* **2014**, *224*, 108–113. [CrossRef] [PubMed]
34. Szewczyk, B.; Pochwat, B.; Rafało, A.; Palucha-Poniewiera, A.; Domin, H.; Nowak, G. Activation of mTOR dependent signaling pathway is a necessary mechanism of antidepressant-like activity of zinc. *Neuropharmacology* **2015**, *99*, 517–526. [CrossRef] [PubMed]
35. Xiao, D.; Liu, L.; Li, Y.; Ruan, J.; Wang, H. Licorisoflavan A Exerts Antidepressant-Like Effect in Mice: Involvement of BDNF-TrkB Pathway and AMPA Receptors. *Neurochem. Res.* **2019**, *44*, 2044–2056. [CrossRef]
36. Di Prisco, G.V.; Huang, W.; Buffington, S.A.; Hsu, C.C.; Bonnen, P.E.; Placzek, A.N.; Sidrauski, C.; Krnjević, K.; Kaufman, R.J.; Walter, P.; et al. Translational control of mGluR-dependent long-term depression and object-place learning by eIF2α. *Nat. Neurosci.* **2014**, *17*, 1073–1082. [CrossRef] [PubMed]
37. Billuart, P.; Bienvenu, T.; Ronce, N.; des Portes, V.; Vinet, M.C.; Zemni, R.; Crollius, H.R.; Carrié, A.; Fauchereau, F.; Cherry, M.; et al. Oligophrenin-1 encodes a rhoGAP protein involved in X-linked mental retardation. *Nature* **1998**, *392*, 923–926. [CrossRef]

Publisher's Note: MDPI stays neutral with regard to jurisdictional claims in published maps and institutional affiliations.

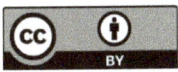

© 2020 by the authors. Licensee MDPI, Basel, Switzerland. This article is an open access article distributed under the terms and conditions of the Creative Commons Attribution (CC BY) license (http://creativecommons.org/licenses/by/4.0/).

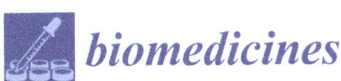

Review

Exploring the Multifaceted Therapeutic Potential of Withaferin A and Its Derivatives

Tapan Behl [1,*], Aditi Sharma [2], Lalit Sharma [2], Aayush Sehgal [1], Gokhan Zengin [3], Roxana Brata [4], Ovidiu Fratila [4] and Simona Bungau [5,*]

1. Chitkara College of Pharmacy, Chitkara University, Punjab 140401, India; aayushsehgal00@gmail.com
2. School of Pharmaceutical Sciences, Shoolini University, Solan, Himachal Pradesh 173229, India; aditisharma31790@gmail.com (A.S.); lalitluckysharma88@gmail.com (L.S.)
3. Department of Biology, Faculty of Science, Selcuk University Campus, Konya 42250, Turkey; biyologzengin@gmail.com
4. Department of Medical Disciplines, Faculty of Medicine and Pharmacy, University of Oradea, 410073 Oradea, Romania; roxana.gavrila@yahoo.com (R.B.); ovidiufr@yahoo.co.uk (O.F.)
5. Department of Pharmacy, Faculty of Medicine and Pharmacy, University of Oradea, 410028 Oradea, Romania
* Correspondence: tapanbehl31@gmail.com (T.B.); sbungau@uoradea.ro (S.B.); Tel.: +91-852-517-931 (T.B.); +40-726-776-588 (S.B.)

Received: 20 November 2020; Accepted: 4 December 2020; Published: 6 December 2020

Abstract: Withaferin A (WA), a manifold studied, C28-steroidal lactone withanolide found in *Withania somnifera*. Given its unique beneficial effects, it has gathered attention in the era of modern science. Cancer, being considered a "hopeless case and the leading cause of death worldwide, and the available conventional therapies have many lacunae in the form of side effects. The poly pharmaceutical natural compound, WA treatment, displayed attenuation of various cancer hallmarks by altering oxidative stress, promoting apoptosis, and autophagy, inhibiting cell proliferation, reducing angiogenesis, and metastasis progression. The cellular proteins associated with antitumor pathways were also discussed. WA structural modifications attack multiple signal transduction pathways and enhance the therapeutic outcomes in various diseases. Moreover, it has shown validated pharmacological effects against multiple neurodegenerative diseases by inhibiting acetylcholesterinases and butyrylcholinesterases enzyme activity, antidiabetic activity by upregulating adiponectin and preventing the phosphorylation of peroxisome proliferator-activated receptors (PPARγ), cardioprotective activity by AMP-activated protein kinase (AMPK) activation and suppressing mitochondrial apoptosis. The current review is an extensive survey of various WA associated disease targets, its pharmacokinetics, synergistic combination, modifications, and biological activities.

Keywords: Withaferin A; anticancer; autophagy; chaperone

1. Introduction

Phytotherapy is the frequent therapeutic approach in complementary as well as in traditional medicine since time immemorial. It is utilized by 60% of the global population and has a vital role in the health care system due to ease of availability and reduced cost compared with synthetic compounds. The result of screening showed that many synthetic drugs are derived from natural origin, which is now extensively used in pharmacological therapies [1]. Considering the importance and bringing novel therapies into the market, the herbals have always been at the forefront of synthetic drugs with complex molecular diversity and biological function variation.

Herbals are considered as natural chemical factories for manufacturing natural compounds with structural diversity. The secondary metabolites from plant origin have gained renewed attention because they directly or indirectly interact with multiple cell components, mainly lipids and proteins, thereby altering the functions of dysregulated cells [2]. The evaluation of the phytopharmacological effect of potential herbal drugs is essential for drug discovery and development [3–6]. Despite the considerable application of natural compounds in drug development, it is assumed that plant-based sources are still unexplored and can be scrutinized for new therapeutic approaches in the modern era. Artemisia annua can reveal the significance of this field (Quinhaosu) derived artemisinin, the antimalarial drug known for its long history in Chinese traditional medicine in the treatment of fevers. The anti-hypertensive agent reserpine is used to remedy snake bite in Indian traditional medicine [7]. Today medicinal plants are evaluated and explored due to modern technologies, including screening and functional assays [8]. There is an escalating demand for novel therapies to treat diseases. There is a growing interest in naturally extracted herbal constituents as targets for potential treatment.

In the Ayurvedic and Unani systems, over the last 3000 years, the genus Withania (family: Solanaceae) has been used indigenously [9]. The distribution is seen widely in the dry regions of the tropical and subtropical areas, extending from the Canary Islands to the Mediterranean region, North Africa, and ending in Southeast/Southwest Asia. Its numerous therapeutic usages have gained modern scientific attention and emerged in World Health Organization (WHO) monographs on preferred medicinal plants. *Withania Somnifera* (Ashwagandha) belongs to the family Solanaceae. It has local names like asgandh, punir (Hindi), Ghodakun, Ghoda (Gujrati), Ashwagandha (Bengali), amukkura, amkulang (Tamil), Pulivendram (Telugu), etc. In Sanskrit, Ashwagandha means "horse's smell" probably arises from the smell of its root, bear a resemblance to that of a sweaty horse. WS is also known commonly as Indian ginseng and Indian winter cherry. In Latin, *somnifera* is known as "sleep making," which means sedating properties, but it has adaptogenic properties or sexual vitality strength [3]. Ashwagandha roots are constituted in numerous Ayurvedic, Siddha, and Unani formulations [9].

This medicinal plant's therapeutic applications include antidiabetic, anti-epileptic, anti-inflammatory, anti-depressant, anti-arthritic, anticoagulant, antipyretic antioxidant, analgesic, regenerating, rejuvenating, and promoting growth [10,11]. The primary chemical constituents include compounds of varying chemical structures viz. flavonoids, withanolides, tannin, and alkaloids. Of these, withanolides have steroidal lactone triterpenoids at C28 position assembled on a reorganized or integral ergostane framework, of which C22 and C26 are in oxidized form resulting in the lactone ring (six-membered) [11].

Reverse pharmacology approaches implicated WA as a bioactive compound having the maximum pharmacological potential of Ashwagandha [12] (Figure 1). The analysis of the WA chemical structure displayed 3 positions that may interact with target proteins. Alkylation reactions and nucleophilic site binding reactions occurs through the A-ring at position C3 and the epoxide network in C24 (Figure 1). These sites are most vulnerable for the nucleophilic attack and alkylation reaction; WA interacts covalently with the target proteins [13].

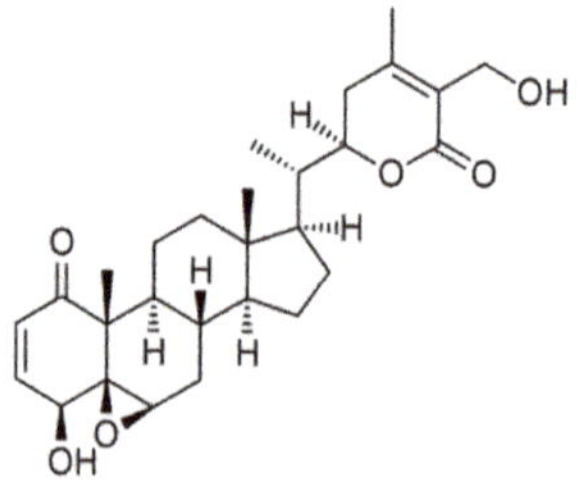

Figure 1. Structure of Withaferin A.

WA evidenced many pharmacological activities, including tumor preventive, antidiabetic, anti-osteoporotic, anti-inflammatory, antiangiogenic effects, cell death inducing, radiosensitizing, and Covid 19 infection. Although the research on molecular mechanisms by which WA attains these pharmacological activities is still going on, various evidence has been indicated, including macromolecules acylation or alkylation or covalent binding to the enzymatic site [13].

The current review is an extensive survey of various WA associated disease targets, summarizing the pharmacokinetics, structural modifications, potential pharmacological activities, and WA formulations, and evaluating also the available evidence to predict the potential targets. More than 150 References, indexed in the most relevant data basis (MDPI, ESEVIER, PubMed, NCBI, Springer, etc.) were found describing parts of our topic.

2. Pharmacokinetics and Bioavailability Studies of Withaferin A

Pharmacokinetic (PK) studies provide valuable information on bioactive compounds of herbal drugs. PK analysis is based upon targeted or untargeted metabolites profiling following the oral administration of a single chemical component of the crude drug. The estimation analysis on mice plasma following oral administration of 1000 mg/kg W. somnifera root aqueous extract showed 0.4585 mg/kg of WA. The PK data displayed rapid oral absorption of WA with C_{max}, T_{max}, and $T_{1/2}$ were 16.69 ± 4.02 ng/mL, 20 min, 59.92 ± 15.90 min, respectively. According to one of the studies WA has one and half times more relative bioavailability than other withanolides in W. somnifera [14]. The permeability was measured and found that the probability (P_{eff}) value of WA was 4.05×10^{-5}, indicating highly impermeable [15]. The oral bioavailability was found to be 32.4 ± 4.8% after 5 mg/kg intravenous and 10 mg/kg oral WA administration. The in vitro analysis indicated that WA could transport across colorectal adenocarcinoma (Caco-2) cells, and it also shows the absence of a P-glycoprotein substrate. The stability studies of WA in gastric fluid, liver microsomes, and intestinal microflora solution showed similar results in male rats and humans with a half-life of 5.6 min.

Moreover, WA reduced quickly, and 27.1% left within 1 h [16]. PK and safety studies of WA advanced stage of cancer were also seen. The phase I study on WA showed that formulation at dose 4800 mg having equivalent to 216 mg of WA, was tolerated well without showing any dose-limiting toxicity. The maximum dose received by cohort patients was four capsules of the WA regimen (TID) [17]. Taken together, the data showed that the administration of WA in advanced stage high grade osteosarcoma patients results in rapid oral absorption and has a good safety profile. Moreover, Phase II clinical trials can be carried at the dose of 216 mg/day [17]. Thus, this natural compound has enormous potential. So, novel targeted drug delivery strategies can be designed to treat various human diseases.

3. Structural Modifications of Withaferin A

The pharmacological activity is enhanced by chemical modifications such as hydroxylation or acetylation. Thus, the knowledge of the structure-function association may motivate new drug development [18]. More significant bioactivity, chemoprotective potential, and stability are acquired by alkylated (methyl or ethyl) secondary metabolites [19,20]. Mortalin is a chaperone that inactivates tumor suppressor protein p53 and induces apoptosis deregulation by promoting carcinogenesis. Stimulation of p53 through its complex abrogation with mortalin arrests cancer cell growth in various studies [21,22]. WA interferes with the interaction of mortalin with p53. The docking of 3β-methoxy-Withaferin-A with the binding domain of the mortalin substrate was done. Methylation of WA exerts a crucial influence on its protein binding efficacy, resulting in chemotherapeutic potency attenuation besides developing drug potency [23].

Another study showed that two WA conjugates, namely cysteine (CR-591) and glutathione (CR-777) conjugates indicated neuroprotective properties in various neurodegenerative disorders. A nanomolar dose of WA CR-777conjugate reversed mesencephalic neuron injury caused by (1-methyl-4-phenylpyridinium (MPP+), alpha-synuclein (α-Syn), 6-hydroxydopamine (6-OHDA).

Moreover, WA CR-777 conjugate maintains neurite integrity, and the overexpression of α-Syn caused by 6-OHDA was reduced. These compounds activate the PI3K/mTOR pathway, which downregulates the oxidative stress, suppresses the TAU phosphorylation, caspase three expression, and aggregation of α-Syn exhibiting neuroprotective properties [24]. An analogue of WA, 2, 3-dihydro-3β-methoxy (3βmWi-A) having β-methoxy group substitution showed no cell cytotoxicity and at higher concentrations well tolerated. It has a protective action in normal cells against ultra-violet (UV), oxidative and chemical stresses and through pro-survival signaling [25]. Another analogue, 2,3-dihydrowithaferin A-3β-O-sulphate, showed a 35-fold increase in vitro cytotoxicity compared to WA against various human cancer cell lines [26]. The different analogues of WA are shown in Figure 2.

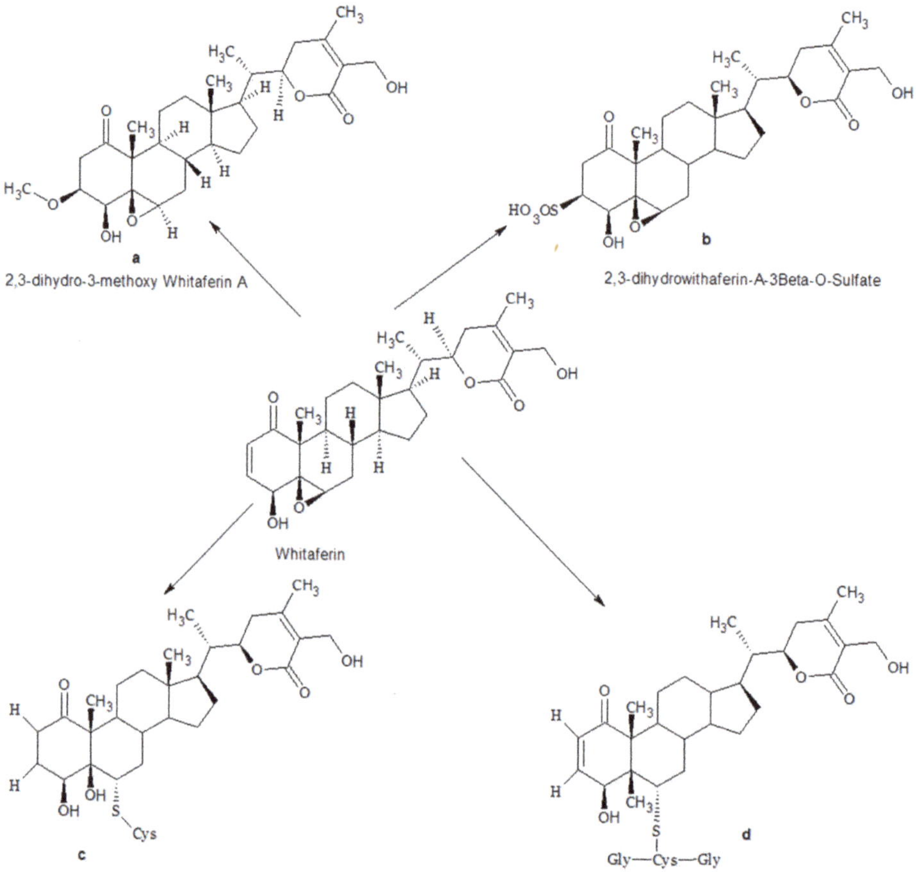

Figure 2. Metabolites of Withaferin A (**a**) 2,3-dihydro-3β-methoxy Withaferin A; (**b**) 2,3-Dihydrowithaferin A-3β-O-sulphate; (**c,d**) cysteine and glutathione conjugates of Withaferin A.

4. Pharmacological Activities of Withaferin A

4.1. Anti-Cancer Activity

The anticancer activity on WA was commenced around the 1970s [27]. Since then, WA's anticancer activity was demonstrated in many cancer cells such as multiple myeloma, neuroblastoma, leukemia, glioblastoma, ovarian, breast, colon head, and neck cancer [12]. The various molecular mechanisms involved target cytoskeleton structure and proteasomal pathway by altering oxidative stress, promoting apoptosis, and autophagy, inhibiting cell proliferation, reducing angiogenesis and metastasis progression. It regulates heat shock proteins, nuclear factor kappa B (NF-κB), and other oncogenic events [28]. Here, we discuss the chemo-preventive effects of WA on multiple organs.

4.1.1. Breast Cancer

Breast cancer is a severe malignancy affecting thousands of women globally. More than 40,000 women in the United States alone are expected to have breast cancer in 2020 [29]. The onset of breast cancer depends on the sex hormone estrogen, participating in tumor growth (by its receptor nuclear estrogen receptor). The two types of estrogen receptor (ER) genes are involved in tumor formation, namely ERα and ERβ. In breast cancer, the critical role is played by ERα. Thereby it is targeted by many pharmacological therapies. Endocrine treatment may reduce the tumor progression by decreasing the endogenous estrogen levels or interfere with ERα stimulation (e.g., by inhibiting enzyme aromatase). This results in tumor disappearance [30,31]. A study on mice with breast cancer revealed WA cytoplasmic action through compacting DNA molecule and splitting the enzyme poly-(ADP-ribose)-polymerase [32]. Another study has demonstrated that WA regulates the signal transducer pathway and activates transcription 3, attenuates IL-6 in inducible (MCF-7 and MDA-MB-231), and constitutive (MDA-MB-231) cell lines. In MDA-MB-231 and MCF-7 cells exposed, WA displayed downregulation of STAT3 transcriptional activity with/without stimulation of interleukin 6 (IL-6) in both cells. The apoptosis was also triggered by WA and can impede cell migration by regulating STAT 3, thus showing therapeutic effect [33]. Another study showed that WA when investigated in mitochondrial dysfunction associated with reactive oxygen species (ROS) generation, resulted in apoptosis of cells. The WA treatment decreases the oxidative phosphorylation as well as also suppresses the activity of complex III. On treatment with WA, DNA impaired variant mitochondrial Rho 0 cell line and 40 embryonic fibroblast-derived from Bax/Bak knockdown cells displayed more resistance than wild-type cells [34]. WA suppresses human breast cells' proliferation by decreasing the proliferating cell nuclear antigen (PCNA) expression [35]. WA enhances the vimentin phosphorylation at serine-56 residue, thereby inhibiting the proliferation in 4T mouse mammary tumor cells [36]. WA in DNA double-strand break (DSB) inhibits the single-strand annealing sub-pathway (SSA) through heat shock protein (HSP90) downregulation [37]. To block autophagy flux, WA inhibits lysosomal activity and induces apoptosis of breast cancer cells [38]. WA action leads to the aggregation of autophagosomes (protein expressions associated with autophagy). The inadequate fuel recycling and tricarboxylic acid substrate results due to the autophagic flux inhibition inducing phosphorylation impairment. WA treatment decreases the lactate dehydrogenase (LDH) expression, increases AMP protein kinase activation, and reduces adenosine triphosphate [39].

4.1.2. Ovarian Cancer

In human ovarian cancer cell lines (SKOV3 and CaOV3), WA arrest the G2/M phase cell cycle [40]. It downregulated the Notch-3/Akt/Bcl-2 signaling mediated cell survival, thereby causing caspase-3 stimulation, which induces apoptosis. Withaferin-A, combined with doxorubicin, and cisplatin at suboptimal dose generates ROS and causes cell death [41–43]. In another study using the A2780 cell line, Xenografting resulted in mortality decreased by WA. It reduces the cytosolic and nuclear levels of NF-κB-related phospho-p65 cytokines in xenografted tumors [44]. Another study showed that ovarian cancer xenografting induced cardiac cachexia, causing loss of the heart's normal functioning, systolic, and diastolic dysfunction. WA treatment improved heart weight and preserved systolic function, but the partial improvement was seen in diastolic dysfunction. Tumor cells induce AT_1R pathway mediated pro-inflammatory markers and formation of MHCβ isoform, which was ameliorated by WA [45]. In nude mice, securin overexpression leads to cellular transformation and tumor development. Knockout securin mice show no tumor development and reverse the cancer phenotype. WA alone or with Cisplatin decreases the expression of securin and showing antitumor effects [46].

4.1.3. Prostate Cancer

Initially, the pathogenesis linked with prostate tumors is an androgen; however, numerous patients also progresses to androgen-independent (metastatic castration-resistant) [47]. The stem-like characteristics are shown by androgen-independent PCa cells (mCRPC) DU-145 and PC-3), whereas exhibited by androgen-dependent PCa cells (e.g., LNCaP) [48–50]. The side populating cells of xenograft tissues and human PCa cell lines exhibited more epithelial-mesenchymal transition (EMT) and comparably more violent than homologous bulk population cells [51]. Thereby, EMT is very closely linked with the mCRPC formation. In prostate tumor cells, WA binds vimentin and induces cell death, but no cell death was seen in normal fibroblasts. It raises the level of c-Fos and ROS generation and decreases the FLIP level, probably resulting in cytoskeletal architecture degradation. Thus, WA can be used as a pharmaceutical agent that effectively kills cancer stem cells (CSCs). These CSCs are different from other cancer cells, as their presence within the tumor mass mediates chemoresistance by regenerating tumors [52]. WA interacts directly with vimentin by causing an alteration in cysteine residue (Cys328), forming an aggregation of vimentin filaments and together with F-actin, causing disruption of vimentin cytoskeleton [53,54]. This is followed by alteration in cell shape, reduced motility, and upregulated phosphorylation of vimentin at Ser38 [55].

The observations evidenced that WA can efficiently target metastatic tumor cells [36]. In cell lines of pancreatic cancer, Panc-1, BxPc3, and MiaPaCa2, WA inhibit Hsp90 chaperone activity, disrupting Hsp90 client proteins, thus showing antiproliferative effects [56]. Another study has shown the efficacy of WA against the CaP iPten-KO model. The role of the metastatic process Akt pathway, Pten deletion, mutation, EMT was seen commonly in metastatic prostate tumors. WA abrogated HG-PIN formation and ameliorated the progression of the Pten-deficient tumor to adenocarcinoma. WA inhibited PI3K/AKT pathway. The AKT-mediated Par-4 and FOXO3A proapoptotic proteins were increased in Pten-KO mice supplemented with WA. Immunohistochemical analysis displayed decreased pAKT expression and the β-catenin and N-cadherin epithelial-to-mesenchymal transition markers in WA-treated tumors control [57]. DNA damage response is initiated by Telomere shortening, which results in senescence and apoptosis [58,59]. The cancer cells run away from the shortening of telomere by enzyme telomerase [60,61]. In ALT cells, WA caused severe damage to telomere by downregulation of shelterin proteins (TRF2 and POT1). It was observed that WA caused cytotoxicity to ALT cells with no effect on telomere and telomerase activity length. By telomerase-independent mechanisms, it kills TEP cells, as reported previously [62]. Another study showed that WA significantly inhibited pAKT expression and facilitated FOXO3a/Par-4 mediated tumor inhibition in TRAMP mice [63]. One of the critical sources of Cancer is mutations in the Wnt pathway that control cancer hallmarks like metastasis and immune evasion [64–67]. Wnt signaling pathway hyperactivation triggers the transformation of normal cells to malignant [68,69].

Interestingly, WA analog 3-azido WA can suppress the Wnt pathway indirectly and thus prevent the transformation of Cancer [70]. WA and its metabolite 3-azido-WA also increase protein, namely proapoptotic prostate cancer response-4 (PAR-4) in androgen-refractory prostate cancer cells [71]. It modulates the β-catenin phosphorylation in the Wnt pathway. In particular, an increased amount of PAR-4 downregulates the Akt kinase activity induces the glycogen synthase kinase 3 beta (GSKβ) activation. This phosphorylates βcatenin is known to obstruct the Wnt signaling pathway [70]. Another study showed WA intraperitoneal administration (0.1 mg) resulted in significant suppression of circulatory free fatty acid and fatty acid synthase expression, ATP citrate lyase, and carnitine palmitoyl transferase 1A proteins in vivo prostate studies [72].

4.1.4. Colorectal Cancer

Another common cancer is colorectal cancer (CRC), the fourth leading cause of mortality worldwide [73]. Despite the incredible progress of efficient chemotherapeutic agents, the drug resistance occurred, determining the non-success of chemotherapy, with escalated toxicity to the gastrointestinal tract, skin, and bone marrow [74,75]. In human colorectal cancer cells, WA generates

ROS followed by the activation of Nrf2, HO-1, NQO1 pathways, and upregulating the expression of the c-Jun-N-terminal kinase (JNK), the upstream regulator of Nrf2. This resulted in cell death induction by blocking the disruption of tumor suppressor geneTAp73. WA induces in G2/M phase cell cycle arrest in HCT116 and SW480 cells of colorectal cancer [76]. It delayed mitosis by interfering with the proteasomal disruption of Mad2 and Cdc20, necessary constituents of the spindle complex [76].

Moreover, it decreased expression and proliferation of Notch-1 in human colon cancer cells [77]. In colorectal cancer, EMT causes AKT and Notch1 activation. As EMT leads to this type of cancer, therapies that target AKT/Notch1 pathways and prevent metastasis are at the top of the current research paradigm. The WA effect was studied on colitis regulated colon mouse model and other mouse models of spontaneous intestinal carcinogenesis. WA effectively inhibits the development of intestinal polyp and colon carcinogenesis; it showed also the downregulation of pro-survival signaling markers (NFκB, Notch1, and pAKT) and reduced the proliferative markers [78]. The chemoprotective action on spontaneous and inflammatory colon carcinogenesis patterns was performed on transgenic mice models; WA treatment demonstrated declined tissue inflammation and adenomas. In the molecular analysis, WA down-regulates the expression of Notch1, pAKT, and NF-κB and other markers of inflammation (interleukin-6 (IL-6), tumor necrosis factor alpha (TNFα), and cyclooxygenase-2) [79], highlighting that this therapeutic agent has a vital role in colon carcinogenesis prevention. Thus, it can be further explored for clinical utility.

4.1.5. Lung Cancer

In lung cancer cells (A549 and H1299), WA pre-treatment showed suppressed cell adhesion, migration, and invasion. Using immunofluorescence, qRT-PCR, and western blot analysis, it was proved that WA downregulated EMT induced by tumor growth factor beta 1 (TGFβ1) and TNFα expression in both cells. WA also suppresses Smad2/3 and NF-κB phosphorylation and nuclear translocation [80]. In another study on A549 cells, WA causes dose-dependent apoptosis. JC-1 staining of cells treated with WA showed declined MMP and was accompanied by caspase-9 and caspase-3 activation, the apoptosis leading players [81]. WA arrested the G0/G1 phase of lung cancer (A549) cells, which further suppresses phosphatidyl inositol-3 kinase (PI3K)/Akt pathway and decrease the Bcl-2expression. WA also displayed a dose-dependent decrease of metastatic lung nodules. WA is an effective anti-lung cancer agent as well as also controls the growth of CSC. It also inhibits the spheroid formation in lung cancer by suppressing the mTOR/STAT3 pathway [81].

4.2. WA-Responsive Proteins in Cancer

Carcinogenesis is a process with multiple stages that involve the deregulation of various physiological and biochemical cascades that control cells' growth and survival and their apoptosis. In this context targeting various signaling mediators that lead to tumor growth is advantageous to be discussed. The electrophilic nature and its interaction with the nucleophilic group results in inducing electrophilic stress, thereby it shows WA as a Michael addition electron acceptor. These free radicals will cause damage to the mitochondria leading to its apoptosis. There is an increase in the exogenous ROS levels dramatically during drug uptake or environmental stress, such as UV radiation [82]. WA treatment forms ROS in various models of Cancer. WA interaction to Keap1 causes increased NRF2 protein levels, which mediate the antioxidant protein expression protecting the cell against the effect of oxidative damage [83].

Meanwhile, various proteins are targeted by WA from the anti-stress pathway and increasing the ROS level. This augmented ROS level further activates antioxidant pathways and causing ROS/cyto-protection imbalance. This finally decides the fate of cancer cells. WA treatment enhances four oxidative stress response proteins that decrease the oxidative damage following WA treatment and re-establish homeostasis. The upregulated proteins in oxidative stress response upon WA treatment include heme oxygenase, one iron-sulfur, aldose reductase, and sepiapterin reductase. Various proteins are downregulated glutathione peroxidase 1, phospholipid hydroperoxide [84,85].

Following oxidative stress and activation of the ubiquitin-proteasome system (UPS) is activated by the Nrf2 transcription factor to remove oxidized proteins and restore homeostasis. Targeting UPS induces more proteotoxic stress in cancer cells. WA treatment upregulates five proteins related to ubiquitin-proteasome includes beta type-1 (PSB1 human), Proteasome subunit alpha type-2 (PSA2 human), 26S proteasome regulatory subunit 10B, Ubiquitin carboxyl-terminal hydrolase (UBP24 human), and Proteasome activator complex subunit-4 (PSME4 human). The WA-target proteins that degrade include Proteasome subunit beta type-10 and type-5, AAA+ chaperone p97, USP24 human isozyme L5 [86,87].

UPS is responsible for cellular removal of proteins, although cells also have an extra protein removal system known as autophagy that disrupts cellular components and the deposited aggregates of protein during UPS attenuation [88]. Autophagy is an adaptive cellular stress response. The treatment with WA disrupts and block autophagy functions [38]. Therefore, autophagy markers that upregulate during WA treatment include mitochondrial import receptor subunit TOM22 homolog, SNARE-associated protein Snapin, ras-related protein Rab-24, tubulin beta chain, histone deacetylase 6, Annexin A4, Tubulin Beta [89,90].

Another transcription factor known as heat shock factor-1 (HSF-1) regulates protein folding and repair [91]. This factor induces stress and also binds with DNA and causes the stimulation of heat shock response elements. WA has a potential antitumor activity, indicating very powerful ER-stress causing properties, assumed from HSF1 reporter assay [92]. HSF1 is marked as a promising WA binding target, further leading to the suppression of genes controlled by HSF-1, such as FKBP4 HSP13 and DJC10. The proteins exaggerated treatment with WA includes chaperone, ER-associated degradation, and protein folding enzymes (isomerase and reductase). Proteins associated with chaperone related protein unc-45 homolog A, heat shock 70 kDa protein 1A; 1B; 13, DnaJ homolog subfamily A member 2, BAG family molecular chaperone regulator 2. The protein targeted by WA and linked with the enzymatic activity of isomerase and reductase include Peptidyl-prolyl cis-trans isomerase, Peptidyl-prolyl isomerase domain, NIMA-interacting 1, and WD repeat-containing protein 1. Proteins that target ER-associated degradation include alpha-mannosidase protein 3, Homocysteine inducible ER, AAA+ chaperone p97, transport and golgi organization protein 1 homolog [84]

At the time of weak cellular stress response initiated by WA, Protein translation must be restrained to avoid new misfolded proteins' aggregation. WA has a role in protein translation machinery, which increases eukaryotic translation initiation factor (IF) 2A, which inhibits cancer cells' proliferation. However, subsequent interaction of WA with IF5A1 (the eIF5A regulon) and IF4B triggers cell death [93].

Moreover, WA also targets the cytoskeleton properties, which include Vimentin, annexin A2, and β-tubulin. Vimentin (VIM) plays the leading role in holding and anchoring organelles by making connections of the nucleus, mitochondria, and endoplasmic reticulum in the cytosol. Various kinases have shown binding with vimentin such as ROKa, Raf-1, phosphorylated ERKs, PKCe [94–96]. Alternatively, vimentin interacts with 14-3-3 proteins that might obstruct signaling cascades that mediate cell cycle progression, signal transduction, and apoptosis; it also binds with HSP90. Furthermore, there is an enhanced vimentin expression in cancerous cells, and it is correlated with EMT, metastasis with poor prognosis thereby resulting in reduced patient survival [54,97]. When binds with vimentin, it inhibits the assembly and intermediate filament network and leads to eventual viability [98]. Annexin A2 (ANXA2) is a calcium-dependent protein, supporting endocytosis, adhesion, and metastasis. It is present abundantly in a broad range of cancers. WA, when binds to annexin A2 core domain, causes suppression of actin polymerization and subsequent limit the migration of the cancer cells [99,100]. Literature also reports that WA arrests the G2/M and G1/S transition cell cycle phase [32].

The targets identified are Dual specificity protein kinase TTK, Nucleoporin Nup43, Protein phosphatase 1B SRRT human, WAPL human, NIPA human, MCMBP human [84]. WA also disrupts of NFκB signaling pathways. It is an important pathway that is dysregulated in various types of Cancer [101]. This suppresses the gene transcription of many downstream genes involved in inflammation includes MCP1, Interleukin-1 (IL6), and IL8, etc. The proteins participated in

NFκB signaling and downregulated by WA include nuclear factor NFκB p105 subunit, Transcription factor p65, signal co-integrator one complex subunit 2, Coiled-coil domain-containing protein 22, COMD3 human. NF-kB participates in the activation of proteins involved in cell growth, cell survival, angiogenesis, and decrease vulnerability to apoptosis [84,102]. NF-kB driven proteins expression stimulation is controlled tightly. Under quiescent conditions, it is an inactive form in the cytoplasm with its inhibitor IkB, masking the nuclear localization process. Inflammatory mediators, and microbial pathogens trigger specific cognate receptors and stimulate NF-kB. This event induces the stimulation of the IkB-kinase (IKK) complex leading to its proteasomal degradation [102]. WA inhibited NF-kB signaling, which includes chronic lymphocytic leukemia (CLL), acute myeloid leukemia (AML), and multiple myeloma (MM) [13].

Cancer stem cells (CSC) are the self-renewal and tumor-initiating cells. The rising trend in the failure of chemotherapeutic drugs and the reappearance of cancer has contributed to cancer stem cells' growth in growing tumors. The main priority is the eradication of these cancer stem cells in modern endeavors of anticancer drug discovery. In the cells of pancreatic ductal adenocarcinoma nestin overexpression, a stem cell marker rises cell motility and results in phenotypic changes, whereas endogenous nestin knockdown decreases cell migration well as cells also retain its epithelial phenotype. WA possesses anti-nestin activity, which suggests its potential in targeting pancreatic CSC [103]. Another study reported [104] the suppression of mammosphere activity, the aldehyde dehydrogenase 1 (ALDH1) activity, elevated CD44, and reduced CD24 levels in breast cancer cells (MCF-7 and SUM159). This poly-pharmaceutical response rationalizes its anticancer mechanism. Chemo proteomic approach shows WA binds and interacts with numerous proteins targeting various protein signaling cascades of cancer. The various anticancer targets are shown in Figure 3.

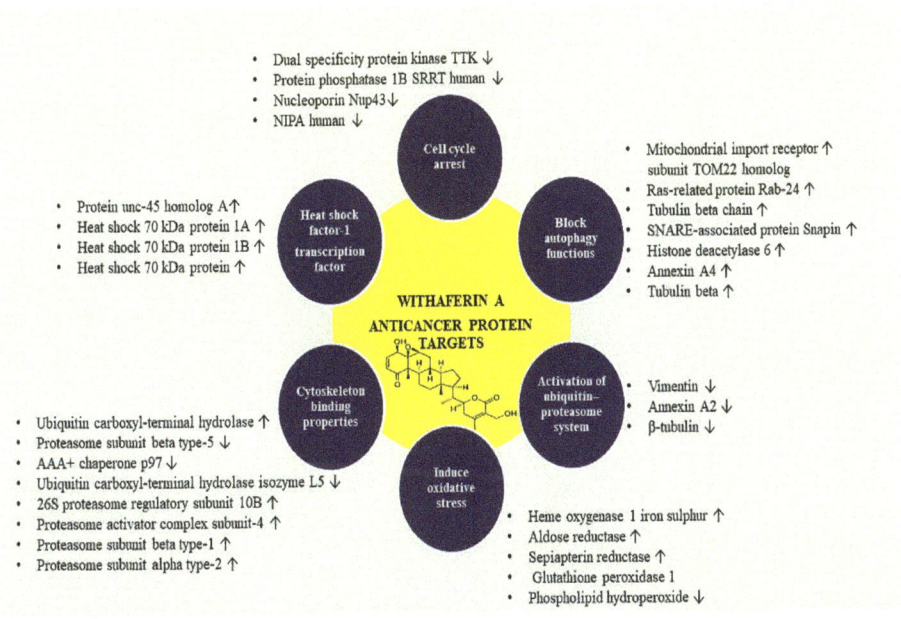

Figure 3. Withaferin A associated anticancer protein targets.

Oxidative Stress Response and Red Cell Proteins

WA was reported to induce ROS production causing oral and colon cancer cells apoptosis [105,106]. In cancer cells, WA induces G2/M cell cycle arrest, antiproliferation, apoptosis, mitochondrial membrane depolarization, caspase activation, migration inhibition and phosphorylated histone H2A.X based damage to DNA [107]. WA inhibits the activities of MMP-2, MMP-9, causing antioxidant gene expression and activation of MAPK. In oral cancer cells N N-acetylcysteine (NAC) pre-treatment suppressed the inhibitory migration alteration and various pathways activated following the WA treatment proving that ROS plays a crucial role in inhibitory migration induced by WA [108].

Moreover, in tumor cells, the cell surface glycoproteins and glycolipids have changed composition of carbohydrates causing aberrant cell-cell recognition, antigenicity, cell adhesion, and malignant cells invasiveness [109]. Glycosyl residues present on the cell surface controls epithelial growth and cell proliferation [110]. During carcinogenesis, the levels of plasma glycoconjugates are elevated at the expense of erythrocyte membranes with the depletion in epithelial cell surface carbohydrates [109]. The loss of erythrocyte membrane glycoproteins was due to increased degradation or due to increased shedding into circulation or reduced synthesis. Neoplastic transformation causes increased levels of plasma sialic acid through the secretion or shedding from the tumor cell [111,112]. As the tumor mass grows, it may contribute to elevated fucose concentrations as a result of glycoproteins release or due to host treatment causing cell damage. WA treatment protected the red blood cell membrane integrity by maintaining glycoconjugates level during carcinogenesis. Oxidative stress alters the membrane bound enzymes, which is important for cell lysis [113]. It has been showed that any changes in red cell fragility induces change in Na^+/K^+-ATPase activity [114]. Tumor bearing hamster's red blood cells were more fragile when compared with control hamsters. This increased fragility may be due to their lipid content alteration and increased oxidative stress. WA significantly restored membrane TBARS levels, Na^+/K^+-ATPase activity and osmotic fragility in red cell [115]. Human umbilical vein endothelial cells (HUVECs) as well as endothelial cell line (EA.hy926) when treated with WA showed increased heme oxygenase (HO-1) expression, an antioxidant gene. This gene is transcriptionally regulated by NF-E2-related factor 2 (Nrf2) transcription factor which senses chemical alteration in the cell and regulates transcriptional responses thus maintaining chemical homeostasis via antioxidant gene expression. WA upregulates and increase the nuclear translocation of Nrf2, inducing HO-1 expression in endothelial cells thereby re-establish cell homeostasis [116].

4.3. Anti Diabetic Activity

Diabetes is a metabolic, endocrine disease where the glucose supply and utilization are mismatched. The pathogenesis includes elevated oxidative stress, which disrupts the pancreas histology and causes beta-cells destruction. Insulin-dependent or type I diabetes mellitus depends totally on insulin replacement therapy as the therapeutic strategy. There are various parts and parcel complications of diabetes, such as obesity, organ sepsis, and microvascular and macro-vascular diabetic complications [117,118]. Another evidence reported that WA leads to potential alteration in glucose metabolism and lipid profiles. In diabetic mice, it suppresses inflammation and stimulates weight loss, contributing to elevated insulin sensitivity [119]. WA attenuated mouse hepatic steatosis, although antidiabetic drug rosiglitazone has a beneficial effect on insulin sensitivity but does not show improved liver and weight loss effects. Inflammatory mediators (TNF-α, IL6, and resistin) play a significant role in obesity. They promote insulin receptor substrates 1 (IRS-1) phosphorylation that negatively controls the signaling of insulin. They were significantly decreased by WA treatment. Previous literature has shown the downregulation of insulin signaling gene expression (insr, pi3k irs1, slc2a4, and irs2) in diabetes. WA treatment upregulated the mRNA expression of insr, insr, pi3k, and irs1 while treatment with rosiglitazone increased insr, irs1, and slc2a4 expression. WA insulin-sensitizing potential seems to have occurred due to its anti-inflammatory action that indirectly affects insulin signaling events, upregulating adiponectin, preventing the phosphorylation of PPARγ [119]. The studies reported attenuation of streptozotocin-induced type 1 diabetes by WA. Oxidative stress stimulates the NF-κB axis, following inflammatory mediators' production that induces pancreatic islet cell destruction. STZ induces alkylation of DNA that ultimately leads to the β-cell dysfunction. Apoptotic morphological changes occur by Caspase 3 upregulation, including DNA fragmentation, membrane blebbing, apoptotic body formation, and cytoplasmic and nuclear condensation [120]. This results in the disruption of pancreatic insulin-secreting β-cells, resulting in hyperglycemia [121,122]. WA intervention abrogates nitrosative stress by lowering tissue nitrile levels. WA was considered as a potential molecule to ameliorate T1DM by caspase three expression, reduction in fragmented DNA, decrease in the concentration of TNF-α, and IL-6 [122]. In acute liver injury induced by acetaminophen, WA activates the Keap1/Nrf2 pathway and mediates the hepatoprotective effect. The Nrf-2/NFκB signaling imbalance leads to a cascade of oxidative stress causing liver damage [123]. Moreover, in another study, also WA proved to be anti-inflammatory and antioxidant. It restores the impaired insulin resistance and corrects the endothelial function [124]. Taken together, these results implicated that TNF-α, IL6, and Nrf-2/NFκB are an essential target of WA.

4.4. Neuroprotective Activity

In the central nervous system (CNS), Aβ accumulation contributes to neurodegeneration. WA 0.5–2 µM decreases the amyloid beta (Aβ) aggregation induced by Tat and cocaine with no cytotoxicity in the cell cultures. WA treatment decreases cytoplasmic vacuoles and dendritic beading. Moreover, this Aβ accumulation in an HIV patient's brain contributes to cascades of neurological disorders that drive aging or related dementias [125]. Moreover, WA is reported to block the acetylcholesterinases and butyrylcholinesterases enzyme activity in in vitro assay.

The hydrolytic activity acetylcholinesterase disrupts neurotransmitter acetylcholine, thereby forming choline and acetate. The role of butyrylcholinesterase still to be explored. As acetylcholine has a significant role in cognitive diseases, acetylcholine's upregulation ameliorates the cognitive deficits in Alzheimer's disease (AD) [126]. The neuroprotective ability of WA (50 mg/kg b.w) demonstrated a resurge of dopamine (DA) and homo vanillic acid (HVA) in substantia nigra and striatum. The reduced level of these catecholamines leads to motor deficits. The increased level of DA and HVA suggest the neuroprotective potential of WA [127]. Traumatic brain injury (TBI) has increased morbidity and mortality rates worldwide, making it a significant public health concern. WA significantly enhanced neurobehavioral function and reduced histological alteration in tissues after injury; it reduces the disruption in the blood-brain barrier and edema in the brain via decreasing apoptosis in endothelial cells. WA attenuate the levels of neuroinflammatory mediators (TNF-α, IL-1β, and IL-6). This regulation regulating microglial activation can be used as a therapeutic regimen for recovery after traumatic brain injury [128].

In AD, activation of microglia is achieved by interaction with Aβ oligomers and Aβ fibrils, which causes an inflammatory reaction by stimulating NLRP3 and nuclear factor NF-κB pathway inducing the release of pro-inflammatory cytokines and chemokines [129,130]. By phagocytosis, Aβ fibrils are engulfed by microglia, and these fibrils are degraded by neprilysin and insulin-degrading enzyme. In patients of AD, stimulation of NLRP3 and NF-κB pathway block the Aβ phagocytosis causing increased Aβ fibrils accumulation, thereby forming a self-perpetuating loop, resulting in neuroinflammation [130]. NF-κB expression was inhibited with WA's treatment, which plays a vital role in the cascade of inflammatory cytokines. The downregulation of JAK and STAT and upregulation of IKBKB and IKBKG was seen [131].

Leucine-rich repeat kinase 2 is a massive protein mutated in neurological patients with Alzheimer's disease and Parkinson's disease (PD). This protein is stabilized by chaperone HSF90 and also with co-chaperone Cdc37. When treated with WA, the N9 microglial cell line decreases the LRRK2 and disrupts the HSP90, Cdc37, which results in destabilization and reduced concentration of LRRK2 [86]. A more beneficial anti-inflammatory role of WA was seen in transgenic mice with TAR–DNA binding protein (TDP43). These mice have a neurodegenerative disease similar to amyotrophic lateral sclerosis and indicate activated microglia with neurotoxic and pro-inflammatory phenotypes. TDP43 expression, NF-kB subunit p65 expression, was found to be increased in the spinal cord. WA treatment improved motor neuron deficits and decreased NF-kB dependent inflammation and thereby decreasing the disease phenotype. WA (10 to 40 mg/kg ip) also displayed anxiolytic efficacy, as measured by increased exploratory time in the open arm in the elevated plus-maze [132]. Altogether this data confirms that

WA has enormous potential as a natural neurotherapeutic agent in ameliorating cognitive deficits associated with AD, PD, ALS; thus, its application in other models of neurodegenerative diseases deserves to be investigated.

4.5. Cardioprotective Activity

Myocardial infarction (MI) is a significant health problem globally and the leading cause of death. WA 1mg/kg decreased the apoptotic cell death, upregulation of protein Bcl-2, and thereby stimulating the mitochondrial antiapoptotic pathway. The in vivo study evidenced WA low dose 1 mg/kg, in mice has a beneficial effect against MI injury, but a higher dose of 5 mg/kg, in mice was not at all protective and deteriorated cardiac cells. WA may affect the Bcl-2/Bax ratio, induced AMPK activation suppressing mitochondrial apoptosis, and thus showed protective cardiac function. Thus, WA has therapeutic usage in patients having cancer enduring cardiovascular system disorders [133].

Fibroproliferative disorders are a type of tissue injury linked with stimulation of collagen synthesizing cells, inducing type I collagen synthesis and deposition [134]. This result due to collagen I gene expression transcription and the escalated collagen I mRNAs half-life [135]. WA disrupts the vimentin filament network in endothelial cells and astrocytes. Vimentin filaments interact and stabilize the type I collagen. WA participates in the regulation of transcriptional and posttranscriptional type I collagen and inhibits the stimulation of TGF, block activation of NF-kB.

Myocardial fibrosis is linked with the accumulation of collagen fibers in the cardiac interstitium, seen in various cardiac disorders: myocardial infarction, hypertensive heart disease, idiopathic interstitial cardiac fibrosis, hypertrophic cardiomyopathy, and decompensated congestive heart failure. The fibrosis disrupts cardiac function resulting in heart failure [136–139]. The studies also showed the antiplatelet, profibrinolytic, and anticoagulant WA (0.09 ug to 4.71 ug/mouse). In TNF-α stimulated human umbilical vein endothelial cells, WA's effect was evidenced on the plasminogen activator inhibitor type 1 (PAI-1/t) expressions and tissue-type plasminogen activator (t-PA). WA blocked thrombin-catalyzed fibrin polymerization and also the platelet aggregation induced by ferric chloride. WA increased bleeding time and also suppressed TNF-α induced PAI-1 synthesis in vivo and ex vivo studies. Moreover, the PAI-1/t-PA ratio was reduced by WA [140]. Altogether, these results evidenced that WA has cardioprotective potential; considering its safety and efficacy, there is a need for clinical trials to support its therapeutic role in heart diseases.

4.6. COVID 19

The proper treatment of cancer patients with the potentially compromised immune system and SARS-CoV2 infection is a serious issue faced by oncologists [141]. Data from four hot spots regions, namely China, United States, Italy, and Spain, showed that patients are admitted to the intensive care unit (ICU) and need mechanical ventilation for life support [142–145]. Covid 19 infection is associated with life-threatening immune reaction, and there is a release of pro-inflammatory cytokines termed as cytokine storm [146]. In a metastatic ovarian cancer model, WA decreases the pro-inflammatory cytokines (IL-6, TNFα, IL-8, IL-18) [44]. The realm of possibility showed that WA reduces the cytokine storm intensity due to its anti-inflammatory properties reported. Two research groups demonstrated that withanolides (such as WA) can bind with the S protein receptor-binding domain of virus, thereby inhibiting the viral binding with the host's ACE2 receptor [147,148]. Another group indicated that WA and withanone bind with coronavirus's main protease, but WA has low a binding affinity compared to an established inhibitor of N3 protease in docking scores [149]. WA treatment decreases the angiotensin II receptor type 1 mRNA expression compared to control groups. Based on these findings and previously reported studies, WA treatment was observed to alter lungs' ACE2 expression under tumor-free and bearing states. No significant results in lungs ACE2 mRNA expression were there. TMPRSS2 is involved in S protein priming, which causes the cleavage of S protein and thereby allowing viral and cellular membranes fusion. SARS-COVID enters via interacting with angiotensin-converting enzyme 2 (ACE2) WA bind at the catalytic site of TMPRSS2 and able to alter its allosteric site. Therefore,

WA can be a potential therapeutic compound to prevent the COVID-19 spread by blocking ACE 2 expression and reducing pro-inflammatory cytokines [150].

4.7. Anti Hepatitis Activity

Nonalcoholic steatohepatitis (NASH) is known as the advanced form of nonalcoholic fatty liver disorders that collectively results in the risk of liver cirrhosis and carcinoma [151,152]. Over intake of fatty acids leads to the formation of toxic lipids inducing inflammation, ER stress, hepatic oxidative stress, and hepatic cell death [153]. Out of all the lipids, ceramides get accumulated in the blood and tissues. WA decreases oxidative stress, displayed by its nuclear factor erythroid related factor 2 pathway and heme oxygenase (HO-1) expression, thereby also ameliorating acetaminophen-induced liver injury. WA 5 mg/kg improved pathologies associated with NASH, such as hepatic steatosis, fibrosis, and inflammation. Various pathways involve kelch like ECH associated protein 1, glycogen synthase kinase 3 [154]. These findings suggest that WA effectively protects cells from NASH, although further studies are still required to know the exact mechanism. This could help in the repurposing of this WA with its potential role in treating NASH.

4.8. Osteoporosis

Osteoporosis is a skeletal bone disorder characterized by an imbalance in bone resorption and formation [155]. WA (5 and 10 mg/kg) upregulates the osteoblast-specific transcription factor expression, promoting osteoblast proliferation and differentiation. WA down-regulates the inflammatory cytokines. In osteoclast, also known as bone-resorbing cells, WA suppresses osteoclast number by downregulating the expression of tartrate-resistant acid phosphatase (TRAP) and receptor activator of nuclear factor kappa-B ligand (RANKL) and osteoprotegerin (OPG). Furthermore, WA also inhibits NF-kB signaling, activated nuclear p65-subunit of NF-kB, and stabilizes RunX2. Thus, promoting the activity of osteoblastic bone-forming cells [156]. These findings indicated that WA prevents osteoporosis by downregulating TRAP and RANKL, thereby inhibiting osteoclast differentiation.

5. Formulations Prepared from Withaferin A

Dexamethasone and WA gold nanoparticles were able to inhibit the epithelial-mesenchymal transition in tumor cells, preventing metastasis by inhibiting mouse melanoma tumors, thereby reducing mice's mortality rate Glucocorticoids receptor-dependent selective cytotoxicity occurs using this metallic nanoparticle formulation [157]. In one study, mannosylated liposomes (ML) were used for encapsulation of WA (adjuvant-induced) for targeting synovial macrophages in a rat model of arthritis. With the help of confocal microscopy, ML-WA showed robust internalization of synovial macrophages. Moreover, osteoprotegerin production was upregulated after the treatment, and there was no degradation of cartilage and bone erosion. The study suggested, ML-WA has enormous potential for reducing bone resorption and inflammation [158].

A new liposomal efficient drug delivery system was developed to target angiogenic endothelial cells and CD13 positive cancer epithelial cells using homing peptide (NGR). NGRKC16-lipopeptide liposomes are encapsulated with WA, which leads to the apoptosis of CD13-positive pancreatic cancer cells and angiogenic endothelial cells. Therefore, reported WA-encapsulated liposomal formulation could be used as a therapeutic strategy to treat aggressive pancreatic Cancer [159]. WA nano vesicular system noisome formulation showed higher anticancer activity against HeLa cells in the SRB assay followed by flow cytometry and comet assays. So, this study provides an opportunity to use natural materials as cancer treatment agents [160]. Polycaprolactone implants embedded with WA was prepared for controlled systemic release to overcome the problems associated with oral bioavailability and decreasing the dose requirement. WA implant inhibits nearly 60% of lung cancer in A549 cell xenografts, but no suppression of Cancer was there when the same dose was given intraperitoneally [161]. WA formulation has proved beneficial in arthritis and Cancer, although this formulation still requires more process optimization for efficient clinical translation. This could also be beneficial for pharmaceutical and translational researchers.

6. Synergistic Combination of Withaferin A

The radiosensitizing combination effect of WA and hyperthermia (HT) or radiotherapy (RT) was studied (acute and fractionated) on B16F1 mouse tumors propagated in C57BL mice and Swiss albino mice [42]. Fractionated radiotherapy with WA increased the complete response (CR) of both the tumors synergistically compared to hyperthermia, further enhancing these effects. Therefore, when used with radiotherapy, WA suggested being a promising radiosensitizer. WA and myricetin (MY) combination act against the growth of pancreatic cancer. It decreased IC_{50} of WA (2.19, 2.65, 3.93 folds) compared to alone WA in PC cells (Panc-1, MiaPaca-2, BxPc-3). 1 µM of WA and 5 µM of MY, when combined, induced an increase in caspase-3 activity by 4-fold as compared to alone treatment of WA (1 µM) (2.3-fold) or MY (5 µM) (1.4-fold), which had shown less effect on the activity of caspase-3. As a whole, WA and MY's synergism caused apoptosis in pancreatic cells [162].

The in vitro co-treatment efficacy of sorafenib (SO) and withaferin A was synergistically evaluated against papillary and anaplastic thyroid cancers. Cell viability reduced significantly from 50% (alone with each drug) to 19% (in combination). G2/M cell-cycle arrest caused by SO+WA combination in anaplastic cells and induces apoptosis (PARP cleavage and inactivation of caspase-3), down-regulating the client proteins like BRAF, Raf-1, and ERK when combined drugs were given. This research provided an approach for maintaining anticancer efficacy with a combination of SO and WA [163]. Antiproliferative and apoptotic effects were evoked by co-treatment of WA and doxorubicin in many cell lines of ovarian cancer (A2780, A2780/CP70, and CaOV3). This resulted in a reduced chemotherapeutic dose of doxorubicin, and even the doxorubicin-induced side effects were also minimized. A significant increment in the production of ROS by co-treatment resulted in damage to DNA and autophagy induced (by increased expression of autophagy marker LC3B), also through caspase-3 cleavage cell death induced. 70–80% reduction was examined in ovarian tumor cells growth xenograft of nude mice generated by synergistic WA. There was a rise in autophagy as seen by LC3B autophagy marker expression and via cleavage of caspase-3 inducing cell death. The combination regimen of WA and cisplatin at suboptimal dose generates ROS and causes cell death [41]. The actions of this combination is attributed by eradicating cells, revealing markers of cancer stem cells like CD34, CD44, Oct4, CD24, and CD117 and downregulation of Hes, Hey, and Notch genes [42].

The synergistic effect of WA and oxaliplatin combination in vitro and in vivo studies on human pancreatic cells was studied. This combination results in inhibition of proliferation and caspase-regulated apoptosis. The dysfunction of mitochondria and PI3K/AKT inhibition generates intracellular ROS through which the proapoptotic effect occurred synergistically. While in vivo methodology evaluated high synergistic antitumor activity in PC xenografts [81]. Hence, a novel pharmaceutical approach for pancreatic cancer treatment could be a cocktail of oxaliplatin and WA.

Effects of both DOXIL (liposomal preparation of doxorubicin) and WA, alone and in combination form was investigated on cell lines of ovarian cancer (A2780) and tumor growth in SCID mice. In vitro spheroids formation assay was used for studying the combinatorial effect of DOXIL and WA on the tumorigenic function of ALDH1 cells (A2780 isolated). Alone treatment of WA (dose-dependent) inhibited both ALDH1 and Notch 1 gene expression, and DOXIL (200 nM) remained ineffective. When treated in a combination of WA+DOXIL, ovarian cancer cell proliferation and ALDH1 protein expression were inhibited with a significant synergistic effect. A robust significant reduction (60% to 70%) in the growth of the tumor, as well as complete metastasis inhibition, was seen in SCID mice (with the ovarian tumor) when co-treated with DOXIL (2 mg/kg) and WA (2 mg/kg). Altogether, it was determined that WA+DOXIL (co-treatment) could be a potable factor for ovarian cancer treatment [164].

Recently, researchers investigated the WA (alone) and the combination of Paclitaxel (PAC) and WA on non-small cell lung cancer (NSCLC) cells growth, proliferation, migration, and invasion. They deceived in vitro probable effects of PAC, Cis-Pt, and WA synergistically in H1299 and A549 cells.

1:40, 1:100 and 10:1 were the combinations of ratios of PAC: WA, PAC: Cis-Pt, and Cis-Pt: WA respectively for examining synergism and further found highly synergistic, showing greater sensitivity of H1299 and A549 cells with co-treatment (PAC and WA). Colony formation, migration, the inversion was inhibited with co-treatment of PAC+WA synergistically and cause apoptosis in H1299 and A549 cells. It was demonstrated that WA targeted both drug-resistant and drug-sensitive NSCLC cells along with PAC's synergistic effects. Hence, the anticancer role of WA alone or with PAC opposing human NSCLC cell lines was investigated, and PAC+WA combination on NSCLC provided a therapeutic strategy [165].

A study found the antitumor effect of WA with 5-fluorouracil (5-FU) by modulating endoplasmic reticulum (ER) stress feasible for cell death and inducing a significant effect antiproliferation. Autophagy and apoptosis were induced by ER stress. Co-treatment of WA and 5-FU arrested G_2M phase cell cycle triggered due to phosphorylation of β-catenin/Wnt signaling (essential proteins). The combination treatment decreased the cell viability in colon cancer cells resulting in more robust efficacy and safe toxicity profile [166]. In the recent outbreak of SARS-CoV-2 disease, an in-silico study reported the antiviral role of within one-N combined with caffeic acid phenethyl ester and WA inhibits SARS-CoV-2 protease M^{pro} functional activity [149]. This study can lead to drug discovery for the treatment of the COVID-19 pandemic. These synergistic combinations of WA reduce toxicity associated with synthetic drugs and help design clinical chemotherapeutic strategy for human carcinoma.

7. Conclusions and Future Perspectives

This review has thrown light on WA pharmacokinetics, its structural modifications, and potential pharmacological activities and formulations. The pharmacokinetics studies revealed that WA's oral absorption is rapid and can be used to design drug delivery systems targeting various diseases. The molecule is attaining global attention as it is a promising anticancer compound with many other therapeutic benefits, including AD, cardioprotective, neuroprotective, osteoporotic, and antiviral effects. In the present review, WA regulates multiple antitumor pathways, including oxidative stress, promoting apoptosis, autophagy, inhibiting cell proliferation, reducing angiogenesis progression, and metastasis progression. Identifying new proteins with significant effects on tumor progression can target future drug discovery of chemotherapeutic agents. The molecular roadmap of WA can also help us select other anticancer compounds, and their synergistic combination can boost clinical efficacy.

The combined activities of WA with radiotherapy and other chemotherapeutic drugs and the analogs of WA have shown beneficial therapeutic outcomes, thereby exploring disease-altering therapies. Moreover, an additional novel target can be designed based on the target cascade of WA; this could further have the potential for novel antitumor therapies. A single target drug develops escape pathways and has more chances to develop resistance and disease relapse. WA acts on multi targets, improves therapeutic outcomes, and overcome drug resistance.

Moreover, in-depth research on pharmacokinetics and bioavailability is needed to establish the active dose of this compound. An extensive toxicological evaluation is needed to determine the safety profile of WA. The tissue exposure of WA by pharmacodynamics biomarkers and even in vivo and in vitro studies could be performed at the same time for significant outcomes. The review evidenced that WA is a potential therapeutic approach that should be considered a potential therapeutic medicine. Validated, planned, and comprehensively designed clinical trials are imperatively needed on various cancers studies before conversion into the clinical realm.

Author Contributions: All authors have equal contribution to this paper, read and agreed with its final content. Conceptualization, T.B. and A.S. (Aayush Sehgal); validation, T.B. and L.S.; data curation, T.B., R.B. and O.F.; writing—original draft preparation, T.B. and A.S. (Aayush Sehgal); writing—review and editing, T.B., O.F. and S.B.; visualization, A.S. (Aditi Sharma) and R.B.; supervision, T.B., G.Z. and S.B.; project administration, T.B. and S.B. All authors have read and agreed to the published version of the manuscript.

Funding: This research received no external funding.

Acknowledgments: The authors are thankful to Chitkara University, Punjab, India, for providing the facilities and online access for the literature.

Conflicts of Interest: The authors declare no conflict of interest.

References

1. Maurya, R. Chemistry and pharmacology of *Withania coagulans*: An Ayurvedic remedy. *J. Pharm. Pharmacol.* **2010**, *62*, 153–160. [CrossRef] [PubMed]
2. Reddy, A.S.; Zhang, S. Polypharmacology: Drug discovery for the future. *Expert Rev. Clin. Pharmacol.* **2013**, *6*, 41–47. [CrossRef] [PubMed]
3. John, J. Therapeutic potential of *Withania somnifera*: A report on phytopharmacological properties. *Int. J. Pharm. Sci. Res.* **2014**, *5*, 2131–2148.
4. Ríos, J.L.; Rec9io, M.C. Medicinal plants and antimicrobial activity. *J. Ethnopharmacol.* **2005**, *100*, 80–84. [CrossRef]
5. Lemma, M.T.; Ahmed, A.M.; Elhady, M.T.; Ngo, H.T.; Vu, T.L.H.; Sang, T.K.; Campos-Alberto, E.; Sayed, A.; Mizukami, S.; Na-Bangchang, K. Medicinal plants for in vitro antiplasmodial activities: A systematic review of literature. *Parasitol. Int.* **2017**, *66713*–*66720*.
6. Naghibi, F.; Esmaeili, S.; Abdullah, N.R.; Nateghpour, M.; Taghvai, M.; Kamkar, S.; Mosaddegh, M. In vitro and in vivo antimalarial evaluations of myrtle extract, a plant traditionally used for treatment of parasitic disorders. *Biomed. Res. Int.* **2013**, *2013*, 316185. [CrossRef]
7. Cragg, G.M.; Newman, D.J. Natural products: A continuing source of novel drug leads. *Biochim. Biophys. Acta* **2013**, *1830*, 3670–3695. [CrossRef]
8. Orlikova, B.; Diederich, M. Power from the garden: Plant compounds as inhibitors of the hallmarks of cancer. *Curr. Med. Chem.* **2012**, *19*, 2061–2087. [CrossRef]
9. Mirjalili, M.H.E.; Moyano, M.; Bonfill, R.M.; Palazon, C.J. Steroidal lactones from Withania somnifera, an ancient plant for novel medicine. *Molecules* **2009**, *14*, 2373–2393. [CrossRef]
10. Dutta, R.; Khalil, R.; Green, R.; Mohapatra, S.S.; Mohapatra, S. *Withania Somnifera* (Ashwagandha) and Withaferin A: Potential in Integrative Oncology. *Int. J. Mol. Sci.* **2019**, *20*, 5310. [CrossRef]
11. Huang, M.; He, J.X.; Hu, H.X.; Zhang, K.; Wang, X.N.; Zhao, B.B.; Lou, H.X.; Ren, D.M.; Shen, T. Withanolides from the genus *Physalis*: A review on their phytochemical and pharmacological aspects. *J. Pharm. Pharmacol.* **2020**, *72*, 649–669. [CrossRef]
12. Hassannia, B.; Wiernicki, B.; Ingold, I.; Qu, F.; Van Herck, S.; Tyurina, Y.Y.; Bayir, H.; Abhari, B.A.; Angeli, J.P.F.; Choi, S.M.; et al. Nano-targeted induction of dual ferroptotic mechanisms eradicates high-risk neuroblastoma. *J. Clin. Invest.* **2018**, *128*, 3341–3355. [CrossRef] [PubMed]
13. Berghe, W.V.; Sabbe, L.; Kaileh, M.; Haegeman, G.; Heyninck, K. Molecular insight in the multifunctional activities of Withaferin, A. *Biochem. Pharmacol.* **2012**, *84*, 1282–1291. [CrossRef] [PubMed]
14. Patil, D.; Gautam, M.; Mishra, S.; Karupothula, S.; Gairola, S.; Jadhav, S.; Pawar, S.; Patwardhan, B. Determination of withaferin A and withanolide A in mice plasma using high-performance liquid chromatography-tandem mass spectrometry: Application to pharmacokinetics after oral administration of *Withania somnifera* aqueous extract. *J. Pharmaceut. Biomed.* **2013**, *80*, 203–212. [CrossRef] [PubMed]
15. Devkar, S.T.; Kandhare, A.D.; Sloley, B.D.; Jagtap, S.D.; Lin, J.; Tam, Y.K.; Katyare, S.S.; Bodhankar, S.L.; Hegde, M.V. Evaluation of the bioavailability of major withanolides of *Withania somnifera* using an in vitro absorption model system. *J. Adv. Pharm. Technol. Res.* **2015**, *6*, 159–164. [PubMed]
16. Dai, T.; Jiang, W.; Guo, Z.; Wang, Z.; Huang, M.; Zhong, G.; Liang, C.; Pei, X.; Dai, R. Studies on oral bioavailability and first-pass metabolism of withaferin A in rats using LC-MS/MS and Q-TRAP. *Biomed. Chromatogr.* **2019**, *33*, e4573. [CrossRef]
17. Pires, N.; Gota, V.; Gulia, A.; Hingorani, L.; Agarwal, M.; Puri, A. Safety and pharmacokinetics of Withaferin-A in advanced stage high grade osteosarcoma: A phase I trial. *J. Ayurveda Integr. Med.* **2020**, *11*, 68–72. [CrossRef]
18. Wijeratne, E.M.; Xu, Y.M.; Scherz-Shouval, R.; Marron, M.T.; Rocha, D.D.; Liu, M.X.; Costa-Lotufo, L.V.; Santagata, S.; Lindquist, S.; Whitesell, L.; et al. Structure-activity relationships for withanolides as inducers of the cellular heatshock response. *J. Med. Chem.* **2014**, *57*, 2851–2863. [CrossRef]

19. Sy-Cordero, A.A.; Graf, T.N.; Runyon, S.P.; Wani, M.C.; Kroll, D.J.; Agarwal, R.; Brantley, S.J.; Paine, M.F.; Polyak, S.J.; Oberlies, N.H. Enhanced bioactivity of Silybin B methylation products. *Bioorg. Med. Chem.* **2013**, *21*, 742–747. [CrossRef]
20. Walle, T. Methylation of dietary flavones increases their metabolic stability and chemopreventive effects. *Int. J. Mol. Sci.* **2009**, *10*, 5002–5019. [CrossRef]
21. Deocaris, C.C.; Lu, W.J.; Kaul, S.C.; Wadhwa, R. Druggability of mortalin for cancer and neuro-degenerative disorders. *Curr. Pharm. Des.* **2013**, *19*, 418–429. [CrossRef]
22. Sane, S.; Abdullah, A.; Boudreau, D.A.; Autenried, R.K.; Gupta, B.K.; Wang, X.; Wang, H.; Schlenker, E.H.; Zhang, D.; Telleria, C.; et al. Ubiquitin-like (UBX)-domain-containing protein, UBXN2A, promotes cell death by interfering with the p53-Mortalin interactions in colon cancer cells. *Cell Death Dis.* **2014**, *5*, 1–14. [CrossRef] [PubMed]
23. Huang, C.; Vaishnavi, K.; Kalra, R.S.; Zhang, Z.; Sekar, K.; Kaul, S.C.; Wadhwa, R. 3β-Methoxy Derivation of Withaferin-a attenuates its anticancer Potency. *Bioinfo Mol. Evid. Med. Aromat. Plants* **2015**, *4*, 1–8.
24. Rabhi, C.; Arcile, G.; Goff, G.L.; Noble, C.D.C.; Ouazzan, J. Neuroprotective effect of CR-777, a glutathione derivative of Withaferin A, obtained through the bioconversion of *Withania somnifera* (L.) Dunal extract by the fungus *Beauveria bassiana*. *Molecules* **2019**, *24*, 4599. [CrossRef] [PubMed]
25. Chaudhary, A.; Kalra, R.S.; Malik, V.; Katiyar, S.P.; Sundar, D.; Kaul, S.C.; Wadhwa, R. 2, 3-Dihydro-3β-methoxy Withaferin-A Lacks Anti-Metastasis Potency: Bioinformatics and experimental evidences. *Sci. Rep.* **2019**, *9*, 17344. [CrossRef]
26. Yousuf, S.K.; Majeed, R.; Ahmad, M.; Sangwana, P.L.; Purnimaa, B.; Saxsena, A.K.; Suri, K.A.; Mukherjeea, D.; Tanejaa, S.C. Ring A structural modified derivatives of Withaferin A and the evaluation of their cytotoxic potential. *Steroids* **2011**, *76*, 1213–1222. [CrossRef]
27. Shohat, B.; Gitter, S.; Abraham, A.; Lavie, D. Antitumor activity of withaferin-A (NSC-101088). *Cancer Chemother. Rep.* **1967**, *51*, 271–276.
28. Sanchez-Martin, M.; Ambesi Impiombato, A.; Qin, Y.; Herranz, D.; Bansal, M.; Girardi, T.; Paietta, M.S.; Tallman, E.; Rowe, J.M.; De Keersmaecker, K.; et al. Synergistic antileukemic therapies in NOTCH1-induced T-ALL. *Proc. Natl. Acad. Sci. USA* **2017**, *114*, 2006–2011. [CrossRef]
29. Siegel, R.L.; Miller, K.D.; Jemal, A. Cancer statistics. *CA Cancer J. Clin.* **2020**, *70*, 7–30.
30. O'Regan, R.M.; Jordan, V.C. The evolution of tamoxifen therapy in breast cancer: Selective oestrogen-receptor modulators and down regulators. *Lancet Oncol.* **2002**, *3*, 207–214. [CrossRef]
31. Simpson, E.R.; Dowsett, M. Aromatase and its inhibitors: Significance for breast cancer therapy. *Recent Prog. Horm. Res.* **2002**, *57*, 317–338. [CrossRef]
32. Stan, S.D.; Hahm, E.R.; Warin, R.; Singh, S.V. Withaferin A causes FOXO3a- and Bim-dependent apoptosis and inhibits growth of human breast cancer cells in vivo. *Cancer Res.* **2008**, *68*, 7661–7669. [CrossRef] [PubMed]
33. Lee, J.; Hahm, E.R.; Singh, S.V. Withaferin A inhibits activation of signal transducer and activator of transcription 3 in human breast cancer cells. *Carcinogenesis* **2010**, *31*, 1991–1998. [CrossRef] [PubMed]
34. Hahm, E.R.; Moura, M.B.; Kelley, E.E.; Van Houten, B.; Shiva, S.; Singh, S.V. Withaferin A induced apoptosis in human breast cancer cells is mediated by reactive oxygen species. *PLoS ONE* **2011**, *6*, 68–72. [CrossRef] [PubMed]
35. Stan, S.D.; Zeng, Y.; Singh, S.V. Ayurvedic medicine constituent withaferin a causes G2 and M phase cell cycle arrest in human breast cancer cells. *Nutr. Cancer* **2008**, *60*, 51–60. [CrossRef] [PubMed]
36. Thaiparambil, J.T.; Bender, L.; Ganesh, T.; Kline, E.; Patel, P.; Liu, Y.; Tighiouart, M.; Vertino, P.M.; Harvey, R.D.; Garcia, A.L.; et al. Withaferin-A inhibits breast cancer invasion and metastasis at sub-cytotoxic doses by inducing vimentin disassembly and serine 56 phosphorylation. *Int. J. Cancer* **2011**, *129*, 2744–2755. [CrossRef] [PubMed]
37. Liu, W.; Wang, G.; Palovcak, A.; Li, Y.; Hao, S.; Liu, Z.J.; Landgraf, R.; Yuan, F.; Zhang, Y. Impeding the single-strand annealing pathway of DNA double-strand break repair by withaferin A-mediated FANCA degradation. *DNA Repair.* **2019**, *1*, 10–17. [CrossRef]
38. Muniraj, N.; Siddharth, S.; Nagalingam, A.; Walker, A.; Woo, J.; Győrffy, B.; Gabrielson, E.; Saxena, N.K.; Sharma, D. Withaferin A inhibits lysosomal activity to block autophagic flux and induces apoptosis via energetic impairment in breast cancer cells. *Carcinogenesis* **2019**, *40*, 1110–1120. [CrossRef]

39. Sivasankarapillai, V.S.; Nair, R.; Rahdar, A.; Bungau, S.; Zaha, D.C.; Aleya, L.; Tit, D.M. Overview of the anticancer activity of withaferin A, an active constituent of the Indian ginseng *Withania somnifera*. *Environ. Sci. Pollut. Res.* **2020**, *27*, 26025–26035. [CrossRef]
40. Fong, Y.; Jin, S.; Rane, M.; Singh, R.K.; Gupta, R.; Kakar, S.S. Withaferin A Synergizes the Therapeutic Effect of Doxorubicin through ROS-Mediated Autophagy in Ovarian Cancer. *PLoS ONE* **2012**, *7*, e42265. [CrossRef]
41. Kakar, S.S.; Jala, V.R.; Fong, M.Y. Synergistic cytotoxic action of cisplatin and Withaferin-A on ovarian cancer cell lines. *Biochem. Biophys. Res. Commun.* **2012**, *423*, 819–825. [CrossRef]
42. Devi, P.U.; Kamath, R.; Rao, B.S. Radiosensitization of a mouse melanoma by withaferin A: In vivo studies. *Indian J. Exp. Biol.* **2000**, *38*, 432–437. [PubMed]
43. Zhang, X.; Samadi, A.K.; Roby, K.F.; Timmermann, B.; Cohen, M.S. Inhibition of cell growth and induction of apoptosis in ovarian carcinoma cell lines CaOV3 and SKOV3 by natural withanolide Withaferin-A. *Gynecol. Oncol.* **2012**, *124*, 606–612. [CrossRef] [PubMed]
44. Straughn, A.R.; Kakar, S.S. Withaferin A ameliorates ovarian cancer-induced cachexia and proinflammatory signaling. *J. Ovarian Res.* **2019**, *12*, 1–14. [CrossRef]
45. Kelm, N.Q.; Straughn, A.R.; Kakar, S.S. Withaferin A attenuates ovarian cancer-induced cardiac cachexia. *PLoS ONE* **2020**, *15*, e0236680. [CrossRef] [PubMed]
46. Kakar, S.S.; Parte, S.; Carter, K.; Joshua, I.G.; Worth, C.; Rameshwar, P.; Ratajczak, M.Z. Withaferin A (WFA) inhibits tumor growth and metastasis by targeting ovarian cancer stem cells. *Oncotarget* **2017**, *26*, 74494–74505. [CrossRef]
47. Cereda, V.; Formica, V.; Massimiani, G.; Tosetto, L.; Roselli, M. Targeting metastatic castration-resistant prostate cancer: Mechanisms of progression and novel early therapeutic approaches. *Expert Opin. Investig. Drugs* **2014**, *223*, 469–487. [CrossRef]
48. Fan, X.; Liu, S.; Su, F.; Pan, Q.; Lin, T. Effective enrichment of prostate cancer stem cells from spheres in a suspension culture system. *Urol. Oncol.* **2012**, *30*, 314–318. [CrossRef]
49. Sheng, X.; Li, Z.; Wang, D.L.; Li, W.B.; Luo, Z.; Chen, K.H.; Cao, J.J.; Yu, C.; Liu, W.J. Isolation and enrichment of PC-3 prostate cancer stem-like cells using MACS and serum-free medium. *Oncol. Lett.* **2013**, *5*, 787–792. [CrossRef]
50. Wang, L.; Huang, X.; Zheng, X.; Wang, X.; Li, S.; Zhang, L.; Yang, Z.; Xia, Z. Enrichment of prostate cancer stem like cells from human prostate cancer cell lines by culture in serum-free medium and chemoradiotherapy. *Int. J. Biol. Sci.* **2013**, *9*, 472–479. [CrossRef]
51. Luo, Y.; Cui, X.; Zhao, J.; Han, Y.; Li, M.; Lin, Y.; Jiang, Y.; Lan, L. Cells susceptible to epithelial-mesenchymal transition are enriched in stem-like side population cells from prostate cancer. *Oncol. Rep.* **2014**, *31*, 874–884. [CrossRef]
52. Kreso, A.; Dick, J.E. Evolution of the Cancer Stem Cell Model. *Cell Stem Cell* **2014**, *14*, 275–291. [CrossRef] [PubMed]
53. Bargagna-Mohan, P.; Deokule, S.P.; Thompson, K.; Wizeman, J.; Srinivasan, C.; Vooturi, S.; Wendschlag, N.; Liu, J.; Evans, R.M.; Markovitz, D.M.; et al. Withaferin A effectively targets soluble vimentin in the glaucoma filtration surgical model of fibrosis. *PLoS ONE* **2013**, *8*, e63881. [CrossRef] [PubMed]
54. Bargagna-Mohan, P.; Hamza, A.; Kim, Y.E.; Khuan Abby Ho, Y.; Mor-Vaknin, N.; Wendschlag, N.; Liu, J.; Evans, R.M.; Markovitz, D.M.; Zhan, C.G.; et al. The tumor inhibitor and antiangiogenic agent withaferin A targets the intermediate filament protein vimentin. *Chem. Biol.* **2007**, *14*, 623–634. [CrossRef]
55. Grin, B.; Mahammad, S.; Wedig, T.; Cleland, M.M.; Tsai, L.; Herrmann, H.; Goldman, R.D. Withaferin alters intermediate filament organization, cell shape and behavior. *PLoS ONE* **2012**, *7*, e39065. [CrossRef] [PubMed]
56. Yu, Y.; Hamza, A.; Zhang, T.; Gu, M.; Zou, P.; Newman, B.; Li, Y.; Leslie Gunatilaka, A.A.; Whitesell, L.; Zhan, C.G.; et al. Withaferin A targets heat shock protein 90 in pancreatic cancer cells. *Biochem. Pharmacol.* **2010**, *79*, 542–551. [CrossRef]
57. Moselhy, J.; Suman, S.; Alghamdi, M.; Chandarasekharan, B.; Das, T.P.; Houda, A.; Murali Ankem, M.; Damodaran, C. Withaferin A inhibits prostate carcinogenesis in a PTEN-deficient Mouse Model of Prostate Cancer. *Neoplasia* **2017**, *19*, 451–459. [CrossRef]
58. Deng, Y.; Chan, S.S.; Chang, S. Telomere dysfunction and tumour suppression: The senescence connection. *Nat. Rev. Cancer* **2008**, *8*, 450–458. [CrossRef]

59. Bartkova, J.; Horejsi, Z.; Koed, K.; Kramer, A.; Tort, F.; Zieger, K.; Guldberg, P.; Sehested, M.; Nesland, J.M.; Lukas, C.; et al. DNA damage response as a candidate anti-cancer barrier in early human tumorigenesis. *Nature.* **2005**, *434*, 864–870. [CrossRef]
60. Bryan, T.M.; Englezou, A.; Gupta, J.; Bacchetti, S.; Reddel, R.R. Telomere elongation in immortal human cells without detectable telomerase activity. *EMBO J.* **1995**, *14*, 4240–4248. [CrossRef]
61. Greider, C.W.; Blackburn, E.H. Identification of a specific telomere terminal transferase activity in Tetrahymena extracts. *Cell* **1985**, *43*, 405–413. [CrossRef]
62. Yu, Y.; Katiyar, S.P.; Sundar, D.; Kaul, Z.; Miyako, E.; Zhang, Z.; Kaul, S.C.; Reddel, R.R.; Wadhwa, R. Withaferin-A kills cancer cells with and without telomerase: Chemical, computational and experimental evidences. *Cell Death Disease* **2017**, *8*, 1–12. [CrossRef] [PubMed]
63. Suman, S.; Das, T.P.; Moseley, J.; Pal, D.; Kolluru, V.; Alatassi, H.; Ankem, M.K.; Damodaran, C. Oral administration of withaferin A inhibits carcinogenesis of prostate in TRAMP model. *Oncotarget* **2016**, *7*, 53751–53761. [CrossRef] [PubMed]
64. Cai, J.; Guan, H.; Fang, L.; Yang, Y.; Zhu, X.; Yuan, J.; Wu, J. MicroRNA-374a activates Wnt/beta-catenin signaling to promote breast cancer metastasis. *J. Clin. Invest.* **2013**, *123*, 566–579.
65. Du, Y.; Wang, Y.; Zhang, F.; Wu, W.; Wang, W.; Li, H.; Xia, S.; Liu, H. Regulation of metastasis of bladder cancer cells through the WNT signaling pathway. *Tumour. Biol.* **2015**, *36*, 8839–8844. [CrossRef]
66. Ormanns, S.; Neumann, J.; Horst, D.; Kirchner, T.; Jung, A. WNT signaling and distant metastasis in colon cancer through transcriptional activity of nuclear beta-Catenin depend on active PI3K signaling. *Oncotarget* **2014**, *5*, 2999–3011. [CrossRef]
67. Weeraratna, A.T.; Jiang, Y.; Hostetter, G.; Rosenblatt, K.; Duray, P.; Bittner, M.; Trent, J.M. Wnt5a signaling directly affects cell motility and invasion of metastatic melanoma. *Cancer Cell* **2002**, *1*, 279–288. [CrossRef]
68. Fu, C.; Liang, X.; Cui, W.; Ober-Blobaum, J.L.; Vazzana, J.; Shrikant, P.A.; Lee, K.P.; Clausen, B.E.; Mellman, I.; Jiang, A. Beta-Catenin in dendritic cells exerts opposite functions in cross-priming and maintenance of CD8+ T cells through regulation of IL-10. *Proc. Natl. Acad. Sci. USA* **2015**, *112*, 2823–2828. [CrossRef]
69. Spranger, S.; Gajewski, T.F. A new paradigm for tumor immune escape: Beta-catenin-driven immune exclusion. *J. Immunother. Cancer* **2015**, *3*, 43. [CrossRef]
70. Amin, H.; Nayak, D.; Ur Rasool, R.; Chakraborty, S.; Kumar, A.; Yousuf, K.; Sharma, P.R.; Ahmed, Z.; Sharma, N.; Magotra, A.; et al. Par-4 dependent modulation of cellular beta-catenin by medicinal plant natural product derivative 3-azido Withaferin A. *Mol. Carcinog.* **2016**, *55*, 864–881. [CrossRef]
71. Srinivasan, S.; Ranga, R.S.; Burikhanov, R.; Han, S.S.; Chendil, D. Par-4-dependent apoptosis by the dietary compound Withaferin A in prostate cancer cells. *Cancer Res.* **2007**, *67*, 246–253. [CrossRef]
72. Kim, S.H.; Hahm, E.R.; Singh, K.B.; Shiva, S.; Ornstein, J.S. Singh SV RNA-seq reveals novel mechanistic targets of withaferin A in prostate cancer cells. *Carcinogenesis* **2020**, *41*, 778–789. [CrossRef] [PubMed]
73. Ferlay, J.; Shin, H.R.; Bray, F.; Forman, D.; Mathers, C.; Parkin, D.M. Estimates of worldwide burden of cancer in 2008: GLOBOCAN 2008. *Int. J. Cancer* **2010**, *127*, 2893–2917. [CrossRef] [PubMed]
74. Gusella, M.; Frigo, A.C.; Bolzonella, C.; Marinelli, R.; Barile, C.; Bononi, A.; Crepaldi, G.; Menon, D.; Stievano, L.; Toso, S.; et al. Predictors of survival and toxicity in patients on adjuvant therapy with 5-fluorouracil for colorectal cancer. *Br. J. Cancer* **2009**, *100*, 1549–1557. [CrossRef] [PubMed]
75. Pallag, A.; Rosca, E.; Tit, D.M.; Mutiu, G.; Bungau, S.G.; Pop, O.L. Monitoring the effects of treatment in colon cancer cells using immunohistochemical and histoenzymatic techniques. *Rom. J. Morph. Embriol.* **2015**, *56*, 1103–1109.
76. Das, T.; Roy, K.S.; Chakrabarti, T.; Mukhopadhyay, S.; Roychoudhury, S. Withaferin-A modulates the Spindle assembly checkpoint by degradation of Mad2-Cdc20 complex in colorectal cancer cell lines. *Biochem. Pharmacol.* **2014**, *91*, 31–39. [CrossRef]
77. Koduru, S.; Kumar, R.; Srinivasan, S.; Evers, M.B.; Damodaran, C. Notch-1 inhibition by Withaferin-A: A therapeutic target against colon carcinogenesis. *Mol. Cancer Ther.* **2010**, *9*, 202–210. [CrossRef]
78. Pal, D.; Tyagi, A.; Chandrasekaran, B.; Alattasi, H.; Murali, K.; Sharma, A.K.; Damodaran, C. Suppression of Notch1 and AKT mediated epithelial to mesenchymal transition by Verrucarin J in metastatic colon cancer. *Cell Death Disease* **2018**, *9*, 1–11. [CrossRef]
79. Chandrasekaran, B.; Pal, D.; Kolluru, V.; Tyagi, A.; Baby, B.; Dahiya, N.R.; Youssef, K.; Alatassi, H.; Ankem, M.K.; Sharma, A.K.; et al. The chemopreventive effect of withaferin a on spontaneous and inflammation-associated colon carcinogenesis models. *Carcinogenesis* **2018**, *39*, 1537–1547. [CrossRef]

80. Kyakulaga, A.H.; Aqil, F.; Munagala, R.C.; Gupta, R. Withaferin A inhibits Epithelial to Mesenchymal Transition in Non-Small Cell Lung Cancer Cells. *Sci. Rep.* **2018**, *15737*, 1–13. [CrossRef]
81. Li, X.; Zhu, F.; Jiang, J.; Sun, C.; Wang, X.; Shen, M.; Tian, R.; Shi, C.; Xu, M.; Peng, F.; et al. Synergistic antitumor activity of withaferin A combined with oxaliplatin triggers reactive oxygen species-mediated inactivation of the PI3K/AKT pathway in human pancreatic cancer cells. *Cancer. Lett.* **2014**, *357*, 219–230. [CrossRef]
82. Moloney, J.N.; Cotter, T.G. ROS signalling in the biology of cancer. *Semin. Cell. Dev. Biol.* **2018**, *80*, 50–64. [CrossRef] [PubMed]
83. Huang, Y.; Li, W.; Su, Z. AN Kong T The complexity of the Nrf2 pathway: Beyond the antioxidant response. *J. Nutr. Biochem.* **2015**, *26*, 1401–1413. [CrossRef] [PubMed]
84. Dom, M.; Offner, F.; Vanden Berghe, W.; Van Ostade, X. Proteomic characterization of Withaferin A-targeted protein networks for the treatment of monoclonal myeloma gammopathies. *J. Proteom.* **2018**, *179*, 17–29. [CrossRef] [PubMed]
85. Narayan, M.; Seeley, K.W.; Jinwal, U.K. Identification and quantitative analysis of cellular proteins affected by treatment with withaferin a using a SILAC-based proteomics approach. *J. Ethnopharmacol.* **2015**, *175*, 86–92. [CrossRef] [PubMed]
86. Narayan, M.; Zhang, J.; Braswell, K.; Gibson, C.; Zitnyar, A.; Lee, D.C.; Gupta, S.V.; Jinwal, U.K. Withaferin A Regulates LRRK2 Levels by Interfering with the Hsp90- Cdc37 chaperone complex. *Curr. Aging Sci.* **2015**, *8*, 259–265. [CrossRef]
87. Zhang, L.; Nemzow, L.; Chen, H.; Lubin, A.; Rong, X.; Sun, Z.; Harris, T.K.; Gong, F. The Deubiquitinating Enzyme. USP24 Is a Regulator of the UV Damage Response. *Cell. Rep.* **2015**, *10*, 140–147. [CrossRef]
88. Mizushima, N.; Komatsu, M. Autophagy: Renovation of cells and tissues. *Cell* **2011**, *147*, 728–741. [CrossRef]
89. Glick, D.; Barth, S.; Macleod, K.F. Autophagy: Cellular and molecular mechanisms. *J. Pathol.* **2010**, *221*, 3–12. [CrossRef]
90. Monastyrska, I.; Rieter, E.; Klionsky, D.J.; Reggiori, F. Multiple roles of the cytoskeleton in autophagy. *Biol. Rev. Camb. Philos Soc.* **2009**, *84*, 431–448. [CrossRef]
91. Dokladny, K.; Myers, O.B.; Moseley, P.L. Heat shock response and autophagy cooperation and control. *Autophagy* **2015**, *11*, 200–213. [CrossRef]
92. Santagata, S.; Xu, Y.; Wijeratne, E.M.K.; Kontnik, R.; Rooney, C.; Perley, C.C.; Kwon, H.; Clardy, J.; Kesari, S.; Whitesell, L.; et al. Using the Heat-Shock response to discover anticancer compounds that target protein homeostasis. *ACS Chem. Biol.* **2012**, *7*, 340–349. [CrossRef] [PubMed]
93. Kwon, O.S.; An, S.; Kim, E.; Yu, J.; Hong, K.Y.; Lee, J.S.; Jang, S.K. An mRNA-specific tRNAi carrier eIF2A plays a pivotal role in cell proliferation under stress conditions: Stress-resistant translation of c-Src mRNA is mediated by eIF2A. *Nucleic Acids Res.* **2017**, *45*, 296–310. [CrossRef] [PubMed]
94. Ivaska, J.; Vuoriluoto, K.; Huovinen, T.; Izawa, I.; Inagaki, M.; Parker, P.J. PKC epsilon mediated phosphorylation of vimentin controls integrin recycling and motility. *EMBO J.* **2005**, *24*, 3834–3845. [CrossRef] [PubMed]
95. Janosch, P.; Kieser, A.; Eulitz, M.; Lovric, J.; Sauer, G.; Reichert, M.; Gounari, F.; Büscher, D.; Baccarini, M.; Mischak, H.; et al. The Raf-1 kinase associates with vimentin kinases and regulates the structure of vimentin filaments. *FASEB J.* **2000**, *14*, 2008–2021. [CrossRef] [PubMed]
96. Perlson, E.; Michaelevski, I.; Kowalsman, N.; Ben-Yaakov, K.; Shaked, M.; Seger, R.; Eisenstein, M.; Fainzilber, M. Vimentin binding to phosphorylated Erk sterically hinders enzymatic dephosphorylation of the kinase. *J. Mol. Biol.* **2006**, *364*, 938–944. [CrossRef] [PubMed]
97. Kidd, M.E.; Shumaker, D.K.; Ridge, K.M. The Role of Vimentin Intermediate Filaments in the Progression of Lung Cancer. *Am. J. Respir. Cell Mol. Biol.* **2014**, *50*, 1–6. [CrossRef] [PubMed]
98. Zhao, J.; Zhang, L.; Dong, X.; Liu, L.; Huo, L.; Chen, H. High Expression of Vimentin is Associated with Progression and a Poor Outcome in Glioblastoma. *Appl. Immunohistochem. Mol. Morphol.* **2018**, *26*, 337–344. [CrossRef] [PubMed]
99. Falsey, R.R.; Marron, M.T.; Gunaherath, G.K.B.; Shirahatti, N.; Mahadevan, D.; Gunatilaka, A.A.L.; Whitesell, L. Actin microfilament aggregation induced by withaferin A is mediated by annexin II. *Nat. Chem. Biol.* **2006**, *2*, 33–38. [CrossRef] [PubMed]
100. Ozorowski, G.; Ryan, C.M.; Whitelegge, J.P.; Luecke, H. Withaferin A binds covalently to the N-terminal domain of annexin A2. *Biol. Chem.* **2012**, *393*, 1151–1163. [CrossRef]

101. Baud, V.; Karin, M. Is NF-[kappa] B a good target for cancer therapy? Hopes and pitfalls. *Nat. Rev. Drug Discov.* **2009**, *8*, 33–40. [CrossRef]
102. Labbozzetta, M.; Notarbartolo, M.; Poma, P. Can NF-κB be considered a valid drug target in Neoplastic Diseases? Our Point of View. *Int. J. Mol. Sci.* **2020**, *21*, 3070. [CrossRef] [PubMed]
103. Su, H.T.; Weng, C.C.; Hsiao, P.J.; Chen, L.H.; Kuo, T.L.; Chen, Y.W.; Kuo, K.K.; Cheng, K.H. Stem cell marker nestin is critical for TGF-β1-mediated tumor progression in pancreatic cancer. *Mol. Cancer Res.* **2013**, *11*, 768–779. [CrossRef] [PubMed]
104. Kim, S.H.; Singh, S.V. Mammary cancer chemoprevention by withaferin-A is accompanied by in vivo suppression of self-renewal of cancer stem cells. *Cancer Prev. Res.* **2014**, *7*, 738–747. [CrossRef] [PubMed]
105. Chang, H.W.; Li, R.N.; Wang, H.R.; Liu, J.R.; Tang, J.Y.; Huang, H.W.; Chan, Y.H.; Yen, C.Y. Withaferin A induces oxidative stress-mediated apoptosis and DNA damage in oral cancer cells. *Front. Physiol.* **2017**, *8*, 634. [CrossRef] [PubMed]
106. Xia, S.; Miao, Y.; Liu, S. Withaferin A induces apoptosis by ROS-dependent mitochondrial dysfunction in human colorectal cancer cells. *Biochem. Biophys. Res. Commun.* **2018**, *503*, 2363–2369. [CrossRef]
107. Kim, G.; Kim, T.H.; Hwang, E.H.; Chang, K.T.; Hong, J.J.; Park, J.H. Withaferin A inhibits the proliferation of gastric cancer cells by inducing G2/M cell cycle arrest and apoptosis. *Oncol. Lett.* **2017**, *14*, 416–422. [CrossRef]
108. Yu, T.J.; Tang, J.Y.; Yang, F.O.; Wang, Y.Y.; Yuan, S.S.F.; Tseng, K.; Lin, L.C.; Chang, H.W. Low Concentration of Withaferin a Inhibits Oxidative Stress-Mediated Migration and Invasion in Oral Cancer Cells. *Biomolecules* **2020**, *10*, 777. [CrossRef]
109. Dabelsteen, E. Cell surface carbohydrates as prognostic markers in human carcinomas. *J. Pathol.* **1996**, *179*, 358–369. [CrossRef]
110. Aranganathan, S.; Senthil, K.; Nalini, N. A case control study of glycoprotein status in ovarian carcinoma. *Clin. Biochem.* **2005**, *38*, 535–539. [CrossRef]
111. Senthil, N.; Manoharan, S.; Balakrishnan, S.; Ramachandran, C.R.; Muralinaidu, R.; Rajalingam, K. Modifying effects of *Piper longum* on cell surface abnormalities in 7,12-dimethylbenz[a]anthracene induced hamster buccal pouch carcinogenesis. *Int. J. Pharmacol.* **2007**, *3*, 290–294.
112. Suresh, K.; Manoharan, S.; Panjamurthy, K.; Senthil, N. Modifying effects of *Annona squamosa* on glycoconjugates levels in 7,12-dimethylbenz(a)anthracene induced hamster buccal pouch carcinogenesis. *J. Med. Sci.* **2007**, *7*, 100–105.
113. Thirunavukarasu, C.; Sakthisekaran, D. Influence of sodium selenite on glycoprotein contents in normal and N-nitrosodiethylamine initiated and phenobarbital promoted rat liver tumors. *Pharmacol Res.* **2003**, *48*, 167–171. [CrossRef]
114. Selvendiran, K.; Sakthisekaran, D. Chemopreventive effect of piperine on modulating lipid peroxidation and membrane bound enzymes in benzo(a)pyrene induced lung carcinogenesis. *Biomed. Pharmacother.* **2004**, *58*, 264–267. [CrossRef] [PubMed]
115. Manoharan, S.; Panjamurthy, K.; Pugalendi, P.; Balakrishnan, S.; Rajalingam, K.; Vellaichamy, L.; Alias, L.M. Protective Role of Withaferin-A on Red Blood Cell Integrity during 7,12-Dimethylbenz[a]anthracene Induced Oral Carcinogenesis. *Afr. J. Tradit Complement. Altern Med.* **2009**, *6*, 94–102. [CrossRef] [PubMed]
116. Heyninck, K.; Sabbe, L.; Chirumamilla, C.S.; Szic, K.S.V.; Veken, P.V.; Lemmens, K.J.A.; Kakkonen, M.L.; Naulaerts, S.; Beeck, K.O.; Laukens, K.; et al. Withaferin A induces heme oxygenase (HO-1) expression in endothelial cells via activation of the Keap1/Nrf2 pathway. *Biochem. Pharmacol.* **2016**, *1*, 48–61. [CrossRef] [PubMed]
117. Rathmann, W.; Giani, G. Global prevalence of diabetes: Estimates for the year 2000 and projections for 2030. *Diabetes Care* **2004**, *27*, 2568–2569. [CrossRef]
118. Vesa, C.M.; Popa, L.; Popa, A.R.; Rus, M.; Zaha, A.A.; Bungau, S.; Tit, D.M.; Aron, R.A.C.; Zaha, D.C. Current Data Regarding the Relationship between Type 2 Diabetes Mellitus and Cardiovascular Risk Factors. *Diagnostics* **2020**, *10*, 314. [CrossRef]
119. Khalilpourfarshbafi, M.; Devi, M.D.; Abdul Sattar, M.Z.; Sucedaram, Y.; Abdullah, N.A. Withaferin A inhibits adipogenesis in 3T3- F442A cell line, improves insulin sensitivity and promotes weight loss in high fat diet-induced obese mice. *PLoS ONE* **2019**, *14*, e0218792. [CrossRef]

120. Riboulet-Chavey, A.; Diraison, F.D.R.; Siew, L.K.; Wong, F.S.; Rutter, G.A. Inhibition of AMP-activated protein kinase protects pancreatic β-cells from cytokine-mediated apoptosis and CD8+ T-Cells induced cytotoxicity. *Diabetes* **2008**, *57*, 415–423. [CrossRef]
121. Vesa, C.M.; Popa, A.R.; Bungau, S.; Daina, L.G.; Buhas, C.; Judea-Pusta, C.T.; Pasca, B.; Dimulescu (Nica), I.; Zaha, D.C. Exploration of insulin sensitivity, insulin resistance, early insulin secretion and β-cell function, and their relationship with glycated hemoglobin level in normal weight patients with newly diagnosed type 2 diabetes mellitus. *Rev. Chim.* **2019**, *70*, 4217–4223.
122. Tekula, S.; Khurana, A.; Anchi, P.; Godugu, C. Withaferin-A attenuates multiple low doses of Streptozotocin (MLD-STZ) induced type 1 diabetes. *Biomed. Pharmacother.* **2018**, *106*, 1428–1440. [CrossRef] [PubMed]
123. Palliyaguru, D.L.; Chartoumpekis, D.V.; Wakabayashi, N.; Skoko, J.J.; Yagishita, Y.; Singh, S.V.; Kensler, T.W. Withaferin A induces Nrf2-dependent protection against liver injury: Role of Keap1-independent mechanisms. *Free Radic. Biol. Med.* **2016**, *101*, 116–128. [CrossRef] [PubMed]
124. Batumalaie, K.; Arif Amin, M.; Murugan, D.D.; Zubaid Abdul Sattar, M.; Abdullah, N.A. Withaferin A protects against palmitic acid-induced endothelial insulin resistance and dysfunction through suppression of oxidative stress and inflammation. *Sci. Rep.* **2016**, *6*, 27236. [CrossRef] [PubMed]
125. Tiwari, S.; Atluri, V.S.R.; Yndart Arias, A.; Jayant, R.D.; Kaushik, A.; Geiger, J.; Nair, M.N. Withaferin A Suppresses Beta Amyloid in APP Expressing Cells: Studies for Tat and Cocaine Associated Neurological Dysfunctions. *Front. Aging Neurosci.* **2018**, *10*, 1–12. [CrossRef]
126. Choudhary, M.I.; Yousuf, S.; Nawaz, S.A.; Ahmed, S.; Rahman, A.U. Cholinesterase inhibiting withanolides from *Withania somnifera*. *Chem. Pharm. Bull. (Tokyo)* **2004**, *52*, 1358–1361. [CrossRef]
127. Banu, M.R.; Ibrahim, M.; Prabhu, K.; Rajasankar, S. Withaferin-A Protects the Nigral Dopamine Neuron and Recovers Motor Activity in Aged Rats. *Cells Tissues Organs* **2019**, *208*, 59–65.
128. Zhou, Z.; Xiang, W.; Jiang, Y.; Tian, N.; Wei, Z.; Wen, X.; Wang, W.; Liao, W.; Xia, X.; Li, Q.; et al. Withaferin A alleviates traumatic brain injury induced secondary brain injury via suppressing apoptosis in endothelia cells and modulating activation in the microglia. *Eur. J. Pharmaco* **2020**, *5*, 1–13. [CrossRef]
129. Mandrekar-Colucci, S.; Landreth, G.E. Microglia and inflammation in Alzheimer's disease. *CNS Neurol. Disord. Drug Targets* **2010**, *9*, 156–167. [CrossRef]
130. Heneka, M.T.; Kummer, M.P.; Stutz, A.; Delekate, A.; Schwartz, S.; Saecker, A.; Griep, A.; Axt, D.; Remus, A.; Tzeng, T.C.; et al. NLRP3 is activated in Alzheimer's disease and contributes to pathology in APP/PS1 mice. *Nature* **2013**, *493*, 674–678. [CrossRef]
131. Rao Atluri, V.S.; Tiwari, S.; Rodriguez, M.; Kaushik, A.; Yndart, A.; Nagesh Kolishetti, N.; Yatham, M.; Nair, M. Inhibition of Amyloid-Beta production, associated neuroinflammation, and Histone Deacetylase 2-mediated epigenetic modifications prevent neuropathology in Alzheimer's disease in vitro Model. *Front. Aging Neurosci.* **2019**, *11*, 1–11. [CrossRef]
132. Khan, Z.H.; Ghosh, A.R. Withaferin-A displays enhanced anxiolytic efficacy without tolerance in rats following sub chronic administration. *Afr. J. Biotechnol.* **2011**, *10*, 12973–12978.
133. Guo, R.; Gan, L.; Lau, W.B.; Yan, Z.; Xie, D.; Gao, E.; Christopher, T.A.; Lopez, B.L.; Ma, X.; Wang, Y. Withaferin A prevents myocardial ischemia/reperfusion injury by upregulating AMP-activated protein kinase dependent B-Cell Lymphoma2 signaling. *Circ. J.* **2019**, *83*, 1726–1736. [CrossRef] [PubMed]
134. Brenner, D.A.; Waterboer, T.; Choi, S.K.; Lindquist, J.N.; Stefanovic, B.; Burchardt, E.; Yamauchi, M.; Gillan, A.; Rinne, R.A. New aspects of hepatic fibrosis. *J. Hepatol.* **2000**, *32*, 32–38. [CrossRef]
135. Rona, G. Catecholamine cardiotoxicity. *J. Mol. Cell. Cardiol.* **1985**, *17*, 291–306. [CrossRef]
136. Diez, J. Mechanisms of cardiac fibrosis in hypertension. *J. Clin. Hypertens. (Greenwich)* **2007**, *9*, 546–550. [CrossRef]
137. Cuspidi, C.; Ciulla, M.; Zanchetti, A. Hypertensive myocardial fibrosis. *Nephrol. Dial. Transplant.* **2006**, *21*, 20–23. [CrossRef]
138. Heling, A.; Zimmermann, R.; Kostin, S.; Maeno, Y.; Hein, S.; Devaux, B.; Bauer, E.; Klövekorn, W.P.; Schlepper, M.; Schaper, W.; et al. Increased expression of cytoskeletal, linkage, and extracellular proteins in failing human myocardium. *Circ. Res.* **2000**, *86*, 846–853. [CrossRef]
139. Lombardi, R.; Betocchi, S.; Losi, M.A.; Tocchetti, C.G.; Aversa, M.; Miranda, M.; Alessandro, G.D.; Cacace, A.; Ciampi, Q.; Chiariello, M. Myocardial collagen turnover in hypertrophic cardiomyopathy. *Circulation* **2003**, *108*, 1455–1460. [CrossRef]

140. Ku, S.K.; Bae, J.S. Antiplatelet, anticoagulant, and profibrinolytic activities of withaferin A. *Vasc. Pharmacol.* **2014**, *60*, 120–126. [CrossRef]
141. Brunetti, O.; Derakhshani, A.; Baradaran, B.; Galvano, A.; Russo, A.; Silvestris, N. COVID-19 infection in Cancer patients: How can oncologists Deal with these patients? *Front. Oncol.* **2020**, *734*, 1–3. [CrossRef]
142. Fratino, L.; Procopio, G.; Di Maio, M.; Cinieri, S.; Leo, S.; Beretta, G. Coronavirus: Older persons with Cancer in Italy in the COVID-19 pandemic. *Front. Oncol.* **2020**, *10*, 1–5. [CrossRef] [PubMed]
143. Dai, M.; Liu, D.; Liu, M.; Zhou, F.; Li, G.; Chen, Z.; Zhang, Z.; You, H.; Wu, M.; Zheng, Q.; et al. Patients with Cancer appear more vulnerable to SARS-COV-2: A multicenter study during the COVID-19 outbreak. *Cancer Discov.* **2020**, *10*, 783–791.
144. Liang, W.; Guan, W.; Chen, R.; Wang, W.; Li, J.; Xu, K.; Li, C.; Ai, Q.; Lu, W.; Liang, H.; et al. Cancer patients in SARS-CoV-2 infection: A nationwide analysis in China. *Lancet Oncol.* **2020**, *21*, 335–337. [CrossRef]
145. Mehta, V.; Goel, S.; Kabarriti, R.; Cole, D.; Goldfinger, M.; Acuna-Villaorduna, A.; Pradhan, K.; Thota, R.; Reissman, S.; Sparano, J.A.; et al. A Case fatality rate of Cancer patients with COVID-19 in a New York hospital system. *Cancer Discov.* **2020**, *10*, 935–941. [CrossRef]
146. Ye, Q.; Wang, B.; Mao, J. The pathogenesis and treatment of the 'cytokine Storm' in COVID-19. *J. Inf. Secur.* **2020**, *80*, 607–613. [CrossRef]
147. Behl, T.; Kaur, I.; Bungau, S.; Kumar, A.; Uddin, M.S.; Kumar, C.; Pal, G.; Shrivastava, K.; Zengin, G.; Arora, S. The dual impact of ACE2 in COVID-19 and ironical actions in geriatrics and pediatrics with possible therapeutic solutions. *Life Sci.* **2020**, *257*, 118075.
148. Maurya, D.K.; Sharma, D. *Evaluation of Traditional Ayurvedic Preparation for Prevention and Management of the Novel Coronavirus (Sars-Cov-2) Using Molecular Docking Approach*; Anushaktinagar: Mumbai, India, 2020.
149. Kumar, V.; Dhanjal, J.K.; Kaul, S.C.; Wadhwa, R.; Sundar, D. Withanone and caffeic acid phenethyl ester are predicted to interact with main protease (Mpro) of SARS-CoV-2 and inhibit its activity. *J. Biomol. Struct. Dyn.* **2020**, 1–13. [CrossRef]
150. Straughn, A.R.; Kakar, S.S. Withaferin A: A potential therapeutic agent against COVID-19 infection. *J. Ovarian Res.* **2020**, *13*, 1–5. [CrossRef]
151. Farrell, G.C.; Larter, C.Z. Nonalcoholic fatty liver disease: From steatosis to cirrhosis. *Hepatology* **2006**, *43*, S99–S112. [CrossRef]
152. Michelotti, G.A.; Machado, M.V.; Diehl, A.M. NAFLD, NASH and liver cancer. *Nat. Rev. Gastroenterol. Hepatol.* **2013**, *10*, 656–665. [CrossRef]
153. Friedman, S.L.; Neuschwander-Tetri, B.A.; Rinella, M.; Sanyal, A.J. Mechanisms of NAFLD development and therapeutic strategies. *Nat. Med.* **2018**, *24*, 908–922. [CrossRef] [PubMed]
154. Patel, D.P.; Yan, T.; Kim, D.; Dias, H.B.; Krausz, K.W.; Kimura, S.; Gonzalez, F.J. Withaferin A improves non-alcoholic steatohepatitis in mice. *J. Pharmacol. Exp. Ther.* **2020**, *2020*, 256792.
155. Tit, D.M.; Bungau, S.; Iovan, C.; Nistor Cseppento, D.C.; Endres, L.; Sava, C.; Sabau, A.M.; Furau, G.; Furau, C. Effects of the hormone replacement therapy and of soy isoflavones on bone resorption in postmenopause. *J. Clin. Med.* **2018**, *7*, 297. [CrossRef]
156. Khedgikar, V.; Kushwaha, P.; Gautam, J.; Verma, A.; Changkija, B.; Kumar, A.; Sharma, S.; Nagar, G.K.; Singh, D.; Trivedi, P.K.; et al. Withaferin A: A proteasomal inhibitor promotes healing after injury and exerts anabolic effect on osteoporotic bone. *Cell Death Dis.* **2013**, *4*, 1–17. [CrossRef] [PubMed]
157. Agarwalla, P.; Mukherjee, S.; Sreedhar, B.; Banerjee, R. Glucocorticoid receptor-mediated delivery of nano gold–withaferin conjugates for reversal of epithelial-to-mesenchymal transition and tumor regression. *Nanomedicine* **2016**, *11*, 2529–2546. [CrossRef]
158. Sultana, F.; Neog, M.K.; Rasool, M.K. Withaferin-A, a steroidal lactone encapsulated mannose decorated liposomes ameliorates rheumatoid arthritis by intriguing the macrophage repolarization in adjuvant-induced arthritic rats. *Colloids Surfaces B Biointerfaces* **2017**, *155*, 349–365. [CrossRef] [PubMed]
159. Jaggarapua, M.M.C.S.; Rachamall, H.K.; Nimmuc, N.V.; Banerjeea, R. NGRKC16-lipopeptide assisted liposomal-withaferin delivery for efficient killing of CD13 receptor-expressing pancreatic cancer and angiogenic endothelial cells. *J. Drug Deliv. Sci. Technol.* **2020**, *58*, 1–12.
160. Shaha, H.S.; Usman, F.; Ashfaq-Khanc, M.; Khalild, R.; Ul-Haqd, Z.; Mushtaqe, A.; Qaiserf, R.; Iqbalg, J. Preparation and characterization of anticancer niosomal withaferin–A formulation for improved delivery to cancer cells: An in vitro and in vivo evaluation. *J. Drug Deliv. Sci. Technol.* **2020**, *59*, 101863. [CrossRef]

161. Gupta, R.C.; Bansal, S.S.; Aqil, F.; Jeyabalan, J.; Cao, P.; Kausar, H.; Russell, G.K.; Munagala, R.; Ravoori, S.; Vadhanam, M.V. Controlled-release systemic delivery—A new concept in cancer chemoprevention. *Carcinogenesis* **2012**, *33*, 1608–1615. [CrossRef]
162. Yu, Y. Withaferin A Targets Hsp90 in Pancreatic Cancer Cells. Ph.D. Thesis, University of Michigan, Ann Arbor, MI, USA, 2011. Available online: https://deepblue.lib.umich.edu/bitstream/handle/2027.42/89629/yorkyu_1.pdf?sequence=1&isAllowed=y (accessed on 20 October 2020).
163. Cohen, S.M.; Mukerji, R.; Timmermann, B.N.; Samadi, A.K.; Cohen, M.S. A novel combination of withaferin A and sorafenib shows synergistic efficacy against both papillary and anaplastic thyroid cancers. *Am. J. Surg.* **2012**, *204*, 895–901. [CrossRef]
164. Kakar, S.S.; Worth, C.A.; Wang, Z.; Carter, K.; Ratajczak, M.; Gunjal, P. DOXIL when combined with Withaferin A (WFA) targets ALDH1 positive cancer stem cells in ovarian cancer. *J. Cancer Stem Cell. Res.* **2016**, *4*, 1–22. [CrossRef] [PubMed]
165. Kyakulaga, A.H.; Aqil, F.; Munagala, R.; Gupta, R.C. Synergistic combinations of paclitaxel and withaferin A against human non-small cell lung cancer cells. *Oncotarget* **2020**, *11*, 1399–1416. [CrossRef] [PubMed]
166. Alnuqaydan, A.M.; Rah, B.; Almutary, A.G.; Chauhan, S.S. Synergistic antitumor effect of 5-fluorouracil and withaferin-A induces endoplasmic reticulum stress-mediated autophagy and apoptosis in colorectal cancer cells. *Am. J. Cancer Res.* **2020**, *10*, 799–815. [PubMed]

Publisher's Note: MDPI stays neutral with regard to jurisdictional claims in published maps and institutional affiliations.

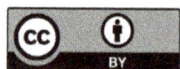

© 2020 by the authors. Licensee MDPI, Basel, Switzerland. This article is an open access article distributed under the terms and conditions of the Creative Commons Attribution (CC BY) license (http://creativecommons.org/licenses/by/4.0/).

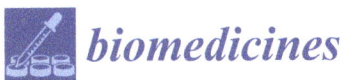

Article

Kahweol Ameliorates Cisplatin-Induced Acute Kidney Injury through Pleiotropic Effects in Mice

Jung-Yeon Kim [1,†], Jungmin Jo [2,†], Jaechan Leem [1,*] and Kwan-Kyu Park [3]

1. Department of Immunology, School of Medicine, Catholic University of Daegu, Daegu 42472, Korea; jy1118@cu.ac.kr
2. Division of Hematology-Oncology, Department of Internal Medicine, Ewha Womans University Mokdong Hospital, Seoul 07985, Korea; 10003kj@ewha.ac.kr
3. Department of Pathology, School of Medicine, Catholic University of Daegu, Daegu 42472, Korea; kkpark@cu.ac.kr
* Correspondence: jcim@cu.ac.kr
† These authors contributed equally to this work.

Received: 14 November 2020; Accepted: 4 December 2020; Published: 6 December 2020

Abstract: Cisplatin is an effective chemotherapeutic agent, but its clinical use is frequently limited by its nephrotoxicity. The pathogenesis of cisplatin-induced acute kidney injury (AKI) remains incompletely understood, but oxidative stress, tubular cell death, and inflammation are considered important contributors to cisplatin-induced renal injury. Kahweol is a natural diterpene extracted from coffee beans and has been shown to possess anti-oxidative and anti-inflammatory properties. However, its role in cisplatin-induced nephrotoxicity remains undetermined. Therefore, we investigated whether kahweol exerts a protective effect against cisplatin-induced renal injury. Additionally, its mechanisms were also examined. Administration of kahweol attenuated renal dysfunction and histopathological damage together with inhibition of oxidative stress in cisplatin-injected mice. Increased expression of nicotinamide adenine dinucleotide phosphate oxidase 4 and decreased expression of manganese superoxide dismutase and catalase after cisplatin treatment were significantly reversed by kahweol. Moreover, kahweol inhibited cisplatin-induced apoptosis and necroptosis in the kidneys. Finally, kahweol reduced inflammatory cytokine production and immune cell accumulation together with suppression of nuclear factor kappa-B pathway and downregulation of vascular adhesion molecules. Together, these results suggest that kahweol ameliorates cisplatin-induced renal injury via its pleiotropic effects and might be a potential preventive option against cisplatin-induced nephrotoxicity.

Keywords: cisplatin; coffee; kahweol; acute kidney injury; oxidative stress; apoptosis; necroptosis; inflammation

1. Introduction

Cisplatin is a platinum-containing chemotherapeutic agent that has been widely used for the treatment of various human cancers [1]. However, its clinical use is frequently limited due to its side effects. Among them, acute kidney injury (AKI) is the most common dose-limiting side effect of cisplatin treatment. Indeed, about a third of patients on cisplatin treatment suffer from the nephrotoxic side effect [1]. However, no effective therapies for cisplatin-induced AKI are currently available. Thus, it is essential to develop therapeutic agents for preventing nephrotoxicity, enabling high-dose chemotherapy using cisplatin.

The pathophysiology of cisplatin-induced renal injury involves multiple mechanisms that are incompletely understood. However, oxidative stress, tubular cell death, and inflammation are considered important contributors to cisplatin-induced renal injury [1–3]. Among them, high levels of oxidative stress are one of the hallmarks of cisplatin-induced renal injury. Numerous studies have reported that cisplatin treatment is associated with increased generation of reactive oxygen species (ROS) and decreased expression of endogenous antioxidant enzymes [4,5]. High levels of oxidative stress can induce tubular cell death [6]. Previous studies have shown that apoptosis of tubular epithelial cells occurs in cisplatin-induced renal injury [1–3]. Apoptosis is a form of programmed cell death and is mediated by caspases, which trigger cell death by catalyzing the specific cleavage of numerous essential cellular proteins. In addition, necrosis, a non-programmed cell death, is also observed in kidneys of rodents treated with cisplatin [1–3]. Recently, a novel type of programmed necrosis, called necroptosis, has emerged as another important type of cell death in cisplatin-induced AKI [7,8]. Indeed, concomitant use of inhibitors of apoptosis and necroptosis presented synergistic renoprotective effects against cisplatin-induced renal injury [9]. Besides direct cellular damage, inflammatory responses are also critical for cisplatin-induced renal injury [1–3]. During cisplatin-induced AKI, excessive amounts of cytokines are produced and secreted from infiltrated pro-inflammatory cells and tubular epithelial cells. Genetic or pharmacological suppression of tumor necrosis factor-α (TNF-α) effectively protected against cisplatin-induced renal injury in mice [10]. Because tubular epithelial cells also secrete a variety of chemokines during cisplatin-induced AKI, pro-inflammatory cells, including neutrophils, macrophages, and CD4$^+$ T cells, are infiltrated into damaged kidneys [11,12]. Excessive accumulation of pro-inflammatory cells can induce additional tissue injury via the generation of cytokines and ROS.

Coffee is the most popularly consumed beverage all over the world after water. A number of epidemiological studies have shown that coffee consumption is inversely proportional to the risk of various human diseases such as cardiovascular disease, cancer, diabetes, and chronic liver disease [13]. Coffee contains a variety of biologically active components. Among them, kahweol is a natural diterpene extracted from coffee beans and has been shown to exhibit anti-oxidative and anti-inflammatory activities [14]. Accumulating evidence suggests that the compound has a beneficial effect on inflammatory conditions of various organs [15–17]. However, whether kahweol has a beneficial effect against cisplatin-induced renal injury has not yet been clarified. The purpose of this study was to evaluate the potential effects of kahweol on cisplatin-induced renal injury and to explore its mechanisms.

2. Materials and Methods

2.1. Animals Procedures

All animal experiments were performed in accordance with the Institutional Animal Care and Use Committee of the Daegu Catholic University Medical Center (Approval number: DCIAFCR-200626-12-Y, approval date: 6 June 2020). Male 7-week-old C57BL/6N mice were acquired from HyoSung Science Inc. (Daegu, Korea) and kept at 20–24 °C and 55% humidity for 1 week. The mice were divided into 3 groups ($n = 8$ per group): vehicle (Veh), cisplatin (CP), and cisplatin plus kahweol (CP+Kah). The CP group was given a single intraperitoneal injection of cisplatin (20 mg/kg in 0.9% saline). An equal volume of the vehicle was injected intraperitoneally into the Veh group. The CP+Kah group was given an intraperitoneal injection of kahweol (20 mg/kg) daily for 4 consecutive days, starting from 1 day prior to cisplatin injection. The doses of kahweol and cisplatin and the treatment protocol were selected based on the results of previous studies [15,18]. Cisplatin was purchased from Sigma-Aldrich (St. Louis, MO, USA) and kahweol was obtained from Abcam (Cambridge, MA, USA). All mice were sacrificed 72 h after cisplatin injection.

2.2. Biochemical Analysis

Plasma creatinine and blood urea nitrogen (BUN) levels were analyzed using a creatinine assay kit (BioAssay Systems, Hayward, CA, USA) and a BUN assay kit (Thermo Fisher Scientific, Waltham, MA, USA), respectively, according to the manufacturer's protocol. A creatinine value more than 0.5 mg/dL [19] or a BUN value more than 33 mg/dL [20] was considered as acute renal failure. Plasma TNF-α and interleukin-6 (IL-6) levels were measured using standard quantitative sandwich ELISA kits (R&D Systems, Minneapolis, MN, USA) according to the manufacturer's protocol. Renal malondialdehyde (MDA) levels were measured using a colorimetric/fluorometric assay kit (Sigma-Aldrich, St. Louis, MO, USA) according to the manufacturer's protocol. Renal levels of reduced glutathione (GSH) and oxidized glutathione (GSSG) were analyzed using a colorimetric detection kit (Enzo Life Sciences, Farmingdale, NY, USA) according to the manufacturer's protocol.

2.3. Histological Analysis, Immunohistochemical Staining, and Immunofluorescent Staining

Isolated kidney tissues were immediately fixed in 10% formalin and then dehydrated in graded series of ethanol. After dehydration, the tissues were cleared in xylene and embedded in paraffin. Thin sections (4 µm) were mounted on glass slides and stained with hematoxylin and eosin (H&E) or periodic acid-Schiff (PAS). The severity of tubular injury was scored semiquantitatively by estimating the percentage of damaged area: 0, 0%; 1, ≤10%; 2, 11–25%; 3, 26–45%; 4, 46–75%; and 5, 76–100% [21,22]. Tubular injury was assessed in 5 arbitrarily chosen fields at ×400 magnification per kidney sample. For immunohistochemical staining, the sections were incubated with a primary antibody overnight and then probed with a secondary antibody. The primary antibodies used for immunohistochemical staining were as follows: anti-neutrophil gelatinase-associated lipocalin (NGAL; Santa Cruz Biotechnology, Santa Cruz, CA, USA), anti-kidney injury molecule-1 (KIM-1; Abcam, Cambridge, MA, USA), anti-galectin-3 (Abcam, Cambridge, MA, USA), anti-CD4 (Abcam, Cambridge, MA, USA), or anti-4-hydroxynonenal (4-HNE; Abcam, Cambridge, MA, USA) antibodies. Images were visualized and captured using a confocal microscope (Nikon, Tokyo, Japan). The percentage of stained areas was determined in 5 arbitrarily chosen fields at ×400 magnification per kidney sample using the i-Solution DT software (IMTechnology, Vancouver, BC, Canada). The number of cells stained with anti-galectin-3 or anti-CD4 antibody was counted in 5 arbitrarily chosen fields at ×400 magnification per kidney sample.

Lotus tetragonolobus lectin (LTL) is a well-known marker for detecting the proximal tubule brush border [22]. The kidneys sections were stained with fluorescein isothiocyanate (FITC)-labeled LTL (Vector Laboratories, Burlingame, CA, USA). Additionally, to identify neutrophils, the sections were probed with anti-Ly6B.2 antibody (Abcm, Cambridge, MA, USA) and then incubated with a secondary antibody. The percentage of stained areas or the number of cells stained with anti-Ly6B.2 antibody was determined in 5 arbitrarily selected fields at ×400 magnification per kidney sample. To stain nuclei, 4′,6-diamidino-2-phenylindole (DAPI) was used.

2.4. Western Blot Analysis

Total proteins were extracted from kidney tissues with a lysis buffer and then loaded onto precast gradient polyacrylamide gels (Thermo Fisher Scientific, Waltham, MA, USA). Separated proteins were transferred from gels to nitrocellulose membranes. The membranes were probed with primary antibodies against nicotinamide adenine dinucleotide phosphate oxidase 4 (NOX4), catalase, manganese superoxide dismutase (MnSOD), cleaved caspase-3, cleaved poly(ADP-ribose) polymerase-1 (cleaved PARP-1), receptor-interacting serine/threonine protein kinase 1 (RIPK1), RIPK3, mixed lineage kinase domain-like protein (MLKL), p-MLKL, nuclear factor-κB (NF-κB) p65, p-NF-κB p65, intercellular adhesion molecule-1 (ICAM-1), and glyceraldehyde-3-phosphate dehydrogenase (GAPDH), followed by incubation with horseradish peroxidase-conjugated secondary antibodies. Primary antibodies against cleaved caspase-3, cleaved PARP-1, RIPK1, RIPK3, MLKL, p65, p-p65, and GAPDH were purchased from Cell Signaling (Danvers, MA, USA). Primary antibodies against catalase, MnSOD, and p-MLKL were acquired from Abcam. Anti-NOX4 antibody was obtained from Novus Biologicals (Littleton, CO, USA), and anti-ICAM-1 antibody was purchased from Santa Cruz Biotechnology. GAPDH was used as an internal control. The protein bands were visualized using enhanced chemiluminescence (ECL) reagents (Thermo Fisher Scientific, Waltham, MA, USA). The signal intensity was analyzed using the iBright™ CL1500 Imaging System (Thermo Fisher Scientific, Waltham, MA, USA).

2.5. Real-Time Reverse Transcription-Polymerase Chain Reaction (RT-PCR)

Total RNA was extracted from kidney tissues using the TRIzol reagent (Thermo Fisher Scientific, Waltham, MA, USA). Reverse transcription was carried out using the RNA to cDNA EcoDry™ Premix Kit (TaKaRa, Tokyo, Japan) according to the manufacturer's protocol. Real-time RT-PCR reactions were performed using the Thermal Cycler Dice Real Time System III (TaKaRa, Tokyo, Japan) and the Power SYBR Green PCR Master Mix (TaKaRa, Tokyo, Japan). Primers used in this study are listed in Table 1. The internal reference gene was GAPDH.

Table 1. List of primers used in this study.

Gene	Primer Sequence (5'→3')	Accession No.
NOX4 [1]	Forward: GAACCCAAGTTCCAAGCTCATT Reverse: GGCACAAAGGTCCAGAAATCC	NM_015760
Catalase	Forward: CAAGTACAACGCTGAGAAGCCTAAG Reverse: CCCTTCGCAGCCATGTG	NM_009804
MnSOD [2]	Forward: AACTCAGGTCGCTCTTCAGC Reverse: CTCCAGCAACTCTCCTTTGG	NM_013671
TNF-α [3]	Forward: GACGTGGAACTGGCAGAAGAG Reverse: CCGCCTGGAGTTCTGGAA	NM_013693
IL-6 [4]	Forward: CCAGAGATACAAAGAAATGATGG Reverse: ACTCCAGAAGACCAGAGGAAAT	NM_031168
E-selectin	Forward: AGCTACCCATGGAACACGAC Reverse: ACGCAAGTTCTCCAGCTGTT	NM_011345
VCAM-1 [5]	Forward: CCCAGGTGGAGGTCTACTCA Reverse: CAGGATTTTGGGAGCTGGTA	NM_011693
ICAM-1 [6]	Forward: TTCACACTGAATGCCAGCTC Reverse: GTCTGCTGAGACCCCTCTTG	NM_010493
GAPDH [7]	Forward: ACTCCACTCACGGCAAATTC Reverse: TCTCCATGGTGGTGAAGACA	NM_001289726

[1] Nicotinamide adenine dinucleotide phosphate oxidase 4. [2] Manganese superoxide dismutase. [3] Tumor necrosis factor-α. [4] Interleukin-6. [5] Vascular cell adhesion molecule-1. [6] Intercellular adhesion molecule-1. [7] Glyceraldehyde-3-phosphate dehydrogenase.

2.6. TdT-Mediated dUTP Nick End Labeling (TUNEL) Assay

Apoptosis was assessed using a TUNEL assay kit (Roche Diagnostics, Indianapolis, IN, USA) according to the manufacturer's protocol. Nuclei were stained with DAPI. Images were visualized and captured using a confocal microscope (Nikon, Tokyo, Japan). The number of cells stained with TUNEL was counted in 5 randomly chosen fields at ×400 magnification per kidney sample.

2.7. Statistical Analysis

Data are presented as mean ± standard error of the mean (SEM) and analyzed with one-way analysis of variance (ANOVA), which was followed by Bonferroni's *post hoc* tests. A p value less than 0.05 was considered statistically significant.

3. Results

3.1. Kahweol Attenuated Cisplatin-Induced Kidney Injury

Mice were administered 20 mg/kg of cisplatin for inducing AKI. All mice survived until 72 h after cisplatin injection. As shown in Figure 1A,B, cisplatin treatment increased plasma BUN and creatinine levels, indicating the development of acute renal failure in cisplatin-injected mice. However, administration of kahweol largely decreased the elevated levels of both markers of renal function (Figure 1A,B).

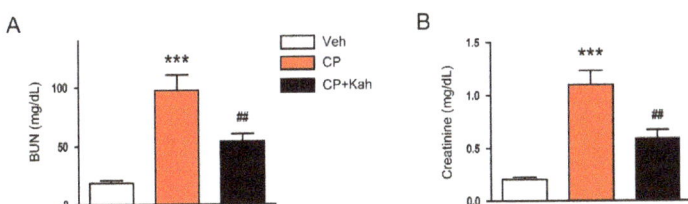

Figure 1. Effect of kahweol on plasma blood urea nitrogen (BUN) and creatinine levels in cisplatin-injected mice. Mice were given an intraperitoneal administration with kahweol (20 mg/kg; Kah) daily for 4 consecutive days, starting from 1 day prior to cisplatin injection. All mice were sacrificed 72 h after cisplatin injection and the blood was collected. (**A**) BUN levels. (**B**) Plasma creatinine levels. $n = 8$ per group. *** $p < 0.001$ vs. the vehicle-treated control group (Veh). ## $p < 0.01$ vs. the cisplatin-injected group (CP).

Next, the effects of kahweol on cisplatin-induced histological changes were analyzed. H&E and PAS staining showed that cisplatin-injected mice exhibited obvious histological injury, as reflected by tubular dilation and cast formation (Figure 2A,B). These histological alterations were significantly attenuated by kahweol (Figure 2A,B).

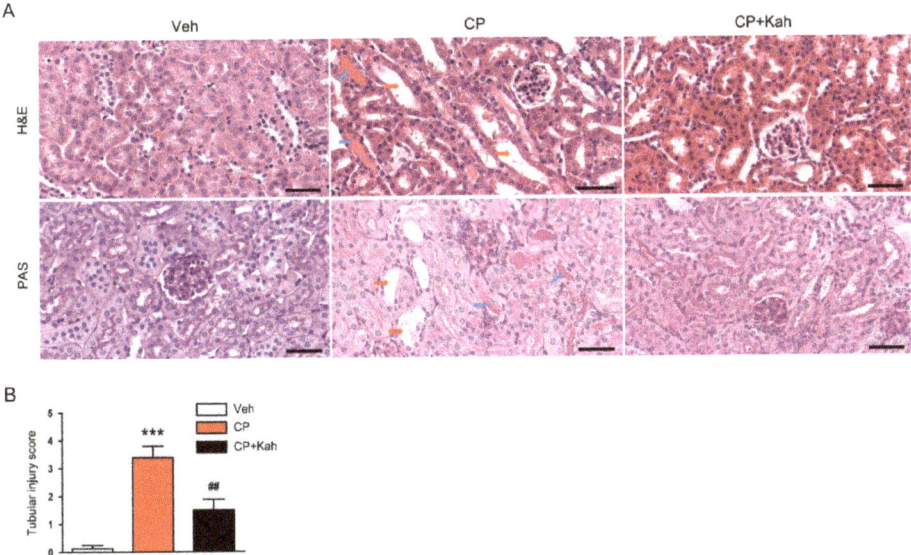

Figure 2. Histological features of the kidneys in all experimental groups. (**A**) Hematoxylin and eosin (H&E) and periodic acid-Schiff (PAS) staining of kidney tissues. Scale bar = 40 μm. Red arrows indicate dilated tubules. Blue arrows indicate tubular cast deposition. (**B**) Tubular injury score. n = 8 per group. *** $p < 0.001$ vs. Veh. ## $p < 0.01$ vs. CP.

Brush border loss in proximal tubules after cisplatin treatment was also demonstrated by LTL staining (Figure 3A,B). However, the administration of kahweol significantly alleviated the brush border loss (Figure 3A,B).

Further, expression of KIM-1 and NGAL, tubular injury markers, was examined using immunohistochemical staining. Cisplatin treatment markedly increased renal expression of both markers (Figure 4A–C). These changes with cisplatin treatment were reduced after administration of kahweol (Figure 4A–C). Together, these results suggest that administration of kahweol ameliorated functional and structural renal injury, especially tubular injury, after cisplatin treatment.

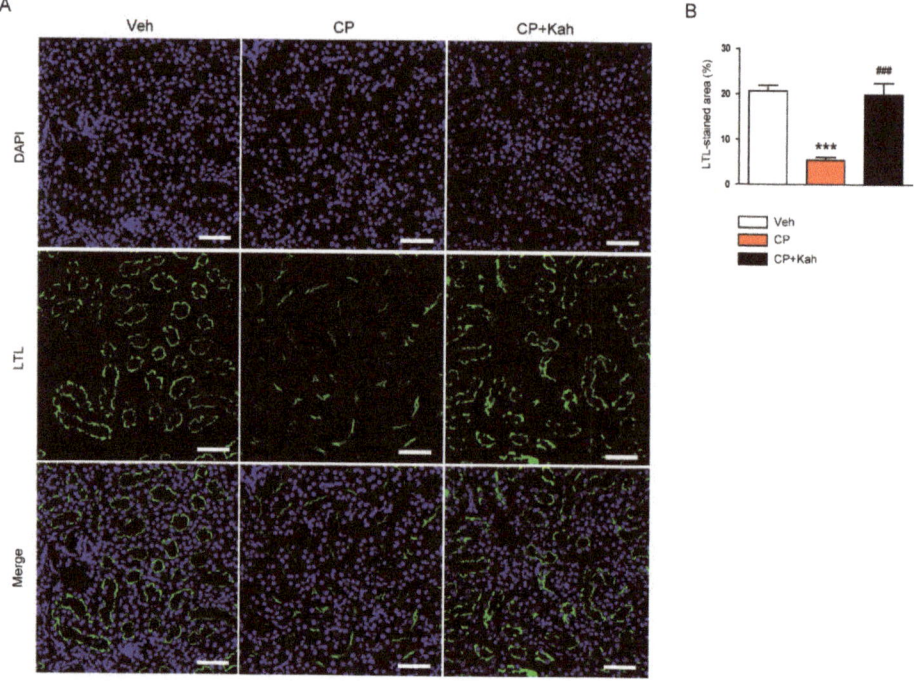

Figure 3. Effect of kahweol on brush border in proximal tubules. (**A**) Lotus tetragonolobus lectin (LTL) staining of kidney tissues. Nuclei were stained with 4′,6-diamidino-2-phenylindole (DAPI). Scale bar = 50 μm. (**B**) Percentage of stained areas for LTL. n = 8 per group. *** $p < 0.001$ vs. Veh. ### $p < 0.001$ vs. CP.

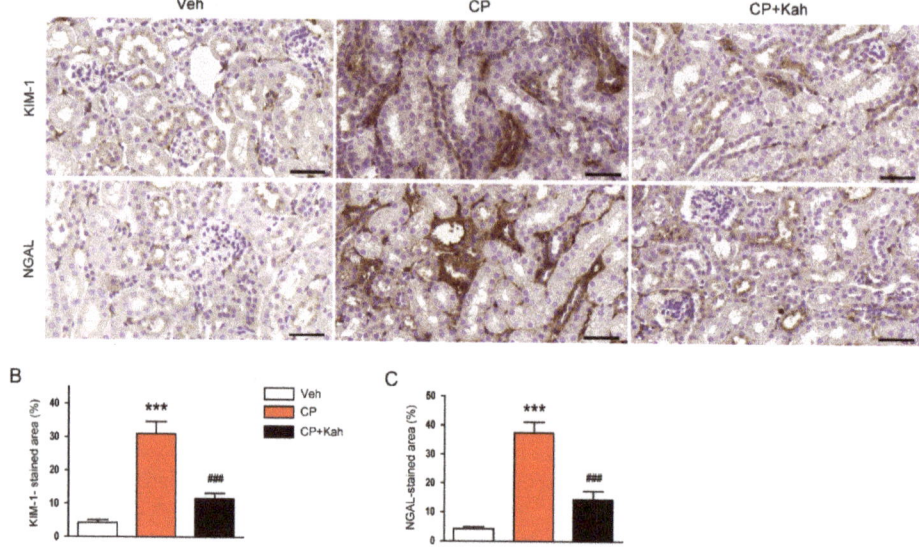

Figure 4. Effect of kahweol on tubular injury markers in cisplatin-injected mice. (**A**) Immunohistochemical staining of kidney tissues for kidney injury molecule-1 (KIM-1) or neutrophil gelatinase-associated lipocalin (NGAL). Scale bar = 50 μm. (**B**) Percentage of stained area for KIM-1. (**C**) Percentage of stained areas for NGAL. n = 8 per group. *** $p < 0.001$ vs. Veh. ### $p < 0.001$ vs. CP.

3.2. Kahweol Inhibited Cisplatin-Induced Oxidative Stress

Oxidative injury is a hallmark of cisplatin-induced renal injury [1–3]. Previous studies have shown that kahweol has anti-oxidant effects [23,24]. To investigate the effects of kahweol on oxidative stress in kidney tissues of cisplatin-injected mice, the kidney sections were stained with anti-4-HNE antibody. 4-HNE is a by-product of lipid peroxidation and is widely used as a marker of oxidative stress [25,26]. As shown in Figure 5A,B, the percentage of the 4-HNE-stained area was markedly increased after cisplatin treatment. Renal levels of MDA (Figure 5C) and GSSG (Figure 5D) were also increased in the cisplatin-injected mice. However, these increases were significantly alleviated by the administration of kahweol (Figure 5A–D). In addition, kahweol attenuated GSH depletion (Figure 5E) and a reduction of GSH/GSSG ratio (Figure 5F) in the kidneys of cisplatin-injected mice.

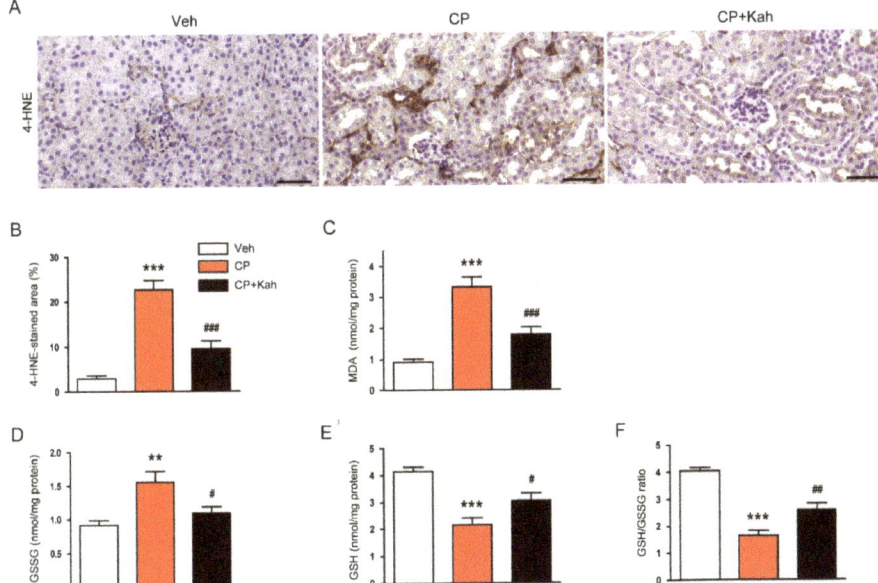

Figure 5. Effect of kahweol on cisplatin-induced renal oxidative stress. (**A**) Immunohistochemical staining of kidney tissues for 4-hydroxynonenal (4-HNE). Scale bar = 100 μm. (**B**) Percentage of stained areas for 4-HNE. (**C**) Malondialdehyde (MDA) levels. (**D**) Oxidized glutathione (GSSG) levels. (**E**) Reduced glutathione (GSH) levels. (**F**) GSH/GSSG ratio. $n = 8$ per group. ** $p < 0.01$ and *** $p < 0.001$ vs. Veh. # $p < 0.05$, ## $p < 0.01$, and ### $p < 0.001$ vs. CP.

It has been shown that NOX4 is a major source of ROS in the kidney and plays a critical role in kidney diseases including cisplatin-induced AKI [27,28]. Thus, we next evaluated the effects of kahweol on NOX4 expression. Elevated mRNA (Figure 6A) and protein (Figure 6B,C) levels of NOX4 after cisplatin injection were largely reduced by kahweol. Further, decreased mRNA (Figure 6D) and protein (Figure 6E,F) expression of antioxidant enzymes, catalase, and MnSOD after cisplatin injection was also largely restored by kahweol.

3.3. Kahweol Suppressed Cisplatin-Induced Tubular Cell Death

Tubular cell apoptosis also plays a crucial role in cisplatin-induced renal injury [1–3]. Therefore, we next examined the effects of kahweol on apoptotic death of tubular epithelial cells in cisplatin-injected mice. A marked increase in the number of cells stained with TUNEL was observed after cisplatin treatment (Figure 7A,B). However, kahweol inhibited the cisplatin-induced tubular cell apoptosis, as demonstrated by a reduction in the number of cells stained with TUNEL (Figure 7A,B). Increased cleavage of caspase-3 and PARP-1 were also largely decreased by kahweol, indicating that kahweol suppressed caspase-3 activation (Figure 7C,D).

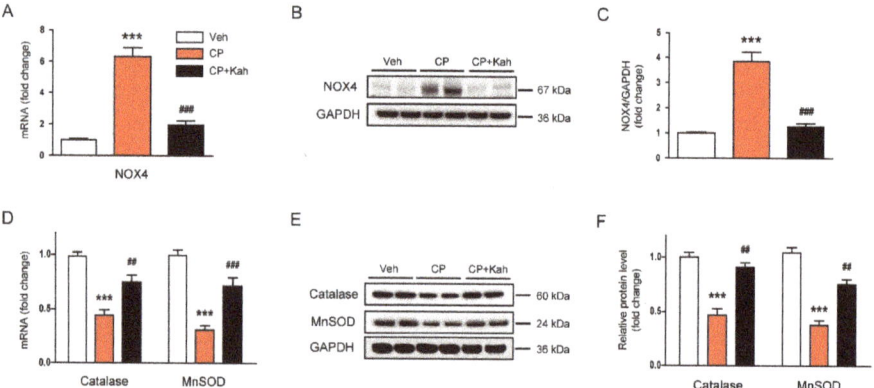

Figure 6. Effect of kahweol on oxidative stress-related enzymes in cisplatin-injected mice. (**A**) The mRNA levels of nicotinamide adenine dinucleotide phosphate oxidase 4 (NOX4). (**B**) Western blotting of NOX4. (**C**) Quantification of Western blot for NOX4. Glyceraldehyde-3-phosphate dehydrogenase (GAPDH) was used as an internal control. (**D**) The mRNA levels of catalase and manganese superoxide dismutase (MnSOD). (**E**) Western blotting of catalase and MnSOD. (**F**) Quantification of Western blots for catalase and MnSOD. GAPDH was used as an internal control. $n = 8$ per group. *** $p < 0.001$ vs. Veh. ## $p < 0.001$ and ### $p < 0.001$ vs. CP.

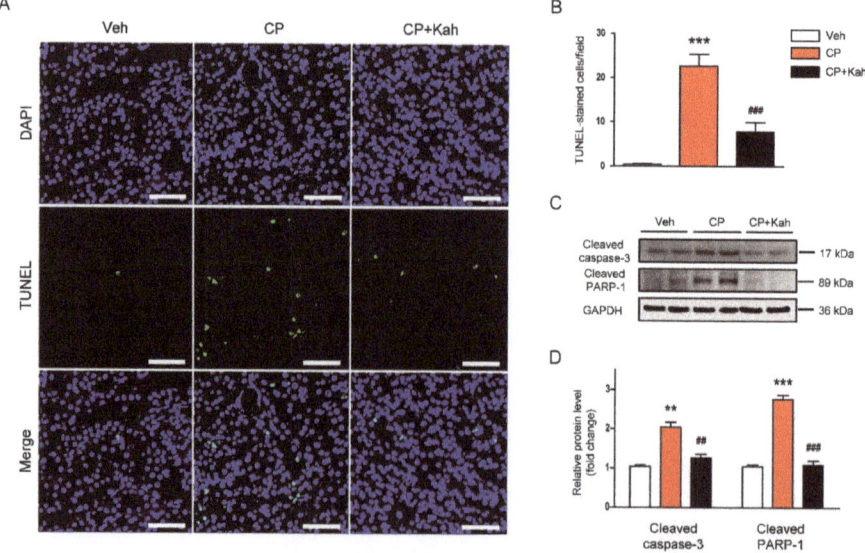

Figure 7. Effect of kahweol on apoptotic cell death in cisplatin-injected mice. (**A**) TdT-mediated dUTP nick end labeling (TUNEL) assay on kidney tissues. Scale bar = 50 μm. To stain nuclei, DAPI was used. (**B**) Number of positively stained cells. (**C**) Western blotting of the proteolytic cleavage of caspase-3 and poly(ADP-ribose) polymerase-1 (PARP-1) proteins. (**D**) Quantification of Western blots for the proteolytic cleavage of caspase-3 and PARP-1. GAPDH was used as an internal control. $n = 8$ per group. ** $p < 0.01$ and *** $p < 0.001$ vs. Veh. ## $p < 0.01$ and ### $p < 0.001$ vs. CP.

Emerging evidence has suggested that necroptosis, a programmed necrosis, also plays a critical role in the pathophysiology of cisplatin-induced AKI [7,8]. To evaluate the effects of kahweol on cisplatin-induced necroptosis, protein levels of RIPK1, RIPK3, and p-MLKL were analyzed by Western blot analysis. Cisplatin treatment largely increased protein expression of RIPK1, RIPK3, and p-MLKL in kidneys (Figure 8A,B). However, this change was significantly inhibited by kahweol (Figure 8A,B).

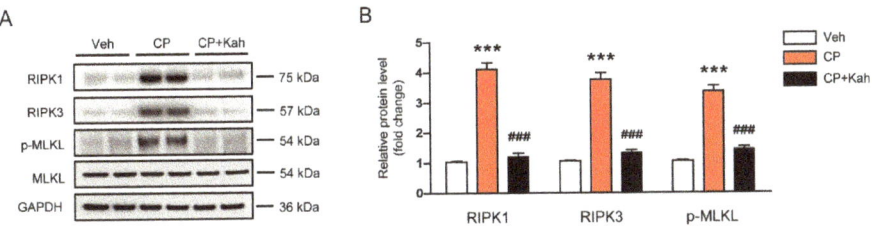

Figure 8. Effect of kahweol on tubular cell necroptosis in cisplatin-injected mice. (**A**) Western blotting of receptor-interacting serine/threonine protein kinase 1 (RIPK1), RIPK3, mixed-lineage kinase domain-like protein (MLKL), and p-MLKL. (**B**) Quantification of Western blots for RIPK1, RIPK3, and p-MLKL. GAPDH was used as an internal control. $n = 8$ per group. *** $p < 0.001$ vs. Veh. ### $p < 0.001$ vs. CP.

3.4. Kahweol Alleviated Cisplatin-Induced Inflammatory Responses

Accumulating evidence suggests that cisplatin treatment triggers an acute inflammatory response by inducing the secretion of cytokines in immune cells [1–3]. Kahweol has also been known to display anti-inflammatory effects [15–17]. Thus, we next examined the effects of kahweol on an inflammatory response induced by cisplatin. Cisplatin treatment increased plasma levels of TNF-α and IL-6 (Figure 9A,B), indicating cisplatin-induced systemic inflammation. Renal mRNA levels of these cytokines were also markedly increased in cisplatin-injected mice (Figure 9C). However, these increases were significantly attenuated by kahweol (Figure 9A–C). Because NF-κB plays an essential role in the production of cytokines, we next examined the effects of kahweol on NF-κB signaling. Khaweol significantly reduced the levels of phosphorylated NF-κB p65 in the kidneys of cisplatin-injected mice (Figure 9D,E). Collectively, these results suggest that kahweol suppressed cisplatin-induced systemic and local inflammation.

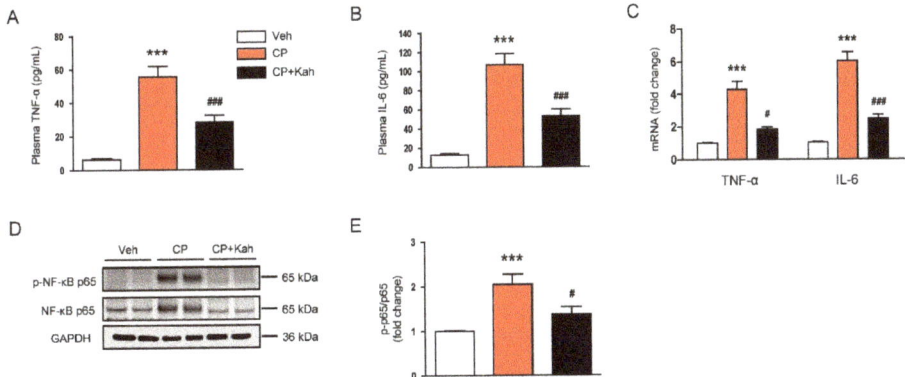

Figure 9. Effect of kahweol on inflammatory cytokine production and nuclear factor-κB (NF-κB) signaling in cisplatin-injected mice. (**A**) Plasma tumor necrosis factor-α (TNF-α) levels. (**B**) Plasma interleukin-6 (IL-6) levels. (**C**) The mRNA levels of TNF-α and IL-6. (**D**) Western blotting of p-NF-κB p65. (**E**) Quantification of Western blot for p-NF-κB p65. GAPDH was used as an internal control. $n = 8$ per group. *** $p < 0.001$ vs. Veh. # $p < 0.05$ and ### $p < 0.001$ vs. CP.

Previous studies have reported that increased accumulation of neutrophils, macrophages, and CD4$^+$ T cells was observed in kidney tissues after cisplatin treatment [11,12]. As expected, cisplatin-injected mice displayed an increase in the numbers of cells stained with anti-Ly6B.2 (Figure 10A,B) or anti-galectin-3 (Figure 10C,D) antibody, compared with control mice. Interestingly, these changes were significantly alleviated by kahweol (Figure 10A–D). It has been well known that vascular adhesion molecules drive the recruitment of immune cells to inflamed tissues [2,3]. Thus, we next examined their renal expression levels in all experimental groups. We found that renal mRNA levels of E-selectin, vascular cell adhesion molecule-1 (VCAM-1), and ICAM-1 were markedly increased after cisplatin injection, which was significantly reduced by kahweol (Figure 10E). Western blot analysis also confirmed that increased ICAM-1 protein level after cisplatin injection was reduced by kahweol (Figure 10F,G).

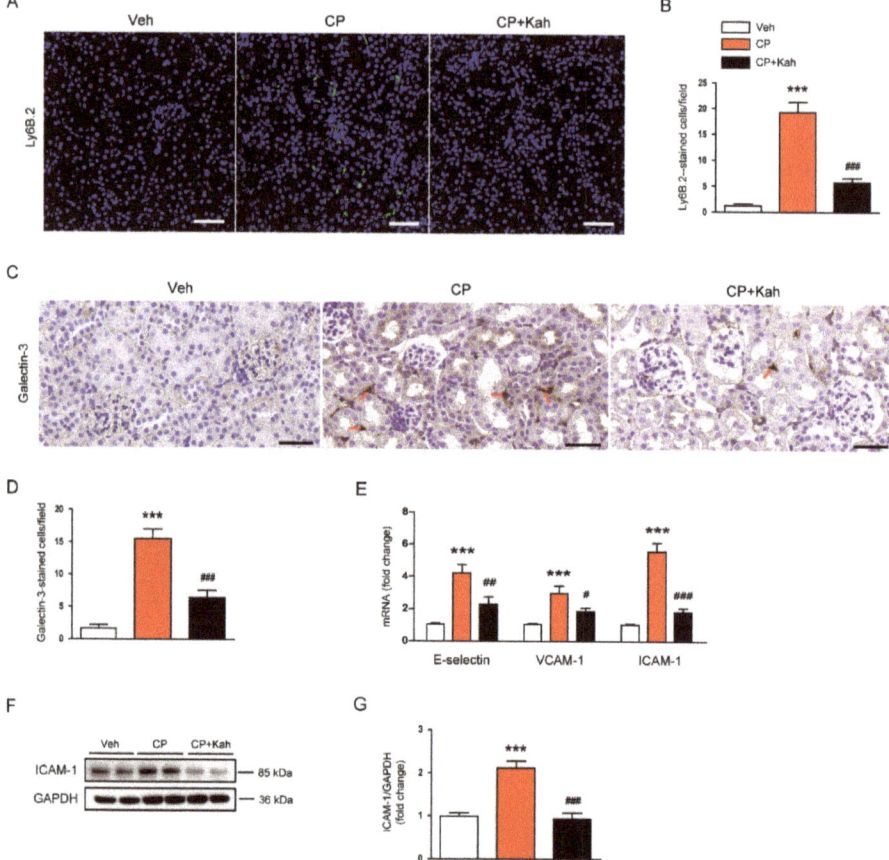

Figure 10. Effect of kahweol on immune cell accumulation in cisplatin-injected mice. (**A**) Immunofluorescent staining of kidney tissues for Ly6B.2. Scale bar = 50 µm. (**B**) Number of Ly6B.2-stained cells. (**C**) Immunohistochemical staining of kidney tissues for galectin-3. Red arrows indicate positively stained cells. Scale bar = 100 µm. (**D**) Number of galectin-3-stained cells. (**E**) The mRNA levels of E-selectin, vascular cell adhesion molecule-1 (VCAM-1), and intercellular adhesion molecule-1 (ICAM-1). (**F**) Western blotting of ICAM-1. (**G**) Quantification of Western blot for ICAM-1. GAPDH was used as an internal control. n = 8 per group. *** $p < 0.001$ compared with Veh. $^\#$ $p < 0.05$, $^{\#\#}$ $p < 0.01$ and $^{\#\#\#}$ $p < 0.001$ compared with CP.

4. Discussion

Cisplatin-induced nephrotoxicity, such as AKI, is a major hurdle in the clinical use of cisplatin. Because there has been no effective treatment for cisplatin-induced nephrotoxicity, the development of novel preventive strategies for preventing cisplatin-induced AKI is important and urgent. Recently, many researchers and pharmaceutical companies are paying much attention to the development of new drugs using substances derived from plants [29]. Kahweol is a natural diterpene extracted from coffee beans and has been shown to exhibit a therapeutic effect against several inflammatory diseases [15–17]. However, whether kahweol has a beneficial effect on cisplatin-induced AKI remains undetermined. In this study, we showed that administration of kahweol prevented the development of renal dysfunction and histopathological abnormalities in cisplatin-injected mice. Especially, tubular injuries were markedly attenuated by kahweol. Our findings suggest that kahweol has a renoprotective effect against cisplatin-induced functional and structural injury.

High levels of oxidative stress are one of the hallmarks of cisplatin-induced renal injury [1–3]. Cisplatin treatment induces excessive ROS generation in kidneys, leading to apoptotic death of tubular epithelial cells [6]. It has been shown that kahweol ameliorated liver injury induced by carbon tetrachloride in mice mainly through suppressing oxidative stress [23]. Kahweol also protected human dopaminergic neurons from oxidative stress-induced apoptosis [24]. In this study, we found that kahweol significantly suppressed cisplatin-induced oxidative stress and resultant tissue injury. TUNEL staining showed that a marked increase in tubular cell death after cisplatin treatment was significantly attenuated by kahweol. Caspase-3 activation was also inhibited by kahweol, indicating that kahweol attenuated cisplatin-induced apoptosis of tubular epithelial cells. Together, our findings suggest that kahweol inhibited oxidative stress and thereby inhibited tubular cell apoptosis in cisplatin-induced renal injury. In good agreement with these results, current evidence suggests that dietary antioxidants such as capsaicin, curcumin, quercetin, and resveratrol exert a protective effect against cisplatin-induced renal injury via inhibition of oxidative stress and apoptosis [30]. Importantly, these dietary antioxidants potentiate the anti-cancer action of cisplatin. Kahweol has been also shown to induce apoptosis in various types of cancer cells [31,32], indicating that the compound exerts different effects on normal cells and cancer cells.

In this study, we also found that kahweol suppressed NOX4 expression in the kidneys of cisplatin-injected mice. NOX4 is a major source of ROS in the kidney and plays a critical role in cisplatin-induced AKI [27,28]. Therefore, it seems that kahweol-induced downregulation of NOX4 mainly contributed to the suppression of oxidative stress in cisplatin-injected mice. Previous studies also have shown that cisplatin treatment reduced the expression and activity of antioxidant enzymes [5,33]. Consistent with these findings, we observed that mRNA and protein levels of MnSOD and catalase were largely decreased in the kidneys after cisplatin treatment. Importantly, this change was significantly inhibited by kahweol. Altogether, these findings suggest that kahweol inhibited cisplatin-induced oxidative stress by modulating pro-oxidant and antioxidant enzymes.

Necroptosis is a programmed form of necrosis and plays an essential role in AKI [34]. RIPK1, RPK3, and MLKL are key players in the process of necroptosis. Upon induction of necrosis, RIPK1 binds to RIPK3 and forms a multi-protein complex, leading to the phosphorylation and oligomerization of MLKL [34]. Oligomerized MLKL translocate to the plasma membrane and induces the membrane rupture and cell lysis. A previous study has demonstrated that cisplatin-induced renal injury was significantly attenuated in RIPK3 or MLKL knockout mice compared to wild-type mice [7]. Recent studies also reported that pharmacological inhibition of RIPK1 effectively attenuated necroptosis of tubular epithelial cells and renal injury in cisplatin-injected mice [35,36]. Consistently, we observed elevated renal expression of RIPK1, RIPK3, and p-MLKL after cisplatin injection. Interestingly, this change was significantly inhibited by kahweol, suggesting that the compound has an anti-necroptosis effect, in addition to the anti-apoptosis effect.

Inflammation also plays a crucial role in cisplatin-induced renal injury [1–3]. During cisplatin treatment, excessive amounts of cytokines are produced and secreted from infiltrated pro-inflammatory cells and tubular epithelial cells. It has been demonstrated that genetic or pharmacological suppression of TNF-α ameliorated cisplatin-induced AKI in mice [10]. In this study, we found that kahweol significantly reduces plasma levels of TNF-α and IL-6 in cisplatin-injected mice. Renal levels of cytokines were also decreased by kahweol. The compound also inhibited the NF-κB signaling pathway that plays an important role in the production of cytokines. Consistent with our findings, previous studies have shown that kahweol suppressed cytokine production and inflammatory responses in animal models of several inflammatory diseases [15–17]. It has been also known that immune cells, including neutrophils, macrophages, and CD4$^+$ T cells, are infiltrated into injured kidneys, inducing additional damage [11,12]. In this study, we also observed that the number of neutrophils, macrophages, and CD4$^+$ T cells were increased in the kidneys of cisplatin-injected mice compared to control mice. Kahweol significantly suppressed the excessive accumulation of these cells. We also found that increased expression of E-selectin, VCAM-1, and ICAM-1 after cisplatin injection was also inhibited by kahweol. These vascular adhesion molecules are primarily expressed in endothelial cells and promotes immune cell infiltration into the tissues [2,3]. In good agreement with our results, previous studies have reported that cisplatin treatment induced upregulation of vascular adhesion molecules in cisplatin-induced AKI [18,37]. Taken together, these results suggest that kahweol inhibited immune cell accumulation presumably through downregulation of vascular adhesion molecules. Further, when the plasma membrane ruptures during the necroptosis process, the contents of the cells leak, causing and exacerbating the inflammatory response [34]. Therefore, the suppressive effects of kahweol on cisplatin-induced necroptosis also may contribute, at least in part, to the inhibition of inflammatory responses.

5. Conclusions

In conclusion, these results suggest that kahweol protects against cisplatin-induced AKI through inhibiting oxidative stress, tubular cell death, and inflammation. Kahweol might be a potential preventive agent against cisplatin-induced AKI, enabling the high-dose use of cisplatin. Our data prompt clinical researchers to investigate the effect of kahweol against cisplatin-induced AKI in humans.

Author Contributions: Conceptualization, J.-Y.K., J.J., and J.L.; formal analysis, J.-Y.K. and J.J.; funding acquisition, J.L.; investigation, J.-Y.K.; methodology, K.-K.P.; supervision, J.L.; visualization, J.-Y.K. and J.J.; writing—original draft, J.-Y.K., J.J., and J.L.; writing—review and editing, J.L. and K.-K.P. All authors have read and agreed to the published version of the manuscript.

Funding: This work was supported by research grants from Daegu Catholic University in 2020 (No. 20205001).

Acknowledgments: We thank Kiryeong Kim for her technical support.

Conflicts of Interest: The authors have no conflicts of interest to declare.

References

1. Holditch, S.J.; Brown, C.N.; Lombardi, A.M.; Nguyen, K.N.; Edelstein, C.L. Recent Advances in Models, Mechanisms, Biomarkers, and Interventions in Cisplatin-Induced Acute Kidney Injury. *Int. J. Mol. Sci.* **2019**, *20*, 3011. [CrossRef] [PubMed]
2. Pabla, N.; Dong, Z. Cisplatin nephrotoxicity: Mechanisms and renoprotective strategies. *Kidney Int.* **2008**, *73*, 994–1007. [CrossRef] [PubMed]
3. Sánchez-González, P.D.; López-Hernández, F.J.; López-Novoa, J.M.; Morales, A.I. An integrative view of the pathophysiological events leading to cisplatin nephrotoxicity. *Crit. Rev. Toxicol.* **2011**, *41*, 803–821. [CrossRef] [PubMed]
4. Trujillo, J.; Molina-Jijón, E.; Medina-Campos, O.N.; Rodríguez-Muñoz, R.; Reyes, J.L.; Barrera, D.; Pedraza-Chaverri, J. Superoxide anion production and expression of gp91(phox) and p47(phox) are increased in glomeruli and proximal tubules of cisplatin-treated rats. *J. Biochem. Mol. Toxicol.* **2015**, *29*, 149–156. [CrossRef]
5. Kim, J.-Y.; Park, J.-H.; Kim, K.; Jo, J.; Leem, J.; Park, K.-K. Pharmacological inhibition of caspase-1 ameliorates cisplatin-induced nephrotoxicity through suppression of apoptosis, oxidative stress, and inflammation in mice. *Mediat. Inflamm.* **2018**, *2018*, 6571676. [CrossRef]

6. Jiang, M.; Wei, Q.; Pabla, N.; Dong, G.; Wang, C.Y.; Wang, T.; Smith, S.B.; Dong, Z. Effects of hydroxyl radical scavenging on cisplatin-induced p53 activation, tubular cell apoptosis and nephrotoxicity. *Biochem. Pharmacol.* **2007**, *73*, 1499–1510. [CrossRef]
7. Xu, Y.; Ma, H.; Shao, J.; Wu, J.; Zhou, L.; Zhang, Z.; Wang, Y.; Huang, Z.; Ren, J.; Liu, S.; et al. A Role for Tubular Necroptosis in Cisplatin-Induced AKI. *J. Am. Soc. Nephrol.* **2015**, *26*, 2647–2658. [CrossRef]
8. Kim, J.W.; Jo, J.; Kim, J.-Y.; Choe, M.; Leem, J.; Park, J.-H. Melatonin Attenuates Cisplatin-Induced Acute Kidney Injury through Dual Suppression of Apoptosis and Necroptosis. *Biology* **2019**, *8*, 64. [CrossRef]
9. Tristão, V.R.; Pessoa, E.A.; Nakamichi, R.; Reis, L.A.; Batista, M.C.; Durão Junior Mde, S.; Monte, J.C. Synergistic effect of apoptosis and necroptosis inhibitors in cisplatin-induced nephrotoxicity. *Apoptosis* **2016**, *21*, 51–59. [CrossRef]
10. Ramesh, G.; Reeves, W.B. TNF-alpha mediates chemokine and cytokine expression and renal injury in cisplatin nephrotoxicity. *J. Clin. Invest.* **2002**, *110*, 835–842. [CrossRef]
11. Miao, N.; Yin, F.; Xie, H.; Wang, Y.; Xu, Y.; Shen, Y.; Xu, D.; Yin, J.; Wang, B.; Zhou, Z.; et al. The cleavage of gasdermin D by caspase-11 promotes tubular epithelial cell pyroptosis and urinary IL-18 excretion in acute kidney injury. *Kidney Int.* **2019**, *96*, 1105–1120. [CrossRef] [PubMed]
12. Miyagi, M.Y.S.; Latancia, M.T.; Testagrossa, L.A.; Andrade-Oliveira, V.; Pereira, W.O.; Hiyane, M.I.; Enjiu, L.M.; Pisciottano, M.; Seelaender, M.C.L.; Camara, N.O.S.; et al. Physical exercise contributes to cisplatin-induced nephrotoxicity protection with decreased CD4+ T cells activation. *Mol. Immunol.* **2018**, *101*, 507–513. [CrossRef] [PubMed]
13. Poole, R.; Kennedy, O.J.; Roderick, P.; Fallowfield, J.A.; Hayes, P.C.; Parkes, J. Coffee consumption and health: Umbrella review of meta-analyses of multiple health outcomes. *BMJ* **2017**, *359*, j5024. [CrossRef] [PubMed]
14. Ren, Y.; Wang, C.; Xu, J.; Wang, S. Cafestol and Kahweol: A Review on Their Bioactivities and Pharmacological Properties. *Int. J. Mol. Sci.* **2019**, *20*, 4238. [CrossRef]
15. Lee, H.-F.; Lin, J.S.; Chang, C.-F. Acute Kahweol Treatment Attenuates Traumatic Brain Injury Neuroinflammation and Functional Deficits. *Nutrients* **2019**, *11*, 2301. [CrossRef]
16. Seo, H.-Y.; Kim, M.-K.; Lee, S.-H.; Hwang, J.S.; Park, K.-G.; Jang, B.K. Kahweol Ameliorates the Liver Inflammation through the Inhibition of NF-κB and STAT3 Activation in Primary Kupffer Cells and Primary Hepatocytes. *Nutrients* **2018**, *10*, 863. [CrossRef]
17. Kim, J.Y.; Kim, D.H.; Jeong, H.G. Inhibitory effect of the coffee diterpene kahweol on carrageenan-induced inflammation in rats. *Biofactors* **2006**, *26*, 17–28. [CrossRef]
18. Tanimura, S.; Tanabe, K.; Miyake, H.; Masuda, K.; Tsushida, K.; Morioka, T.; Sugiyama, H.; Sato, Y.; Wada, J. Renal tubular injury exacerbated by vasohibin-1 deficiency in a murine cisplatin-induced acute kidney injury model. *Am. J. Physiol.-Ren. Physiol.* **2019**, *317*, F264–F274. [CrossRef]
19. Dunn, S.R.; Qi, Z.; Bottinger, E.P.; Breyer, M.D.; Sharma, K. Utility of endogenous creatinine clearance as a measure of renal function in mice. *Kidney Int.* **2004**, *65*, 1959–1967. [CrossRef]
20. Kim, S.H.; Jung, G.; Kim, S.; Koo, J.W. Novel Peptide Vaccine GV1001 Rescues Hearing in Kanamycin/Furosemide-Treated Mice. *Front. Cell. Neurosci.* **2018**, *12*, 3. [CrossRef]
21. Kim, J.-Y.; Leem, J.; Jeon, E.J. Protective Effects of Melatonin Against Aristolochic Acid-Induced Nephropathy in Mice. *Biomolecules* **2020**, *10*, 11. [CrossRef] [PubMed]
22. Kim, J.-Y.; Leem, J.; Hong, H.-L. Protective Effects of SPA0355, a Thiourea Analogue, Against Lipopolysaccharide-Induced Acute Kidney Injury in Mice. *Antioxidants* **2020**, *9*, 585. [CrossRef] [PubMed]
23. Lee, K.J.; Choi, J.H.; Jeong, H.G. Hepatoprotective and antioxidant effects of the coffee diterpenes kahweol and cafestol on carbon tetrachloride-induced liver damage in mice. *Food Chem. Toxicol.* **2007**, *45*, 2118–2125. [CrossRef] [PubMed]
24. Hwang, Y.P.; Jeong, H.G. The coffee diterpene kahweol induces heme oxygenase-1 via the PI3K and p38/Nrf2 pathway to protect human dopaminergic neurons from 6-hydroxydopamine-derived oxidative stress. *FEBS Lett.* **2008**, *582*, 2655–2662. [CrossRef] [PubMed]
25. Kim, J.-Y.; Jo, J.; Kim, K.; An, H.-J.; Gwon, M.-G.; Gu, H.; Kim, H.-J.; Yang, A.Y.; Kim, S.-W.; Jeon, E.J.; et al. Pharmacological Activation of Sirt1 Ameliorates Cisplatin-Induced Acute Kidney Injury by Suppressing Apoptosis, Oxidative Stress, and Inflammation in Mice. *Antioxidants* **2019**, *8*, 322. [CrossRef] [PubMed]
26. Kim, J.-Y.; Lee, S.-J.; Maeng, Y.-I.; Leem, J.; Park, K.-K. Protective Effects of Bee Venom against Endotoxemia-Related Acute Kidney Injury in Mice. *Biology* **2020**, *9*, 154.

27. Yang, Q.; Wu, F.R.; Wang, J.N.; Gao, L.; Jiang, L.; Li, H.D.; Ma, Q.; Liu, X.Q.; Wei, B.; Zhou, L.; et al. Nox4 in renal diseases: An update. *Free Radic. Biol. Med.* **2018**, *124*, 466–472. [CrossRef]
28. Meng, X.M.; Ren, G.L.; Gao, L.; Yang, Q.; Li, H.D.; Wu, W.F.; Huang, C.; Zhang, L.; Lv, X.W.; Li, J. NADPH oxidase 4 promotes cisplatin-induced acute kidney injury via ROS-mediated programmed cell death and inflammation. *Lab. Invest.* **2018**, *98*, 63–78.
29. Lien, E.J.; Lien, L.L.; Wang, R.; Wang, J. Phytochemical analysis of medicinal plants with kidney protective activities. *Chin. J. Integr. Med.* **2012**, *18*, 790–800. [CrossRef]
30. Gómez-Sierra, T.; Eugenio-Pérez, D.; Sánchez-Chinchillas, A.; Pedraza-Chaverri, J. Role of food-derived antioxidants against cisplatin induced-nephrotoxicity. *Food Chem. Toxicol.* **2018**, *120*, 230–242. [CrossRef]
31. Oh, S.H.; Hwang, Y.P.; Choi, J.H.; Jin, S.W.; Lee, G.H.; Han, E.H.; Chung, Y.H.; Chung, Y.C.; Jeong, H.G. Kahweol inhibits proliferation and induces apoptosis by suppressing fatty acid synthase in HER2-overexpressing cancer cells. *Food Chem. Toxicol.* **2018**, *121*, 326–335. [CrossRef] [PubMed]
32. Jeon, Y.J.; Bang, W.; Cho, J.H.; Lee, R.H.; Kim, S.H.; Kim, M.S.; Park, S.M.; Shin, J.C.; Chung, H.J.; Oh, K.B.; et al. Kahweol induces apoptosis by suppressing BTF3 expression through the ERK signaling pathway in non-small cell lung cancer cells. *Int. J. Oncol.* **2016**, *49*, 2294–2302. [CrossRef] [PubMed]
33. Rjeibi, I.; Feriani, A.; Ben Saad, A.; Sdayria, J.; Saidi, I.; Ncib, S.; Souid, S.; Allagui, M.S.; Hfaiedh, N. *Lycium europaeum* Extract: A New Potential Antioxidant Source against Cisplatin-Induced Liver and Kidney Injuries in Mice. *Oxid. Med. Cell. Longev.* **2018**, *2018*, 1630751. [CrossRef]
34. Anders, H.J. Necroptosis in Acute Kidney Injury. *Nephron* **2018**, *139*, 342–348. [CrossRef] [PubMed]
35. Kuang, Q.; Xue, N.; Chen, J.; Shen, Z.; Cui, X.; Fang, Y.; Ding, X. Necrostatin-1 Attenuates Cisplatin-Induced Nephrotoxicity Through Suppression of Apoptosis and Oxidative Stress and Retains Klotho Expression. *Front. Pharmacol.* **2018**, *9*, 384.
36. Wang, J.N.; Liu, M.M.; Wang, F.; Wei, B.; Yang, Q.; Cai, Y.T.; Chen, X.; Liu, X.Q.; Jiang, L.; Li, C.; et al. RIPK1 inhibitor Cpd-71 attenuates renal dysfunction in cisplatin-treated mice via attenuating necroptosis, inflammation and oxidative stress. *Clin. Sci. (Lond.)* **2019**, *133*, 1609–1627. [CrossRef]
37. Salem, N.; Helmi, N.; Assaf, N. Renoprotective effect of platelet-rich plasma on cisplatin-induced nephrotoxicity in rats. *Oxid. Med. Cell. Longev.* **2018**, *2018*, 9658230. [CrossRef]

Publisher's Note: MDPI stays neutral with regard to jurisdictional claims in published maps and institutional affiliations.

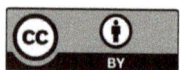

© 2020 by the authors. Licensee MDPI, Basel, Switzerland. This article is an open access article distributed under the terms and conditions of the Creative Commons Attribution (CC BY) license (http://creativecommons.org/licenses/by/4.0/).

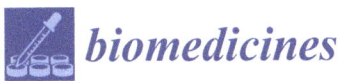

Article

Plumericin Protects against Experimental Inflammatory Bowel Disease by Restoring Intestinal Barrier Function and Reducing Apoptosis

Shara Francesca Rapa [1], Rosanna Di Paola [2], Marika Cordaro [3], Rosalba Siracusa [2], Ramona D'Amico [2], Roberta Fusco [2], Giuseppina Autore [1], Salvatore Cuzzocrea [2], Hermann Stuppner [4] and Stefania Marzocco [1,*]

[1] Department of Pharmacy, University of Salerno, Via Giovanni Paolo II 132, 84084 Fisciano, Italy; srapa@unisa.it (S.F.R.); autore@unisa.it (G.A.)
[2] Department of Chemical, Biological, Pharmaceutical and Environmental Sciences, University of Messina, 98168 Messina, Italy; dipaolar@unime.it (R.D.P.); rsiracusa@unime.it (R.S.); rdamico@unime.it (R.D.); rfusco@unime.it (R.F.); salvator@unime.it (S.C.)
[3] Department of Biomedical, Dental, Morphological and Functional Imaging Sciences, University of Messina, Via Consolare Valeria, 98125 Messina, Italy; cordarom@unime.it
[4] Institute of Pharmacy/Pharmacognosy, Center for Molecular Biosciences Innsbruck (CMBI), University of Innsbruck, Innrain 80/82, 6020 Innsbruck, Austria; Hermann.Stuppner@uibk.ac.at
* Correspondence: smarzocco@unisa.it; Tel.: +89-969159

Abstract: Intestinal epithelial barrier impairment plays a key pathogenic role in inflammatory bowel diseases (IBDs). In particular, together with oxidative stress, intestinal epithelial barrier alteration is considered as upstream event in ulcerative colitis (UC). In order to identify new products of natural origin with a potential activity for UC treatment, this study evaluated the effects of plumericin, a spirolactone iridoid, present as one of the main bioactive components in the bark of *Himatanthus sucuuba* (Woodson). Plumericin was evaluated for its ability to improve barrier function and to reduce apoptotic parameters during inflammation, both in intestinal epithelial cells (IEC-6), and in an animal experimental model of 2, 4, 6-dinitrobenzene sulfonic acid (DNBS)-induced colitis. Our results indicated that plumericin increased the expression of adhesion molecules, enhanced IEC-6 cells actin cytoskeleton rearrangement, and promoted their motility. Moreover, plumericin reduced apoptotic parameters in IEC-6. These results were confirmed in vivo. Plumericin reduced the activity of myeloperoxidase, inhibited the expression of ICAM-1, P-selectin, and the formation of PAR, and reduced apoptosis parameters in mice colitis induced by DNBS. These results support a pharmacological potential of plumericin in the treatment of UC, due to its ability to improve the structural integrity of the intestinal epithelium and its barrier function.

Keywords: plumericin; inflammatory bowel disease; intestinal epithelial cells; experimental colitis; intestinal barrier; apoptosis

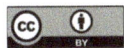

1. Introduction

Inflammatory bowel diseases (IBD), mainly including ulcerative colitis (UC) and Crohn's disease (CD), are complex chronic inflammatory conditions that can be debilitating and sometimes lead to life-threatening complications [1,2]. The IBD pathogenesis is complex and multifactorial (e.g., environmental, infectious, immunological, psychological, and genetic) [3].

UC is characterized by continuous colonic inflammation with loss of normal vascular pattern, erythema, erosions, granularity, bleeding, friability, and ulcerations, with distinct demarcation between inflamed and non-inflamed bowel [4]. The classical histological changes in UC include decreased crypt density, crypt architectural distortion, irregular mucosal surface, and heavy diffuse transmucosal inflammation and impairments in intestinal epithelial barrier function [4].

The intestinal epithelial barrier plays a pivotal role in maintaining intestinal homeostasis. The epithelial layer, in conjunction with the mucosal layer and specialized cells, forms a well-equipped, intricately regulated, and stringent barrier with continuous scrutiny by immune cells to create an immune-silent environment [5]. The intestinal epithelial barrier disruption allows the entry of pro-inflammatory molecules, such as pathogens, toxins, and antigens, from the luminal environment into the mucosal tissues and circulatory system [6]. Thus, it contributes to the development of intestinal inflammation, as in IBD and in particular in UC [7]. In this scenario, intestinal epithelial cells (IECs) play a pivotal role responding to microbial stimuli to reinforce the barrier function and participating in the coordination of an appropriate immune and inflammatory response [8].

The single layer of IECs, forming the intestinal barrier, are sealed by the intracellular junctions that modulate intestinal permeability by regulating the paracellular transport of water and ions. Intracellular junctions also represent the first line of defense against the entry of noxious agents that, once transported via the paracellular route, can initiate local inflammation, and, once in the circulation, they can also promote systemic tissue inflammation and damage [9–11]. Junctions' barrier disruption and increased paracellular permeability, followed by permeation of luminal pro-inflammatory molecules, can induce activation of the mucosal immune system, contributing to sustained inflammation, tissue damage during colitis, and other related complications [12–14]. The sustained inflammation induces IECs apoptosis suggesting that TNF-mediated pathways play key roles in inducing this programmed cell death [15].

Standard UC therapies including anti-inflammatory, immunosuppressive, and biological treatments are widely used, but due to the low remission rate and the severe side effects of these therapies, there is increasing interest in new therapeutic interventions in IBD patients [7,16,17].

Plant-derived natural products significantly contributed to drug discovery in the past and still provide an effective source for lead structure identification [18]. In South America, preparations of the stem bark and latex of the Amazonian tree *Himatanthus sucuuba* (Spruce ex Müll.Arg.) Woodson (Apocynaceae) have been traditionally used as anti-inflammatory, antitumor, analgesic, and antiulcer agents [19]. Plumericin, a major bioactive constituent of *H. sucuuba*, is a spirolactone iridoid and has been shown to exhibit antiparasitic [20], antimicrobial [21], and antifungal [22] activities. Plumericin has been shown to be a potent NF-κB pathway inhibitor [23], to have antiproliferative properties in the vasculature [24], and to reduce TNF-α-induced senescence of endothelial cells [25]. More recently this natural compound has been reported to reduce inflammation and oxidative stress during intestinal inflammation [26]. Thus, in order to further characterize the plumericin potential in IBD, in this study, we evaluated its effect on intestinal barrier and apoptosis in a model of intestinal inflammation both in vitro and in vivo.

2. Experimental Section

2.1. Reagents

Unless otherwise specified, all reagents and compounds were purchased from Sigma Chemicals Company (Sigma, Milan, Italy).

2.2. Plant Material

Plumericin was isolated from the bark of *H. sucuuba*. Detailed description of the phytochemical work including the isolation and identification of plumericin and other compounds from *H. sucuuba* has previously been provided elsewhere [27]. Details about the storage, stability, and purity of the plumericin have previously been described [26].

2.3. In Vitro Studies

2.3.1. Cell Culture

Intestinal epithelial cells, IEC-6 (CRL-1592), was purchased from the American Type Culture Collection (ATCC). IEC-6 cell line, deriving from rat small intestinal crypt, was cultured using Dulbecco's modified Eagle's medium (4 g/L glucose) supplemented with 10% (v/v) fetal bovine serum, 2 mM L-glutamine, 1.5 g/L NaHCO$_3$, and 0.1 U/mL bovine insulin. Cells were grown at 37 °C in a humidified atmosphere of 5% CO$_2$/95% air, and the viability was monitored using phase contrast microscopy and trypan blue staining. Cells were used at the 16–19th passage.

2.3.2. Establishment of An In Vitro IEC-6 Cell Model of Inflammatory Injury

In order to establish a cellular model of inflammatory damage, IEC-6 cells were plated and, after 24 h of adhesion, at right confluence, were treated with plumericin (0.5–2 µM) for 1 h and then co-exposed to plumericin and two pro-inflammatory stimuli, such as lipopolysaccharides from *E. coli* (LPS; 10 µg/mL) plus interferon-γ (IFN; 10 U/mL) for different times, based on the mediator to evaluate [28].

2.3.3. Measurement of Claudin-1, Occludin, E-Cadherin, Bax, Bcl-2, Bcl-xL and Caspase-3 Expression by Cytofluorimetry

IEC-6 cells were plated into 96-well plates (2.0 × 10^3 cells/well) and treated with plumericin (0.5–2 µM), as previously indicated, for 24 h. For this analysis, IEC-6 cells were then collected and washed with phosphate buffered saline (PBS). Fixing solution was added to cells for 20 min and then IEC-6 cells were incubated in fix perm solution for a further 30 min. Anti-Claudin-1 (Thermofisher Scientific, Waltham, MA, USA), anti-Occludin (Thermofisher Scientific, Waltham, MA, USA), anti-E-cadherin (Cell Signaling Technology, Dellaertweg, The Netherlands), anti-Bax (Santa Cruz Biotechnologies, Dallas, TX, USA), anti-Bcl-2 (Santa Cruz Biotechnologies, Dallas, TX, USA), anti-Bcl-xL (Thermofisher Scientific, Waltham, MA, USA), or anti-caspase 3 (Thermofisher Scientific, Waltham, MA, USA) antibodies were then added for 1 h. The secondary FITC-conjugated antibody, in fixing solution, was added to IEC-6 cells and cell fluorescence was then evaluated by a fluorescence-activated cell sorter (FACSscan; Becton Dickinson, Milan, Italy) and analyzed by Cell Quest software (version 4; Becton Dickinson, Milan, Italy), as formerly reported [29].

2.3.4. Immunofluorescence Assay for Cytoskeleton Analysis by Confocal Microscopy

To evaluate plumericin effects on cellular cytoskeleton, IEC-6 cells were seeded on coverslips in 12 well plate (2.0 × 10^5 cells/well) and treated with plumericin (1 µM) alone or in combination with LPS + IFN, for 24 h. Cells were fixed with 4% paraformaldehyde in PBS for 15 min and permeabilized with 0.1% saponin in PBS for 15 min. Slides were then incubated with FITC-conjugated anti-F-actin (Phalloidin-FITC, Sigma, Milan, Italy) at the concentration of 1 mg/mL in PBS for 30 min. The slides were then washed three times with PBS and DAPI was used for counterstaining of nuclei. Coverslips were finally mounted in mounting medium and fluorescent images were taken under the Laser Confocal Microscope (Leica TCS SP5, Wetzlar, Germany), as previously described [30].

2.3.5. Wound Healing Assay

In order to evaluate IEC-6 cellular migration a wound-healing assay was performed, as previously reported [31]. IEC-6 cells (1.0 × 10^5 cells/well, 24-well plates) were allowed to adhere for 24 h. After 100% of confluence, a mechanical scratch was induced at the center of the IEC-6 monolayer by gently scraping cells with a sterile plastic p10 pipette tip. Cells were then washed with PBS and treated with plumericin (0.5–2 µM) alone or in combination with LPS + IFN for 24 h. After the scratch, IEC-6 cells were placed in a humidified and equilibrated (5% v/v CO$_2$) incubation chamber of an Integrated Live Cell Workstation Leica AF-6000 LX at 37 °C for 24 h. A 10× phase contrast objective was used in order to record cell movements, with a frequency of acquisition of 10 min. To determine the migration rate of individual cells, we considered the distances covered from the initial time to the selected time points (bar of distance tool, Leica AF software, 2.3.5 build 5379, Leica, Wetzlar, Germany). For each scratch, at least three different positions were registered and, to measure the migration distances, for each position, at least 10 different cells were randomly selected. GraphPad Prism 5 software (GraphPad, San Diego, CA, USA) was used to perform the statistical analyses.

2.3.6. Analysis of Apoptosis

The anti-apoptotic activity of plumericin was analyzed by evaluating the percentage of hypodiploid DNA, using propidium iodide (PI) staining by flow cytometry [32]. Briefly, IEC-6 cells (3.5×10^5) were grown in 24-well plates and allowed to adhere. Thereafter cells were exposed to plumericin (0.5–2 µM) for 1 h and then co-exposed to plumericin and LPS + IFN for further 24 h. Following treatment, culture medium was removed, cells washed once with PBS, and then resuspended in 500 µL of a solution containing 0.1% (w/v) sodium citrate and 50 µg/mL PI. Culture medium and PBS were centrifuged, and cell pellets were pooled with cell suspension to retain both dead and living cells for analysis. After incubation at 4 °C for 30 min in the dark, cell nuclei were analyzed with a Becton Dickinson FACScan flow cytometer (FACSscan; Becton Dickinson, Milan, Italy) using the CellQuest program (version 4; Becton Dickinson, Milan, Italy).

2.4. In Vivo Studies

2.4.1. Animals

Male CD1 mice (20–25 g, Harlan Nossan, Milan, Italy) were housed in a controlled environment, maintained on a 12-h light/dark cycle, and received a standard rodent chow and water, available ad libitum. The University of Messina Review Board for Animal Care (OPBA) approved the study (650/2017-PR). Animal care was in conformity with current legislation of the EU for the protection of animals used for scientific purposes (Directive 2010/63/EU).

2.4.2. Induction of Experimental Colitis

Colitis was induced by intrarectal administration of 2,4,6-dinitrobenzene sulfonic acid (DNBS, 4 mg per mouse) [33]. In preliminary experiments, this dose of DNBS was found to induce reproducible colitis without mortality. Mice were anesthetized by Enflurane. Subsequently, DNBS (4 mg in 100 µL of 50% ethanol/50% saline, v/v) was injected into the rectum through a catheter inserted 4.5 cm proximally to the anus. Vehicle alone (100 µL of 50% ethanol/50% saline) was administered in control experiments (control). Thereafter, the animals were kept for 15 min in a Trendelenburg position. After colitis induction, the animals were observed for 4 days. On day 4, the animals were weighed and anaesthetized with chloral hydrate, and the abdomen was opened by a midline incision. The colon was removed, freed from surrounding tissues, opened along the antimesenteric border, washed, weighed, and processed for histologic and biochemical studies. Plumericin (3 mg/kg; 0.2% DMSO) was intraperitoneally (i.p.) administered.

2.4.3. Experimental Groups

Animals were casually divided into several groups ($n = 10$ for each group):
- Control + vehicle group: Vehicle solution was given by i.p. administration each day for 4 days;
- Control + plumericin (3 mg/kg) group: Plumericin was administered i.p. each day for 4 days (data not shown);
- DNBS + vehicle group: DNBS was injected to the mice as described, subsequently, vehicle solution was administered i.p. each day for 4 days; the first dose was injected 1 h after the injection of DNBS;
- DNBS + plumericin (3 mg/kg) group: DNBS was injected to the mice as described, subsequently, plumericin (3 mg/kg) was given i.p. each day for 4 days; the first dose was injected 1 h after the administration of DNBS.

2.4.4. Immunohistochemical Localization of ICAM-1, P-Selectin and PAR

At 4 days after DNBS administration, colon tissues were fixed in 10% (w/v) PBS-buffered formaldehyde and 7 µm sections were prepared from paraffin embedded tissues. After deparaffinization, endogenous peroxidase was quenched with 0.3% (v/v) H_2O_2 in 60% (v/v) methanol for 30 min. The sections were permeabilized with 0.1% (w/v) Triton X-100 in PBS for 20 min. Non-specific adsorption was minimized by incubating the section in 2% (v/v) normal goat serum in PBS for 20 min. Endogenous biotin or avidin binding sites were blocked by sequential incubation for 15 min with biotin and avidin (Vector Laboratories, Burlingame, CA, USA), respectively. Colon tissue sections were incubated overnight with anti-ICAM-1 (Santa Cruz Biotechnology, Dallas, TX, USA), anti-P-selectin 1 (Santa Cruz Biotechnology), or anti-PARP (Santa Cruz Biotechnology). Colon sections were rinsed with PBS and incubated with peroxidase-conjugated bovine anti-mouse immunoglobulin G (IgG) secondary antibody or peroxidase-conjugated goat anti-rabbit IgG (Jackson Immuno Research, West Grove, PA, USA). Specific labelling was detected with a biotin-conjugated goat anti-rabbit IgG or biotin-conjugated goat anti-mouse IgG and avidin-biotin peroxidase complex (Vector Laboratories, Burlingame, CA, USA). To verify the binding specificity for all antibodies, control slices were incubated with only primary antibody or secondary antibody. In these controls, no positive staining was detected. Immunohistochemical images were collected using a Zeiss microscope and Axio Vision software. For graphic display of densitometric analyses, the intensity of positive staining (brown staining) was measured by computer-assisted color image analysis (Leica QWin V3, London, UK). The percentage area of immunoreactivity (determined by the number of positive pixels) was expressed as percent of total tissue area (red staining). Replicates for each experimental condition and histochemical staining were obtained from each mouse in all experimental groups. All immunohistochemical analyses were carried out by 2 observers blinded to the treatment [34].

2.4.5. Myeloperoxidase Assay

Neutrophil infiltration in the colon was examined by measuring tissue myeloperoxidase (MPO) activity using a spectrophotometric assay with tetramethylbenzidine as substrate, according to a previously published method [35]. After DNBS injection, colon tissues were collected and weighed. Each piece of tissue was homogenized in a solution containing 0.5% hexa-decyl-trimethyl-ammonium bromide dissolved in 10 mM potassium phosphate buffer pH 7 and centrifuged for 30 min at $20{,}000 \times g$ at 4 °C. An aliquot of the supernatant was then allowed to react with a solution of 1.6 mM tetramethylbenzidine and 0.1 mM hydrogen peroxide (H_2O_2). The rate of change in absorbance was measured spectrophotometrically at 650 nm. MPO activity was described as the quantity of enzyme degrading 1 µmol of peroxide per min at 37 °C and was expressed in U/g wet tissue.

2.4.6. Bax and Bcl-2 Determination by Western Blot Analysis from Colon Tissue

Tissue samples from the terminal colon were suspended in extraction Buffer A containing 0.2 mM PMSF, 0.15 µM pepstatin A, 20 µM leupeptin, 1 mM sodium orthovanadate, homogenized at the highest setting for 2 min, and centrifuged at $1000 \times g$ for 10 min at 4 °C. Supernatants represented the cytosolic fraction. The pellets, containing enriched nuclei, were re-suspended in Buffer B containing 1% Triton X-100, 150 mM NaCl, 10 mM Tris-HCl pH 7.4, 1 mM EGTA, 1 mM EDTA, 0.2 mM PMSF, 20 µM leupeptin, and 0.2 mM sodium orthovanadate. After centrifugation for 30 min at $15{,}000 \times g$ at 4 °C, the supernatants containing the nuclear protein were stored at −80 °C for further analysis. The following primary antibodies were used: anti-Bax (Santa Cruz Biotechnology), anti-Bcl-2 (Santa Cruz Biotechnology) at 4 °C overnight in 1 × PBS, 5% (w/v), non-fat dried milk, and 0.1% Tween-20. After, membranes were incubated with peroxidase-conjugated bovine anti-mouse IgG secondary antibody or peroxidase-conjugated goat anti-rabbit IgG (Jackson ImmunoResearch, West Grove, PA, USA) for 1 h at room temperature. To ascertain that blots were loaded with equal amounts of protein lysates, they were also incubated in the presence of the antibody against β-actin (Santa Cruz Biotechnology). Signals were detected with enhanced chemiluminescence detection system reagent according to manufacturer's instructions (Super Signal West Pico Chemiluminescent Substrate, Pierce, Altrincham, UK). The relative expression of the protein bands was quantified by densitometry with Bio-Rad ChemiDoc XRS + software and standardized to β-actin levels. Images of blot signals (8-bit/600-dpi resolution) were imported to analysis software (Image Quant TL, v2003, Altrincham, UK), as previously reported [36].

2.5. Data Analysis and Statistical Evaluation

Data are reported as mean ± standard error of the mean (SEM) of at least three independent experiments. Each experiment was conducted in triplicate. For the in vivo studies, N represents the number of animals used. In the experiments involving histology or immunohistochemistry, the figures shown are demonstrative of at least three experiments. Statistical analyses were performed using the variance test. Bonferroni's test was used to make multiple comparisons. A p-value of less than 0.05 was considered significant.

3. Results

3.1. Plumericin Increased Adhesion Molecules Expression in LPS + IFN-Stimulated IEC-6

Mucosal inflammation as observed in colitis compromises the epithelial barrier, resulting in the exposure of lamina propria to luminal antigens and microbes that further contribute to the inflammatory response and barrier defects [37]. Adhesion proteins play a key role in maintaining the integrity of the intestinal epithelial barrier. However, several studies have reported differential effects of inflammatory mediators on adhesion proteins during IBD [38]. In order to assess plumericin's ability to modulate the expression of adhesion molecules, such as Claudin-1, Occludin, and E-cadherin, in inflammatory conditions, we analyzed their expression by flow cytometry. Our results indicated that plumericin (0.5–2 μM) significantly increased Claudin-1 ($p < 0.001$ vs. LPS + IFN; Figure 1a), Occludin ($p < 0.001$ vs. LPS + IFN; Figure 1b), and E-cadherin ($p < 0.001$ vs. LPS + IFN; Figure 1c) expression, in LPS + IFN stimulated IEC-6.

3.2. Plumericin Enhanced IEC-6 Cells Actin Cytoskeleton Rearrangement Induced by LPS + IFN

During the restitution of IECs, extensive reorganization of the actin cytoskeleton is necessary. For this reason, confocal microscopy was used to examine the effect of plumericin (1 μM) in normal and in inflammatory conditions on the assembly of actin stress fibres, that play a crucial role in the remodeling, stretching, and migration of epithelial cells. Untreated cells showed an intact actin cytoskeleton and its fibers traversing the cytosol. Addition of LPS + IFN caused a weak reorganization of actin filaments characterized by their redistribution to the cell subcortical compartment and subsequent cell. Moreover, in the presence of LPS + IFN, plumericin produced a reversion of this effect (Figure 2).

3.3. Plumericin Promoted IEC-6 Motility

During colitis, intestinal wound healing is dependent on the precise balance of migration, proliferation, and differentiation of the epithelial cells adjacent to the wounded area. In order to assess the effect of the plumericin on the reconstitution process at the intestinal level, we carried out a wound-healing assay, to evaluate cellular migration, on treated IEC-6 monolayers. Our results indicated that plumericin (0.5–2 μM) alone did not significantly alter IEC-6 migration speed compared to untreated cells ($p < 0.001$ vs. control; Figure 3a,c). However, in inflammatory conditions, plumericin demonstrated significant improvement in the speed of IEC-6 migration, compared to LPS + IFN-treated cells ($p < 0.001$ vs. LPS + IFN; Figure 3b,c).

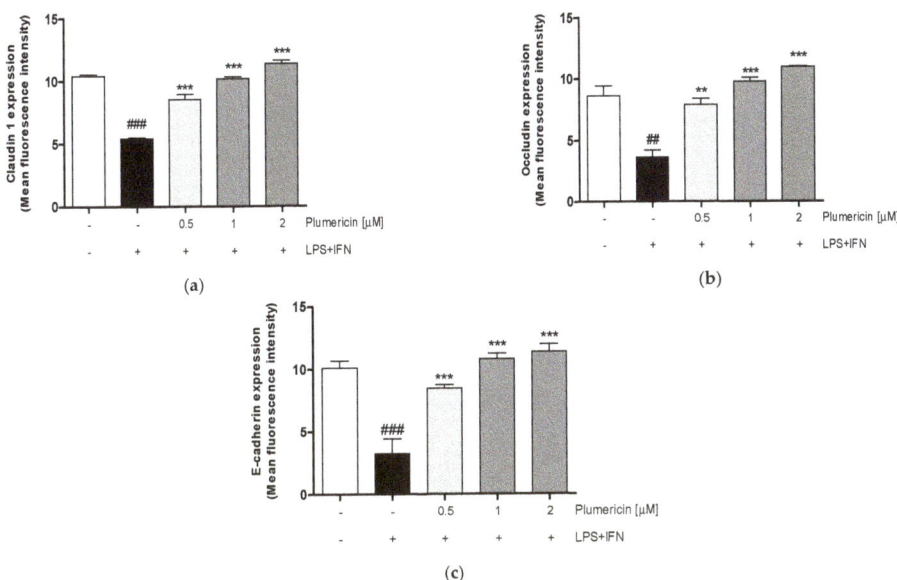

Figure 1. Effect of plumericin on adhesion molecules: Claudin 1 (**a**), Occludin (**b**), and E-cadherin (**c**) expression in LPS + IFN-stimulated IEC-6, evaluated by flow cytometry. Values are expressed as mean ± SEM of mean fluorescence intensity. ### and ## denote, respectively, $p < 0.001$ and $p < 0.01$ vs. untreated cells; *** and ** indicate, respectively, $p < 0.001$ and $p < 0.01$ vs. LPS + IFN.

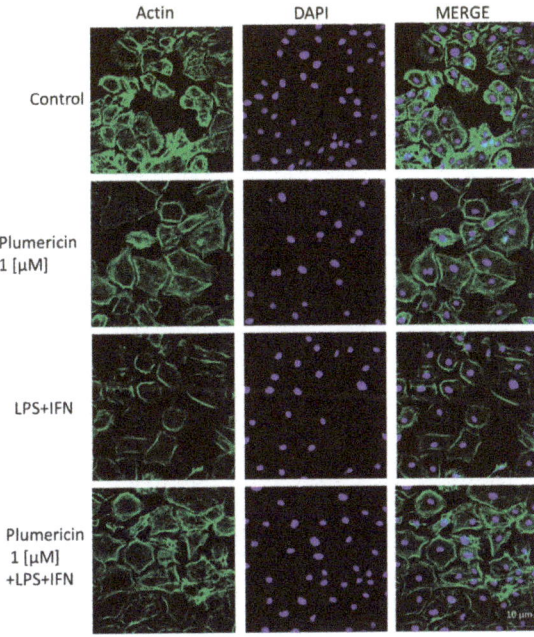

Figure 2. Effect of plumericin (1 μM) on the actin stress fibers assembly in IEC-6 cells. Immunofluorescence analysis was performed using immunofluorescence confocal microscopy. Scale bar = 10 μm. Green fluorescence indicated the localization of actin stress fibers and blue fluorescence indicated the localization of nuclei (DAPI). The MERGE indicates an overlap of the two fluorescences.

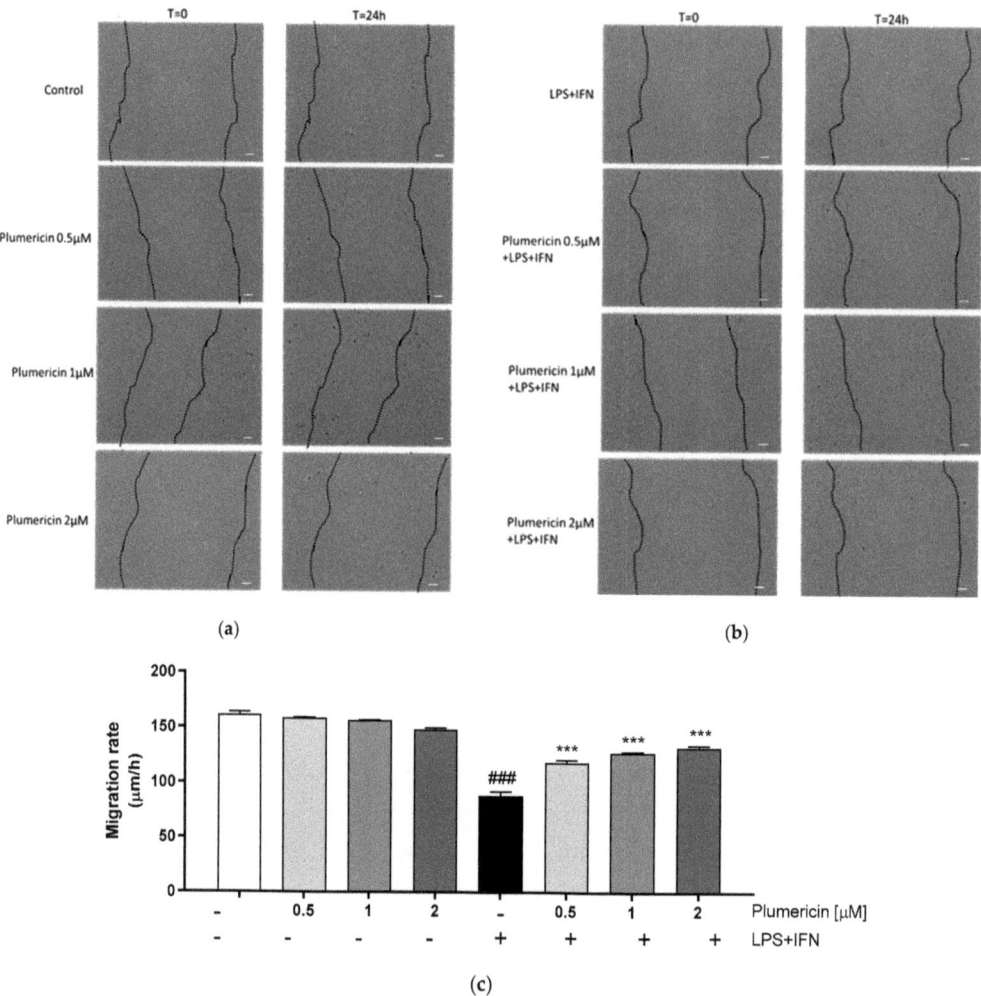

Figure 3. Effect of plumericin alone and in presence of LPS + IFN on cellular migration, evaluated by wound-healing assay. Pictures representing the wound repair, induced by mechanical scratch in IEC-6, from plumericin treatment alone (**a**) and in combination with LPS + IFN (**b**). Bar = 150 µm. (**c**) representing the quantitative analysis expressed as IEC-6 migration rate after 24 h. Values are expressed as migration rate (µm/h). ### indicates $p < 0.001$ vs. untreated cells; *** indicates $p < 0.001$ vs. LPS + IFN.

3.4. Plumericin Reduced LPS + IFN-Induced Apoptosis

In order to investigate the mechanisms underlying the gastroprotective effect of plumericin, we evaluated apoptosis, by cytofluorimetric analysis of PI stained hypodiploid nuclei. Our results indicated that plumericin (0.5–2 µM) significantly reduced LPS + IFN-induced apoptosis in IEC-6 cells, at higher concentrations tested (Figure 4a; $p < 0.001$ vs. LPS + IFN).

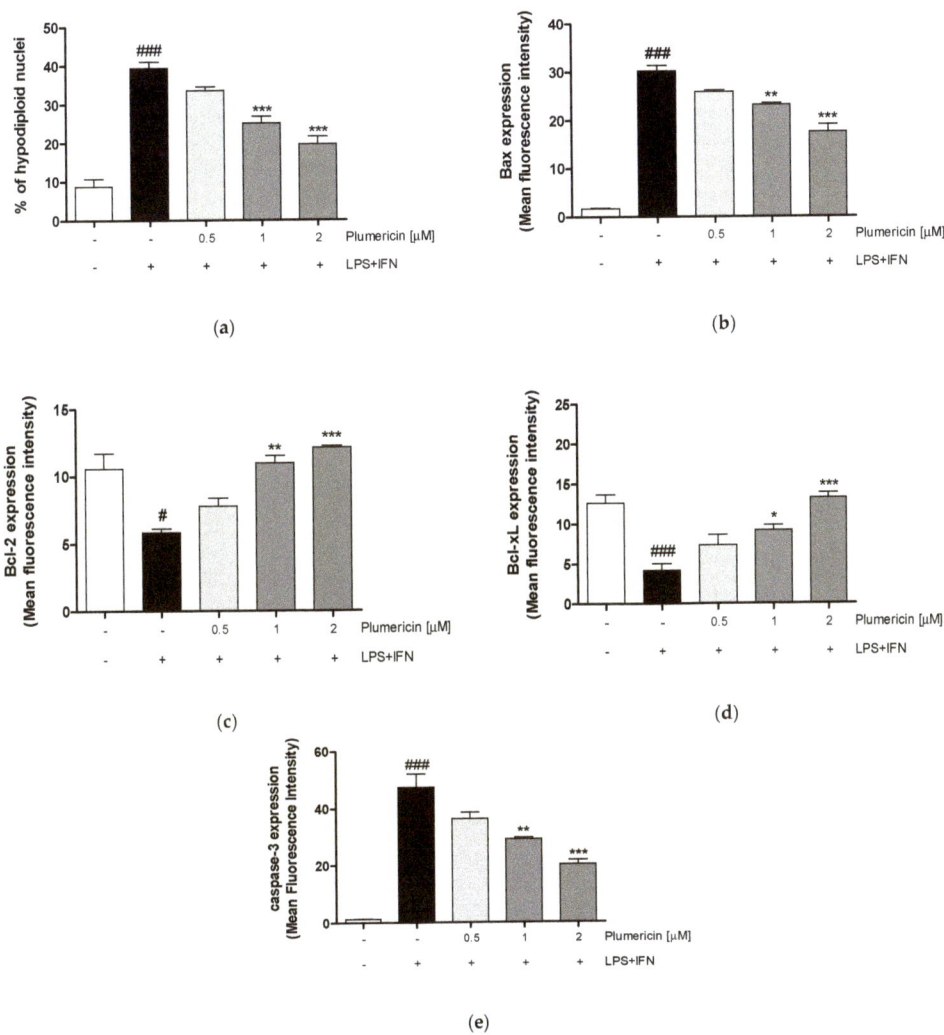

Figure 4. Apoptosis detection by propidium iodide (PI) staining of hypodiploid nuclei (**a**), and effect on Bax (**b**), Bcl-2 (**c**), Bcl-xL (**d**), and Caspase-3 (**e**), after IEC-6 incubation with plumericin. Data are expressed as mean ± S.E.M. of % of hypodiploid nuclei or as mean of fluorescence intensity. ### and # denote, respectively, $p < 0.001$ and $p < 0.05$ vs. untreated cells; ***, **, and * denote, respectively, $p < 0.001$, $p < 0.01$, and $p < 0.05$ vs. LPS + IFN.

To further investigate the anti-apoptotic ability of plumericin, we evaluated the expression of Bax, a pro-apoptotic protein, and Bcl-2 and Bcl-xL, two anti-apoptotic proteins, by cytofluorimetric analysis. Our results indicated that plumericin (0.5–2 µM) significantly reduced Bax expression ($p < 0.01$ vs. LPS + IFN; Figure 4b) and increased Bcl-2 and Bcl-xL expression in LPS + IFN-stimulated IEC-6 ($p < 0.01$ vs. LPS + IFN; Figure 4c,d), at higher concentrations tested.

Plumericin's anti-apoptotic ability was further demonstrated by evaluating caspase-3 expression, with flow cytometry. Our results have shown that plumericin significantly reduced the expression of caspase-3, compared to LPS + IFN-treated cells ($p < 0.01$ vs. LPS + IFN; Figure 4e)

3.5. Effect of Plumericin on ICAM-1 and P-Selectin Expression in DNBS-Induced Colitis

In this study, we also evaluated the intestinal expression of ICAM-1 and P-selectin that contribute to cell recruitment during colon inflammation. Positive staining for ICAM-1 (Figure 5b) and for P-selectin (Figure 5e) was substantially increased in the vessels of the lamina propria and submucosa as well as in epithelial cells of injured colon and in infiltrated inflammatory cells in damaged tissues from DNBS-injected mice. Treatment with plumericin (3 mg/kg; i.p.) reduced the staining for ICAM-1 (Figure 5c) and for P-selectin (Figure 5f) in the colon tissues collected from DNBS-injected mice. No positive staining for ICAM-1 and for P-selectin was observed in the colon tissues collected from control mice (Figure 5a,d, respectively), as you can see from the densitometric analyses, respectively, in Figure 5g,h.

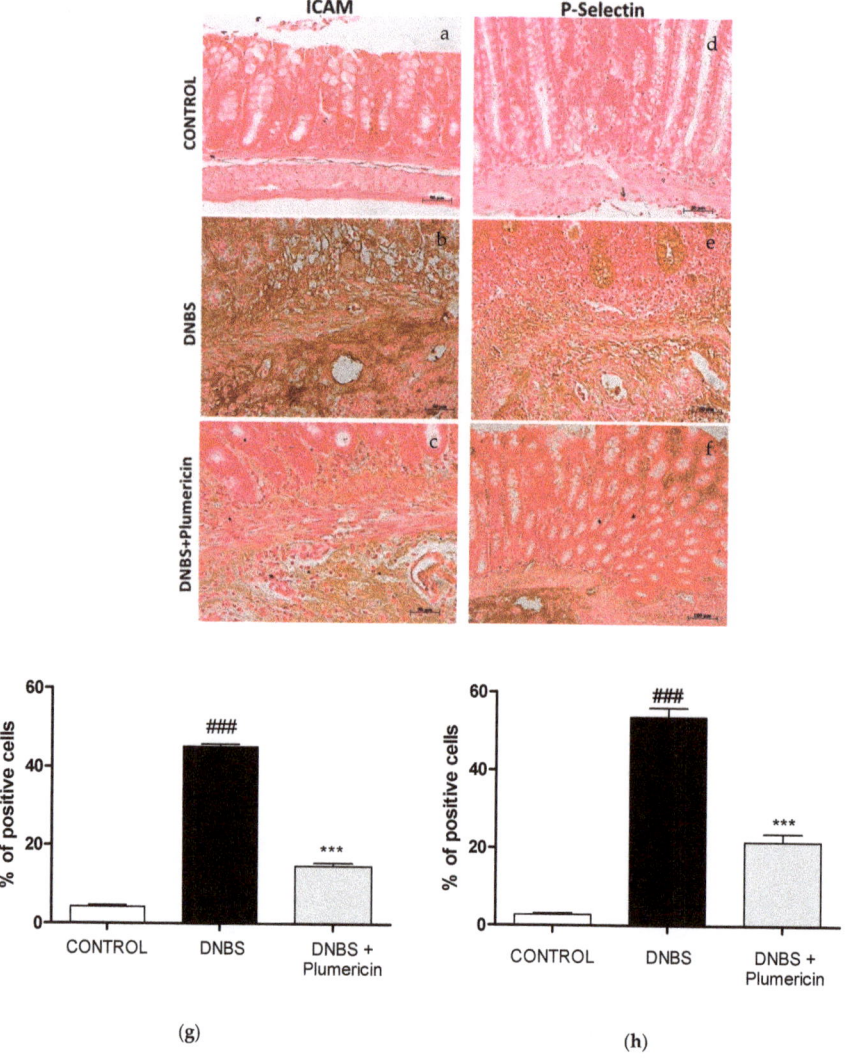

Figure 5. Effect of plumericin on ICAM-1 (**a–c**) and P-selectin (**d–f**) expression. (**g,h**) represent, respectively, densitometric analysis expressed as percentage of total tissue area. Photographs are representative of all animals in each group and data are means ± S.E.M. of 10 mice for each group. ### denotes $p < 0.001$ vs. control; *** denotes $p < 0.001$ vs. DNBS.

3.6. Plumericin Treatment Reduced MPO Activity in DNBS-Induced Colitis

DNBS intrarectally administration was characterized by an augmentation in MPO activity, an indicator of neutrophil accumulating in the colon. This was consistent with light microscopic observations showing the colon of vehicle-treated DNBS mice to contain a large number of neutrophils. In contrast, plumericin (3 mg/kg, i.p.) significantly reduced the degree of polymorphonuclear cell infiltration (determined as reduction in MPO activity) in inflamed colon ($p < 0.001$ vs. DNBS; Figure 6).

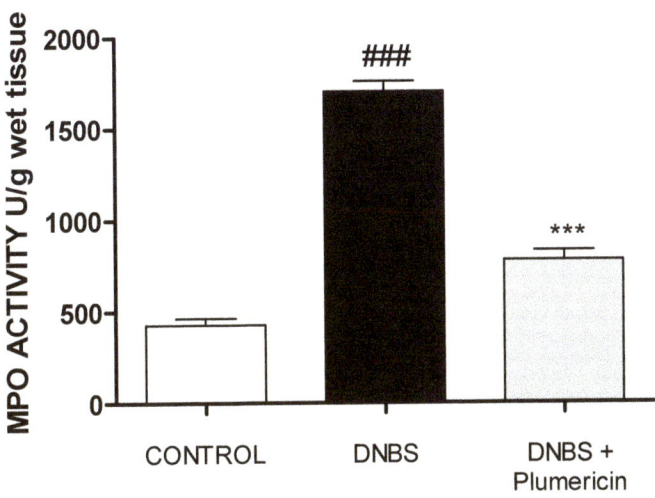

Figure 6. Effect of plumericin on myeloperoxidase (MPO) activity. Data are expressed as the mean ± S.E.M. of 10 mice for each group. ### denotes $p < 0.001$ vs. control group; *** denotes $p < 0.001$ vs. DNBS.

3.7. Effect of Plumericin Treatment on PAR Formation in Colitis Induced by DNBS

Immunohistochemistry for PAR, as an indicator of in vivo PARP activation, revealed positive staining localized in the nuclei of inflammatory cells in colon tissues from DNBS-injected mice (Figure 7b). Plumericin (3 mg/kg, i.p.) significantly reduced the extent of PAR immunoreactivity in the colon (Figure 7c), four days after DNBS administration. No positive staining for PAR was found in the colon tissues from control mice (Figure 7a), as you can see from the densitometric analyses (Figure 7d).

3.8. Effect of Plumericin on Apoptotic Damage in DNBS-Induced Colitis

To test whether colon damage was also associated with apoptosis, four days after DNBS, the appearance of proteic effectors of canonical mitochondrial apoptosis such as pro-apoptotic (Bax) protein and anti-apoptotic (Bcl-2) protein, was investigated by Western blot analysis. The balance of Bax levels was appreciably increased in the colon from mice subjected to DNBS. On the contrary, plumericin treatment (3 mg/kg; i.p.) prevented DNBS-induced Bax expression ($p < 0.001$ vs. DNBS; Figure 8a). Moreover, in the control groups, a basal level of Bcl-2 was detected. In DNBS-injected mice, Bcl-2 expression was reduced, but plumericin administration showed an increase in Bcl-2 expression ($p < 0.001$ vs. DNBS; Figure 8b).

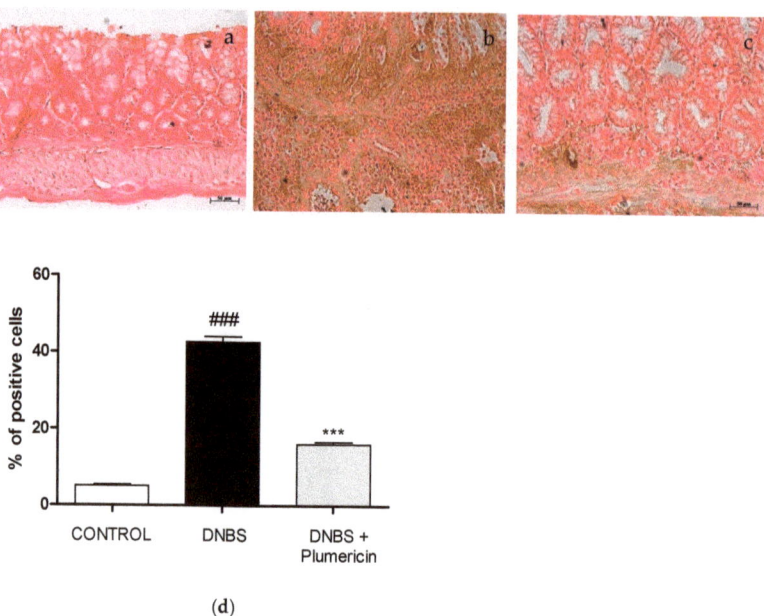

Figure 7. Effects of plumericin treatment on PAR formation (**a**–**c**) in colitis induced by DNBS. These data are also visible in graph of the percentage of total tissue area (**d**). Photographs are representative of all animals in each group. Data are expressed as the mean ± S.E.M. of 10 mice for each group. ### denotes $p < 0.001$ vs. control; *** denotes $p < 0.001$ vs. DNBS.

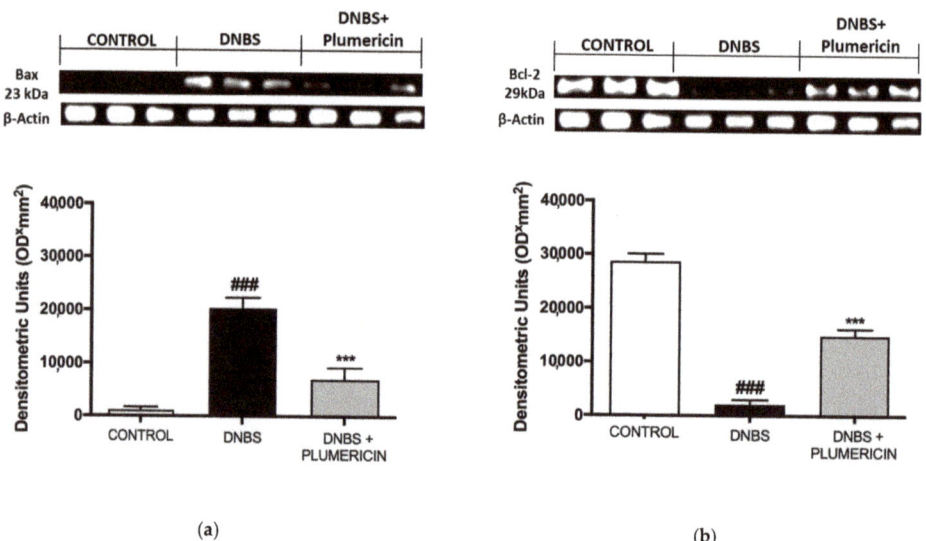

Figure 8. Bax (**a**) and Bcl-2 (**b**) expression was measured by Western blot. Densitometric analysis of protein bands was normalized to the level of β-actin. Data are representative of at least three independent experiments and are expressed as mean ± S.E.M. from 10 animals for each experimental group. A representative blot is shown and densitometric analysis is reported. ### denotes $p < 0.001$ vs. control; *** denotes $p < 0.001$ vs. DNBS.

4. Discussion

UC is a chronic progressive condition and impose significant multidimensional burdens on patients and health care systems. At the turn of the 21st century, IBDs as UC have become a global disease with accelerating incidence in newly industrialized countries whose societies have become more westernized [1–4]. A great interest is focused on new therapies that may be beneficial in treating these chronic diseases and the use of plant products for treating UC has increased, as many of them are known to act on different targets of the pathology process such as inflammation, oxidative stress, and intestinal barrier function [39,40]. In this study, we focused the attention on the effect of plumericin, an iridoid spironolactone isolated from *H. sucuuba*, on the management of the intestinal barrier impairment and apoptosis during intestinal inflammation.

A "leaky gut" may be an initial event in the pathogenesis of IBDs and it may also perpetuate chronic mucosal inflammation in UC flaring up uncontrollable inflammatory signal cascades and the altered expression of intracellular junction proteins is observed in patients with UC [41]. Epithelial tight junctions (TJs) and adherens junctions (ADJ) forms a selectively permeable seal between adjacent epithelial cells and define the limit between the apical and basolateral membrane domain. Their impairment allows the passage of pro-inflammatory molecules and can induce a mucosal immune system activation finally resulting in a sustained inflammation and tissue damage [5,42]. Accordingly, in our experimental model, we observe an impaired claudin-1, occludin, and E-cadherin expression in LPS + INF treated IEC-6. Plumericin treatment was able to avoid this impairment, reducing the decrease of these junction proteins expression in treated IEC-6 respect to the pro-inflammatory stimulus.

The actin cytoskeleton is a master regulator of the assembly and remodeling of epithelial junctions and establishment of tissue barriers. The interaction of intracellular junction with the actin cytoskeleton is vital to the maintenance of junction structure and allow the barrier integrity regulation by cytoskeleton [43]. During inflammation, it is known that a reorganization of the apical junctions mediate epithelial barrier dysfunction and the actin cytoskeleton plays a pivotal role in regulating junctional integrity and remodeling under physiological and pathological states [44]. IEC-6 cells, when confluent, produce monolayers that resemble normal small intestinal cells and show an organized actin cytoskeleton [45,46]. In our experiments, we found that plumericin ameliorated the marked reduction of actin stress fibers and the corresponding increase of the cortical actin density observed in LPS + IFN-treated IEC-6. Recent studies suggest that balanced actin filament turnover protects epithelial barriers and attenuates tissue injury during mucosal inflammation in vivo [47].

A reorganization of the actin cytoskeleton is fundamental during IECs' restitution. The healing process is initiated by migration of intestinal epithelial cells residing near the wounded area to the injury in order to fill up defects in the intestinal barrier. However, in various intestinal diseases, the intestinal healing is impaired, leading to persistent mucosal defects and potential consequences for the entire organism [48]. Thus, healing of the inflamed mucosa is considered a key step to achieve clinical remission in UC [41,49,50]. By means of a wound healing assay, we observed that plumericin improved cellular migration speed in IEC-6, thus increasing the restitution process.

Apoptosis regulates the replacement rate of the epithelial cells, and an increase of epithelial cell apoptosis, as occurs in IBD and in colitis in particular, disrupts mucosal epithelial differentiation [51]. Our data indicate that plumericin inhibited the IEC-6 apoptosis. This effect was associated with a reduction in pro-apoptotic proteins, such as Bax, and with an increase in antiapoptotic factors, such as Bcl-2 and Bcl-xL. Moreover, in plumericin-treated IEC-6, a reduction in caspase-3 was also observed, thus further proving the anti-apoptotic effect of plumericin.

In order to also confirm these effects observed in IECs in an in vivo model, we evaluated the effect of plumericin in a model of DNBS-induced colitis in mice.

DNBS administration induced P-selectin expression on the endothelial vascular wall and up-regulated the surface expression of ICAM-1 on endothelial cells. In plumericin-treated mice, we observed a lower expression of P-selectin and an up-regulation of ICAM-1, without affecting constitutive levels of ICAM-1 on endothelial cells. The absence of an increased expression of the adhesion molecule in the colon tissue in plumericin-treated animals was associated with the reduction of leukocyte infiltration, as assessed by the specific granulocyte enzyme MPO, which is also an oxidative stress marker.

ROS can cause DNA damage, leading to poly ADP ribose synthase activation and cell death [52]. Plumericin inhibited the positive staining for PAR compared to the DNBS-group. Epithelial cell damage in the inflamed colonic mucosa has been stated to involve the apoptotic process. In the DNBS group, we observed a significant increase in the pro-apoptotic protein Bax and a reduction in the antiapoptotic Bcl-2. Plumericin treatment induced both an inhibition of Bax expression and a parallel increase in Bcl-2, thus contributing to reducing the apoptotic process.

Plumericin shares its effects on these pathways with several other electrophilic compounds of high pharmaceutical and nutraceutical interest including dimethylfumarate and curcumin, which have also been reported to be effective on colitis [36,53,54]. This evidence further supports the pharmacological potential of plumericin as an adjuvant in IBDs.

5. Conclusions

The results of this study provide evidence, both in vitro and in vivo, that support the potential effect of plumericin on IBDs contributing to the maintenance of intestinal epithelial barrier and to reducing apoptosis. These findings together with the anti-inflammatory and antioxidant potential previously reported, strongly support the therapeutical potential of plumericin both in the acute phase of colitis, mainly acting on inflammation and oxidative stress, and also in the relapsing phase, where the restitution of intestinal barrier integrity seems to play a pivotal role.

Author Contributions: S.M. conceived and designed the study, S.F.R., R.D.P., R.S., R.D., M.C., and R.F. performed the experiments, S.M., S.F.R., and R.D.P. analyzed and interpreted the data, S.M. and S.F.R. drafted the manuscript, G.A., S.C., and H.S. critically revised the manuscript. All authors have seen and approved the manuscript.

Funding: This research was founded by University of Salerno (FARB 2018-ORSA180779 and FARB 2019-ORSA180779) to S.M. and by funds of the Austrian Science Fund (FWF) under the National Research Network (NFN)-project "Drugs from Nature Targeting Inflammation" (DNTI) to H.S. (subprojects S10703 and S10713).

Institutional Review Board Statement: The study was conducted according to the guidelines of the Declaration of Helsinki, and the University of Messina Review Board for Animal Care (OPBA) approved the study (650/2017-PR).

Informed Consent Statement: Not applicable.

Data Availability Statement: The data presented in this study are available on request from the corresponding author.

Acknowledgments: The authors thank Denise Notaro (University of Salerno) for the technical assistance.

Conflicts of Interest: The authors declare no conflict of interest.

References

1. Hugh, T. IBD: Functional characterization of an IBD risk gene. *Nat. Rev. Gastroenterol. Hepatol.* **2018**, *15*, 190–191. [CrossRef]
2. Ananthakrishnan, A.N.; Bernstein, C.N.; Iliopoulos, D.; Macpherson, A.; Neurath, M.F.; Ali, R.; Vavricka, S.R.; Fiocchi, C. Environmental triggers in IBD: A review of progress and evidence. *Nat. Rev. Gastroenterol. Hepatol.* **2018**, *15*, 39–49. [CrossRef] [PubMed]
3. Deng, Y.; Han, X.; Tang, S.; Li, C.; Xiao, W.; Tan, Z. Magnolol and honokiol attenuate apoptosis of enterotoxigenic Escherichia coli-induced intestinal epithelium by maintaining secretion and absorption homeostasis and protecting mucosal integrity. *Med. Sci. Monit.* **2018**, *24*, 3348–3356. [CrossRef]
4. Gajendran, M.; Loganathan, P.; Jimenez, G.; Catinella, A.P.; Ng, N.; Umapathy, C.; Ziade, N.; Hashash, J.G. A comprehensive review and update on ulcerative colitis. *Dis. Mon.* **2019**, *65*, 12. [CrossRef] [PubMed]

5. Chelakkot, C.; Ghim, J.; Ryu, S.H. Mechanisms regulating intestinal barrier integrity and its pathological implications. *Exp. Mol. Med.* **2018**, *50*, 103. [CrossRef] [PubMed]
6. Turner, J.R. Intestinal mucosal barrier function in health and disease. *Nat. Rev. Immunol.* **2009**, *9*, 799–809. [CrossRef]
7. Xu, P.; Becker, H.; Elizalde, M.; Masclee, A.; Jonkers, D. Intestinal organoid culture model is a valuable system to study epithelial barrier function in IBD. *Gut* **2019**, *67*, 1905–1906. [CrossRef]
8. Peterson, L.W.; Artis, D. Intestinal epithelial cells: Regulators of barrier function and immune homeostasis. *Nat. Rev. Immunol.* **2014**, *14*, 141–153. [CrossRef]
9. Horton, F.; Wright, J.; Smith, L.; Hinton, P.J.; Robertson, M.D. Increased intestinal permeability to oral chromium (51Cr) -EDTA in human Type 2 diabetes. *Diabet. Med.* **2014**, *31*, 559–563. [CrossRef]
10. Piya, M.K.; Harte, A.L.; McTernan, P.G. Metabolic endotoxaemia: Is it more than just a gut feeling? *Curr. Opin. Lipidol.* **2013**, *24*, 78–85. [CrossRef]
11. Spruss, A.; Kanuri, G.; Stahl, C.; Bischoff, S.C.; Bergheim, I. Metformin protects against the development of fructose-induced steatosis in mice: Role of the intestinal barrier function. *Lab. Investig.* **2012**, *92*, 1020–1032. [CrossRef] [PubMed]
12. Brudek, T. Inflammatory Bowel Diseases and Parkinson's Disease. *J. Parkinsons Dis.* **2019**, *9*, S331–S344. [CrossRef] [PubMed]
13. Axelrad, J.E.; Lichtiger, S.; Yajnik, V. Inflammatory bowel disease and cancer: The role of inflammation, immunosuppression, and cancer treatment. *World J. Gastroenterol.* **2016**, *22*, 4794–4801. [CrossRef] [PubMed]
14. Cianchi, F.; Cuzzocrea, S.; Vinci, M.C.; Messerini, L.; Comin, C.E.; Navarra, G.; Perigli, G.; Centorrino, T.; Marzocco, S.; Lenzi, E.; et al. Heterogeneous expression of cyclooxygenase-2 and inducible nitric oxide synthase within colorectal tumors: Correlation with tumor angiogenesis. *Dig. Liver Dis.* **2010**, *42*, 20–27. [CrossRef]
15. Goretsky, T.; Dirisina, R.; Sinh, P.; Mittal, N.; Managlia, E.; Williams, D.B.; Posca, D.; Ryu, H.; Katzman, R.B.; Barrett, T. p53 mediates TNF-induced epithelial cell apoptosis in IBD. *Am. J. Pathol.* **2012**, *181*, 1306–1315. [CrossRef]
16. Bryant, R.V.; Brain, O.; Travis, S.P. Conventional drug therapy for inflammatory bowel disease. *Scand. J. Gastroenterol.* **2015**, *50*, 90–112. [CrossRef]
17. Chudy-Onwugaje, K.O.; Christian, K.E.; Farraye, F.A.; Cross, R.K. A State-of-the-Art Review of New and Emerging Therapies for the Treatment of IBD. *Inflamm. Bowel Dis.* **2019**, *25*, 820–830. [CrossRef]
18. Newman, D.J.; Cragg, G.M. Natural products as sources of new drugs over the 30 years from 1981 to 2010. *J. Nat. Prod.* **2012**, *75*, 311–335. [CrossRef]
19. Amaral, A.; Ferreira, J.L.; Pinheiro, M.L.; Silva, J. Monograph of Himatanthus sucuuba, a plant of Amazonian folk medicine. *Pharmacogn. Rev.* **2007**, *1*, 305–313.
20. Sharma, U.; Singh, D.; Kumar, P.; Dobhal, M.P.; Singh, S. Antiparasitic activity of plumericin & isoplumericin isolated from Plumeria bicolor against Leishmania donovani. *Indian J. Med. Res.* **2011**, *134*, 709–716. [CrossRef]
21. Kuigoua, G.M.; Kouam, S.F.; Ngadjui, B.T.; Schulz, B.; Green, I.R.; Choudhary, M.I.; Krohn, K. Minor secondary metabolic products from the stem bark of Plumeria rubra Linn. displaying antimicrobial activities. *Planta Med.* **2010**, *76*, 620–625. [CrossRef] [PubMed]
22. Singh, D.; Sharma, U.; Kumar, P.; Gupta, Y.K.; Dobhal, M.P.; Singh, S. Antifungal activity of plumericin and isoplumericin. *Nat. Prod. Commun.* **2011**, *6*, 1567–1568. [CrossRef] [PubMed]
23. Fakhrudin, N.; Waltenberger, B.; Cabaravdic, M.; Atanasov, A.G.; Malainer, C.; Schachner, D.; Heiss, E.H.; Liu, R.; Noha, S.M.; Grzywacz, A.M.; et al. Identification of plumericin as a potent new inhibitor of the NF-κB pathway with anti-inflammatory activity in vitro and in vivo. *Br. J. Pharmacol.* **2014**, *171*, 1676–1686. [CrossRef] [PubMed]
24. Heiss, E.; Liu, R.; Waltenberger, B.; Khan, S.; Kollmann, P.; Zimmermann, K.; Cabaravdic, M.; Uhrin, P.; Stuppner, H.; et al. Plumericin inhibits proliferation of vascular smooth muscle cells by blocking STAT3 signaling via S-glutathionylation. *Sci. Rep.* **2016**, *6*, 20771. [CrossRef]
25. Khan, S.Y.; Awad, E.M.; Oszwald, A.; Mayr, M.; Yin, X.; Waltenberger, B.; Stuppner, H.; Lipovac, M.; Uhrin, P.; Breuss, J.M. Premature senescence of endothelial cells upon chronic exposure to TNFα can be prevented by N-acetyl cysteine and plumericin. *Sci. Rep.* **2017**, *7*, 39501. [CrossRef]
26. Rapa, S.F.; Waltenberger, B.; Di Paola, R.; Adesso, S.; Siracusa, R.; Peritore, A.F.; D'Amico, R.; Autore, G.; Cuzzocrea, S.; Stuppner, H.; et al. Plumericin prevents intestinal inflammation and oxidative stress in vitro and in vivo. *FASEB J.* **2020**, *34*, 1576–1590. [CrossRef]
27. Waltenberger, B.; Rollinger, J.M.; Griesser, U.J.; Stuppner, H.; Gelbrich, T. Plumeridoid C from the Amazonian traditional medicinal plant Himatanthus sucuuba. *Acta Crystallogr. C* **2011**, *67*, o409–o412. [CrossRef]
28. Adesso, S.; Autore, G.; Quaroni, A.; Popolo, A.; Severino, L.; Marzocco, S. The Food Contaminants Nivalenol and Deoxynivalenol Induce Inflammation in Intestinal Epithelial Cells by Regulating Reactive Oxygen Species Release. *Nutrients* **2017**, *9*, 1343. [CrossRef]
29. Adesso, S.; Russo, R.; Quaroni, A.; Autore, G.; Marzocco, S. Astragalus membranaceus Extract Attenuates Inflammation and Oxidative Stress in Intestinal Epithelial Cells via NF-κB Activation and Nrf2 Response. *Int. J. Mol. Sci.* **2018**, *19*, 800. [CrossRef]
30. Adesso, S.; Ruocco, M.; Rapa, S.F.; Dal Piaz, F.; Di Iorio, R.B.; Popolo, A.; Autore, G.; Nishijima, F.; Pinto, A.; Marzocco, S. Effect of Indoxyl Sulfate on the Repair and Intactness of Intestinal Epithelial Cells: Role of Reactive Oxygen Species' Release. *Int. J. Mol. Sci.* **2019**, *20*, 2280. [CrossRef]

31. Basilicata, M.G.; Pepe, G.; Rapa, S.F.; Merciai, F.; Ostacolo, C.; Manfra, M.; Di Sarno, V.; Autore, G.; De Vita, D.; Marzocco, S.; et al. Anti-Inflammatory and Antioxidant Properties of Dehydrated Potato-Derived Bioactive Compounds in Intestinal Cells. *Int. J. Mol. Sci.* **2019**, *20*, 6087. [CrossRef] [PubMed]
32. Pepe, G.; Rapa, S.F.; Salviati, E.; Bertamino, A.; Auriemma, G.; Cascioferro, S.; Autore, G.; Quaroni, A.; Campiglia, P.; Marzocco, S. Bioactive polyphenols from pomegranate juice reduce 5-Fluorouracil-induced intestinal mucositis in intestinal epithelial cells. *Antioxidants* **2020**, *9*, 699. [CrossRef] [PubMed]
33. Cordaro, M.; Impellizzeri, D.; Gugliandolo, E.; Siracusa, R.; Crupi, R.; Esposito, E.; Cuzzocrea, S. Adelmidrol Reduces Colitis. *Mol. Pharmacol.* **2016**, *90*, 549–561. [CrossRef] [PubMed]
34. Paterniti, I.; Impellizzeri, D.; Cordaro, M.; Siracusa, R.; Bisignano, C.; Gugliandolo, E.; Carughi, A.; Esposito, E.; Mandalari, G.; Cuzzocrea, S. The Anti-Inflammatory and Antioxidant Potential of Pistachios (Pistacia vera L.) In Vitro and In Vivo. *Nutrients* **2017**, *9*, 915. [CrossRef] [PubMed]
35. Impellizzeri, D.; Bruschetta, G.; Di Paola, R.; Ahmad, A.; Campolo, M.; Cuzzocrea, S.; Esposito, E.; Navarra, M. The anti-inflammatory and antioxidant effects of bergamot juice extract (BJe) in an experimental model of inflammatory bowel disease. *Clin. Nutr.* **2015**, *34*, 1146–1154. [CrossRef]
36. Casili, G.; Cordaro, M.; Impellizzeri, D.; Bruschetta, G.; Paterniti, I.; Cuzzocrea, S.; Esposito, E. Dimethyl Fumarate Reduces Inflammatory Responses in Experimental Colitis. *J. Crohn's Colitis* **2016**, *10*, 472–483. [CrossRef]
37. Schmitz, H.; Barmeyer, C.; Fromm, M.; Runkel, N.; Foss, H.D.; Bentzel, C.J.; Riecken, E.O.; Schulzke, J.D. Altered tight junction structure contributes to the impaired epithelial barrier function in ulcerative colitis. *Gastroenterology* **1999**, *116*, 301–309. [CrossRef]
38. Oshima, T.; Miwa, H.; Joh, T. Changes in the expression of claudins in active ulcerative colitis. *J. Gastroenterol. Hepatol.* **2008**, *23* (Suppl. 2), S146–S150. [CrossRef]
39. Farzaei, M.H.; Rahimi, R.; Abdollahi, M. The role of dietary polyphenols in the management of inflammatory bowel disease. *Curr. Pharm. Biotechnol.* **2015**, *16*, 196–210. [CrossRef]
40. Da Silva, V.C.; de Araújo, A.A.; de Souza Araújo, D.F.; Souza Lima, M.; Vasconcelos, R.C.; de Araújo Júnior, R.F.; Langasnner, S.; de Freitas Fernandes Pedrosa, M.; de Medeiros, C.; Guerra, G. Intestinal Anti-Inflammatory Activity of the Aqueous Extract from Ipomoea asarifolia in DNBS-Induced Colitis in Rats. *Int. J. Mol. Sci.* **2018**, *19*, 4016. [CrossRef]
41. Michielan, A.; D'Incà, R. Intestinal Permeability in Inflammatory Bowel Disease: Pathogenesis, Clinical Evaluation, and Therapy of Leaky Gut. *Mediat. Inflamm.* **2015**, *2015*, 628157. [CrossRef] [PubMed]
42. Lechuga, S.; Ivanov, A.I. Actin cytoskeleton dynamics during mucosal inflammation: A view from broken epithelial barriers. *Curr. Opin. Physiol.* **2021**, *19*, 10–16. [CrossRef] [PubMed]
43. González-Mariscal, L.; Betanzos, A.; Nava, P.; Jaramillo, B.E. Tight junction proteins. *Prog. Biophys. Mol. Biol.* **2003**, *81*, 1–44. [CrossRef]
44. Lee, S.H. Intestinal permeability regulation by tight junction: Implication on inflammatory bowel diseases. *Intest. Res.* **2015**, *13*, 11–18. [CrossRef]
45. McGuire, P.G.; Seeds, N.W. The interaction of plasminogen activator with a reconstituted basement membrane matrix and extracellular macromolecules produced by cultured epithelial cells. *J. Cell. Biochem.* **1989**, *40*, 215–227. [CrossRef]
46. Quaroni, A.; Wands, J.; Trelstad, R.L.; Isselbacher, K.J. Epithelioid cell cultures from rat small intestine. Characterization by morphologic and immunologic criteria. *J. Cell Biol.* **1979**, *80*, 248–265. [CrossRef]
47. Chen, B.; Yang, Z.; Yang, C.; Qin, W.; Gu, J.; Hu, C.; Chen, A.; Ning, J.; Yi, B.; Lu, K. A self-organized actomyosin drives multiple intercellular junction disruption and directly promotes neutrophil recruitment in lipopolysaccharide-induced acute lung injury. *FASEB J.* **2018**, *32*, 6197–6211. [CrossRef]
48. Leaphart, C.L.; Qureshi, F.; Cetin, S.; Li, J.; Dubowski, T.; Baty, C.; Beer-Stolz, D.; Guo, F.; Murray, S.A.; Hackam, D.J. Interferon-gamma inhibits intestinal restitution by preventing gap junction communication between enterocytes. *Gastroenterology* **2007**, *132*, 2395–2411. [CrossRef]
49. Neurath, M.F. New targets for mucosal healing and therapy in inflammatory bowel diseases. *Mucosal. Immunol.* **2014**, *7*, 6–19. [CrossRef]
50. Colombel, J.F.; Rutgeerts, P.; Reinisch, W.; Esser, D.; Wang, Y.; Lang, Y.; Marano, C.W.; Strauss, R.; Oddens, B.J.; Feagan, B.G.; et al. Early mucosal healing with infliximab is associated with improved long-term clinical outcomes in ulcerative colitis. *Gastroenterology* **2011**, *141*, 1194–1201. [CrossRef]
51. Blander, J.M. On cell death in the intestinal epithelium and its impact on gut homeostasis. *Curr. Opin. Gastroenterol.* **2018**, *34*, 413–419. [CrossRef]
52. Impellizzeri, D.; Siracusa, R.; Cordaro, M.; Peritore, A.F.; Gugliandolo, E.; Mancuso, G.; Midiri, A.; Di Paola, R.; Cuzzocrea, S. Therapeutic potential of dinitrobenzene sulfonic acid (DNBS)-induced colitis in mice by targeting IL-1β and IL-18. *Biochem. Pharmacol.* **2018**, *155*, 150–161. [CrossRef]
53. He, Y.; Yue, Y.; Zheng, X.; Zhang, K.; Chen, S.; Du, Z. Curcumin, inflammation, and chronic diseases: How are they linked? *Molecules* **2015**, *20*, 9183–9213. [CrossRef] [PubMed]
54. Burge, K.; Gunasekaran, A.; Eckert, J.; Chaaban, H. Curcumin and intestinal inflammatory diseases: Molecular mechanisms of protection. *Int. J. Mol. Sci.* **2019**, *20*, 1912. [CrossRef]

MDPI
St. Alban-Anlage 66
4052 Basel
Switzerland
Tel. +41 61 683 77 34
Fax +41 61 302 89 18
www.mdpi.com

Biomedicines Editorial Office
E-mail: biomedicines@mdpi.com
www.mdpi.com/journal/biomedicines

www.ingramcontent.com/pod-product-compliance
Lightning Source LLC
LaVergne TN
LVHW070227100526
838202LV00015B/2100